AF526682

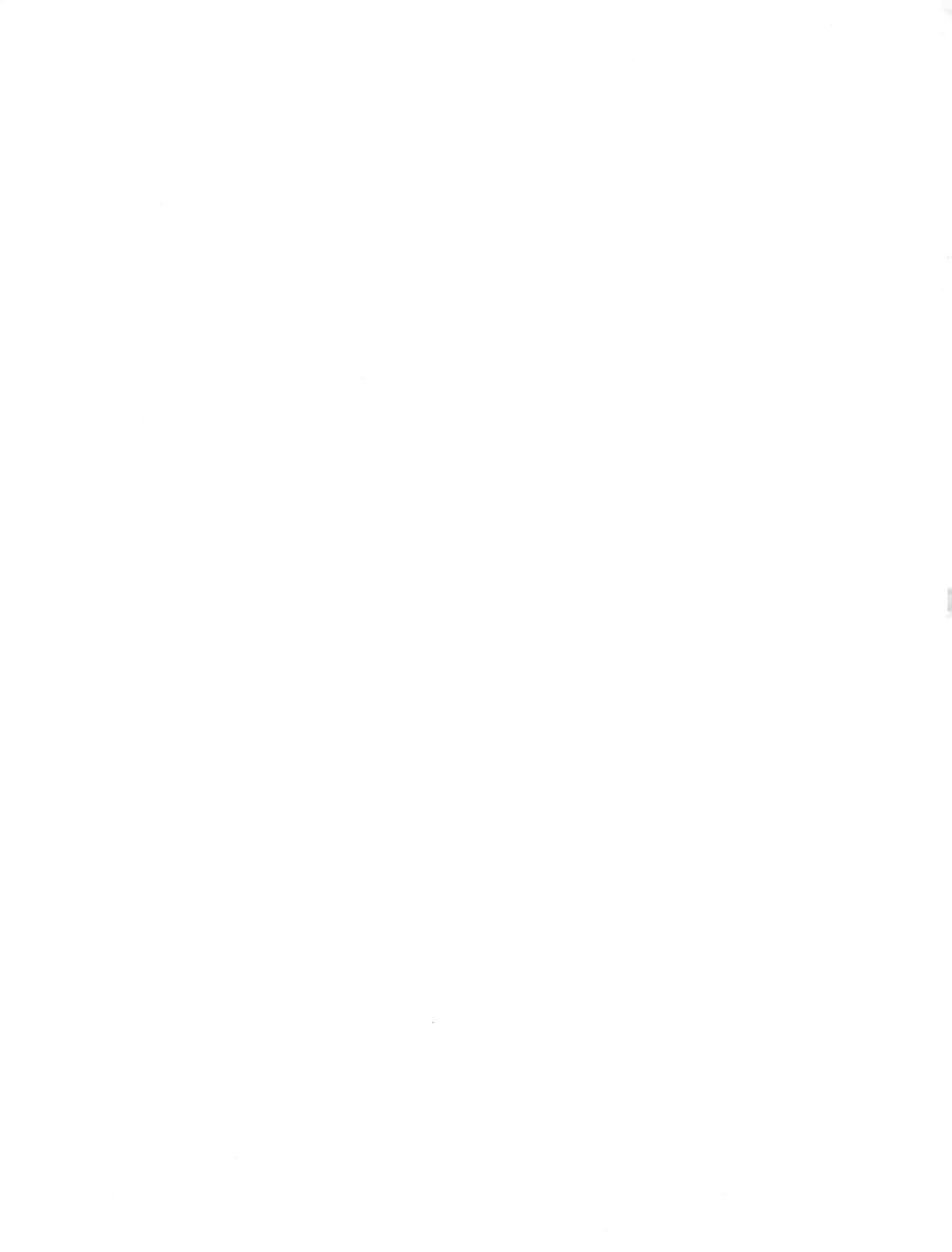

Handbook of
Materials Management in Healthcare Industry

Handbook of Materials Management in Healthcare Industry

Prof. V. Venkat Reddy
Ph.D.
Honorary Director,
Indian Institute of Materials Management
Formerly Vice President
Ivax Paper Chemicals Ltd.
(An Indo-British Joint Venture)
Hyderabad.

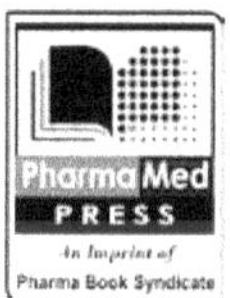

PharmaMed Press
An imprint of Pharma Book Syndicate
A unit of BSP Books Pvt. Ltd.
4-4-309/316, Giriraj Lane,
Sultan Bazar, Hyderabad - 500 095.

Handbook of Materials Management in Healthcare Industry by
V. Venkat Reddy

Published by

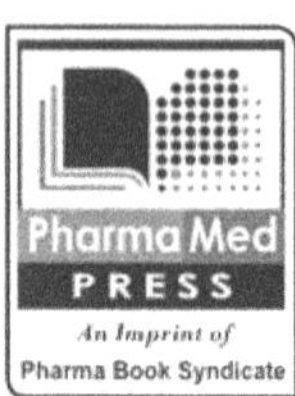

PharmaMed Press
An imprint of Pharma Book Syndicate
A unit of BSP Books Pvt. Ltd.
4-4-309/316, Giriraj Lane, Sultan Bazar, Hyderabad - 500 095.
Phone: 040-23445605, 23445688; Fax: 91+40-23445611
E-mail: info@pharmamedpress.com

ISBN: 978-93-5230-105-8 (HB)

Dedication

Dedicated to my Parents

My father, former Secretary, Board of Revenue, Government of Andhra Pradesh and an administrator par excellence who always insisted that we must pursue excellence in whatever avocation we choose.

and

My mother, who wished that I pursue the medical profession. Though destiny made me an Industrial Engineer, her wish, is partially fulfilled now through this handbook for benefit of healthcare professionals.

Preface

Healthcare facilities in India have seen rapid growth and improvement post-liberalization of Indian economy. The volume and complexity of Materials Management (MM) has increased due to the rapidly changing technology in healthcare, regulatory measures, and the impact of economic factors, both within and beyond the control of the hospitals, nursing homes and clinics. This book is written as a ready reference for all those who are directly or indirectly interested in MM in healthcare for better patient care.

In recent years, materials function has undergone a complete revolution. Indeed, it is the last of the specialized business functions to be centralized and given the responsibility and the authority for making major contributions to profits. Yet progress in this area of business management in healthcare industry is just beginning. There can be little doubt that the materials function is destined to make an increasing contribution to the success of most healthcare enterprises.

There are two compelling reasons why MM will play an increasingly important role in most businesses. The first reason stems from the current emphasis on scientific research. Skyrocketing expenditures for research produces a large number of new and complex products that are manufactured by increasingly specialized methods and processes. New products in turn often demand new materials and new sources of supply. Increased specialization in the field of healthcare typically necessitates discovery or development of special suppliers who can provide unique materials and services at low costs. This pattern expands and intensifies the economic and technical problems associated with procurement. The second reason for the increasing importance of this function centres on the changes that are taking place in the organizational structure. Since the time of Frederick W. Taylor, business managers have become increasingly aware of the benefits of work specialization.

Industrial MM principles and practices are similar to a great extent to those of the healthcare MM, with some differences in the services oriented healthcare and the manufacturing or production line. Industrial principles and practices apply more directly to the non-patient, support areas of the hospital while principles and practices of healthcare MM are geared toward patients, physicians, and technicians. This book brings out these differences in a descriptive and objective manner.

Because of the growth of the concept of MM, hospitals began to promote untrained staff who had little or no formal training in basic procedures. Secretaries became buyers overnight sans training. In an effort to supplement the available staff, hospitals began hiring people from the industries who are not familiar with hospital routine. And the problem compounded itself because there were no theoretical references to provide answers to their questions. People in such situations would find this handbook tremendously needy.

The main thrust of the book is on integrated MM in Indian healthcare industry, where there is an acute paucity of authentic literature. This book deals with the management of materials and the control of material costs in a healthcare enterprise. It emphasizes purchasing as the primary materials activity. The book views materials function in the context of total business operation.

Because of the growing importance of institutional MM in healthcare institutions, an effort has been made to cover the basic principles and practices of this field from an institutional approach. This book has been written primarily for the materials managers, the purchasing managers and the hospital administrators. It should serve as a professional practice reminder for hospital and nursing home administrators, clinic managers, departmental heads, and others supervising healthcare centres, whatever the size, control or kind. Postgraduate students of healthcare administration like M.B.A (MM), MHM, business administration, and related fields may also find this handbook helpful. In addition, it can serve as a reference for the hospital supply industry including vendors, manufacturing representatives, and distributors, and all those who directly serve material managers and indirectly, the patients.

Handbook of MM in Healthcare Industry is an adaptable reference book. It provides a sound and complete indispensable introduction to the materials function. It includes descriptions of how to accomplish a wide variety of MM objectives and provides assessment tools, such as checklists and specific action plans, for improving operational performance. It has the best thoughts of experienced managers around the world concerning the various aspects of hospital MM in one volume. This provides quick access to working managers regarding everyday issues without having to do extensive research. Efforts have been made to strike a balance between the overview approach and the treatment of specific details.

In developing this text, content has drawn freely from the research and experiences of scholars and business executives who have knowledge in the field of Healthcare MM, besides my personal managerial and research experience at the Indian Institute of Materials Management (IIMM) giving the book crucial practical outlook.

The book is divided into five parts, which are further sub-divided into 25 chapters. A logical build-up has been ensured so as to enable the reader to gain a clear insight of the integrated MM function. Wherever necessary, examples and illustrations have been provided. Part I deals with origin and growth of MM in Indian healthcare industry, integrated hospital MM, and MM for hospital pharmacy. Part II covers purchasing function, origin, scope and objectives, organization, purchasing cycle, parameters, negotiations, and comparison of hospital purchasing with industrial purchasing including special features of hospital purchasing. Part III is devoted to inventory control, scope, costs associated with inventories, economic order quantity, selective controls of inventory and lead-time designing of inventory models. Part IV is about stores organization, building, layout, physical verification and valuation of inventories and supply and distribution management. The last part, V deals with the topics of value analysis/value engineering, supply chain management including its relevance to healthcare industry and concludes with information technology applications in healthcare. The chapters 24 and 25 in part V present only general concepts in brief. For schools that include the topic of purchasing and MM as part of a course in production or marketing or industrial engineering, the first four parts of the text will provide the introduction to the comprehensive concepts of purchasing and MM.

The management of this handbook project has been a challenging logistical task, but at the same time, it has also been extremely rewarding. It has allowed me to synthesize my grasp of individual aspects of the field into an integrated whole. It has also given me an opportunity to work with colleagues around the country and learn from their experience. In fact, it has done for me what I hope it will do for every person who reads the book.

Everyone who uses this book will benefit, either by reading it in its entirety or individual chapters of concern in daily operations. Readers' suggestions on additional topics for future editions are always welcome. Please feel free to share your thoughts.

- V. VENKAT REDDY

Acknowledgement

I am grateful to a number of individuals who were instrumental in designing and writing this book from an idea stage to completion. It is difficult to express my gratefulness to all those who have directly or indirectly enthused me in this endeavour. I am indebted to every one of them.

This book could not have been materialized without the direct involvement, support and help of the following individuals, whom I wish to thank.

My Guru, Prof. P. Gopalakrishnan, former professor, Administrative College of India, who taught me the nuances of materials management and guided my thoughts, concepts and perspectives.

Shri T. Rama Mohana Rao, IAS (Retd.), my mentor, former Director of industries, who guided me in my career. His belief in my capabilities helped me to reach where I am today.

I thank Shri Kuldip Rai, former Deputy General Manager, ECIL for the contribution of the chapter "Information Technology (IT) Applications in Healthcare".

I thank Mr. Nikhil shah and Mr. Anil shah, Directors of BSP Books Pvt. Ltd. Hyderabad for having consented to publish this book in spite of tight production schedules. My thanks also goes to Naresh Davergave, Production Manager, Ms. Rajitha and other members of the staff for their meticulous work.

In writing this book relevant material were culled out from different sources like journals, articles, reports and books. Where ever published materials are discussed in this book, the authors and publication details have been mentioned in the list of bibliography. If the related information and facts have been mentioned from internet source, website have also been acknowledged.

My overriding indebtedness to my wife Smt. V. Raja Kumari, who provided me with time, and support needed to prepare this handbook. I am thankful to my daughters Usha, Sandhya and Veena who encouraged me to bring out this handbook. My special thanks goes to Sandhya for providing a lot of input on hospital administration in the US.

Last but not the least; I thank my former and present students, hospital administrators and teachers of Healthcare Management, who helped me in shaping my thoughts.

- V. VENKAT REDDY

About the Author

Dr. VENKAT REDDY VAGVALA, an Industrial Engineer with an MBA in Marketing and Doctorate in Faculty of Management, worked at Chief Executive level in public and private sector organizations for over 12 years after his stints as Head of Materials Department in various public and private sector industries for a period of 14 years and earlier in the Department of Industries, Government of AP for over a decade. He has a passion for academics. He was ratified as Professor Osmania University (OU) by the duly constituted committee chaired by the Vice-Chancellor. He has so far published about 25 papers on various facets of Materials Management (MM), Inventory Management, and Supply Chain Management (SCM), many of these in the journal Materials Management Review. He is paper setter/examiner for M.Tech (IEM), M.Tech (PEM), MBA, MHM, GDMM and PGDMM Programmes of Jawaharlal Nehru Technological University (JNTU), OU, NIMS and IIMM and is Approved Guide/examiner for Dissertation/Thesis for PhD., M.Tech and MBA programs of JNTU, IGNOU, IIMM, AIMA etc., and supervised more than one hundred students' dissertations. He served as visiting Professor, JNTU for M.Tech and MBA Programs at their Center for Management Studies and School of Management Studies and also Apollo Institute of Hospital Administration, Hyderabad, School of Agricultural Business Management, AP Agriculture University, Badruka Institute of Foreign Trade, Hyderabad. He also served as Director/Professor, RISHI UBR College for Women, Hyderabad.

He is presently Visiting Professor, Nizam's Institute of Medical Sciences, and Institute of Public Enterprise Hyderabad. He is guest speaker at Administrative Staff College of India, Engineering Staff College of India, Centre of Plant Engineering Services, (COPES), Hyderabad Management Association, National Institute of Micro, Small and Medium Enterprises (NIMSME), Central Institute of Rural Electrification (CIRE), Government of India, and many other institutions of repute. He is Member, Board of Studies, Indian Institute of Materials Management (IIMM) since 1982. He was the 9th in the country and the first from erstwhile Andhra Pradesh to be awarded the Distinguished Membership - the highest award for outstanding services rendered to MM profession, besides other awards such as “Best Faculty Award”, “Best Materials Manager of the year 1983-84 Award” and “Member of the year 1988-89 Award” by IIMM. He is Life Fellow of IIMM and Indian Institution of Plant Engineers and has been the Hon. Course Director, IIMM, Hyderabad since 1980. Presently he is a Management Consultant and has been teaching subjects such as MM, Operations Management, Product Management, Industrial Marketing, Services Marketing, SCM, Inventory Management, Purchase Management, World Class Manufacturing, Global Sourcing, International Trade etc., at various Management Institutes.

He worked as Chief Executive of a public sector company and also in private sector for more than a decade. His experience of teaching and practising ran concurrently.

Contents

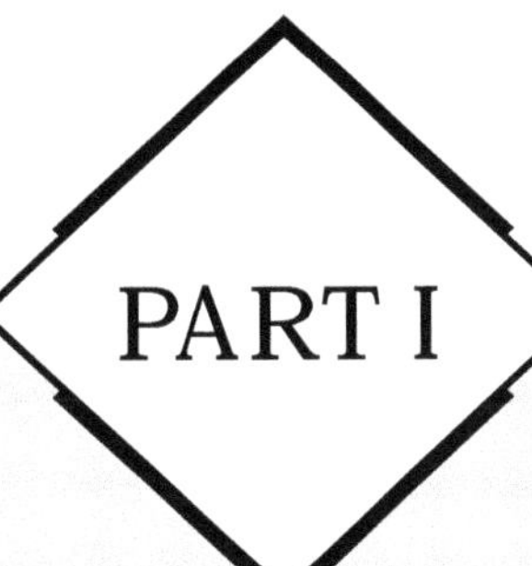

Chapter-1: Origin and Growth of Materials Management in Indian Healthcare Industry

Chapter-2: Integrated Hospital Materials Management

Chapter-3: Materials Management in Hospital Pharmacy

PART - I

Origin and Growth of Materials Management in Indian Healthcare Industry

Contents

CHAPTER - 1

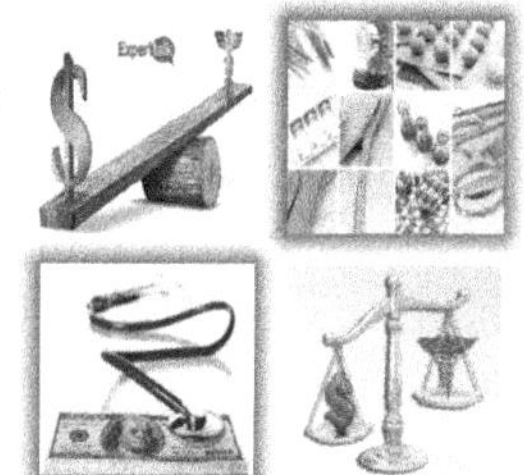

Origin and Growth of Materials Management in Indian Healthcare Industry

INTRODUCTION

Change is the only constant in the life. A dynamic profession like Materials Management evolves continuously and absorbs new ideas, concepts and philosophies. It also develops new tools and techniques to cope with the ever changing environment. In fact, the resilience of a profession or academic discipline stems from its ability to continuously adapt and improvise. Over the past quarter of a century, materials management in India has witnessed changes in cataclysmic propositions and transformed from a mere clerical, administrative function into a strategic business initiative. However, between David's slingshot and an intercontinental ballistic missile, the industrial Materials Management was scientifically systemized. The future - The confluence of bio-technology and Information Technology is the harbinger of the future. It will make way for neural networks and systems-on-chips embedded into human skin to transform the capability of managers beyond comprehension; with bated breath, we await the exciting future.

ORIGIN OF MATERIALS MANAGEMENT

Men need goods and services from others in order to live in comfort. As a matter of fact, that is what distinguishes the human beings from animals. The more they are civilized, the more such needs arise. At the beginning of human history, the basic needs that were in demand were met by usurpation or theft and services through slavery. Unfortunately, these practices are still in existence in some parts of the world. When mankind became more civilized and less barbaric, the needs were met at first stage by barter or by donation. Man spent millions of years hunting for his food. Then he learnt to use the skin of the animals for clothing. Slowly he found the advantages of agriculture. Some became adept at weaving, others in pottery, and a few in metal working. The medium of exchange was represented by standard objects such as food grains, animals, metals, precious stones, etc. the "Nexum" or Manicipatio the Greeks used 'cattle' as medium of exchange. The Manicipatio in Rome was accomplished through the "Libripens", who could be considered as the material administrators. To facilitate exchange, the libripens introduced metals which later lead to minting of coins that they called 'Pecunia' ('cattle' in Latin). Hence, it has been observed that we owe the coin to the Materials Manager and thus he became more and more necessary. During the third stage, the Romans considered the "Emptio Venditio" i.e., instead of coin at sight, a combined price; and the contract of effective barter became consensual contract of sales and purchases. There was no industry in an organized manner in the medieval ages. The purchase function achieved specialization quite early in man's history. The development of man can be directly correlated to the development of the purchasing function. In due course, man realized that it would be to his advantage, if instead of learning all the trades, he specialized in one trade and purchased the other products in return for what he produced, and thus the barter system developed. As the specialization increased, he found it difficult to fix values for the products to facilitate exchange. To ease the transactions, money came in to existence. In fact, money itself has come to represent only what it can buy. Once specialization in trade was developed and money was introduced, the development of mankind was really rapid. Man could purchase his requirement of goods and services and gain satisfaction. This process was extended to the organizations he built. As there was a ready market for specialized goods and services, economic development became viable that resulted in the growth of technology. Thus purchasing is always an essential part of man's activities and it forms the very basis of his development. The earliest example of purchase order dates back to 2500 BC. It was a clay tablet of Babylonian origin and was meant for supply of fragrant oil to be delivered in lots of 50 JARS at 15 days interval. **(Menon K.S., Purchasing and Inventory Control, A.H. Wheeler and Co. 1993)**

Towards the end of 17th century, King Louis XIV of France created a new position in French army; "Marechal General des Logis" (General Marshall of logistics), who was responsible for supply and transport of materials including selection of routes. Therefore, the term 'Logistics' approximately corresponds to the modern concept of materials management. The importance of position can be noticed from the title "Marechal" (Marshall). The entrepreneur created new ideas and put to practice by mobilizing himself the necessary capital, and managed personnel, production, sales and finance. **Later on, over a period of time, he divested himself one after other functions to others in the following fashion:**

- Finance Department including accounting and auditing took care of the finances.
- Human Resources Department or Personnel Department took care of personnel staff control and industrial relations.
- The relative importance of sales, production, finance and staff managers has varied according to economic cycles, kind of businesses and the culture of enterprises.

However, the materials function was not delegated to others and he managed it himself as he considered it vital. Thus the four areas established themselves as basic functions. Materials today are the life blood of industry without which no organization can operate.

In the initial stages of industrial evolution, productivity hardly increased. Availability of manpower far exceeded machine power. Emphasis was on men as the first source of productive

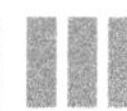

power. Before the 20th century, machines and the manufacturing processes were simple, uncomplicated, though slow. Materials were simple and available in plenty and at low costs. Distribution was confined to a limited area. Location of manufacturing units close to the sources of cheap raw materials was one of pre-requisites to production. Introduction of better and newer machines coupled with scientific management to arrange and schedule them led to the factory system, which in turn resulted in many industrial changes and inventions, changing the whole complex of manufacturing. Gradually materials became more complex, labour more specialized and mechanization increased continuously. The growing complexity of materials combined with its scarcity and high cost and the increasing volume of production naturally shifted the importance to "Materials" as it became the largest element in the total cost of the product. This shift in the relative value of materials making it the largest single element in the total cost of production continues even today.

In India, the concept of materials management was in vogue several centuries back. Kautilya's Arthashastra is one such work of literature wherein the Indians were said to have mastered the art of materials management. In his great work "Ashtadhyayi", Panini the ancient Indian grammarian referred to many great storage vessels like the 6 foot high cylindrical vessel made of earth called 'kusala', 'kumba', with a narrow mouth, 'Kupa' resembling a well, 'Sala' a masonry structure with an opening called 'Bila' etc. In 'Arthasastra', **Kautilya, the famous Raj guru of King Chandragupta Maurya** gives a detailed description of the storage practices followed during the latter's reign. The Mauryan regime had constructed ships with facilities to store huge quantities of food grains, which were also engaged in foreign trade. The renowned minister set out well defined duties of the keepers of the Crown storehouses. The principle keeper was called 'Dhanyadhipa' and the qualification needed to hold that position was to be an expert in determining the varieties and grades of the grains as also the techniques to store them in a healthy state and to protect them from pests, rodents etc.

In the 19th century, Napoleon carried all of his supplies, including food, in the form of dried products. His armies were spread out and communication methods had to be devised to coordinate the movement of men, equipment, and supplies. He used sophisticated methods for the same. He never would have achieved the success that he had if he had not been concerned with the logis-tics of obtaining and moving supplies. Thus was born the concept of "material". Modern armies still practice this logistics of material.

Industry before the 19th century was confined to the home. Each family was either given or bought supplies from which it created desired products. Mechanization began in that century and gave rise to factories, with people leaving their homes to work in central locations. Textile mills of this era were to be the home of the first primitive computer. This was not successful, but the need had been identified.

In Indian industry, the concept of Stores Management did not receive its due recognition till 1980's though the concepts of scientific stores management were in vogue during the Gupta period. The new marketing concepts such as **customer satisfaction, customer delight, customer surprise brought in their way that industry has to deliver "more for less".** Customers are demanding, no

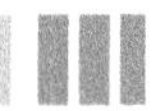

Stock outs, shorter lead times, frequent deliveries and delivery within specified time frame. In addition, the customers are expecting value added services such as bar coding of secondary containers, shrink warping pallets, drop shipment and even direct door delivery at the same cost or even lower cost. This pressure heightens service from stores manager for improvement, cost and service not only from customers but also from top managers.

In the early days of the industrial revolution, the industrialists were not formally acquainted with the principles of materials management. The three decades that followed industrial revolution marked the advent of modern production. The introduction of artificial source of power meant that factories could be located away from rivers and coastal areas. Electricity, Steel and Gas energy could run large number of machines. A deluge of inventions viz., the automobiles and trucks, radio, telephone, airplane and sophistication of machine tools has brought new vistas to industry and commerce. Mass production was incorporated in the factories all over and these soon developed into well designed plants. Production increased in complexity and labour took on new importance.

The most significant concept evolved in that period was the recognition of need for an operating line and servicing staff. **F W Taylor,** the father of scientific or modern management took the first major step towards functional organization and staff specialist. Taylor provided for the materials management function a long range planning, production control and scheduling, as well as other operational tools, such as quality control, industrial engineering, cost control and standardization of operations and procedures *(Ballot 1971). HL Gangt, refined Taylor's production control.*

There are quite a few authors who believe that materials management is an extension of purchasing function and they say " when most of the functions related to materials management are grouped together organizationally, the purchasing manager becomes a materials manager in fact, if not entitled. Eventually management recognized that function being performed in each of all departments is no longer purchasing, but something else; materials management. They recognized this by changing purchase manager to the title of materials managers." **(Hammer 1970).**

Most of the present materials managers have developed from purchasing executives. It is not surprising therefore that they regard materials management is logical extension of purchasing function *(Datta 1978).*

Even as late as 1900, when the United States and the leading European nations were already established as industrialized nations, the concept of separate and independent materials activity was novel to most managers. Of course, subsequent research by **Harold E. Fearon and John H. Hoagland** showed that, in mining firms at least, purchasing existed as a separate activity as early as 1832, and was very common in railroad firms by 1887. However, it came to manufacturing firms somewhat later and unfortunately some firms did not have strong independent purchasing or materials activities as late as the 1950's. By the end of 50's, the concept of coordinated administration of materials function became overwhelmingly important, placing heavy emphasis on both value and control.

 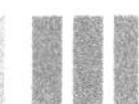

During World War II, industries had no selling problem. Their success depended very much on their ability to obtain raw materials to keep their factories working. This has lead to recognition of materials management as a specialized managerial function. The fact was no longer contested. It allowed considerable improvement of materials management staff. "Materials Management" gained new prestige with the book **"Crusade in Europe"** written by **General Eisenhower,** former President of U.S.A. He states that, "The complete success in modern industries depends on efficient organization of the materials service; an efficient material service is one of the most astonishing of all brilliant achievements".

In the middle of the 1960's, bank interest rates began to rise all over the world from 3 to 4 percent in 1950's to 9 to 16 percent. Keeping excessive inventory under such circumstances was a luxury that leads many companies to bankruptcy. Inventory management became an indispensable item in competition. The Japanese were the precursors. During the golden jubilee convention of National Association of Purchasing Agents of USA held in 1965, the US Secretary of Commerce called "Purchasing" a major factor keeping the country competitive in an increasingly tough old market. Materials management is termed as **"The last gold mine"** for business executives. It is indeed the last of specialized functions to be given the responsibility and authority for making major contributions to business profits. And the efficiency or the lack of it, with which this vital function is carried out, will make or mark the success of the organization.

In 1970's, commodities were still in shortage and prices increased abnormally culminating with oil embargo in 1973. Source marketing appeared. It became evident that **systemized scientific materials management was in unquestionable function in overall management.**

This led to:

- Progressive elimination of subordination.
- Evolution of materials management in several aspects, professional and functional.
- Historical evolution within wider context

Evolution of Materials Management

Table 1.1 Evolution of materials management function

Perception of	Primitive	1st evolution	2nd evolution	Present development
Status of materials management	Errand boy	Serving production	Market experts	Managers of 60 percent of total expenses
Materials management staff	Glorified office boy	Bureaucrat	Commerce expert in marketing	Negotiator engineer economist lawyer
Possibilities of improvement in Materials Management	Dead end	Purchasing aid, buyer senior buyer	Section chief Dept chief Manager	Executive Director Vice President
Usefulness of Materials Management	Expenses only	Avoid shortage, demobilize inventory	Source marketing strategic planning	Contributor for profit

Thus today materials are life blood of an industry. Materials management is basic part of any organization that produces a product or service of economic value. It is not only essential for profit making industries but also for service enterprises, both in public and private sectors of economy.

Very soon, materials managers will have a career superior to a vice president. The decades of sixties was an era of industrialization, India saw a trend towards improvement in production capabilities. In seventies, major emphasis shifted to marketing and selling. The decade of eighties rediscovered need for resources conservation. It brought a realization that commodity shortages have a severe impact on profitability. In the current decade, the economic scenario in India is changing at breathtaking pace. The changes in various areas such as fiscal, trade policy reforms, industrial reforms etc., are aimed at stimulating growth.

The opening up of the economy to global competition is bound to throw up unforeseen challenges to Materials Management professionals in this country. As the walls of protectionism are demolished, the foreign technology and goods flow in. Materials Management will perform a more and more important role in the future. Today's entrepreneur emphasizes "Research and Modernization". New products will demand new suppliers; new technical and economical supply problems will have to be solved. Tendency to concentration, assisted by fusions, amalgamation and takeovers, etc. will demand better negotiators and a high level relationship, of the same status as those of suppliers.

Complexity of organizations and the use of IT has increased, thus increasing the need for well trained and competent Materials Managers. Shortage of many primary materials and sources of energy will demand alternatives. These may be found through "Value Analysis". Industry and commerce will not only need more Material Managers, but also those who are better prepared and more efficient and agile. The young managers will have good opportunities for progressing, according to their ambitions, ability and efforts. Well trained and efficient Material Managers will earn higher salaries and perks because they are important executives. Considering the nature and complexities of modern day materials management, it is difficult to lay down any particular academic qualification as a necessary professional requirement of a good materials manager.

National Association of Purchasing Agents appointed **Harbridge House Consultants Boston,** Massachusetts in the year 1960 to make a study on Materials Management. Harbridge Consultants made a study and were unable to arrive at comprehensive definition of Materials Management and concluded that, "too many managers simply do not know what materials management was". **Dean S. Ammer says, "Every study that has been made indicated that there is no agreement as to precisely what activities should be undertaken by the materials manager."**

A survey of literature on Materials Management indicates that there are as many definitions of Materials Management. Different authors included different functions in materials management. However all the authors are unanimous in Materials Management include basic three functions purchasing, stores, inventory control (which includes sub functions of planning, handling, and distribution).

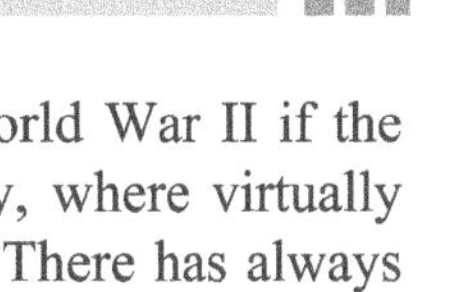

There are those who say the United States would not have won the World War II if the concept of materials management had not been used in the aircraft industry, where virtually overnight the nation was able to develop and build warplanes by thousands. There has always been this connection between the military and distribution of supplies. Today, modern industries could not realize profits, and thus could not survive, if not for the use of sophisticated forms of materials management, such as materials requirements planning.

EVOLUTION OF PURCHASING IN INDIAN INDUSTRY

In order to have a better appreciation of evolution of purchasing function in Indian industry, it is helpful to first understand the historical role of purchasing and its development. At the turn of the twentieth century, in small or newer businesses, the owners controlled all buying. It was one of the many duties they performed. Clerical detail is inherent in buying. As the company expanded, it was necessary to have someone pick up this clerical workload; however buying authority remained with the owner. As the operations of companies increased; the buying function was assigned to the production department, since it consumed most purchased materials in the manufacturing process. The clear trend to bifurcate purchasing from production was evidenced in 1940's. Studies towards the end of this period show the purchasing officer reporting to the president or a vice president in 70 percent of the firms surveyed. By the late 1950's, the trend is even clearer. A survey of 350 companies shows the purchasing head reporting to top management; about 95 per cent of the time to the president, a vice president or executive vice president (38 per cent), the general manager (36 per cent), the treasurer (15 per cent), the production vice president (3 per cent), or to the controller (3 per cent), director of manufacturing, production manager, or plant supervisor (5 per cent). There has been little understanding of purchasing role by non purchasing executives. This was probably because the function previously had not been so important, and purchasing people were generally not considered the top talent in an organization. Purchasing therefore has been relegated to a position subordinate to other departments, especially production. Now, fortunately, this practice is changing due to a gradual recognition that effective purchasing requires individuals with specialized skills, knowledge, and ability to cope with the changing conditions that beset modern business.

"The key to efficient and effective industrial marketing is not the supplier but the buyer." This statement by **Peter F Drucker,** one of America's foremost management spokesmen, highlights a growing awareness of the role of purchasing activities in our business society. Yet for all the thousands of books written on marketing, there is but a handful on the buying function. (Peter Drucker, "The Economies of Dark Continent;" fortune magazine, 1962) Mr. Drucker says further, "The industrial purchaser has to know his own business, of course, and the progress made here in the last few years is all to the good. He has to know what the product or supply he buys is supposed to contribute to his company's end results, has to buy it at cost per unit of his own output rather than just by the price tag. But he also needs to know just as much about the structure of the supplier industry and its economics." Pointing a finger at purchasing performance, he continues, "... The buyer of industrial product and supplies is in many cases semi literate, or even illiterate, in a business

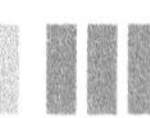

sense." Although these words reflect an oversimplification of the state of the purchasing art, here is an awareness both of the tremendous value of the purchasing function, and of the limitation of those in the field. Hospitals subscribe to the importance of good purchasing, yet must admit to an overall weakness on the part of individuals practising its skills. One may argue that it isn't necessary to have a purchasing department. Whether, one exists or not, the buying function must be performed. Buying can be done by anyone in engineering, production, finance, or management. However, during the first half of the 20th century, most businesses found, through experience, that it is desirable to establish a separate department, known as purchasing, to handle procurement activity.

One more proof of top management's recognition of the purchasing function is to be found in recent statements by several of industry's foremost statesman. **Roge M. Blough,** Chairman of the board of United States Steel, has said: "It seems to me that you [purchasing men] hold one of the master keys to progress and growth in American industry.... You spend nearly a quarter trillion dollars each year in the market place. Can we hope even to comprehend the effect that your purchasing decisions actually have upon the nation and its economy, the spur that you along with others in your organization can give, or fail to give, to the processes of innovation, and the power you have to influence America's competitive position in the world ?"

Today's purchasing manager must be one of the most knowledgeable managers in his company. Unless he understands enough design, engineering, production, and marketing and related functions in sufficient detail, he can't possibly do his job. Purchasing people must be brought into the picture in the earliest stages of design, engineering, and production. Frequently, they are able to make creative suggestions and studies that result in improved products, faster production schedules, even better design and appearance. Realistically, the hard necessities of price considerations will probably always come first. But, more and more companies are realizing that creative purchasing practices can result in more than just saving money. They can make money as well. Top management will give purchasing more authority as it comes to realize that, without control, purchasing can't take the necessary action to prevent unnecessary costs and losses.

RECENT TRENDS IN MATERIALS MANAGEMENT IN THE INDIAN CONTEXT

During the second half of the 1970's, the country was still with the mindset of 'License, Quota, and Permit Raj'. National planning was based on the 5-year plans as per the blueprint given by the first Prime Minister of India Shri Jawaharlal Nehru. We were trying to practise the socialistic pattern of economy as in the erstwhile USSR. The western ideas of capitalism, free competition and market driven economy were considered too imperialistic and materialistic for our society. At the national level, **the Indian National Congress (INC)** was the sole ruling party up to 1977 and its leader, the charismatic **Mrs. Indira Gandhi,** the ideal Prime Minister. All this suddenly changed due to the backlash of national emergency in 1977. The first opposition coalition came to power at the centre in the national elections that followed the lifting of emergency. It can be said to be the beginning of coalition politics at the national level. During this period of political upheavals and

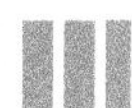

uncertainty, the corporate managers had to evolve the strategic plans within the framework of national policy making. Import licensing restrictions had to be contended with. Industrial licensing was a very complicated exercise in the labyrinth of corridors of power. Hence in 1976, the theme of national planning in so far as it concerned Materials Management was industrial licensing.

All the while it was also being felt that bureaucratic controls were throttling national growth and preventing the country from achieving prosperity and higher standard of living for its teeming millions. Hence in the year 1977, the predominant theme was national growth and the contributions which the profession of MM could possibly make to accelerate the process of growth, by augmenting utilization of installed capacity and improvement in industrial productivity.

There was a strong perception in the Planning Commission at that time that the twin problems of underdevelopment and unemployment could be solved by encouraging ancillaries and small scale industries. When the Janata Party came to power, post emergency, they gave a further fillip to the national endeavour for small scale sector by reserving many more items for exclusive manufacture by Small Scale Industries (SSI) and creating a new 'tiny' sector. 'MM and ancillary Development' was the major issue.

Around this time, severe materials shortages began to be felt by several sectors of the Indian industry, particularly those that are dependent on petroleum products and petrochemicals. The challenge to MM in the years ahead was perceived as coping with materials shortages. The Government in 1979 and 1980 tried to take a peek at the immediate future and evolve strategies for procurement of hard-to-buy materials.

Materials Management during 1981-85

At the commencement of the decade of 80's, the Materials Management (MM) professionals in India and all over the world started taking a fresh look at the relevance of their profession to the overall objectives of the corporations which they were working for. It was realized that MM cannot exist only in an intellectual plane and insulate itself from the mainstream of corporate life. MM in 1981 concentrated on the theme of "Materials Management and Corporate Objectives". The professionals strongly urged the Materials Managers to be conscious to the constraints imposed on their profession by the corporate objectives. One of the important objectives that emerged was in the area of cost control. With double digit inflation all around, costs were rapidly getting out of control. This led to rising prices of finished products and thus came into existence the upward price spiral. The theme of "Curbing Inflation by Efficient Materials Management" was the flavour of the day. It soon became apparent that cost control of incoming materials was desirable but just not sufficient. If the companies were to prosper and be competitive too, the productivity must be maintained at a higher level and improved upon continuously. This can be possible only by making the inputs available at the right time and right place. In capital intensive industries, spare parts play a very important role in utilization of plant and machinery and in productivity enhancement. It was rightly felt that effective MM could boost productivity. By 1984, the theme was "Inventory

Management for Corporate Results". It clearly concluded that corporate results could only be achieved through efficient and effective Materials Management.

Materials Management during 1986 - 1990

By the year 1986, it was evident to the materials managers and to corporate think tanks that the old order was inexorably changing. The 21st century would be drastically different from anything witnessed in the history of mankind. MM professionals deliberated up on the theme of "Materials Management Challenges of 21st Century". The vital role that MM can play towards corporate profitability came to be the most important. Around that time, the impact of Information Technology was being felt on Materials Management, Information Systems throughout the world. Digital communications and Internet started penetrating in the Indian psyche. The World Wide Web was perceived as a source of all information, communication, advertising and source of potential suppliers of future. Keeping this in mind, the various aspects of Materials Management in the hi tech environment became important to materials managers of that time.

Materials Management during 1991 to 1996

Materials in the manufacturing sector constitute 50 to 70 percent of the total cost and savings would make the product competitive in the market. Wages and infrastructure facilities like power, freight and so on will continue to escalate; thus bringing pressure on controlling the cost of materials. Until total costs are controlled, the exports of our products will suffer, as they will not be internationally competitive. This will deny us the economies of scale. It has to be remembered that incentives for exports like cash compensatory support, duty drawbacks and so on will remain temporary palliatives, since the pressure on the government to reduce subsidy will remain strong.

Globalization essentially means that economic activity and business of a country do not remain confined within its political boundaries. Its companies have operations in several other countries and at the same time, they are not protected from external competition from other global companies. Such transnational companies (or stateless corporations) invest or carry on business in whichever part of the world where it is most profitable and not necessarily in the country of their origin.

This new trend has transformed the world economy. Economic globalization now marries the cheap capital of rich countries with the cheap skilled labour of developing countries to produce the most competitive goods. The great opportunity provided by globalization should combine cheap global capital with inexpensive Indian skills to take India to march ahead strategy.

The main challenge for Indian industry is to become globally competitive in terms of costs, quality, and delivery performance. **Today, it is not enough to be "First Class", our companies have to become "World Class".**

From the year 1994 onwards, Materials Management started relying more and more on Information Technology and the relationships among Information Technology, Materials Management, and corporate competitiveness. Information Technology can be of help to an organization

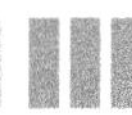

in many areas. The first of these areas is in cycle time reduction. Information Technology can do a great deal in speeding up business. Secondly, it can enhance service levels and is the best tool in improving customer satisfaction. Thirdly, world class manufacturing organizations would not have been possible without the advancements that have taken place in Information Technology, which is the prime mover to bring the corporate competitiveness and lastly, the decentralization of power.

SUPPLY CHAIN MANAGEMENT IN THE CYBER AGE

Supply Chain Management encompasses all elements of sourcing, indenting, procuring, production scheduling, order processing, inventory management, transportation, warehousing and customer service as well as the information and monitoring system. Supply Chain Management coordinates and integrates all these activities into a seamless process where all "partners" of the chain like vendors, carriers and third party logistic companies are 'links' in the chain. Chief executives are hard pressed to optimize sales growth, reduce costs, secure better working capital management and improve overall performance, productivity and profitability. Production should not rely solely on sales forecasts, but instead by synchronizing closely with customer orders. It is here that Information Technology has to play a significant role by giving an edge to logistics and link individual parts with the whole chain.

In the cyber age, cyber highways have become as important, if not more important than our highways. Worldwide websites E-mails and E-commerce will be the order of the day. Citizens are become worldwide citizens. E-commerce has matured and Information Technology companies are the new creators of economic value when supply chains will now become intelligent supply chains.

Increased use of Information Technology to enhance commerce and communication is predicted. This has enabled global sourcing, increased transaction speed and made geographical distance inconsequential. It enables each element of value chain to enhance customer's delight. Successful enterprises identify the potential of Supply Chain Management, taking the supplier base as partners of progress.

EVOLUTION OF MATERIALS MANAGEMENT IN THE HEALTHCARE INDUSTRY

Healthcare provision must be viewed as an industry like any other. Its products and underlying value systems are somewhat different but the basic managerial structures are no different. Techniques that improve performance in one industry must be evaluated for feasibility in others. Materials Management has been recognized as an effective tool in other industries for years. It is only a matter of time before its value is fully realized in healthcare. Hospitals should be viewed not only as a group of coordinated activities in a structure but also as a series of neighbor hoods, each concerned with the acquisition, processing, and distribution of materials, as well as with the provision of diagnostic and treatment services related to patient care. These neighbourhoods, or departments, are relatively autonomous; yet exist together as if they were in a city. They all have the same underlying objective, which is to care for patients' medical needs. Their common goal must be to find the most efficient and effective way of achieving this basic objective:

At one time, hospital supplies were limited. Bed linen was changed infrequently. Food was brought to large patient wards in buckets. Each patient had a plate and a spoon, recyclable dressings, and a few medications. To complicate matters, supplies that were used on patients had to be cleaned, packaged, and sterilized for reuse. The need for these manufacturing functions led to the development of laundries and small, decentralized processing areas. As technology grew, a myriad of tests and procedures developed as a result of advances in anaesthesia, microbiology, and radiology. Each technological advance spawned a new stock of supplies necessary to support it. The need for supplies and equipment unique to healthcare gave rise to a profusion of manufacturers anxious to meet these requirements. Their needs and objectives sometimes were at odds with those of healthcare providers themselves. This led to high prices and unnecessarily large stocks of supplies. To cope with this situation, a new activity arose in healthcare institutions: the acquisition, storage, and distribution of materials. Unfortunately, these activities were often performed by persons who were neither trained nor interested in doing them effectively. However, in the 1970s, the sheer volume and cost of these activities reached a point where some hospitals began to adopt Materials Management concepts and practices. The single-source control system of inventory management, processing, and distribution of materials became the key to bringing order out of chaos.

A system can be defined as a logical sequence of concepts or components designed to accomplish a specific function efficiently. Material Management, therefore, qualifies as a system. Systems have the following components:

1. Inputs
2. Processes
3. Outputs
4. Controls

These components may be envisioned within the four Materials Management sub systems of procurement, inventory management, including acquisition, processing, and distribution. Feedback on the performance of this system needs to be monitored, and adjustments are to be made to its design and operation, so that a continuing cycle of logical and effective material related behaviour is established. This system of materials management is one of the elements that tie the total organization together. The concept of materials management must be integrated into the total operating philosophy of a hospital if that facility is to be efficient.

HOSPITAL MATERIALS MANAGEMENT AT PRESENT

A few years ago, it was common to find hospitals that did not use centralized Materials Management. As the economy tightened and regulatory and consumer constraints on the healthcare industry increased, more and more MM programmes came into existence. However, MM in the healthcare industry is still in the early stages of development in terms of being recognized as a

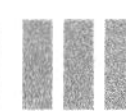

specific and credible discipline. It is true that increasing numbers of managers have graduate and postgraduate degrees and have studied the managerial and logistical techniques developed in other industries. However, the actual time spent in specifically studying healthcare MM has been generally insignificant. More materials managers are now reading books and journals devoted to this subject, attending seminars, joining professional associations, and taking certifying examinations. Thus, much of the structure and foundation of this discipline is in place. However, **materials managers still consider themselves as order takers, not direction setters.** They accept the idea that departments such as surgery, radiology, and laboratory are outside the realm of MM and that MM is only based on the implementation end of the hospital's long-range plan instead of being involved in its development. All the information and techniques related to the management of materials in this specific industry has not been synthesized into a common body of knowledge that can be identified and taught in colleges and universities. Next, the disparate professional organizations that represent the various aspects of healthcare MM have not been integrated into one unified professional body. There must always be effective representation of the specific interests of the special areas such as central processing, laundry, purchasing, etc. which are the different aspects of MM. If these managers are to obtain the required broad recognition and deep support, a unified body must represent them. Finally, materials managers, in the aggregate, have not been successful in proving to administrators, physicians, and board of directors that they are qualified, competent, and have earned the right to participate in the broad direction-setting process for their organizations. Many of them can effectively manage routine daily operations. They must also acquire the vision, expertise, and skill necessary to be accountable for the materials management of the total organization. Then their hospitals will be able to realize the full benefits of effective Materials Management.

FUTURE OF HOSPITAL MATERIALS MANAGEMENT

Great strides have been made since the mid 1980s in India. This field is at a normal, healthy point in its development. The levels of education and expertise of its materials managers are increasing. Performance and practices are becoming more standardized and it is gaining recognition. However, the challenges and opportunities of the coming years will be even greater. The measure of how fully managers realize the potential of their field will depend upon how assertively and effectively they grasp these opportunities and make them reality. Some trends are apparent and can serve as starting points for managers as they design future materials management programmes for their facilities.

Top Management Support

Every hospital must have a clear policy statement, issued by the chief executive officer and approved by the board of directors, that establishes firm support for, and a clear expectation that, materials management practices will be carried out effectively. This operating philosophy is to be handed down from the top of the organization. It will serve as the stimulus for all department heads to work with the materials manager in finding ways to improve their operations. It is also the basis

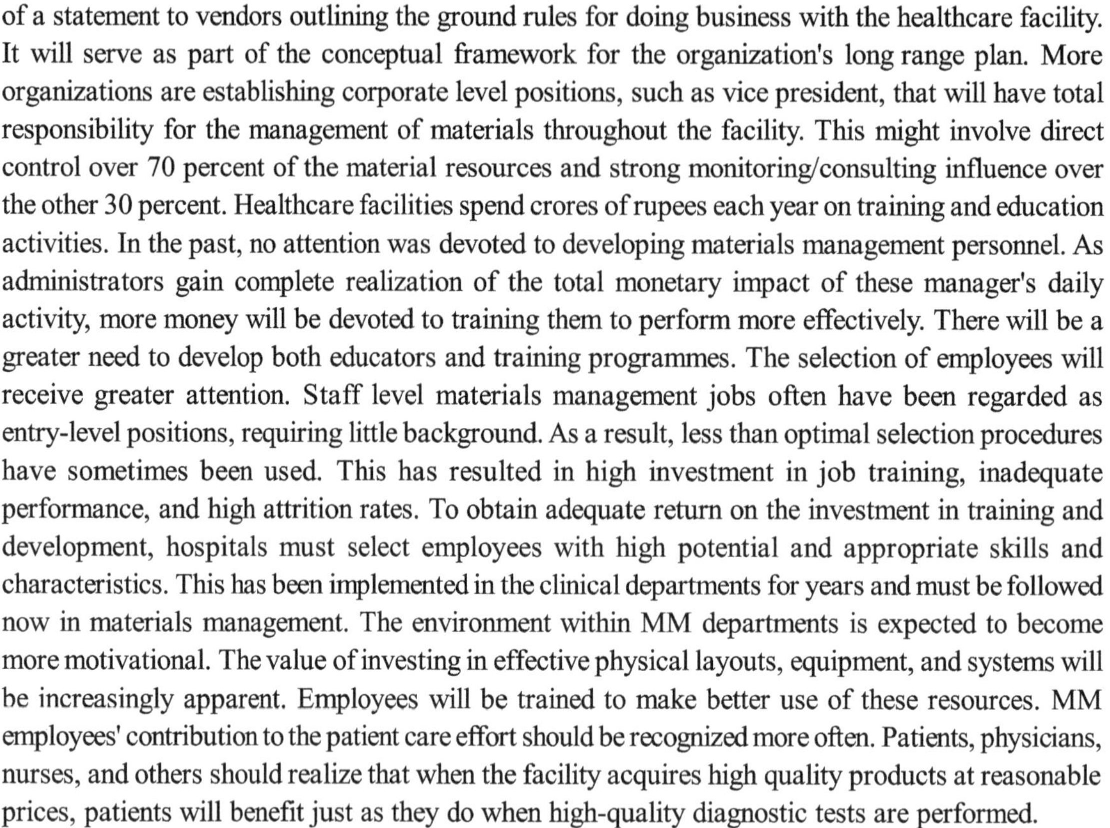

of a statement to vendors outlining the ground rules for doing business with the healthcare facility. It will serve as part of the conceptual framework for the organization's long range plan. More organizations are establishing corporate level positions, such as vice president, that will have total responsibility for the management of materials throughout the facility. This might involve direct control over 70 percent of the material resources and strong monitoring/consulting influence over the other 30 percent. Healthcare facilities spend crores of rupees each year on training and education activities. In the past, no attention was devoted to developing materials management personnel. As administrators gain complete realization of the total monetary impact of these manager's daily activity, more money will be devoted to training them to perform more effectively. There will be a greater need to develop both educators and training programmes. The selection of employees will receive greater attention. Staff level materials management jobs often have been regarded as entry-level positions, requiring little background. As a result, less than optimal selection procedures have sometimes been used. This has resulted in high investment in job training, inadequate performance, and high attrition rates. To obtain adequate return on the investment in training and development, hospitals must select employees with high potential and appropriate skills and characteristics. This has been implemented in the clinical departments for years and must be followed now in materials management. The environment within MM departments is expected to become more motivational. The value of investing in effective physical layouts, equipment, and systems will be increasingly apparent. Employees will be trained to make better use of these resources. MM employees' contribution to the patient care effort should be recognized more often. Patients, physicians, nurses, and others should realize that when the facility acquires high quality products at reasonable prices, patients will benefit just as they do when high-quality diagnostic tests are performed.

Organization of Hospital Delivery System

Hospitals strive to replace declining inpatient revenues with income from alternate delivery systems and services. In this effort, materials managers can play increasingly valuable roles in improving the bottom lines of these services. Hospitals' ability to reduce operating costs while maintaining quality of service will be a vital factor in whether or not these alternate services succeed or fail. The development of centralized material distribution centres to support a facility or group of facilities will accelerate. Well trained specialists would operate these centres round the clock which are designed to fulfill the total supply management needs of the organization. A major emphasis is to ensure that clinical people spend their time in direct patient care and that those who are best able to do so in a cost effective way perform non clinical support functions. Performance targets for MM functions should be established for all operating areas of the organization. For example, the value of inventory to be invested in the surgery department, as well as turnover rates and rates of availability, should be determined jointly by the materials manager and surgery manager, monitored, and adjusted as needed. Emphasis should be on how this investment contributes to the primary goal of patient care and to the organization's total bottom line. Active standardization committees play a great role in the hospital's daily operation. These groups have strong administrative support

 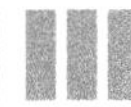

and are involved in the standardization of products, systems, and actual performance. Such a committee may routinely review inventory turnover by department and serve as added support to the materials manager in correcting performance problems. **Nearly 20 percent of the average cost of materials is related to capital equipment that many times has been acquired without adequate involvement from the purchasing department.** Administrators of effectively managed hospitals demand that a triad approach, involving the requesting department, purchasing department, and biomedical engineering department, be used to manage all major capital acquisitions from start to finish.

IMPACT OF INFORMATION TECHNOLOGY

Computer support is the order of the day, even in smaller hospitals. With the continuing expansion of the microcomputer and personal computer markets, many organizations operate online, in a real-time environment. Materials managers will have to stay abreast of changes in computer support systems if they hope to remain competitive in the healthcare industry of the future. Forecasting models and other techniques, such as **Material Requirements Planning (MRP),** which have been well established in other industries, can be modified for use in healthcare.

Standardized material requirements will be established for each diagnosis and procedure. As projected admissions and surgery cases are scheduled, the computer systems generate lists of required materials. These are compared to on hand/on order quantities and replenishment orders are generated automatically. Thus, the flow or consumption of materials is tied directly to the actual workflow of the institution. The need to develop these standard material requirements serve as the springboard for improving communication between material managers and clinical managers. This also accelerates understanding of the interrelated nature of everyone's contribution to direct patient care. Every healthcare facility should also adopt standard cost accounting practices. This will be critical in ensuring that patient care is provided at an acceptable level of quality and at a profit. The mark of the effective organizations is their use of an interdisciplinary team approach to developing standards and managing costs. Team members include representatives from finance, clinical departments, medical records, and materials management.

There has been an increasing use of direct computer-to-computer digital communication between healthcare facilities and major vendors. In addition, bar code and **optical character recognition (OCR)** devices are used routinely in streamlining the handling of the materials. This requires an increasingly effective interface between manufacturers and users of medical products. There will now be more demand on vendors to ship goods just in time. This is based upon the Japanese concept of inventory management and has led to significant reduction in inventory carrying costs for healthcare providers. It will provide a great challenge to material managers to ensure that it does not result in increased stock outs. It will be in the best interests of manufacturers, distributors, and users to work together to find effective systems that can satisfy everyone's profit needs while meeting patients' need for quality care at reasonable cost. Another area in which healthcare providers and vendors ought to work more closely is in the provision of value analysis programmes. Value

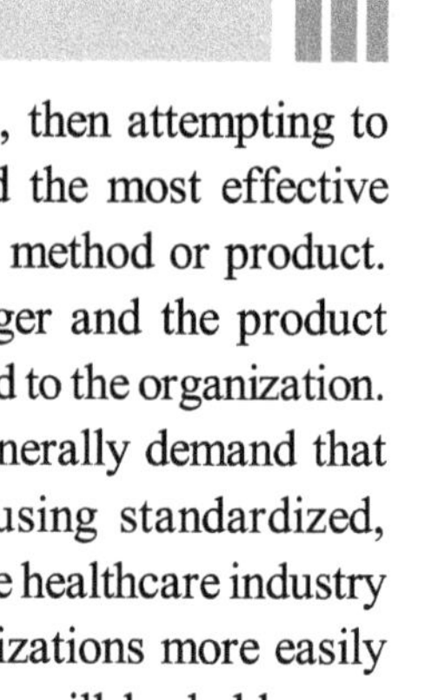

analysis involves analyzing a function or product in terms of its components, then attempting to identify the most effective method of achieving the functional objective and the most effective product for applying that method. The goal is to find the most value efficient method or product. This concept should be implemented on a broad scale. The materials manager and the product standards committee serve as the facilitators for seeing that this service is provided to the organization. Vendors will play a significant role in its actual provision. Administrators generally demand that materials management performance be monitored routinely and reported using standardized, statistically valid protocols. These will become more standardized throughout the healthcare industry so that administrators will be able to measure the performance of their organizations more easily both against themselves and against their competitors. As a result, managers will be held more accountable for the actual performance. As the healthcare industry becomes more competitive, this will be reflected in the emoluments. Thus, the manager's personal bottom line gets linked directly to the organization's bottom line. Effective managers, who can help improve their company's bottom line, will naturally stand out in a quantifiable way and can receive significant rewards. Managers who are not able to do this will be replaced ultimately. This is how it should function in a healthy, economically viable environment.

Bright Future Ahead

Individual material managers can do much to see that the healthcare industry reaps the full benefits of effective materials management. They can become involved in professional associations such as the **Indian Institute of Materials Management** at the local, regional, and, ultimately, national levels. Within this framework, they can strive to see that the groups achieve the following objectives:

- Increased communication between the different disciplines of Materials Management.
- Increased communication between materials management entities and related organization's departments such as those for surgical nurses and infection control practitioners.
- Development of a unified professional body to represent the interests of all materials management specialities, as in the case of National Association of Hospital Purchasing - Material Management in USA.
- Participation in regular educational programmes designed to meet the specific needs of the members.
- Sharing of performance statistics among members with the aim of increasing the average level of performance within the community.
- Increased recognition for individual members and the group for contributions to cost-effective healthcare in the community.

The next step is to establish a personal development plan. This can be enhanced by soliciting suggestions from a superior, the head of the human resource department of the healthcare facility,

 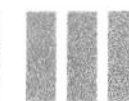

and key people in the professional organization. **Managers should plan specific steps that will lead to measurable improvement in the following three areas:**

1. Knowledge and skill
    - College level courses leading to higher academic attainments and to correct specific deficiencies.
    - Seminars, symposia and workshops.
    - Enriching their knowledge by reading professional journals.
2. Major performance objectives related to their current position.
3. Recognition of the value of their achievements and those of their staff as they relate to an improved bottom line for the organization.

The health care industry is filled with challenges and opportunities. Its future is bright. Materials managers have learnt and grown over the years. In addition, they are in a fortunate position of having expertise in an area that is becoming increasingly vital to the long term success, and even survival, of the healthcare industry. Their success is bounded only by the breadth of their vision and the degree of assertiveness with which they grasp their opportunities.

PROJECTIONS AND TRENDS IN MATERIALS MANAGEMENT

Predicting trends in Materials Management involves the forecasting of trends in society, engineering, business, government, health, education, and life style. A number of separate but interdependent factors affect the lives of material managers and purchasers in the healthcare field. Medicine is one. General economic conditions, social planning, and social relationships are some others. Still another is technology, including architecture, industrial design and engineering and sanitary engineering. There are environmental as well as system changes. Government, and its actions and acts e.g., price controls, the safety and occupational hazards, minimum wages, medicare and medicaid, the transportation, the public health directly affects the hospital purchasing or materials manager's job. Whether the government is spending, and is more liberal with non profit capital improvement or research grants, or whether it is austere, requiring more local and independent financing, the jobs of materials managers are different because of its influence.

There were fewer laws but more regulations in the 1980s, especially in the healthcare field. The 1990s brought a wider range of freedom, more leisure, less social than technological emphasis, and a higher standard of living, despite inflation. The present decade will search for a set of ideals concurrent with less inflation and the attempt to keep employment constant, eliminate socio economic uncertainties, and offer wider latitude for individual, business, and labour growth.

The trend towards improved ecology, conservationism, consumerism, increased freedom and equality between individuals, a search for less materialistic goals, and an increased emphasis on social rather than technological pursuits is likely. The emphasis will be on newer methods of financing healthcare, rising patient costs caused by long term illness, more attempts to save lives by

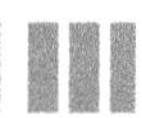

highly sophisticated services, the hospital as the centre of healthcare technology, prospective reimbursement by third party payers and diagnostic related groups, and price competition. The pendulum is swinging back to conservatism, although not, perhaps, to the conservatism of the 1940s because of the social legislation enacted since then. Economists have noted several trends that they say will continue in the new millennium. Inflation will continue throughout the world. With tariffs and the increasing cost of products from countries such as Japan and West Germany, imports into USA may decrease. There will be an improved stabilization of the dollar overseas, after some liberalizing of the tariff rules. There will be improved productivity in manufacturing and service industries. Some form of cost control will continue, at least for the next few years, particularly in healthcare, the oil industry, and certain manufacturing and processing industries.

Hospital costs will increase. Some sort of national health insurance programme is necessary in every country, involving payroll taxes and modification of the present system of healthcare. A package that covers all the healthcare costs of the average working family may bring about economies in healthcare. As the pressure for more efficiency in the hospital and more cost effective healthcare increases, administrators and materials managers will seek group purchasing agreements and shared services with other hospitals and with institutions such as universities and colleges.

Marketing healthcare services is another trend for the present decade. This is a business oriented programme applied to all hospitals in which hospitals attempt to market their services in their city or town and in outlying areas through extension of their services. This would mean arrangement of physicians' team to visit and lecture in small hospitals and clinics in rural areas more popularly known as referral hospitals; distribution of literature throughout the state describing a hospital's spectrum of services; and other direct and indirect marketing efforts.

An emphasis on social attitudes will characterize the hospital and other service institutions. Hospital administrators are aware of the trend towards patients' rights, although it is not yet clear how they relate to the physician patient relationship, the hospital physician patient relationship, or legal considerations involving these. Bio ethical concepts such as the right to life and the right to die are being discussed. Hospitals will be affected by an added dimension i.e., consumer movement in healthcare. There shall be spectacular increases in enrollments in healthcare educational institutions. In the recent past, there have been significant increases in admissions to nursing schools, but there are still shortages of nurses, some other paramedics and technicians. As part of new educational efforts, there will be new techniques and institutions for adult education, such as online colleges.

Engineering and Technology

There will be innovations in facility design and construction, because of cost constraints, energy problems, problems with capital financing due to high, almost prohibitive, interest rates. In package engineering, disposables will continue and escalate in volume, with new adaptations. Some manufacturers are beginning to offer both reusables and disposables as alternates. Pre-pareds, such as blood plasma administration sets, will increase, as will unit doses

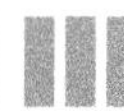

in pharmaceuticals. In sanitation engineering, there will be a major attempt to meet ecological problems of hospitals through improved waste disposal methods. Safety engineering will continue to be important. There will be extensive centralization of information on high speed data processors. The initial cost of computers will continue to decline, and smaller hospitals will tend to switchover to use of computer systems. Computers will continue to be of major interest to the larger hospitals also because their information storage, retrieval, and reporting costs are remarkably low. Computer services that offer application software programmes will interest smaller hospitals. **Medical telemetry, nurtured by space flights engineering, will be extended to the hospital's special care and emergency units.**

There are many developments in biomedical engineering. Hence an outside research laboratory should be used to test and report on new equipment. Testing of an electric wheelchair might be reported by an electrical test centre. Several such private research laboratories in the country offering highly valuable services to hospitals. A major field of endeavour for the hospitals is addiction to alcohol as well as to drugs. This may require utilization of new technology. Improved machinery will be used to handle laundry, shipping and receiving all materials, and their transportation, vertical and horizontal. An example is the electronic cart. Improvements such as automatic loading and unloading devices and automatic lubrication will result in faster functioning and larger capacities.

Government

Government will always continue to influence trends in healthcare. These influences will be of great importance to the Materials Management department, which is one of the few major departments of the hospital that can affect savings, or at least a reduction in costs. It means more and better source selection, more value analysis or value improvement programmes; more interest in shared services and in group or corporative buying; and new trends in dietary and pharmaceutical purchasing e.g., convenience foods and hospitals with no kitchens. The materials or purchasing managers will continue to attempt to obtain the "best" possible purchase with every hospital rupee spent. Pharmaceuticals are expected to experience the greatest developments but with greater restraints. New molecules are generally expensive and purchasing professionals should be involved in their procurement. This will mean more use of generic drugs and formularies in the hospital. There will be an increase in the variety and volume of laboratory procedures, but new tests will be add ons rather than alternatives. There will be increased do-it-yourself test kits for special conditions. The emergency room and ambulatory surgery will expand, requiring specialized personnel and equipment linked to community emergency services, with helicopters, helipads or heliports at hospitals; radio communication ambulances; and a very sophisticated regional or area wide emergency medical service system. Grants are now being made by the government for emergency care improvements. There will be further rapid growth of automatic chemical analyzers in the laboratory. The order of the day will be that tests will be directly linked to computers for rapid transmission - an automated laboratory system for major routine tests.

A competent materials manager will have all procurement functions; will be responsible for the functional flow of all materials to and from all departments, including dietary, central service,

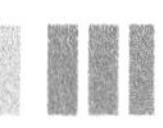

and pharmacy; and supervise laundry, receiving and stores, central communications and dispatch, communications, inventory control, printing, distribution, disposal, and purchasing research and management. He will have expanded responsibilities, more accountability, and become a vital member of the hospital management team. There have been numerous discussions on the subject of the materials manager. In the final analysis, it is his task to bring together divergent capabilities and produce a smoothly functioning human group. Unless the materials manager is a broad gauged manager, the potential benefits from Materials Manager will not be fully realized. His success should be measured not so much by the individual work that he does, but by his ability to work through others.

HEALTHCARE ECONOMICS

The economics of growth will certainly change. The hospital market has shown some definite indications of rising costs. Expenditures for healthcare have increased with the expectations of a population that has become more knowledgeable about its health and that seeks care from a number of sources the private physician's office, the hospital, the clinic, the public health department, the private non profit agency, and the university centre. Hospitals have increased their expenditures at a greater rate than the rest of the healthcare market. Studies have indicated that hospital expenditure as a percentage of total healthcare expenditures increased from 34 percent to 40 percent during the last two decades; rupee expenditures increased phenomenally. The Indian healthcare industry is seen to be growing at a rapid pace and is expected to become a US$280 billion industry by 2020. The Indian healthcare market was estimated at US$35 billion in 2007 and is expected to reach over US$70 billion by 2012 and US$145 billion by 2017. According to the Investment Commission of India, the healthcare sector has experienced phenomenal growth of 12 percent per annum between 2003 and 2007. Rising income levels and a growing elderly population are all factors that are driving this growth. In addition, changing demographics, disease profiles and the shift from chronic to lifestyle diseases in the country has led to increased spending on healthcare delivery.

India faces a huge need gap in terms of availability of number of hospital beds per 1000 population. With a world average of 3.96 hospital beds per 1000 population, India stands just a little over 0.7 hospital beds per 1000 population.[9] . Moreover, India faces a shortage of doctors, nurses and paramedics that are needed to propel the growing healthcare industry. India is now looking at establishing **academic medical centres (AMCs)** for the delivery of higher quality care with leading examples of **Manipal Group & All India Institute of Medical Sciences (AIIMS)** already in place. As incomes rise and the number of available financing options in terms of health insurance policies increase, consumers become more and more engaged in making informed decisions about their health and are well aware of the costs associated with those decisions. In order to remain competitive, healthcare providers are now not only looking at improving operational efficiency but are also looking at ways of enhancing patient experience overall. India has approximately 600,000 allopathic doctors registered to practice medicine. This number however, is higher than the actual number practising because it includes doctors who have emigrated to other countries as well as doctors

 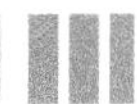

who have expired licenses. India licenses 18,000 new doctors a year. [Healthcare in India Source: http://en.wikipedia.org/w/index.php old id=369970093.]

As on today, it appears that the hospital industry is less affected by recession than industry as a whole. Use of hospital services has grown steadily. This was also true during the recession of 1975. Hospitals are healthier than ever today. Most of them are enjoying a greater cash flow because of increased utilization of existing facilities; this, in turn, results in increased income.

The use of outpatient facilities is growing even faster than that of the hospital as a whole. This could be as a result of (a) a greater acceptance of outpatient surgery and (b) the fact that unlike physicians' clinics, emergency rooms both for trauma and medical emergencies are now open for longer hours, at nights, and weekends too. The hospital is playing the role of a family doctor in many urban areas. Outpatient services are accessible: they do not require appointments or involve long period in the waiting room as do physicians' clinics. With the increased use of both inpatient and outpatient facilities, expenditures for hospital supplies, equipment, and services are also increasing. **Richard Dudley and Robert Brouwer** pointed out that "the growth in hospital expenditures is the result of inflation to a great extent, as well as the rise in population, increased use of health resources, and improved procedures for the care of patients." They also commented that "more intensive treatment and new and expensive procedures that contribute to the diagnoses of medical problems and care of patients are now available. These advancements undoubtedly resulted in the broadening of healthcare resources, improved care for the public, and increased revenues." Predicting the future of the healthcare industry is possible if one realizes that the variables may be changed and that, to a great extent, the same variables that changed the healthcare industry earlier will also affect it in the years to come. These changes, in turn, will have a dramatic effect on the field of hospital materials management.

During the decade of 1990's, with the advent of a number of corporate hospitals, the expectations of the patient care have undergone a number of changes.

Important among those are the following:

1. Consumer wants continued high standards of healthcare, but at lower costs.
2. The provider is cast as an adversary of comprehensive national healthcare systems.
3. Business and industry will enter into greater decision making on healthcare changes.
4. Programmes to prevent illness and promote health may follow as ways to reduce costs.
5. Majority of the healthcare institutions are in a most disorganized state.

In order to cope with technological advances in healthcare industry, the hospital purchasing and materials management must understand:

1. The need to avoid dehumanization in the hospital.
2. New biomedical research.

3. Increased medical specialization.
4. A more careful monitoring of new medical technology by the state and central governments.
5. Assessments relating to the efficiency of open heart surgery, foetal monitoring, haemodialysis, and noninvasive radiological and ultrasound diagnostic procedures.
6. The influence of health planning and third party reimbursement on the purchase of new machines: these two factors have been deterrents.
7. Weighing the risks of technology against the benefits.
8. Forecasting requirements.
9. Computers to assist in decision making.

Materials managers have to be aware of the following general trends for hospitals in the next decade:

1. Increased acuity of illness, and increased need for tertiary hospitals.
2. An increase in multi hospital group beds.
3. Cost containment.
4. Increased incentives for ambulatory care.
5. Reemphasis on home care, particularly for the increased aging population.
6. Increase in long term care and facilities.
7. Less technical emphasis on prolonging the life of terminally ill patients.
8. New arrangements in healthcare delivery.
9. Shorter lengths of stay (more utilization review).
10. A decline in residency programmes.
11. New developments in hospital programmes for promoting health, health education, screening for targeted illnesses indicative of high morbidity, and industrial medicine (all outreach programmes and available in both investor owned and non profit facilities).

Following economic trends have been predicted:

1. Inflation
2. Malpractice lawsuits
3. Cost containment
4. Constraints such as less cash flow, less money for modernization, a slower rate of increase for technological advances, priority given to revenue producing activities over service activities, and pressures to limit staffing, new jobs, and pay levels.

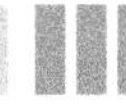

5. Increased emphasis on regionalization of patient services.
6. Increased insurance coverage.

STRATEGIES FOR OVERCOMING THE PROBLEMS

1. Creation of holding companies.
2. Broadened financial bases, through contracts with industry, and other organizations, not just insurance firms.
3. Development of marketing strategy new revenues from sale of services and from complementary hospital business activities.
4. The use of political pressure to fight adversaries.
5. More participation by hospitals in the regulatory process.
6. Adoption of new organizational strategies namely multi hospital arrangements such as shared services.
7. Gaining more support from philanthropic organizations and individuals from state and central governments.

FUTURE OF HEALTHCARE INDUSTRY

The future holds increased inflation, more use of Information Technology, changing lifestyles, increased governmental control, and continuing financial problems. All these affect the hospital and, therefore, the materials manager. There will be increased litigation for liability against hospitals and doctors. Safety measures in the hospital will be stressed. There will be increased need for the hospital buyer to resort to group purchasing and shared services and to explore new marketing techniques. The materials manager of future will require more technical knowledge of products and equipment that he is asked to purchase. He will need to establish an affinity with the physicians on the staff and with the heads of the various specialized departments in hospital care. The materials manager will need to be better educated, not only in materials management, but in those businesses and clinical areas that are related to his work. More people with master's degrees in healthcare administration are expected to become materials managers. Materials manager needs to take a human relations approach to building up and nurturing relationships, and understand the need to work well with people at all levels. In short, the materials manager of the future should be very well qualified so that he or she can move from the materials management position to that of assistant administrator, associate administrator, or administrator. There are indications that this is already happening in several of the larger hospitals throughout the country. Materials manager needs to see his work in relation to his institution, the community, and the political, social, and economic trends. His goal is to keep pace with advances in procurement techniques and goals; many that have been tested and adopted in manufacturing and service industries are applicable to the healthcare field. If the administration of healthcare is to provide improved quality care at less cost, under new forms of organization, the purchaser must be in the forefront of these new healthcare developments, both for the benefit of his institution and ultimately for the benefit of the patients.

Medical humanism is beginning to emerge. This humanism is a challenge to the materials manager. Instead of buying products primarily to meet day to day logistical demands, he or she is required to manage the materials function as part of overall healthcare. The materials manager can be part of an emerging cadre of healthcare people who are bringing about a partnership for health.

Thus the future materials manager in a hospital should be at once a doctor, on engineer, a chemist, on economist and on accountant with through grounding in costs and its applications. He would be a good diplomat too and above all a sharp all a sharp and shrews administrator endowed with quick wit. **His effectiveness often makes the difference between life and death.**

EPILOGUE

The future - The confluence of bio technology and Information Technology is the harbinger of the future. It will make way for neural networks and systems on chips embedded into human skin to transform the capability of managers beyond comprehension; with bated breath, we await the exciting future.

SUMMARY

A dynamic profession like the Materials Management evolves continuously absorbs new ideas, concepts and philosophies. Materials today are the life blood of industry without which no organization can operate. The growing complexity of materials combined with its scarcity and high cost and the increasing volume of production naturally shifted the importance to "materials" as it became the largest element in the total cost of the product.

In India, the concept of materials management was in vogue several centuries back. Modern armies still practice this logistics of material. There are quite a few authors who believe that Materials Management is a logical extension of purchasing function. This has lead to recognition of materials management as a specialized managerial function. It allows considerable improvement of materials management staff. Materials management is termed as **"The last Gold Mine"** for business executives. Materials management is basic part of any organization that produces a product or service of economic value. Very soon, materials managers will have a career superior to a vice president. Materials Management will perform a more and more important role in the future.

The complexity of organizations and the use of IT have increased, thus increasing the need for well trained and competent Materials Managers. Industry and commerce will need not only more Materials Managers, but also better prepared and more efficient and agile ones. Well-trained and efficient Material Managers will earn higher salaries and perks because they are important executives.A survey of literature on Materials Management indicates that there are many definitions of Materials Management. Different authors included different functions in Materials Management. However all the authors are unanimous in Materials Management, basic three functions - purchasing, stores, inventory control (which includes sub functions of planning, handling, and distribution).

Modern industries cannot realize profits, and thus cannot survive, without the use of sophisticated forms of materials management, such as material requirements planning. There has been little understanding of role of purchasing by non-purchasing executives. Today's purchasing manager must be one of the most knowledgeable managers in his company.

MM in 1981 concentrated on the theme of "Materials Management and Corporate Objectives". The theme of 'Curbing Inflation by efficient Materials Management" was the flavor of the day. By 1984, the theme was "Inventory Management for Corporate Results". It clearly came out that corporate results could only be achieved through efficient and effective Materials Management .Materials in the manufacturing sector constitute 50 to 70 percent of the total cost and savings would make the product competitive in the market. From the year 1994 onwards, Materials Management started relying more and more on Information Technology and the relationships among, Information Technology, Materials Management, and corporate competitiveness.

Supply Chain Management encompasses all elements of sourcing, indenting, procuring, production scheduling, order processing, inventory management, transportation, warehousing and customer service as well as the information and monitoring system.

Healthcare provision must be viewed as an industry like any other. At one time, hospital supplies were limited. The single-source control system of inventory management, processing, and distribution of materials became the key to bringing order out of chaos .Material Management qualifies as a system. This system of is one of the elements that tie the total organization together. **The concept of material management must be integrated into the total operating philosophy of a hospital if that facility is to be efficient.**

The levels of education and expertise of hospital materials managers are increasing. Some trends are apparent and can serve as starting points for managers as they design future material management programmes for their facilities.More organizations are establishing corporate level positions, such as vice president, that will have total responsibility for the management of materials throughout the facility. In the past, no attention was devoted to developing Materials Management personnel. Staff level Materials Management jobs often have been regarded as entry level positions, requiring little background. Hospitals strive to replace declining inpatient revenues with income from alternate delivery systems and services. In this effort, materials managers can play increasingly valuable roles in improving the bottom lines of these services. The development of centralized material distribution centres to support a facility or group of facilities will accelerate.

Material managers will have to stay abreast of the changes in computer support systems if they hope to remain competitive in the healthcare industry of the future. Forecasting models and other techniques, such as material requirements planning (MRP), which have been well established in other industries, can be modified for use in healthcare. Standardized material requirements will be established for each diagnosis and procedure. The need to develop these standard material requirements serve as the springboard for improved communication between material managers and clinical managers. Every healthcare facility should also adopt standard cost accounting practices.

Team members include representatives from finance, clinical departments, medical records, and Materials Management.

- There is increasing use of direct computer-to-computer digital communication between healthcare facilities and major vendors. It will provide a great challenge to material managers to ensure that it does not result in increased stock outs. The materials manager and the product standards committee serve as the facilitators for seeing that this service is provided to the organization. Administrators generally demand that materials management performance be monitored routinely and reported using standardized, statistically valid protocols. Individual material managers can do much to see that the healthcare industry reaps the full benefits of effective material management. Hospital material managers have learnt and grown over the years.

A number of separate but interdependent factors affect the lives of material managers and purchasers in the healthcare field. Government, and its actions and acts e.g. price controls, the safety and occupational hazards, minimum wages, Medicare and Medicaid, the transportation, the public health directly affect the hospital purchasing or material manager's job. In the years to come, there will be improved productivity in manufacturing and service industries. Some form of cost control will continue, at least for the next few years, particularly in healthcare, the oil industry, and certain manufacturing and processing industries.

- **Hospital costs will increase :** As the pressure for more efficiency in the hospital and more cost effective healthcare increases, administrators and material managers will seek group purchasing agreements and shared services with other hospitals and with institutions such as universities and colleges.

- **Marketing healthcare services is another trend for the present decade :** An emphasis on social attitudes will characterize the hospital and other service institutions. Hospitals will be affected by an added dimension a consumer movement in healthcare.

- **Computer services that offer application software programmes will interest smaller hospitals :** Government will always continue to influence trends in healthcare. The material or purchasing managers will continue to attempt to obtain the "best" possible purchase with every hospital rupee spent. A competent materials manager will have all procurement functions; be responsible for the functional flow of all material to and from all departments, including dietary, central service, and pharmacy; and supervise laundry, receiving and stores, central communications and dispatch, communications, inventory control, printing, distribution, disposal, and purchasing research and management. There have been numerous discussions on the subject of the materials manager. Unless the materials manager is a broad-gauged manager, the potential benefits from MM will not be fully realized.

 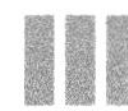

The hospital market has shown some definite indications of rising costs. Hospitals have increased their expenditures at a greater rate than the rest of the healthcare market. Studies have indicated that hospital expenditure as a percentage of total healthcare expenditures increased from 34 percent to 40 percent during the last two decades; rupee expenditures increased phenomenally. With a world average of 3.96 hospital beds per 1000 population, India stands just a little over 0.7 hospital beds per 1000 population. Use of hospital services has grown steadily. Hospitals are healthier than ever today.

The future holds increased inflation, more use of Information Technology, changing lifestyles, increased governmental control, and continuing financial problems. All these affect the hospital and, therefore, the materials manager. There will be increased litigation for liability against hospitals and doctors. There will be increased need for the hospital buyer to resort to group purchasing and shared services and to explore new marketing techniques. The materials manager of the future will require more technical knowledge of the products and the equipment that he is asked to purchase. The materials manager will need to be better educated, not only in materials management, but in those businesses and clinical areas that are related to his work. More people with master's degrees in healthcare administration will become material managers. In short, the materials manager of the future should be so well qualified that he or she can move from the material management position to that of assistant administrator, associate administrator, or administrator. This humanism is a challenge to the materials manager. Instead of buying products primarily to meet day-to-day logistical demands, he or she is required to manage the materials function as part of overall healthcare. The materials manager can be part of an emerging cadre of healthcare people who are bringing about a partnership for health.

REVIEW QUESTIONS

1. Describe briefly the evolution of Materials Management function in hospitals.
2. What would be the future of hospitals Materials Management in India?
3. What are the recent trends in Materials Management in India with particular reference to healthcare industry?
4 Write short notes on
    a) Impact of Information Technology on Materials Management
    b) Impact of engineering and technology on hospitals Materials Management
    c) Healthcare economics
    d) Future of healthcare industry in India
    e) Origin of Materials Management

PART - I

Integrated Hospital Materials Management

Contents

CHAPTER - 2

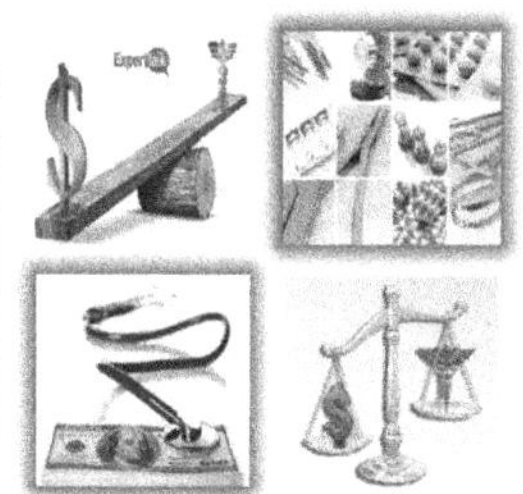

Integrated Hospital Materials Management

INTRODUCTION

Gross national product - the output of goods and services produced by the nation in a given time is the barometer to measure a nation's wealth. Goods are physical objects, something we can touch, feel, or see. Services are the performance of some useful function such as banking, healthcare, restaurants, education, or social services etc.,

Source of wealth is measured by the amount of goods and services produced and derived from the mother earth. Although we may have rich natural resources in our economy such as mineral deposits, farmland and forests, these are only potential sources of wealth. A production or service function is needed to transform our resources into useful goods.

Flow of materials controls the performance of the process. If the right materials in the right quantities are not available at the right time, the process cannot produce what it should. Labour and machinery will be underutilized. The profitability, even the very existence, of an organization will be a threat. Thus materials are essential not only in profit making industries but also in service enterprises, whether the management is in a public sector or private sector. Although Materials Management existed almost in every organization in the past, it was only during the earlier period 40 to 45 years that most organizations started having a separate Materials Management Department.

In India, concept of Materials Management as an **"Integrated Activity"** is relatively recent and its importance began to be realized by industries, during the latter half of 1960's and early 1970's. Materials Management plays a major role in developing our economy, as it controls materials availability, quick turnover of finance to optimize money, production, purchase and commercially viable materials distribution. Awareness of these roles of materials management has grown rapidly during the last two decades.

MATERIALS MANAGEMENT (MM) - AN EVOLVING CONCEPT

Materials Management (MM) is an attempt at evolving a unified approach to managing materials. The concepts and practices of MM developed in United States industry in the 1930s and were refined further in the post-World War II era. Many factories had materials managers in the 1950s and 1960s, but in the industrial hierarchy, the acceptance of this new position was not fully recognized until the mid 1970s. In India, the developments in this profession were sporadic, and definitions of MM remain unclear even to this day. There appears to be one theme woven through all of those definitions. That is the integration of the various processes of planning, acquiring, controlling, moving, and storing materials and final products in order to make the optimum use of all resources including capital, labour, and facilities. Some definitions involve the total control of costs of goods and services from raw materials to products and services supplied to customers. In September 1970, Purchasing provided the following definition of MM: **"An integrated systems approach to material flow, MM is basically oriented to achieving more efficient control of materials from one end of the production line to the other.** Companies who have tried MM agree that it provides more accurate planning and scheduling, tighter inventory control, better cost control, fewer production crises, and more dependable deliveries to customers." Although this is not a recent definition, it still applies.

The definition accepted by International Federation of Purchasing and Materials Management (IFPMM) is: "MM is a total concept involving an organizational structure unifying into a single responsibility, the systematic flow and control of materials from identification of the need through customer delivery. Included within this concept are the material functions of planning, scheduling, buying, moving and distributing. These are logically represented by the disciplines of production, and inventory control, purchasing and physical distribution." Another definition adopted by National Association of Purchasing Management (NAPM) (USA) reads as follows: "MM is an organizational concept in which a single manager has authority and responsibility for all activities principally concerned with the flow of materials into an organization, purchasing, production planning, scheduling, incoming traffic, inventory control, receiving and stores are normally included". One of the clearest definitions of Materials Management was given by **Robert B. Ballot** which is as follows: "MM is a coordinated function, responsible to plan for, acquire, store, move and control materials and final products to optimize usage of facilities, personnel, and capital funds and to provide customer service in line with corporate goals." In these words, consider the key words viz. Coordination, Plan, Acquire, Store, Move and Control. These words are normally included in every definition of MM. **Prof. P. Gopala Krishnan,** Former Professor, Administrative Staff College of India, Hyderabad, defines MM as the function responsible for coordination of planning, sourcing, purchasing, moving, storing and controlling materials in an optimum manner, so as to provide pre decided service level to the customer at a minimum cost. MM as a company's supply system covers a broad spectrum of functions closely related to each other. Even though the broad functions are listed here, one should not conclude, from this that these functions have to be centralized in MM organizationally.

FUNCTIONS OF MATERIALS MANAGEMENT

Functions of MM are broadly classified into two viz., primary and secondary functions.

Primary Functions

- Material planning and control
- Purchasing
- Storing and stock keeping
- Inventory control

Secondary Functions

- Make or buy decision
- Standardization
- Product development and introduction of new products and services
- Product improvement
- Product evaluation
- Reciprocity

MM is a body of knowledge which helps the manager to improve productivity of capital by reducing material cost, preventing large amounts of capital being locked up for longer periods than necessary in inventory and improving capital turnover ratio. **The basic goal of any industrial or service organization is development and manufacture of goods or services that can be sold at profit.**

This goal is accomplished by judicious blending of what are called the 5 M's i.e.:

1. Men
2. Machines
3. Money
4. Materials and
5. Management

Materials today are the life blood of every organization, without which no organization operates. The relative importance of these 5 M's continuously shifted during the process of Industrial Revolution and thereafter.

Six major areas are covered by the function of MM: purchasing, production control, inventory control, materials handling, traffic, and physical distribution. Materials manager usually does not have responsibility for production. From a departmental organization that viewed purchasing as

 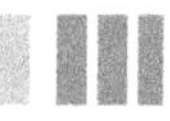

a second or third line responsibility, where the department's responsibility for material acquisition stopped once the product left the general stores area, MM now functions in industry in four jurisdictional areas, to a greater or lesser line degree, as follows.

Process 1 - Forecasting and planning

Process 2 - Procurement and stores

Process 3 - Deliveries to production and using departments

Process 4 - Budgets credit and controls

Industry has recognised the newly developed status and importance of MM by placing the materials manager directly under the top executive. One of the clearest definitions of MM was given by **Robert W. Christian: "MM is a concept based on organization groupings of the corporate functions primarily concerned with the acquisition, storing, handling, distribution, and control of materials."**

When the Journal of Purchasing, published by the National Association of Purchasing Management was renamed in February 1974 as the Journal of Purchasing and Material Management, the change was described as one indication of the broadened scope of modern purchasing management. This statement reflected the possible bias of the purchasing manager. Earlier the people involved in MM and Production Control were seen as rivals. Further, the success or failure of the materials manager was seen as a result of how important that position was in management. The materials manager was seldom given authority commensurate with his responsibility as part of the top executive echelon. Failure to consider this job important meant the difference between success and failure many times. Many of the problems in the early growth of this new position centred on the perception of the executive suite, and those in the traditional vice-presidential or other top positions looked at the materials manager as a lesser functionary. This attitude later changed a great deal, although materials managers are still proving themselves in industry.

It is acknowledged that there are some pitfalls in the adoption of MM. These include the fact that conflicts over this new, centralized, executive position could increase costs instead of assuring savings. Further, the new division of responsibility may cause submerged hostilities between people to surface. Moreover, if the position of materials manager and his functions are structured too rigidly, those positions may be difficult to adapt, modify, or change when needed.

Ron Baer and John Centamore reported the confusion over MM. They organized a survey and concluded: "There is no typical MM organization. There are a variety of structures used by different companies. Managers evidently approach the materials concept pragmatically, choosing the organization that suits their particular needs." The writers go on to say, however, that **"the materials system is based on functions, rather than structure. It is a totally integrated approach to material control, not a rigorous form of managerial organization."**

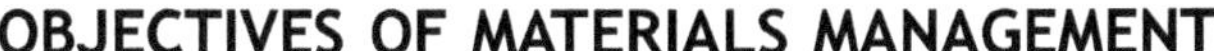

OBJECTIVES OF MATERIALS MANAGEMENT

Functions of MM are basically economic in nature even in non to profit organizations. The most fundamental objective is survival. MM function therefore has to support objectives of the undertaking as a whole.

Would include among other things:

- Maximum service to customers
- Survival and growth
- Good working conditions
- Advancement to employees
- Technological lead over the competitors

Modern trend is strong materials department with jurisdiction over almost all functions that effect availability, flow, conservation, utilization, quality and cost of materials. MM, an economic activity, in a hospital setting, serves functions whose goals are not really economic. When MM is delegated to the user by custom or neglect, it is almost inevitable that resources will not be used in the most rational fashion.

Primary Objectives

- To ensure continuity of supply, manage and control the flow of equipment and supplies from acquisition to disposal.
- To operate with minimum investment in inventory and other assets.
- To meet or exceed all of the requirements of the prudent buyer concept. To purchase all supplies and equipment prudently with consideration for cost, service and quality.
- To control the amounts of unofficial inventory (that which has been expensed and dispensed) by quarterly physical inventories and stockless purchasing.
- To pay the lowest possible price for purchased materials without compromising the other objectives.
- To effect economies in cost of materials and cost on materials.
- High inventory turnover.
- Lowest acquisition and possession cost.
- Consistency in quality of materials.
- To remain awake to the changes in the market with respect to new materials and services.
- To improve the quality of service in patient care by use of better materials or components and thereby increase the competitiveness of such services.

- To increase competitiveness of hospital services by reducing their prices through cost reduction and value analysis.
- Ensuring co operation among all heads of departments of the organization.
- Conservation of materials resources.
- Good vendor/ vendee relationship through centralized contacts and sales representative orientation to the hospital materials management philosophy.
- To save foreign exchange through import substitution and economize on foreign purchases.
- To improve the department's efficiency.
- To apply management methods such as value analysis, cost analysis, and product utilization studies to the supply, process, and distribution of products and equipment.
- To provide the mechanism whereby, improved patient care will prevail through product standardization and evaluation, with emphasis on quality of care and containment of cost.
- To relieve nursing and other departments of all supply related functions inventories, requisitioning, recording, delivering, and processing supplies and equipments.
- To provide all consumer departments with a total supply system in which the right supply is always available at the right place and right time in right quantities.

Secondary objectives

- Make or buy decisions.
- Product development, improvement and introduction of new products and services due to changes in process diagnosis and treatment.
- Product improvement.
- Favourable reciprocal relationships (reciprocity).
- Interdepartmental harmony.
- To forecast. Because of their intimate knowledge of market through contact with suppliers, materials managers can help to a great extent in forecasting both sales and purchases.
- To keep costs under control.
- To keep administration department heads and other appropriate parties informed of changes in equipment, products and supply methods.

This is the age of very fast technological development. Hence, product obsolescence occurs very fast. Materials department by its efforts will help to reduce cost of materials by buying right quality of materials at the best possible price by making use of modern purchasing techniques. MM is able to directly contribute to profits of the hospital. MM has been recognized as an effective tool in manufacturing industry. It is only a matter of time before its value is fully realized in healthcare.

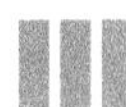

MATERIALS MANAGEMENT IN HOSPITALS

Charles E. Housley and Dean S. Ammer made some interesting comparisons between the theory and concepts of **Hospital Materials Management (HMM).** Housley included pharmacy as one of the major departments to be supervised. Ammer believed that it is a moot point whether HMM would be able to control physical stocks in the pharmacy as the pharmacist is, himself, a materials manager of sorts and he would always have custody of stocks of drugs. Control could be exercised by HMM only if pharmacy was made subordinate to the materials manager. This state of affairs is neither logical nor likely. However, in the case of the food service department, Ammer and Housley both agree that, although the purchase and storage of perishables would be a basic part of the dietitian's job, to which the material manager can make only indirect contributions, most of the canned goods and most of the staples can be controlled by the materials manager. Thus, Housley (who was himself once an associate administrator of a large hospital in USA) puts many more functions under the control of the materials manager than does Ammer. As a backdrop for this text the author interacted with several MM professionals in small, medium and large hospitals located in twin cities of Hyderabad and enquired about the functions and operations of Materials Management in their respective hospitals. For the purpose of study Hospitals were grouped into three groups based on functions and operations of Materials Management. Respondents were invited to comment on each, both in terms of their own hospitals and in general terms on duties they performed. Activities included in group X are purchasing, inventory control, distribution, and traditional purchasing functions in the typical hospital headed by materials manager or general manager materials. In group y materials manager reports directly to hospital Director Operations and involved in controlling all conventional purchasing functions, as well as production and dispatch of all clean and soiled material. Whereas group Z includes all traditional purchasing functions; production and dispatch of all reusable and disposable items; laundry, dietary, and allied services including all internal and external delivery and distribution and other logistical functions, except control over dietary and pharmacy distribution which ought to be part of materials management. Materials manager whose primary function is purchasing and who reports directly to an administrator could just be designated as materials manager. However he could be called as a full-fledged materials manager had he supervised all purchasing, stores, inventories, distribution, production, traffic control, and communications and functionally or organizationally was responsible for all supplies and equipment and for the ordering and processing of all disposables and reusables. Those who responded to the survey were holding titles as materials managers or administrators or directors. All the three groups emphasized that the importance placed on Materials Management in a hospital was related more to who reports to the materials manager than to whom the materials manager reports.

The majority of the respondents responded fall in group X prevalent in small hospitals.

Group Y was found in a limited number of hospitals mostly existing in single location.

Group Z was found in medium and large hospitals in multi locations in twin cities and in the process of adopting or adopted integrated materials management. (The author is indebted to John H. Holmgren Walter J.Wertz. for making use their methodology with suitable modifications to be in consonance with local conditions).

Pitfalls in MM described earlier were also found to apply to the situations observed in hospitals unless the administrators back up their materials managers, giving them the authority to go with their responsibility. Depending on its size and its staff and their qualifications, HMM is organized differently in each hospital. The basic premise of materials management is that the manager should have major control over the receiving, ordering, and distribution and processing of all materials throughout the hospital, whether or not he controls decentralized inventories in departments. Whether or not the materials manager should have functional control over the pharmacy, dietary, and maintenance departments is however considered debatable. It has been noted by researchers that more and more institutions, such as universities and hospitals, that combine many of the Materials Management functions are applying Material Management centralization policies and there is more centralization taking place in such institutions than there is in industry. Many of these institutions have demonstrated operational savings. This might improve further as the government reimbursements for Medicaid and Medicare patients decrease and hospitals begin to look at ways of reducing costs through application of MM practices.

Based on the research studies the following suggestions helps to reduce costs of hospital operations especially during inflationary periods:

1. Committing the hospital fully to Materials Management operations.
2. Stricter inventory control.
3. Group purchasing contracts.
4. Make or buy studies.
5. Standardization of products by a standardization committee.
6. Competitive bidding instead of favouring prime or selective vendors.
7. Centralized purchasing for all hospital departments.
8. Educating user department heads regarding saving on material costs.
9. Value analysis to explore whether other products or procedures can accomplish the same objective.
10. Ensuring proper backup stocking by vendors.
11. Centralized issue of all instruments from one point.
12. Working out consignment arrangements for items the vendor owns them until they are issued to the wards or departments.
13. Utilizing the ABC inventory control system of concentrating purchasing emphasis on those 10 percent of items that account for 70 percent of value of consumption.
14. Educating the medical staff in cost containment, with regard to instruments, equipment, and generic drugs.
15. Negotiating agreements that will take into account fluctuating markets.

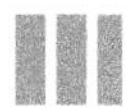

16. Establishing criteria other than brand name for selecting equipment as selection by brand name leaves little room for obtaining a competitive price.
17. Improving maintenance agreements and maintenance of equipment to delay the need for replacement.

The respondents also observed that it would be desirable to turn over all inventories on an average of eight times a year. However, the medical surgical inventory would turn over 10 to 12 times, food and beverages 30 to 45 times and pharmacy 9 to 12 times in a year.

All those surveyed agreed that a strong value analysis and standardization committee was important. Materials manager could help in standardization of supplies and equipment, thus reducing costs and improving inventory control. The key to effective standardization is not the existence of the committee as much as the composition of that committee. Decision makers from all Head of departments, as well as the medical staff, should contribute to the recommendations made to this committee. It should be a cohesive committee. It was suggested that implementation of a standardization programme by which doctors can request equipment and instruments, but requests are held and reviewed monthly by the chairman of each committee through which the requests are routed should encourage standardization.

In India, the healthcare industry has not adopted the group purchasing concept to take advantage of bulk purchases at a competitive price. Group purchasing, if adopted, among nonprofit hospitals and consortiums will result in prudent buying. U.S., **General Accounting Office (GAO)** report to the chairman of the subcommittee on health, committee on finance, U.S. Senate, entitled "Hospitals in the Same Area Often Pay Widely Different Prices for Comparable Supply Items," (Washington, D.C.: Government Printing Office, 1980) also recommended group purchasing.

The GAO's research study in US Hospitals was conducted on the following functional areas:

1. How authority for purchasing and supply functions is delegated.
2. The extent to which sound procurement and materials management practices were followed.
3. A checklist and guidelines for evaluating purchasing and materials management functions.
4. Group purchasing.
5. The degree to which dietary, pharmacy, and maintenance purchasing were part of centralized purchasing.
6. Inventory management.
7. The general cost effectiveness of the purchasing programme, particularly with regard to regional differences in prices paid by hospitals.

The report found that hospitals in the same area often paid widely different prices for comparable items, whereas prices did not seem to vary too widely by region. The GAO observed that some hospitals paid too much for certain items and recommended that purchasing agents share information more than they do. It also found that there were too many extra services provided by certain vendors, thereby increasing costs, and that there were too many price variations among hospitals. GAO study is a valuable background tool for material managers in hospitals in the United States in evaluating their own performance.

GAO does not intend to impose its specific organizational structure upon a hospital or dictate purchasing and Materials Management functions. The study only presents opportunities for improving these functions and allows each hospital to determine which opportunities to use. The study is worth reading as a background and as a basis for comparison. There still needs to be considerably more research and activity to determine the real effectiveness of Materials Management programmes before we can arrive at a time when Material Management is completely understood and applied universally as a concept and as a functional approach in hospitals throughout the world. GAO is attempting to review manners, methods, and practices of purchasing and Materials Management to see if costs could be reduced in purchasing departments in hospitals particularly since the Medicare and Medicaid dollars spent for healthcare amount to 40 to 45 percent of the total hospital dollars spent in USA. The GAO recommendation to Medicare and Medicaid agencies may be helpful in reminding hospitals to do comparative shopping wherever possible, but there needs to be a comparison of "Brand A with Brand A," not "Brand A with Brand B," because two items that have the same function may be very different in quality.

There is no penalizing of hospitals for lack of either group purchasing involvement or investments that are not prudent. The differences in the ways in which HMM is viewed by writers, speakers, and materials managers could be due to a lack of understanding of the functions and operations of Materials Management in the hospital environment, a reflection of their own background, the differences between people and hospitals, the lack of management's understanding, and too much emphasis on purchasing. Perhaps this emphasis is a result of the fact that many material managers rise, like phoenix, out of the purchasing office. The real thrust of Materials Management is managing people, not just supplies and equipment. Originally the materials manager concept was to add additional functions to the purchasing manager's job to better utilize his talents for a better overall lower cost of handling goods and supplies. This point is further accentuated by the belief that there is more room for saving within the hospital itself than in the purchasing function. Materials Management is growing and that is clearly understood by most knowledgeable materials managers. In some of the hospitals in India, there is some impatience and dissatisfaction with those hospitals where Materials Management exists more in name than in fact; and there is a need to strive for increased status and professionalism as materials managers.

Dean S. Ammer has made a distinction between **"Material" and "Materiel" Management.** He mentions that the difference between the terms lies in the emphasis laid on individual materials vs. materials management activities. **The Webster definition of materials relates "to the production and distribution of economic goods and the social relationships of owners and labourers." "Materiel," as**

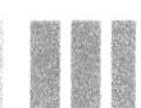

defined by Webster's Collegiate Dictionary, is the "equipment, apparatus, and supplies used by an organization or institution." The same dictionary also describes "materiel" as the French word for "material" and uses the word "materiel" in a definition of "material." **Charles E. Housley** described the fact that Material Management appears to be in its infancy and there are already signs of an ill-prepared birth. There are still purchasing directors struggling with back orders and having an overloaded stock inventory, as compared with a materials manager in full functional control of all supplies, materials, and equipment, both in the acquisition and distribution as well as the control of disposables and reusables. Mismanagement also exists and involves such characteristics as apathy, reticence, disorganization, poor motivation, poor planning, disinterest in education, and a high degree of isolation. Housley cites the failure of certain materials managers to follow up on requests or ideas. A user department may call Materials Management, purchasing, or central supply for an item and receive the response that the item is out of stock, but nothing is ever done about the request and the user is not told anything about it. There also seems to be poor communication and lack of feedback from departments because the Materials Manager does not go out of his way to see how they are reacting to his programmes. The final category of mismanagement is overstock of inventories.

William K. Henning, a major contributor to Hospital Materials Management, stated the case for this relatively new development in hospitals. Although Materials Management was applied on a large scale by the military as early as World War II, the majority of hospitals, even today, apply Materials Management only on a very limited scale. Materials Management is a relatively new concept in the healthcare field. A growing number of hospitals are consolidating central supply to begin the formation of a grouping of central support services. Purchasing and storage have been combined organizationally in most hospitals. Many hospitals are using unit distribution systems: unit dose for pharmaceuticals and exchange cart or par level systems for medical and general items. These distribution systems extend the central service to functional areas such as nursing and permit the daily reconciliation of patient charges related to unit product usage. There is also the impact of data processing on Materials Management, when, as Henning cites, hospitals shifted attention from hand processing reusables to the management of volumes of consumables.

ADVANTAGES OF MATERIALS MANAGEMENT IN MODERN HOSPITALS

Advantages of Materials Management in the modern hospitals include the following:

1. Enhancing the opportunities for both internal (centralized) and external (group) purchasing.
2. Increasing control of billing to patients and departmental cost centres, thereby increasing income with less lost or non reported usage. This is accomplished by virtue of the interface between the responsibilities of the controller and the materials manager in such areas as bids, negotiations, contracts, and inventory controls, patient charging audits, budgeting, cost containment, and systems management.

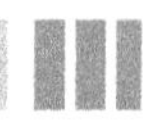

3. Organizing functions so that the administrator can expect results from one person and one department.

4. Reducing inventories resulting from greater centralized control of at least the major material functions, externally and internally.

5. Placing the supply, process, and distribution functions under one manager, thus increasing the productivity of these functions, increasing cost savings, and making it possible to improve cash flow, maximize personnel productivity, and streamline the passage of material to the designated departments.

6. Increasing the opportunity and the demand for standardization and other costsaving techniques.

7. **Improving the method of evaluating Materials Management performances by:**

a. Measuring departmental expenses against total cost of goods purchased, processed, and delivered.

b. Improving interdepartmental communications, speeding up response time, having fewer back orders, and improving surgery scheduling by improving control over supplies and instruments.

c. Measuring quality of products through standardization and testing.

d. Comparing the prices paid for common, expensive items with other hospitals in the region.

e. Measuring the rate of inventory turnover by dividing the annual purchase volume by the investment in inventory.

f. Comparing the difference in costs before and after hospital wide Materials Management was instituted.

g. Improving service levels.

The definitions of Materials Management, as used in hospitals, vary. They usually stress that, when most of the functions related to Materials Management are centralized under the purchasing manager, he then becomes a materials manager. Materials Management is a broad, functional system encompassing more than purchasing alone. It considers the life cycle of materials. Its functions include ordering and scheduling purchase and deliveries, inventory control, incoming traffic control, store-keeping and warehousing, claims administration, receiving and receiving inspection, and in some instances, shipping. They could also include demand forecast, research, expediting, production planning, and interface with data processing. As they adopted other business practices in the second half of 1980s, healthcare institutions have begun to adopt Materials Management too. Although Materials Management in industry emphasizes the production and manufacture of products, the concept would appear to apply equally to an institution whose most important commodity is service. Only about a quarter of a hospital's total operating expenses go to the supply and procurement function.

Hospitals lagged behind industry in adopting Materials Management for reasons other than just their service orientation. The healthcare industry is a non profit one; it is subject to pressures from many different kinds of stake holders, both internally and externally; it deals with professional and medical concerns; and it has an infrastructure of occupations whose members jealously guard what they deem to be their prerogatives-from surgeons to nurses to certified emergency medical assistants.

Automation and the quest for improved efficiency and cost containment have changed hospital organization. Resistance to change is breaking down. Healthcare providers are being forced to find new methods of cost containment because of spiraling health costs, wage and price controls, reported healthcare crises, inflation, decreased length of hospital stay per patient, difficult reimbursement policies under Medicare and Medicaid, increased costs of training and medical technology, and increased patient and doctor demands for services. Materials Management is seen, therefore, as a way of stemming the rising costs of hospital care. This approach assumes that savings can be affected through increased centralization, automation, and control of like functions affecting procurement, storage, and distribution. Next to nursing, materials are the most expensive elements in the hospital.

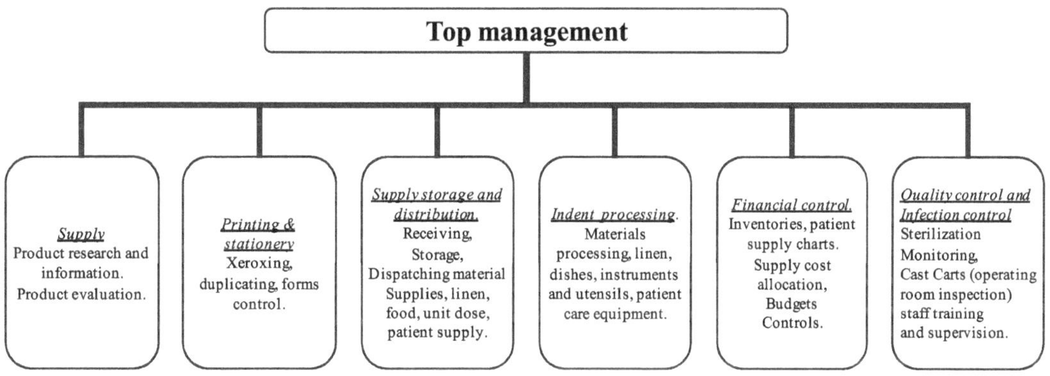

Figure 2.1 Materials Management - Role as a cross function

The battle over what constitutes Materials Management was more intense in industry than it is now in the healthcare field. **John A. O'Connell,** coordinator of the Materials Management services for **Sisters of Holy Cross,** Notre Dame, Indiana, notes that "whereas the purchasing agent in industry has a close working relationship with division heads (such as the sales manager, traffic controller, inventory chief, and production control manager), the hospital's purchasing agent does not have the equivalent close working affinity. Instead, he is often ignored or his advice sought after the fact." He feels that the Materials Management concept applies to the hospital field particularly well. O'Connell believes that this traditional gap between the purchasing agent and top hospital executives can be closed only when the materials manager not only acquires supplies and equipment, but gets involved very early in programming, budgeting, new services, construction, internal operations, and the flow of materials and supplies within the hospital. The materials manager's job is broader than before and includes all hospital purchasing, traffic, inventory control, internal transportation and delivery. It may also involve other logistics: housekeeping, laundry, waste disposal, and reusable processing. The need for a master control point and supervision of all supply deliveries become

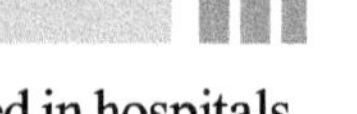

essential as new automatic transportation cart systems (such as AMSCAR) are installed in hospitals, and as newly constructed hospitals establish central production and dispatch centres.

Management by objectives may be the best criterion for organizing a purchasing department, where the organization and personnel are developed after the objectives of procurement and distribution are formulated. These objectives stress on function more than organization. Materials Management has been applied more often in the larger medical complexes, but the ideal organization of a hospital's purchasing depends largely on its concept of administration and the degree to which it accepts newer principles of business administration.

Future developments in the healthcare field are bound to further accelerate the acceptance and implementation of Materials Management. These developments include systems and data processing, managerial competence, increased cost containment and increased complexity of organizations. On the positive side, Materials Management is cited as providing distinct advantages over traditional purchasing: better buying, elimination of problems over responsibility and improved interdepartmental cooperation, faster inventory turn over, improved continuity of material ordering and handling process, decreased transportation costs, improved personnel morale and motivation, less materials obsolescence, improved quality control, and improved relations with vendors.

ORGANIZING MATERIALS MANAGEMENT FUNCTIONS IN HOSPITALS

Organizing Materials Management functions in hospitals involves specialized personnel to a greater or lesser degree, depending on the size of the facility. The organization of most material management activities in U.S. and Canadian hospitals includes all the following activities as the materials managers are involved in all purchasing functions, including dietary and pharmacy.

1. Procurement management purchase order system, source selection, stocking, replacement scheduling, traffic and transportation methods (external).
2. Logistics management inventory control, forecasting and planning; laundry, processing of reusables, value improvement programme.
3. Distribution management distribution of supplies to departments, materials handling, packaging and disposal of disposables.

Management functions have the following objectives:

1. Decontamination, waste disposal, and pollution control.
2. Controlling inventories throughout the hospital.
3. Expediting.
4. Controlling movement of materials to and within the hospital.
5. Overseeing laundry and central supply (these are essentially supply functions).

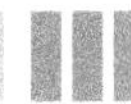

6. Receiving, inspecting, storing, and delivering all supplies.
7. Making forecasts and planning; overseeing systems and procedures.
8. Acting as central agent for all purchase orders, in order to assist in budget control and standardization.
9. Scheduling all purchasing functions.

In a medium sized hospital with three hundred or more beds, Materials Management objectives would be attained through the following breakdown of units of work:

1. The supervising materials manager would be responsible for purchasing, expediting, traffic and transportation, and material control.
2. The purchasing manager, like a buyer in a larger hospital, would negotiate and process all purchases; he would be responsible for the function of systems and procedures relating to the Materials Management division and would work closely with all departments as a management liaison for the department, especially in regard to management reports.
3. The expediter would expedite all back orders and standing purchase orders required within the hospital, some of which would be obtained from local sources.
4. The traffic and transportation supervisor or unit would be responsible for prompt, economical transportation of supplies to the hospital, as well as for internal material handling and physical distribution. This unit would be responsible for decontamination and ecological disposables also.
5. The material control supervisor or unit would be responsible for quality control, evaluation of new products, and control of the processing and distribution of sterile supplies, automatic cart transportation system (or its manual equivalent), and laundry; he is, in one respect, the counterpart of the production control supervisor in industry, and should be trained in scheduling, Performance Evaluation Research and Testing (PERT), critical path method (CPM), and other schedule-monitoring systems. **(John H. Holmgren and Walter J. Wentz)**

More and more healthcare administrators and purchasing managers appear to have accepted the concept of Materials Management. It is, as Paul V. Farrell had indicated, "a fact of life," one that purchasing managers can accept or resist, dependent on their motivation and understanding of this basic approach to improved management of the hospital supply system. Holmgren noted that: "The problem in winning acceptance for this kind of organization is the one posed by the functional takeover by materials management of decentralized, departmental activities."

Despite its importance, Materials Management is still not a clearly identified function simply because it is an activity that is not performed exclusively by the materials manager and his subordinates. Almost every department in the typical healthcare institution dabbles in Materials Management. In earlier years, HMM generally failed to achieve widespread recognition and identification partly because of ignorance, and also there were not so many materials to manage.

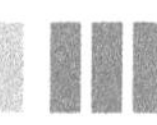

Now, the HMM has developed into a process that is second in economic impact only to the work of the nursing staff. In India the concept of Materials Management as an integrated activity is relatively nascent and its importance began to be realized by Indian healthcare industry, during later half of 1980's or early 1990's. HMM is playing a major role in developing our economy, especially service sector in the recent past as it controls materials availability, quick turnover of finance to optimize investment and healthcare operations. Awareness of these roles of materials function has grown rapidly during last two decades.

NEED FOR INTEGRATED CONCEPT

Within the realms of Materials Management the Purchasing, materials planning, receiving, storage, inventory control, and also scrap and surplus materials disposal organizationally centralized in one department. In the event if some of the activities were to be handled independently, it may lead to clash of interests. Suppose purchasing department is allowed, to function individually, may take decisions, which result in sub-optimization. Purchase department may be tempted to take a myopic decision to buy large quantities to take advantage of quantity discounts without out giving due consideration to increased inventory holding costs. In other words, we need to achieve a good equilibrium between the conflicting objectives from a total organization standpoint so as to achieve most favorable results as a whole.

Example. A hospital intend to add additional facilities to the existing ones will necessitate planning for the increased requirements, developing new sources, of supply, modification in inventory levels apart from the enlarged work load of receipt of equipment and supplies, inspection and storage. In an integrated set up the materials management aims to achieve optimum supply by reconciling the conflicting goals of low materials costs and overheads a high level of customer service and also a very low level of capital tied up in inventories, by the use of EDP supported data, systems and the logistics/materials flow models, in close coordination with other functions in the hospital. The task of EDP here is support data systems and logistics/ materials flow models to resolve the interface problems between the individual functional elements in the overall Materials Management.

ADVANTAGES OF INTEGRATED MM CONCEPT

Organizations, which have gone in a big way for the integrated MM usually, enjoy the following advantages:

1. **Better accountability:** By an effective centralization of authority and responsibility for all aspects of materials function, a specific responsibility is established.

2. **Better coordination**: When a single individual is accountable for all activities in the department, creates a common identity, which in turn results in enhanced support and assistance from staff in materials management function

3. **Better performance**: Integrated materials management results in increased Productivity of capital as all the interconnected functions are included organizationally, this leads to better performance and effectiveness through speed and accuracy in communication.

4. Adaptability to EDP

Modern information technology: The materials activities when centralized make possible designing of data processing systems. All information with regard to materials function is centralized under the integrated MM function. This in turn facilitates collection, collation and analysis of data leading to take comprehensive decisions.

5. Miscellaneous advantages: Under a central materials manager, a team spirit is inculcated. This results in better morale and cooperation.

INTEGRATED CONCEPT IN HMM

The whole healthcare industry is changing. In view of these changes, the integrated concept of HMM is essential because of the following reasons:

- Major distributors are cutting back significantly on their sales force.
- Several large national distributors have either closed down or diversified into other areas. Major manufacturers have created new lines and turned away from those for which they were famous.
- Certain drug manufacturers have eliminated major distributors to better position themselves for future hospital markets.
- Some distributors have merged.
- Consortia have been developed to provide regional geographic coverage in response to corporate hospital requirements.
- Equipment manufacturers are engaged in intense competition. They are now stressing the more important advantages of their products in terms of future productivity and cost effectiveness as opposed to revenue potential and the simple addition of frills.

Diagnostic Related Groups (DRGs) imply the requirement that managers stay abreast of the above mentioned and other changes and gauge their ramifications. Managers' expertise and the continued development of skills to provide the best possible linkage for the supplies and equipment of all department heads is rapidly becoming part of their future. In summary, the integration effort requires administratively guided teamwork, and today's environment, with its cost restrictions, makes this process mandatory for survival. Healthcare industry is fortunate to have the resources of such important personnel as regional materials managers. These, with a proper blend of panels from dietary, laboratory, and pharmacy, constitute a solid formula for success.

The situation is changing away from an era when few supported integration efforts. The burden of proof is always on materials managers as professionals to gather the evidence and push for control. Materials managers should not let the time pass by them. They must properly identify their responsibilities. They should not be perceived as having authority and responsibility for an integrated system where none exists. It is not uncommon to find a hospital where materials managers' responsibility essentially is limited to general stores. They could be doing an excellent job in general

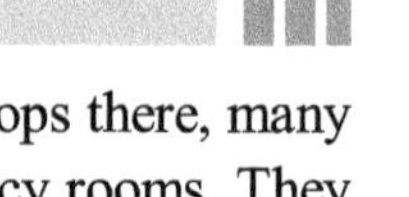

stores and general distribution to nursing units. Even though the span of control stops there, many are held accountable for what goes on in areas such as the operating and emergency rooms. They could, for example, be responsible for inventory held in pharmacy, or the orthopaedic hard goods in the surgery suite. Materials managers must identify both their authority and their responsibility.

A typical example is the case of a materials manager in a non-integrated setting. The total house inventory was worth Rs. 50,00,000. General stores held Rs.12,50,000 worth of inventory, the operating room Rs. 20,00,000, the pharmacy Rs. 7,50,000, and the laboratory Rs. 6,00,000, with the rest spread throughout other departments. This is not an uncommon inventory scenario in many hospitals. The statistics show that only about a fourth of the inventory is indeed under the control of the materials manager; even if that individual were to decrease the general stores inventory by an astounding 50 percent, it would affect only 12 percent of the total house inventory. Indeed, many managers control only 20 percent to 25 percent of the rupee value.

It is this author's belief that the timing is right for managers to lay out a plan to obtain from administration both the authority and the responsibility for house wide management of materials. They cannot be held accountable for what they cannot control. Once integration and control are harnessed, advantages towards true cost containment abound.

SUMMARY

Materials Management is a relatively new field. Richard Tersine and Campbell stated that **"Aggregate Materials Management is a look at the forest as a whole and not each tree."** An organization is an open system, since its constituents have contact not only with each other, but also with external environment consisting of suppliers, customers, competitors, the community and other interested parties. Materials flow from inside, and to those parties and the organizations that require a panoramic view of the whole movement. The significance, relevance and organizational status of MM will increase in the future. Numerous forces are dictating changes in this direction. One force is the trend towards increasing the number of highly specialized and complex products and services. As a result of this development, more organizations will make fewer products in house and buy more of their material requirements. Consequently, materials will represent an increasing percentage of total product costs. Their control, in future, will be even more important than it is today. A second major force is the increasing trend towards use of costly sophisticated equipment for diagnosis and treatment. An uninterrupted flow of material is required for such a facility. A third major force is burgeoning cost of materials. An expanding world population with almost insatiable demand for goods and services is creating shortages in supply, which are bound to cause operating costs to skyrocket. The days of cheap abundant raw materials are a thing of the past. For these reasons and many others, the HMM is no longer a trivial matter relegated to lower managerial levels.

The future holds increased and continuing inflation, changing lifestyles, more sophisticated technology, increased governmental control, and financial problems. All of these affect the hospital and, therefore, the materials manager. There is bound to be increased litigation against hospitals

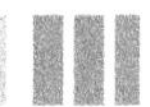

and doctors. Safety measures in the hospital will be stressed. Healthcare organizations will be required to evolve ways of reducing insurance and patient costs. There will thus be an increased need for the hospital buyer to turn to group purchasing and shared services and to explore new marketing techniques. The materials manager of the future will require more technical knowledge of the products and the equipment that are required to be purchased. Materials managers will need to establish an affinity with the physicians on the staff and with the heads of specialized departments in hospital care. The materials manager will need to be better educated, not only in materials management, but in those business and clinical areas that are related to MM. More people with master's degrees in healthcare administration are likely to become material managers. Like all business executives, the materials manager too needs to take a human relations approach to relationships, and understand the need to work well with people at all levels. Materials managers of the future should be so well qualified that they can move from the Materials Management position to that of assistant administrator, associate administrator, or administrator. This is happening in several of the larger hospitals throughout the country. The materials manager needs to see his work in relation to his institution, the community, and in the light of current political, socio-economic trends. His goal will be to keep pace with advances in procurement techniques and goals. Many of those tools and techniques have been tested and adopted in industry and are applicable to the healthcare field. The administration of healthcare is required to provide improved quality care at less cost, under new forms of organization. Hence, the purchaser must be in the forefront of these new healthcare developments, both for the benefit of his institution and for the benefit of the patients at large. The materials manager in future will be part of an emerging cadre of healthcare people who will bring about a truer partnership for health.

In the game of cricket, batsman obtains runs and bowler contains runs and the both are therefore, considered heroes. The game is traditionally assumed to be a battle between bowlers and batsmen. Radio, T.V. commentators and sports critics praise the tight bowling or the prowess of the batsmen. However, there is another great contributor to a match the fielder. A fielder by his excellence in fielding prevents a number of runs from being scored and makes a direct contribution to his team's performance. He is a silent worker. If he is sloppy, the batting side would get more runs and if he is more efficient, they would not get as many runs as they got. However, hardly anyone recognizes him as a hero.

Materials manager is like a fielder. He saves runs. Every run he saves is a run added to his side. Similarly, every rupcc he saves by managing materials is like a rupee added to the profits of the company. This is behind the new concept of MM being a profit centre of the company.

Present liberalized economy is like a 20-20 match of 50 overs version. Every rupee saved in the business through cost containment is a profit added to the company.

REVIEW QUESTIONS

1. How does the Materials Management of hospitals differ from that of industrial organizations?
2. How can the Materials Management function fit into the hospital organization? Delineate an organization chart for your hospital.
3. "Integrated Materials Management aims at cost reduction and integrates, co-ordinates, and entwines. Discuss in light of Hospital Materials Management.
4. Discuss the functions and scope of materials department in both profit and non-profit healthcare organizations.
5. In order to cope up with technological advances and economic trends, what would be the role of Materials Management in hospitals? -Discuss
6. Write short notes on
   a) Primary objectives of Hospital Materials Management
   b) Primary functions of hospital materials manager
   c) Integrated Materials Management concept
   d) Group purchasing
   e) Differentiate between Materials and Materials Management

PART - I

Materials Management in Hospital Pharmacy

Contents

- *Introduction*
- *Functions*
- *Location*
- *Design*
- *Dispensing Area*
- *Manufacturing Area*
- *Administrative Area*
- *Storage Area*
- *Procurement*
- *Prime Vendor Agreements*
- *Competitive Bidding*
- *Inventory Control*
- *Distribution Management*
- *Outpatient Pharmacy*
- *Drug Utilization*
- *Drug Information*
- *Standardization and Treatment Protocols*
- *Drug Utilization Review*
- *Controlling Material Expenses*
- *Other Issues*
- *Summary*
- *Review Questions*

CHAPTER - 3

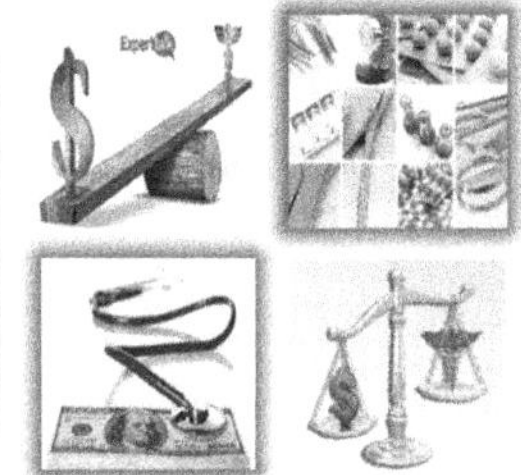

Materials Management in Hospital Pharmacy

INTRODUCTION

Pharmacy is a therapeutic facility of the hospital. It is one of the most extensively used facilities and it is an area, in which large amounts of money are spent on purchases on a recurring basis. It is also one of the highest revenue generating centres. A fairly high percentage of the total expenditure of the hospital goes for the pharmacy services. Hence, planning and designing the pharmacy needs to be done in a manner that results in efficient administrative and clinical services. Very often, pharmacy is not as well organized and well managed in typical hospitals as its importance warrants. **Purchasing and inventory control are often treated as a single entity in pharmacies. They are certainly interrelated.** However, each is a unique function with different objectives. The objective of purchasing is to acquire medicines of acceptable quality while minimizing their expense. The objective of inventory control is to maintain adequate quantities of drugs and pharmaceuticals on hand while minimizing associated expenses. In this management endeavour, planning deserves great time and diligence. Careful planning enhances its effectiveness and minimizes time spent on subsequent phases. The planning stage can be divided into four activities, i.e., determining goals and objectives, establishing organizational and departmental policies, designing systems and finally, organizing the activities.

Quality, service, and price determination are as important to pharmaceuticals as in the case of medical/surgical supplies, housekeeping supplies and everything else procured for use in any organization. Quality is the responsibility of the pharmacy department in conjunction with the therapeutics committee. It is generally not the responsibility of the purchaser or the product utilization committee because pharmaceuticals are medicinal substances including chemical compounds and non-infectious biological substances utilized in diagnosis, treatment, or prevention of abnormal physiological conditions. Quality determination of pharmacy items requires the specialized knowledge of the pharmacist and the medical staff. Hence quality determination by the pharmacist and therapeutics committee is essential. The purchaser's responsibility is to procure the quality product specified, and to accept no substitutes unless they are expressly approved.

Generic equivalents are used in the hospital pharmacy, provided their physical, chemical and biological properties are tested and verified. It is important to understand that many generic equivalents are marketed without research or testing to substantiate their properties. Major pharmaceutical manufacturers expend considerable time and money on research to substantiate their claims. Many generics are simply copies of products repackaged and differently named. Hence, generic equivalents require testing and evaluation prior to their use in healthcare facilities. Physicians always prefer to prescribe branded pharmaceuticals rather than generics. This practice does not preclude generic testing. This also is the responsibility of the pharmacist.

Pharmacy is distinctly different from other hospital departments in its mix of product management services and product based informational services. Departments responsible for product management typically incorporate into their services either comprehensive information about a relatively small spectrum of products (e.g., pulmonary therapy) or only very basic and/or fundamental information about a very broad range of products which are generally held in the central supply. On the other hand, pharmacy must be capable of providing comprehensive and detailed information about many products. The pharmacy, therefore, is torn between the pressures associated with cost effective management of pharmaceuticals and the knowledge based informational responsibilities. The regulatory and legal controls with which the pharmacy must comply impact its distributive aspects. The professional functions of pharmacy involve compilation and dissemination of information about its products. The pharmacy's internal organization often reflects this dual responsibility with separate components for distributive and clinical/drug information functions.

A good pharmacy is a blend of several things i.e., qualified personnel, modern facilities, efficient organization and operations and sound budgeting and operates with the support and cooperation of the medical, nursing and administrative staff of the hospital. Building up a modern and progressive pharmacy calls for introducing new methods of operations, new production approaches and new distribution techniques to achieve reduced costs and increased efficiency. The planners must keep in mind this picture of pharmacy of the future.

FUNCTIONS

Primary functions of pharmacy, some of which may be performed directly by its chief, are as follows.

- Deciding quality and quantity of drugs and pharmaceutical products: After pharmacy decides the list of items to be purchased and their quantities, purchasing handles all requisitions for purchases.
- Maintaining consistency in the purchasing, receiving and accounts payable cycle. Purchasing and accounting provide major assistance to the pharmacy in the management of materials.
- Ensuring that purchasing serves as a resource on systems and procedures and provides an efficient clerical source for purchase order generation that need not be duplicated in the pharmacy. Accounts payable take up the coordinated responsibility.

- Ensure that accurate, timely payments are processed for pharmacy purchases. Accounting must establish budgeting and financial reporting systems for monitoring and evaluating the performance of pharmacy's Materials Management.
- Receiving, storing, compounding, packaging, labelling and dispensing pharmaceutical items.
- Serving as a source of drug information to physicians, pharmacists and other healthcare professionals, as well as patients. This involves compiling, storing, retrieving and disseminating drug information and providing pharmaceutical advice and consultation regarding drug therapy.
- Participating in the hospital's educational programmes.
- Planning and organizing pharmacy department, establishing policies and procedures, and implementing them in accordance with the policies of the hospital.
- Serving as a member of the pharmacy and therapeutics committee, to be actively involved in its functions and activities, and implement its decisions.
- Researching and evaluating new drugs. This involves participating in performing therapeutic assessment of drugs and in the preparation of a hospital formulary so that equally effective but less expensive drugs may be put on the formulary. (A formulary is a list of drugs approved by the medical staff and the pharmacy committee for hospital use and kept in the inventory.)
- Keeping track of drugs and formulations or combinations banned in the country and elsewhere, and keeping abreast of W.H.O.'s revision of "essential list of drugs" and other notifications.
- Carrying out quality assurance programmes to ensure quality by sampling and analyzing it either in the hospital or through an external agency or testing laboratory like the drug inspectorate. This may be done when in doubt of the efficacy or potency of a drug.
- Complying with statutory regulations, initiating licenses to be obtained, and maintaining records as legally required.
- Providing training to pharmacy students. Many hospitals are recognized to provide practical training to pharmacy students in partial fulfillment of their course requirements.
- Utilizing resources effectively. Pharmacy managers should examine economic, personnel, and physical facility resources to identify deficiencies and then take appropriate steps to correct them.

Regardless of pressures to integrate Hospital Materials Management functions, the unique selection, control, and recordkeeping requirements for pharmaceuticals make it difficult and even redundant to transfer from pharmacy more than the purely administrative aspects of procurement, distribution, and disposition of drugs. Pharmacy interacts with many other hospital departments in its performance of Materials Management functions.

LOCATION

Planners must include enough flexibility and expansion potential in initial planning of the pharmacy itself so that expansion programmes can be carried out with minimum disruption to its physical location or without having to move it to an entirely new location at a subsequent date.

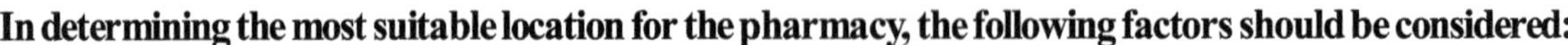

In determining the most suitable location for the pharmacy, the following factors should be considered:

- Flow of drugs and other raw materials into the pharmacy.
- Flow of drugs and services from the pharmacy to the inpatient areas and other departments in the hospital.
- Flow of outpatients' traffic through the hospital.
- Needs for future expansion.

Pharmacy bulk store must be conveniently accessible from the central receiving, inpatient areas and outpatient departments. A ground floor location close to the inpatient areas, outpatient department and to elevators is ideal. In some hospitals, the outpatient and inpatient dispensing activities are combined. When the outpatient department is the overriding consideration in determining the location of the pharmacy, the result is a less than optimal location for the inpatient dispensing activities. They soon start feeling that a separate inpatient pharmacy facility needs to be established. In many hospitals, inpatients are required to buy their requirements of medicines directly from the pharmacy on cash or credit card payment basis. Medicines are not supplied and billed. Much to their consternation, many hospitals sooner than later discover that pharmacy facilities have become woefully inadequate. Keeping this in mind, the pharmacy should have at least one outside wall to allow for expansion. It should also preferably be located adjacent to an area, which can be relocated easily when the need for expansion is felt.

DESIGN

Each hospital must adhere to the accepted norms of good pharmacy practice and the legal requirements. Broadly speaking, the pharmacy has four main functional areas: the dispensing, production (or preparation), administrative and storage areas (Fig. 3.1). These areas must be designed and located for convenient access, staff control and security. Facilities required in these areas are discussed below.

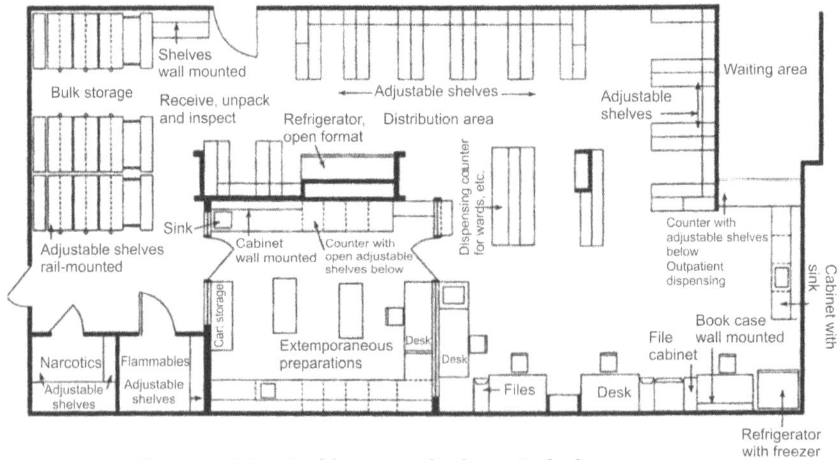

Figure 3.1 Typical layout of a hospital pharmacy

The author is indebted to hospital planning design and management authored by Mr. Kundar and others for use of this diagram

DISPENSING AREA

1. Patient waiting area, preferably air conditioned, with adequate comfortable seating and other facilities.
2. Patient dispensing counters, preferably glass panelled. It must have space earmarked for computer assisted pricing, billing and cash or card payments on one side and for dispensing on the other.
3. Storage area with adequate space for a large number of active drugs stored in routine shelves layout efficiently.
4. Pick up and receiving counter and spare counters for temporary storage of carts.
5. Area for review and recording of drug orders.
6. Compounding area.
7. Working counters and cabinets for pharmacy activities.
8. Refrigerated storage.
9. Secured Storage for narcotics and other controlled drugs.
10. Storage for alcohol and volatile and inflammable substances.
11. Space for maintaining patient medication profiles and cross checking of medication, for providing drug information, and a room for pharmacist to meet with the patient who requires extensive consultation, instructions or counselling, if these functions are performed.

MANUFACTURING AREA

- Bulk compounding area.
- Provision for packaging and labels.
- Provision for quality assurance.
- Clinical sinks and hand washing facilities.

The preparation of parenteral fluids comes under the mandatory regulations of the drug control act which has now been made stricter and more comprehensive. Hospitals wanting to manufacture these fluids are advised to thoroughly study the regulations and procedures.

ADMINISTRATIVE AREA

1. Reception and front office, which may also handle office functions including filing, communications, references, etc.

2. Chief pharmacist's office and office space for assistant chief pharmacist and clinical pharmacist, wherever applicable.
3. Waiting area for visitors, medical representatives and salesmen.
4. Conference room cum library.
5. Staff facilities like lockers, toilets, lounge, duty room for on call duty pharmacist(s), etc. Some or all of these can be offsite.

STORAGE AREA

For convenience, some of the storage requirements already mentioned in other

Sections are repeated here under.

- Bulk storage
- Active storage
- Refrigerated storage
- Volatile and alcohol storage
- Secured storage for narcotics and controlled drugs
- Storage for general supplies, equipment, files, stationery, etc.

PROCUREMENT

In the area of drugs and pharmaceuticals, the same products, or equivalents, are generally available directly from a number of manufacturers or dealers. In some instances, a drug is manufactured by one firm, marketed, labelled, and distributed by several distributors or dealers. Sometimes several distributors compete in the same service segments, handling identical products. Some manufacturers or dealers permit only direct purchasing, others distribute exclusively through distributors. Thus pharmacy frequently has several alternatives for source-of-supply depending upon the product.

Purchasing from Manufacturers

Traditionally, pharmacies purchased most of their requirements directly from manufacturers. This trend is now changing. Direct purchasing eliminates the middlemen and is therefore likely to result in lower prices. It also facilitates the buyers to take advantage of special or promotional pricing, provided storage requirements and projected usage would warrant taking advantage of the sale. It helps buyers to benefit from promotional payment plans, such as delayed payment for specified periods if the order is placed before a designated date. However, direct purchasing is a costly process. There are expenses in terms of both materials and personnel time for purchasing, receiving, and accounts payable departments associated with purchase order processing. Organized recordkeeping is required to keep track of orders in direct purchases from numerous sources.

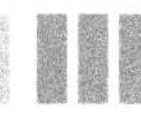

Significant delivery delays are inherent. Time spent in generating purchase orders and time in delivery call for higher safety stocks, thus resulting in increased inventories and lost opportunities to put the cash to other possibly more productive uses for the organization. Any apparent lower prices in direct purchasing must be weighed against those overhead expenses.

Purchasing from Distributors

Primary alternative to direct purchasing from manufacturers is buying from distributors. They obviously charge a little more for providing additional services like warehousing and distribution. This expense typically is built into the price or is identified as an added fee, often stated as percentage of purchases. Procuring from distributors reduces or eliminates generating orders by providing for telephonic or email orders and making payments on the basis of invoices. Frequent ordering and reduced delivery lead times combine to shift a portion of the pharmacy inventory, and the expenses of maintaining it, to the distributor. The distributor often provides additional services on request to the pharmacy that further contribute to inventory control, including:

- Shelf labels for individual product identification.
- Product stickers for individual pricing information.
- Inventory movement reports.
- Notification of price increases and emergency deliveries.
- Physical inventory capabilities.

On the other hand, deficiencies of buying from distributors include inconsistent availability of products and inaccuracies in filling orders. Hospital inventories of critical products can be reduced only if confidence in product availability and timely delivery are high. High order filling rates are in the best interests of both the pharmacy and the distributor. When order filling rates are poor, the distributor forgoes the immediate opportunities to sell out of stock items and also risks loss of business. It is important to monitor performance to ensure that the distributor's commitment is fulfilled.

PRIME VENDOR AGREEMENTS

Advantages of purchasing from distributors are reflected in the progression of individual distributors to the status of prime vendors. In this relationship, the pharmacy commits itself to make all possible purchases through a single distributor in exchange for reduced service fees and lower prices. This benefits both sides. Pharmacy should expect not only the economic advantages of a reduced fee but also a strengthened commitment from the distributor to provide all possible drug inventory management services. The prime vendor concept enhances the value of many services rendered by distributors. For instance, inventory usage reports vastly increase in utility when all, rather than a fraction, of drug purchases are represented in the report.

The direct purchase prices charged by manufacturers from pharmacies are frequently lower than those quoted to distributors. This situation can arise either as a result of the terms of group

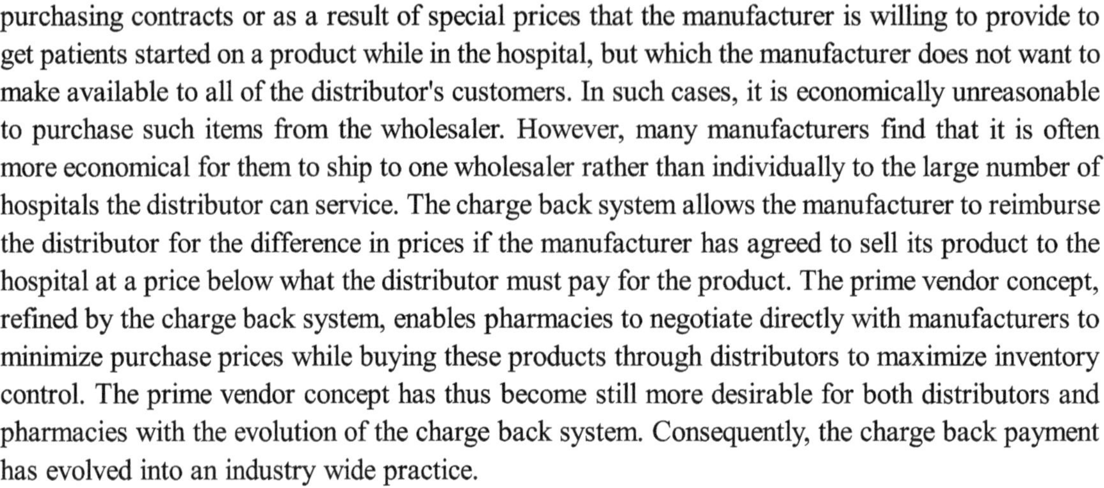

purchasing contracts or as a result of special prices that the manufacturer is willing to provide to get patients started on a product while in the hospital, but which the manufacturer does not want to make available to all of the distributor's customers. In such cases, it is economically unreasonable to purchase such items from the wholesaler. However, many manufacturers find that it is often more economical for them to ship to one wholesaler rather than individually to the large number of hospitals the distributor can service. The charge back system allows the manufacturer to reimburse the distributor for the difference in prices if the manufacturer has agreed to sell its product to the hospital at a price below what the distributor must pay for the product. The prime vendor concept, refined by the charge back system, enables pharmacies to negotiate directly with manufacturers to minimize purchase prices while buying these products through distributors to maximize inventory control. The prime vendor concept has thus become still more desirable for both distributors and pharmacies with the evolution of the charge back system. Consequently, the charge back payment has evolved into an industry wide practice.

COMPETITIVE BIDDING

Competitive bidding from various manufacturers and distributors produces three primary benefits:

1. Identifying the purchase price most advantageous for the pharmacy.
2. Locking in that price for the specified contract period, providing immunity against general price increases.
3. Ensuring the manufacturer of exclusive sales for that product, to the extent that the pharmacy can control drug selection.

However, the clerical and administrative effort required in identifying multiple sources, soliciting and comparing bids, and awarding contracts can be considerable. Therefore, it may be prudent to limit the bid process to products that have the most budgetary impact.

Group Purchase

Manufacturers generally consider two predominant factors while submitting quotations. These factors are the pharmacy's potential purchase volume and its commitment to honour a contract. Pharmacy can increase its potential purchase volume leverage by inviting bids collectively with other pharmacies. Recognition of this leverage, along with the clerical expenses of competitive bidding, has led to the proliferation of organized buying groups. These focus exclusively on drug purchasing or as a part of a larger group programme aimed at purchasing many categories of items. Buying groups typically charge a membership fee as, a fixed amount per annum, a percentage of purchases, or a combination of these to cover its expenses. As the number of members in a group escalates and its purchasing leverage improves, a dichotomy frequently occurs. Group consensus and resulting commitment to honour group contracts may become more and more difficult to achieve. **The sustained success of a growing buying group depends upon how well the individual members maintain the integrity of the contract awards.** Prices are also compared from one group

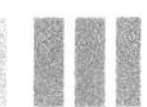

to another. While some groups certainly enjoy greater success than others in obtaining more competitive prices, several other factors must also be considered. Groups may award contracts based on aggregate product line prices rather than on lowest bids for individual items. This could happen for example, when a product available in multiple strengths may receive the award for all strengths in order to maintain consistency in prescriptions for that product, even though the bid for a particular strength of it may not have been the lowest. Prices achieved by buying groups may sometimes leap frog ahead of one another depending upon the cycle of the contract year. The expectations of larger groups to hold down prices are generally greater. Bid prices which they receive can set the new prices in the market. As a result, larger groups drive the prices for purchases outside the group as well as within the group.

Borrowing and Lending

Another source of supply is the potential for a loaned supply from another pharmacy. This is a limited source. Despite a large inventory, a pharmacy may need additional supplies at such times when normal channels are not open, such as on weekends and nights. To ensure that the inter-pharmacy relationship provides the opportunity to borrow when necessary, the pharmacy also must be willing to lend. Of course, thorough documentation of lending and borrowing, and timely replenishments, are essential to minimize abuses. Hospitals find it necessary to utilize each of these drug procurement systems and concepts. Total procurement expenses for each should be analyzed for determining the preferred system. These vary from one institution to another. Even with identification of the preferred system, factors such as cost, delivery time, size of drug lot, etc., frequently determine the type of procurement preferred.

INVENTORY CONTROL

Inventory control encompasses the broader objectives of identifying the appropriate purchase quantity; purchase interval, minimum and maximum stock levels. The goal is to ensure product availability when needed at minimal expense. The discussions of inventory analyses have direct application to pharmacy. Two categories of drugs can be identified from the large spectrum of pharmaceuticals making up the pharmacy inventory. One category is composed of drugs that are used infrequently, are relatively expensive, and are absolutely critical to have on hand. This category requires that adequate inventory levels be maintained at all times. As a result, these drugs generally require higher on hand inventory than their historical usage would appear to justify. The second inventory category is composed of drugs that, when ranked by their unit cost times frequency of use, account for the largest portion of pharmacy expenditures. These drugs are readily identifiable by ABC analysis, one of the most useful inventory control concepts. **An ABC analysis of the pharmacy inventory provides a foundation upon which all other control functions can be built.** ABC analysis provides opportunities to control the inventory by focusing on the A items alone because of the significant time required to monitor all medications, and the limited resources available. The

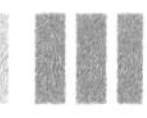

above mentioned two categories of drugs merit close attention in inventory management. Intricacies of hospital inventory management are dealt extensively in Part III.

It is useful to label each product location with the reorder point and quantity. Shelf labels often are included in the services of prime vendors or distributors. Distributor shelf labels typically list minimum quantities, maximum quantities, and product identification numbers. The minimum and maximum stock quantities indirectly provide the same basic information as the reorder point and reorder quantity.

DISTRIBUTION MANAGEMENT

Drug distribution within a hospital should aim for maintaining optimal control and accountability without compromising on the availability of critical medication to patients. These goals require that the pharmacy make drugs available throughout the hospital using multiple distribution systems.

Floor Stock

Floor stock system is the most basic of the drug distribution methods. This ensures optimal availability for patient administration with the least control and accountability. Floor stock medications are not labelled or specified for any particular patient but are stocked in the area because of high probability of use and the need to have those drugs readily available for immediate administration. Medicines designated to be floor stocked in particular areas should have assigned par stock levels. This helps to provide what little control is available with this system. Floor stocked medication can be replaced either by a requisition from the stocking area to pharmacy or by automatic replacement as soon as the pharmacy receives a patient charge for the item.

Accurate patient medication charging is a problem because it relies on initiation of drug charges by the nursing departments. This may not receive a nursing priority because of the multitude of other patient care pressures. Automatic charge replacement combined with designated par stock levels for each medicine offers the ability to monitor the rate of charge capture for the floor stocked medication. Floor stock distribution systems sacrifice the benefits of pharmacy's double check in the dispensing process. Floor stocked medicines are a necessity in limited circumstances. However, the spectrum of drugs that are floor stocked should be minimized and such distribution discouraged because of the inherently minimal control and accountability.

Individual Patient Supply

Individual patient supply distribution closely parallels traditional prescription dispensing in retail pharmacies. Drug distribution systems progressed from floor stock to individual multi day patient supply. This system offers enhanced drug control and accountability since each medication supply is individually labelled and charged to a specific patient. The individual labelling adds the qualitative benefit of a double check on the proper medication for the patient. This double check is further enhanced if the pharmacy dispenses the individual patient medication supply from a direct copy of the physician's original prescription rather than from a drug requisition transcribed from the order. Major disadvantages of this distribution system

 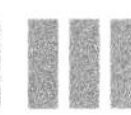

arise from the multiple day or multiple dose supply. The multiple day supply requires the maintenance of a large inventory of drugs in nursing units. This system also necessitates a cumbersome crediting process for returned and unused drugs if an equitable patient charging system is desired. The disposition of these returned and credited medicines also creates a dilemma as to whether these drugs can be uncontaminated and subsequently dispensed to other patients. If they are determined to be so dispensable, they will be temporarily returned to stock. They must however retain identification by manufacturer's lot number in the event of a drug recall. This system is preferred in rehabilitation units where patient self-administration is an objective. Individual multiple day patient supply is considered preferable to floor stock distribution. It is not generally the preferred system for frequently used, routinely administered medications.

Unit Dose

Unit dose drug distribution system is preferred for medications that are ordered and administered routinely. This distribution system addresses some of the shortcomings of floor stock and individual multiple day supply systems. It also retains many of their advantages. Unit dose drug distribution involves the dispensing of not more than a 24-hour individual patient supply of individually packaged and labelled medication in as ready to administer a form, as possible. This system minimizes the drug inventory held in nursing units and also reduces the volume of medication crediting. The individually packaged and labelled medication effectively prevents contamination and safely allows for subsequent re dispensing. The label also provides a source of manufacturer lot number identification. The labelled unit dose medication maintains double check in dispensing administration process and ensures the ability to track the medication up to the patient. A pharmacy patient medication profile may be maintained with floor stock and individual multiple day supply systems. However such profiles are a necessity in providing daily dispensing information with the unit dose system. Patient medication profiles enable pharmacy to monitor total drug therapy to minimize duplications and drug interactions. This system also provides a more efficient system for nursing by significantly reducing dose preparation time.

Adaptations of the unit dose drug system have assigned pharmacists to the nursing units to review original physician orders and dispense initial doses for new orders. This is referred to as a decentralized system and offers improved communication with physicians, nursing personnel, and patients. This system also expedites the availability of first doses and enhances pharmacy's monitoring of drug administration. A comparison of operational expenses for the floor stock, individual supply, and unit dose systems, considering only pharmacy and ignoring revenue capture, would rank floor stock as the least costly. However, in a comparison of global life cycle costs of the systems including consideration of nursing time savings, the unit dose system is the most economical.

Intravenous Solutions

Intravenous solutions as per the Drug Control Administration are broadly classified into two categories. i.e., **Sterile admixture services and Drugs defined by the Drug Control Administration as 'controlled substances.'**

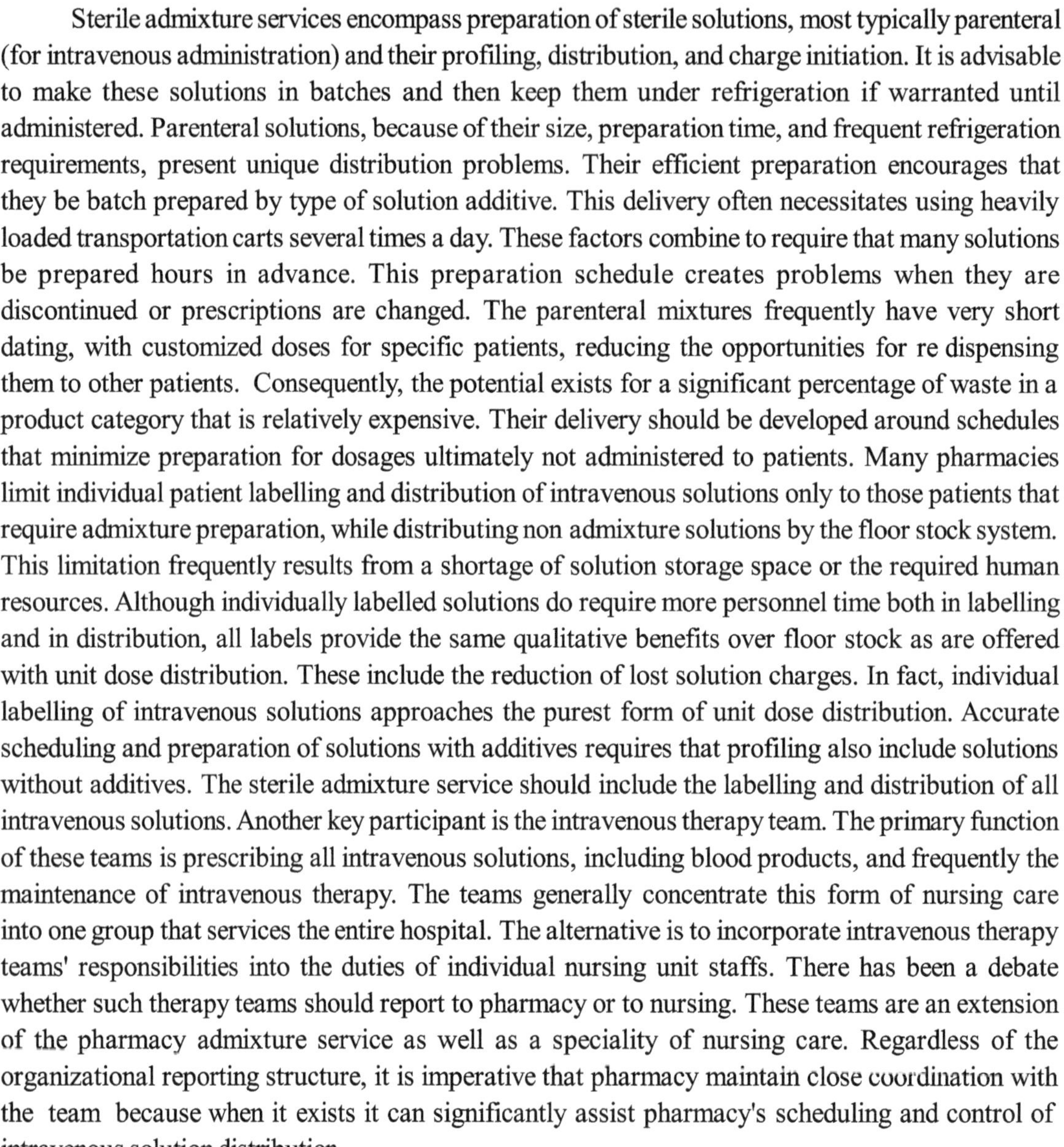

Sterile admixture services encompass preparation of sterile solutions, most typically parenteral (for intravenous administration) and their profiling, distribution, and charge initiation. It is advisable to make these solutions in batches and then keep them under refrigeration if warranted until administered. Parenteral solutions, because of their size, preparation time, and frequent refrigeration requirements, present unique distribution problems. Their efficient preparation encourages that they be batch prepared by type of solution additive. This delivery often necessitates using heavily loaded transportation carts several times a day. These factors combine to require that many solutions be prepared hours in advance. This preparation schedule creates problems when they are discontinued or prescriptions are changed. The parenteral mixtures frequently have very short dating, with customized doses for specific patients, reducing the opportunities for re dispensing them to other patients. Consequently, the potential exists for a significant percentage of waste in a product category that is relatively expensive. Their delivery should be developed around schedules that minimize preparation for dosages ultimately not administered to patients. Many pharmacies limit individual patient labelling and distribution of intravenous solutions only to those patients that require admixture preparation, while distributing non admixture solutions by the floor stock system. This limitation frequently results from a shortage of solution storage space or the required human resources. Although individually labelled solutions do require more personnel time both in labelling and in distribution, all labels provide the same qualitative benefits over floor stock as are offered with unit dose distribution. These include the reduction of lost solution charges. In fact, individual labelling of intravenous solutions approaches the purest form of unit dose distribution. Accurate scheduling and preparation of solutions with additives requires that profiling also include solutions without additives. The sterile admixture service should include the labelling and distribution of all intravenous solutions. Another key participant is the intravenous therapy team. The primary function of these teams is prescribing all intravenous solutions, including blood products, and frequently the maintenance of intravenous therapy. The teams generally concentrate this form of nursing care into one group that services the entire hospital. The alternative is to incorporate intravenous therapy teams' responsibilities into the duties of individual nursing unit staffs. There has been a debate whether such therapy teams should report to pharmacy or to nursing. These teams are an extension of the pharmacy admixture service as well as a speciality of nursing care. Regardless of the organizational reporting structure, it is imperative that pharmacy maintain close coordination with the team because when it exists it can significantly assist pharmacy's scheduling and control of intravenous solution distribution.

Controlled Substances

Distribution of drugs categorized as controlled substances by the Drug Control Administration requires exceptions to normal distribution by the pharmacy because of governmental regulations. The narcotics and psychotropic substance act regulates the manufacture, distribution, dispensing, and delivery of certain drugs or substances that have a high potential for abuse or dependence.

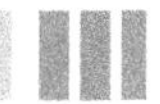

Every hospital must register with drug control authorities as dispenser of controlled substances and keep the following records of such drugs:

- Initial and subsequent biannual inventory
- Receipt
- Dispensing
- Disposal

These records must include the following information:

- Name of controlled drug
- Dosage form
- Strength
- Amount

Dispensing records must include:

- Number or volume of drug dispensed.
- Name and address of the person to whom the drug is dispensed.
- Date of dispensation.
- Name or initials of dispensing pharmacist.

Drug records in hospitals may differ from those in outpatient pharmacies. The latter must fully document the dispensation of controlled drugs individually on prescriptions. Prescriptions for narcotics and psychotropic drugs must bear the original signature of the prescribing physician, cannot be refilled, and must be filed separately in hospitals; the frequency of orders and quantity of doses would make it unduly burdensome for the pharmacy to maintain records for each individual dispensation. Hospital pharmacies also frequently dispense medications, including controlled substances that for legitimate reasons ultimately are not administered to patients. The required prescribing and administration records also are available in patient charts or medical records.

For these reasons, it has become common practice to consolidate such prescription, dispensation, and administration information onto proof of use records for each drug dispensed as floor stock to each nursing unit; these records document the nurse responsible for the administration of each such dose. This document provides not only a concise record of controlled drug disposition throughout the hospital; it also is more easily reconcilable against pharmacy's records of dispensation to each nursing unit.

OUTPATIENT PHARMACY

Outpatient prescription services represent a major distribution system in a hospital pharmacy. Outpatient drug distribution essentially involves dispensing multi-day supplies of individual medication pursuant to a physician's prescription and the pharmacy's earlier dispensing records. Prescriptions must be dated, initialled by the dispensing pharmacist, and serially numbered.

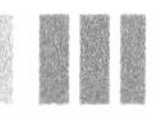

The prescription must be filed as stipulated by government regulatory authorities. The prescription must contain at least the following to comply with statutory requirements:

- Name and address of dispensing pharmacy
- Serial number of the prescription
- Date of prescription filling or refilling
- Name of prescribing physician
- Name of patient
- Directions for medication use.

DRUG UTILIZATION

Drug expenses account for the largest percentage of the hospital pharmacy's operational budget. Thus the budget is material intensive. Although pharmacy cannot directly control this part of its budget, it can certainly influence it. The amounts of money involved, training and character of the pharmacy profession and the essential purpose of pharmacy department have a considerable impact on drug usage in the hospital. **Two concepts of drug equivalency assist the pharmacy in controlling the cost of utilization: 1. generic equivalency and 2. therapeutic equivalency.**

Generic Equivalency

Drug products may be referred to by their chemical names. These names are often long, unwieldy, difficult to pronounce and are therefore frequently altered to a simpler generic term. The generic names may be used by any manufacturer of identical drugs. New drug products frequently are marketed by the manufacturer under an additional trade or brand name to increase patients' and physicians' awareness of that particular item. The trade name is legally protected. Normally it cannot be used by any other manufacturer without specific authorization. Marketing of new drugs is protected by a patent period. When the patent expires, other manufacturers have options to seek permissions to market the same generic drug either under their own trade name or the generic name. Some manufacturers elect to market the drug as a generic, assuming that greater value lies in identification with the proved product rather than a new trade name or its generally lower cost. However regardless of whether or not a trade name is used, all drug products with the same generic name in the same dosage form (e.g. tablet, capsule, suspension) and in the same strength or concentration are generically equivalent.

Therapeutic Equivalency

Therapeutic equivalency is a more subjective concept. Therapeutically equivalent or alternate drugs are not necessarily generically equivalent but elicit a similar response when administered. One of the best and least controversial examples of drugs treated as therapeutic equivalents is vitamin products. Similar combination vitamin products are not identical in chemical composition

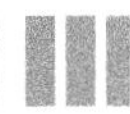

but still produce essentially the same results when administered. Therapeutic equivalency may be somewhat subjective. Variations in formulation of even generically equivalent products may produce differences in bioavailability (defined as the availability of the drug at place of action) that result in therapeutic in equivalence.

Formulary Systems

Generic and therapeutic equivalencies are significant in the drug selection process. It is virtually impossible, as well as waste of resources, to stock every major product brand of pharmaceutical in the pharmacy. Consequently, a drug formulary concept is used to limit stocked medications to non duplicative generically and therapeutically equivalent drugs. **A drug formulary is a healthcare institution's system of selection and stocking of medications, particularly a continuously updated list of items that have been determined to be acceptable for stocking in the pharmacy department.** Pharmacy and therapeutics committee of the medical staff are the appropriate decisionmaking body on drug formulary decisions.

Drug formularies are defined by a number of terms, such as open, closed, and restricted. These terms are defined differently from one institution to another. Closed formularies are those that strictly limit the drug choices. A physician cannot prescribe a non formulary medication in such a situation because such medications are simply not stocked. A closed formulary represents the strictest type, and drugs are added only after a rigorous review by the pharmacy and therapeutics committee is conducted. In an open formulary, drugs are added with only a cursory review or simply based upon the request of one or more than one physicians. Open formulary offers physicians the greatest prescribing freedom, and also poses the largest number of problems in inventory control. A restricted formulary is a compromise between the open and closed systems. Some drugs may be available only after predetermined conditions are satisfied. The most common and lenient form of restriction is that all non-formulary drug orders be clarified by the pharmacist with the physician. This type at a minimum requires the pharmacist to suggest formulary alternatives to the physicians. Physicians are permitted to confirm their desire to have the original order dispensed if they so choose after this said consultation. Another restriction makes non-formulary orders valid only if countersigned by physician at the specified levels. For example, a non formulary antibiotic may require countersignature by a physician member of the infectious disease department or a non formulary pre anaesthetic drug may need countersignature by the director of anaesthesia. A third restriction in some hospitals is to place time limits on non formulary medications. Antibiotics which are non formulary may be permitted for administration only until culture and sensitivity results pinpoint the appropriate formulary selection. There are also many other types of drug formulary restrictions. Administration of formulary decisions carries significant financial impact. Generic substitutions should be preferred when available from reputable manufacturers and therapeutic substitution should be sought for the selected drug categories. The drug formulary is much more than a mere stock list of drugs available in the pharmacy.

DRUG INFORMATION

Closed formularies and restrictions are inadequate without timely provision of information to physicians to support drug decisions. Communication between pharmacists and physicians is imperative, in face-to-face discussion, emails, telephonic communication, or dissemination through house journal. This is the most important and potentially cost effective responsibility of the pharmacy department. The formulary must be readily available to physicians. A copy should be displayed prominently in each patient care area. The provision of drug information, therefore, while normally considered a professional service, is directly related to effective product management in the pharmacy.

STANDARDIZATION AND TREATMENT PROTOCOLS

In addition to drug formulary review, medical staff committees, such as pharmacy and therapeutics, can assist with drug product control in other ways. The committees can endorse and approve drug therapy protocols and standardized formulations. These protocols are pre established order sets that are initiated after strict patient criteria are satisfied. Standardized formulations are beneficial in maximizing the efficient preparation of medications that need to be compounded. Standardized formulations are prepared in larger quantities to allow multiple dispensing from a single batch. Two common examples are oral liquid analgesic preparations for cancer patients and basic hyper alimentation solutions. Standardized hyper alimentation solutions not only reduce dosage calculations associated with the admixture time but also increase the potential to use the expensive solutions for another order if the initial one is discontinued before the solution is used. Another example is standardized medication orders for routine postpartum patients after a delivery. Such drug therapy protocols reduce the potential for inadvertent orders of non formulary medications. These protocols lead to more consistent usage estimates for drug purchasing.

DRUG UTILIZATION REVIEW

Strong formulary policies and effective purchasing and distribution procedures realize only limited success in minimizing drug expenses if physicians prescribe costly medication while more cost effective alternatives are ignored. This reduces effectiveness of drug utilization systems and controls. Drug utilization reviews are required for monitoring the appropriateness of prescribing. Drug utilization review can be accomplished by three methods: retrospective, concurrent, and prospective.

The system of retrospective review requires that appropriate conditions or criteria for the use of a particular drug or treatment protocol be defined in advance. Such criteria must be carefully selected, based on medical knowledge and accepted standards of practice, and agreed upon by audit committee members of the medical staff. Reviews of medical records of patients who have received the drug then are audited against the criteria.

Concurrent review is a specialized form of patient medication profile monitoring conducted by pharmacists in the routine performance of profile maintenance. Concurrent drug utilization review is similar to retrospective review but is conducted during a course of therapy while it is being conducted

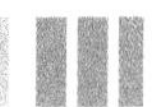

on the audited item. Concurrent review offers several advantages over retrospective reviews. Retrospective reviews rely upon completed medical record documentation and only promise future corrective action if indicated. Concurrent review allows for completion of missing patient information as well as for the opportunity to have a positive influence on drug therapy which is in progress.

Prospective reviews are conducted after a drug has been ordered but before even the first dose is administered. The criteria for prospective reviews are different from those for retrospective and concurrent reviews. They are not as closely correlated to current changes in the patient's condition. Prospective evaluations provide opportunities to influence drug therapy before it is initiated. This has to be accomplished in a limited time frame.

The above mentioned drug utilization review methods have the potential for producing both qualitative and economic advantages. Retrospective reviews are generally the least difficult to perform, prospective reviews the most difficult. The time and effort needed to perform any utilization reviews require that the process be limited to a relatively small number of drugs, selected judiciously. The drug utilization review process is incomplete if it ends at the initial statistical stage. A feedback mechanism to the medical staff must exist in order to identify utilization deficiencies. The deficiencies should be re evaluated later to determine the effect of corrective measures that might have resulted from the review.

Clinical Pharmacy

Clinical pharmacy is an ideology, concepts, and strategies that affect optimal drug utilization. It may be embodied in many activities, including:

- Medication profile review
- Patient medication history
- Dosage calculations
- Participation in cardiopulmonary resuscitation (CPR) efforts
- Rounding with physicians
- Patient education

Clinical pharmacy does not embrace the full scope of Materials Management in that it does not include the acquisition and distribution of drugs. However, it does fully cover drug disposition. Clinical pharmacy derives its purpose from the relationship of drug and patient. It has become a dominant force in the growth of the profession because it addresses directly the need for and use of pharmacy's products.

CONTROLLING MATERIAL EXPENSES

The path of drug products through pharmacy's Materials Management involves many of the same decision points that exist in other material departments:

- Purchase ready packaged or repackage?
- Buy disposables or reusables?
- Elect packaging consistency or lower price?
- Select quality or lower price?
- Risk equipment failure or obtain service contract?
- Emphasize materials savings or labour savings?
- Minimize short term or long term expenses?
- Elect departmental savings or institutional savings?

Many of these decisions offer acceptable alternatives either way. In some instances they may be mutually exclusive. The purchase of unit dose packaged medications versus bulk medications and repackaging into unit doses is an example of acceptable alternatives. Bulk packages (e.g., bottles of 1,000 tablets, 500 ml or 1 litre bottles of liquid) are nearly always far more economical per dose than are unit dose packaged medications. Even after adding the cost of packaging material and labour, per dose expense of repackaging from bulk to unit dose is less expensive. The decision as to which to purchase varies among hospitals and among individual medications. **Reasons for purchasing commercially packaged unit doses, even when more expensive, include the following:**

- Manufacturer's package integrity is maintained, ensuring longer package stability.
- Potential for mislabelling is reduced.
- Labour expenses for repackaging are avoided.
- Manufacturer's packaging material, seal, and label generally are of higher quality.
- The drug product is available more quickly for dispensation.
- Total expense per dose frequently is not significantly greater.

Decisions on purchasing disposables or reusables must be considered in many hospital departments. Nearly all such decisions in pharmacy are related to the use of disposables. The choice between disposables and reusables involves sterile filters, refilling syringes, ointment slab/papers, stock containers, protective gowns, and even towels or linens. Selection of disposables in such situations is preferred. Labour savings and convenience usually more than compensate for the additional expenditure. Packaging consistency is an important component for sterile admixtures. Many medications for intravenous piggyback administration may be added to a piggyback mini bottle or mini bag or may be purchased from the drug manufacturer in an original container suitable for the addition of the solution. The dispensing of medications in the intravenous solution supplier's mini bottle or mini bag offers a consistency in packaging and labelling that may be valuable in pharmacy's preparation and nursing administration. The less consistent packaging in manufacturers'

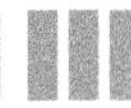

piggyback containers may be less expensive. The selection of these alternatives includes consideration of overall system efficiencies, storage, and delivery requirements as well as costs. The goal is to optimize the balance between quality of care and cost of care.

Increasing availability of generic drugs and the concept of therapeutic substitution are expanding opportunities for selecting drugs on the basis of lower cost. Lower cost does not necessarily mean compromising on quality. Quality must always be considered when comparing drug products. Two products may be chemically or therapeutically equivalent but their bio availabilities (e.g., abilities to be absorbed into the blood stream) may differ because of differences in formulations. Despite increasing pressures to control expenses, cost should continue to rank below efficacy, quality and non toxicity in drug product comparisons. In many instances, the least costly alternative to the pharmacy may not be the least costly to the healthcare institution. The growth and development of hospital pharmacy services have been justified on the basis of improved economy, efficiency, and quality of overall patient care in spite of corresponding increases in operating expenses.

The ever changing healthcare delivery environment requires that throughout drug purchasing, packaging, and distribution systems, pharmacy remains vigilant in analyzing systems and services and their responsiveness to the total needs of the institution. The costs of new drugs, new packaging, and methods of drug distribution and administration must continue to be analyzed with a view to minimize the total expenses to the institution and ultimately to the patient. A more expensive drug or drug package, which adds to pharmacy's expenses, in some instances may have to be accepted for achieving potentially greater savings to the institution. Services with orientation towards both drug distribution and information distribution are provided by the pharmacy department. Either of these elements may be examined independently. The ideal combination elevates the overall quality of pharmacy services. Principles of Materials Management have application in the provision of institutional pharmacy services. Successful management of the pharmacy will be judged increasingly by the degree of proper drug usage and control.

Dual Responsibilities

Pharmacy has dual responsibilities, i.e., providing information about drugs and controlling purchase and distribution of drugs. While Materials Management is focused more on product handling, it must also consider its distributive and informative roles. These two elements can and must mutually coexist.

Materials Management function in pharmacy translates into "management and control of drugs, pharmaceutical services, and pharmacy related equipment from purchase to patient administration or use." This encompasses hospital pharmacy services. The supplies or materials expenses of the typical pharmacy are nearly three times that of its human resource cost. Consequently, it is imperative that the management and control of pharmacy materials be based on the scientific principles of Materials Management. The considerations relating to control of drugs are not new to pharmacy. Pharmacy manages a broad range of products and a correspondingly large inventory. Pharmacy is acutely aware of potential lost opportunity costs when drugs are out-of-stock. The

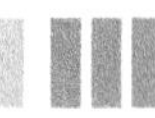

hospital drug distribution systems focus on the need to optimize accuracy and control while minimizing waste. Sterile admixture services incorporate standardization and centralization. Pharmacy's Materials Management responsibilities cannot be absorbed or assigned elsewhere. The practices of pharmacy are regulated by legislative, regulative, and professional bodies through standards, laws, regulations, and guidelines.

Regardless of pressures to centralize MM functions, the selection, control, and recordkeeping requirements for drugs make it difficult to transfer from pharmacy more than the purely clerical aspects of the procurement, distribution, and disposition of drugs. However, the pharmacy does interface with many other hospital departments in its performance of MM functions:

- Purchasing and accounting provide major assistance to the pharmacy.
- Purchasing handles requisitions for direct from manufacturer purchases. This maintains consistency in the purchasing receiving accounts payable cycle.
- Purchasing is a valuable resource on procedures and concepts and provides an efficient clerical source for purchase order generation that need not be duplicated in the pharmacy.
- Accounts payable ensure that accurate, timely payments are processed for pharmacy purchases. Established, fine tuned budgeting and financial reporting systems are vital in monitoring and evaluating the performance of pharmacy's MM.

Nursing and medical staff are also included among interdepartmental relationships. Pharmacy handles product addition, deletion, standardization, and substitution effectively with agreement and cooperation of the groups ultimately responsible for prescribing and administering the products. Therapeutic efficacy and cost effectiveness are essential considerations in product selection discussions with the medical staff. Pharmacy must be sensitive to storage requirements, product stability, final preparation, and ease of administration as vital nursing considerations. These require pharmacy to consider both its business and clinical interests. It is not cost effective to use an expensive antibiotic when a less expensive one should provide adequate treatment. The more expensive one may cover a broader spectrum of bacterial infections which is a valuable benefit to the patient in cases where identification of the disease causing bacteria is uncertain. While dealing with therapeutic effectiveness of medications, it is difficult to serve both economic and clinical interests impartially.

Pharmacy provides multifaceted services. Proper organizational positioning of the pharmacy department as a result of the economic interests associated with Materials Management and the clinical interests of product effectiveness is absolutely essential. Pharmacy handles large inventory and is responsible for the cost of its optimal management. At the same time, pharmacy's professional status is built on its knowledge base of drug information and would be diluted by being in a group identified primarily by products rather than informational services. Performance of pharmacy must be judged on the quality and effectiveness of both types of activities. Its performance suffers if either one is emphasized at the expense of the other. Consequently, pharmacy's positioning depends on the organization's sensitivity to its balance of services. Within any organizational structure, strong interdepartmental relationships, respect, and rapport can be developed and maintained.

OTHER ISSUES

In the dispensing and distribution systems, many innovative approaches and methods have been introduced in recent years. Traditional pharmacy services are rapidly undergoing a change all over the world. Some of the larger and progressive hospitals would introduce and test these newer systems and be pace setters for other hospitals to follow.

SUMMARY

Pharmacy department is one of the many departments in a complex organization the hospital. All departments should have goals and objectives which should be known by the pharmacy chief, in addition, the pharmacy manager should thoroughly understand the hospitals organization in order to integrate the department's goals with those of other departments and the hospital.

Pharmacy is one of the most extensively used facilities and it is an area, in which large amounts of money are spent on purchases on a recurring basis. It is also one of the highest revenue generating centres. A fairly high percentage of the total expenditure of the hospital goes for the pharmacy services. Hence, planning and designing the pharmacy need to be done in a manner that results in efficient administrative and clinical services.

The important primary functions, among others, are as follows:

1. Deciding quality and quantity of drugs and pharmaceutical products.
2. Receiving, storing, compounding, packaging, labelling and dispensing pharmaceutical items.
3. Serving as a source of drug information to physicians, pharmacists and other healthcare professionals, as well as patients.
4. Planning and organizing pharmacy department, establishing policies and procedures, and implementing them in accordance with the policies of the hospital.
5. Serving as a member of the pharmacy and therapeutics committee, to be actively involved in its functions and activitics, and implcmcnt its dccisions.
6. Researching and evaluating of new drugs.
7. Keeping track of drugs and formulations or combinations banned in the country and elsewhere, and keeping abreast of W.H.O.'s revision of "essential list of drugs" and other notifications.
8. Carrying out quality assurance programmes to ensure quality by sampling and analyzing it either in the hospital or through an external agency or testing laboratory like, the drug inspectorate.

9. Complying with statutory regulations, initiating licenses to be obtained, and maintaining records as legally required.

10. Providing training to pharmacy students.

Planners must include enough flexibility and expansion potential in initial planning of the pharmacy. The following factors should be considered: Flow of drugs and other raw materials into the pharmacy; flow of drugs and services from the pharmacy to the inpatient areas and other departments in the hospital; flow of outpatients' traffic through the hospital, and needs for future expansion.

Each hospital must adhere to the accepted norms of designing a good pharmacy and also bear in mind the legal requirements. The pharmacy normally comprises of four areas, viz. dispensing area, manufacturing area, administrative area and storage area.

In the area of drugs and pharmaceuticals, the same products, or equivalents, are generally available directly from a number of manufacturers or dealers. In some instances, a drug is manufactured by one firm, marketed, labelled, and distributed by several distributors or dealers. The pros and cons of purchasing from manufacturers and purchasing from distributors are to be evaluated before coming to a final decision.

Advantages of purchasing from distributors are reflected in the progression of individual distributors to the status of prime vendors. The direct purchase prices charged by manufacturers from pharmacies are frequently lower than those quoted to distributors.

Group purchasing is not very popular in Indian healthcare industry. This is one of the potential sources for obtaining the best value for money, whether it is for small, medium or large hospital.

Borrowing and lending is another source of supply, potential for a loaned supply from another pharmacy. This is a limited source to be used at such times when normal channels are not open, such as on weekends and nights.

Inventory control encompasses the broader objectives of identifying the appropriate purchase quantity; purchase interval, minimum and maximum stock levels. The goal is to ensure product availability when needed at minimal expense.

Drug distribution within a hospital should aim for maintaining optimal control and accountability without compromising on the availability of critical medication to patients. These goals require that the pharmacy make drugs available throughout the hospital using multiple distribution systems.

The floor stock system is the most basic of the drug distribution methods. Floor stocked medication can be replaced either by a requisition from the stocking area to pharmacy or by automatic replacement as soon as the pharmacy receives a patient charge for the item.

Individual patient supply distribution closely parallels traditional prescription dispensing in retail pharmacies. Drug distribution systems progressed from floor stock to individual multi day

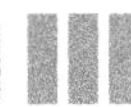

patient supply. This system offers enhanced drug control and accountability since each medication supply is individually labelled and charged to a specific patient. Unit dose drug distribution system is preferred for medications that are ordered and administered routinely. This distribution system addresses some of the shortcomings of floor stock and individual multiple day supply systems.

Intravenous solutions as per the Drug Control Administration are broadly classified into two categories. 1. Sterile admixture services and 2. Drugs defined by the Drug Control Administration as 'controlled substances.' Sterile admixture services encompass preparation of sterile solutions, most typically parenteral (for intravenous administration) and their profiling, distribution, and charge initiation. The distribution of drugs categorized as controlled substances by the Drug Control Administration requires exceptions to normal distribution by the pharmacy because of governmental regulations.

Outpatient prescription services represent a major distribution system in a hospital pharmacy. Outpatient drug distribution essentially involves dispensing multi day supplies of individual medication pursuant to a physician's prescription and the pharmacy's earlier dispensing records. Two concepts of drug equivalency assist the pharmacy in controlling the cost of utilization: 1. generic equivalency and 2. therapeutic equivalency.

Generic equivalency of drug products may be referred to by their chemical names. These names are often long, unwieldy, difficult to pronounce and are therefore frequently altered to a simpler generic term. Generic names may be used by any manufacturer of identical drugs. When the patent expires, other manufacturers have options to seek permissions to market the same generic drug either under their own trade name or the generic name. However regardless of whether or not a trade name is used, all drug products with the same generic name in the same dosage form (e.g. tablet, capsule, suspension) and in the same strength or concentration are generically equivalent.

Therapeutic equivalency is a more subjective concept. Therapeutically equivalent or alternate drugs are not necessarily generically equivalent but elicit a similar response when administered e.g., vitamin products. Therapeutic equivalency may be somewhat subjective.

Drug formularies are defined by a number of terms, such as open, closed, and restricted. These terms are defined differently from one institution to another.

Drug information is the most important and potentially cost effective responsibility of the pharmacy department. Formulary must be readily available to physicians. It is advisable that a copy should be displayed prominently in each patient care area. The provision of drug information, therefore, while normally considered a professional service, is directly related to effective product management in the pharmacy. Standardized formulations are prepared in larger quantities to allow multiple dispensing from a single batch.

Drug utilization review can be accomplished by three methods: retrospective, concurrent, and prospective.

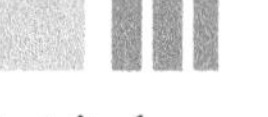

Clinical pharmacy does not embrace the full scope of Materials Management in that it does not include the acquisition and distribution of drugs. However, it does fully cover drug disposition.

Controlling material expenses: The path of drug products through pharmacy's Materials Management involves many of the same decision points that exist in other materials departments.

Pharmacy has dual responsibilities, i.e. providing information about drugs and controlling purchase and distribution of drugs. While MM is focused more on product handling, it also must consider its distributive and informative roles. These two elements can and must mutually coexist.

MM function in pharmacy translates into "management and control of drugs, pharmaceutical services, and pharmacy related equipment from purchase to patient administration or use.

Numerous standards, laws and regulations govern the overall operations of the pharmacy department. They must also be understood by the pharmacy manager and must be compiled with to reduce the hospitals liability, and provide quality pharmaceutical services that meet recognized needs.

In dispensing and distribution systems, many innovative approaches and methods have been introduced in recent years. Traditional pharmacy services are rapidly undergoing a change all over the world. Some of the larger and progressive hospitals would introduce and test these newer systems and be pace setters for other hospitals to follow.

REVIEW QUESTIONS

1. What factors do you take into consideration to locate pharmacy stores in a multispecialty hospital?
2. What are special features of pharmacy procurement?
3. Drug distribution in a hospital aims at maintaining optimum control and accountability-Discuss.
4. What are the facilities required for a good pharmacy practice?
5. Pharmacy has dual responsibilities i.e. providing information about drugs and controlling of purchasingand distribution of drugs. Discuss.
6. Write short notes on

a) Dispensing area	b) Manufacturing area
c) Prime vendor agreements	d) Group purchasing
e) Controlled substances	f) Clinical pharmacy
g) Drug utilisation review	

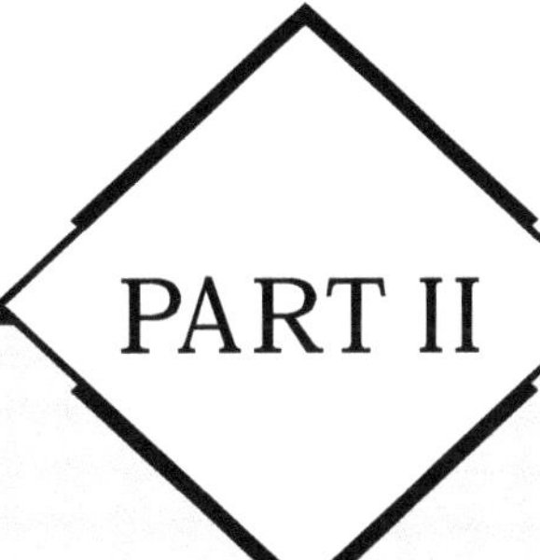
PART II

PART - II

Purchasing Function, Origin, Scope and Objectives

Contents

CHAPTER - 4

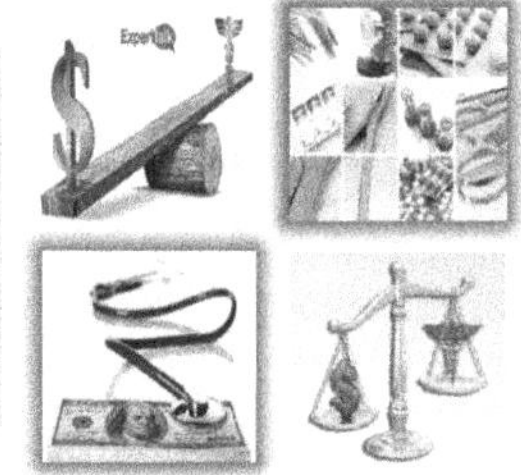

Purchasing Function, Origin, Scope and Objectives

INTRODUCTION

Purchasing is one of the basic functions in any hospital because in any transaction, however primitive, there is always a buyer and a seller. The buyer requires certain goods (materials or services) to satisfy his needs and wants. He seeks a seller who, can and is willing to supply him whatever he needs. Together they negotiate a mutually satisfactory price and the deal is completed. The concept of economic process can be summarized stating that it consists of converting raw materials into goods or services that have a higher commercial value or greater utility for consumer. The difference in costs between the raw materials and the finished products is value addition. In hospitals, the cost element of materials as a percentage of total revenue is between 40 to 45 percent. This means that added value is between 55-60 percent. Materials constitute the largest chunk in creation of value for which the patient is willing to pay a price. It is necessary for the purchaser to exercise utmost prudence in ensuring that best ultimate value is obtained for every rupee spent on materials. **Value for money has to be the principle objective of purchase department.** Today, purchasing is not the same as in yesteryear.

ORIGIN AND GROWTH OF PURCHASING FUNCTION

A large proportion of the total revenue in a hospital comes from sale of medicines. The art of trading materials i.e., the process of buying and selling is nearly as old as man himself. Before the advent of money as medium of exchange, men bartered items, surplus to their requirements for things, which they needed. From the time man discovered that he could put his talents to produce or manufacture things, he began to specialize in whatever was his vocation or distinctive competence since man found it more economical to purchase materials of quality suitable to his needs, at prices, which he considered favourable. Thus, the purchasing function achieved specialization quite early in man's history.

The earliest example of purchase order dates back to 2500 BC. It was on a clay tablet of Babylonian origin. It was meant to supply of fragrant oil to be delivered in lots of fifty jars at fifteen days intervals. Until the turn of the twentieth century, the concept of separate independent function did not exist. In most cases, company owners did their own buying. As the organizations grew larger, the buying jobs were delegated to engineering and manufacturing managers or user departments on the premise that those who specified and used materials knew how best to buy them. The management recognized integrated concept of materials management in which purchasing function plays a pivotal role. **Good purchasing is something more than mere service function called in to perform a more or less clerical task, after important materials decisions were taken elsewhere.** The purchasing management became a profit centre. A saving of 5 - 10 percent in the cost of purchases is equivalent to 2.5 to 5 percent of revenue earned. In contrast, the expenditure on wages, salaries, and other fringe benefits of all employees amount to one third of materials cost or 20 percent of total revenue of a hospital. In service organizations such as hospitals, nursing homes, and various diagnostic and pharmaceutical centres, functioning expenditures usually range between 10 to 35 percent (other than capital equipment).

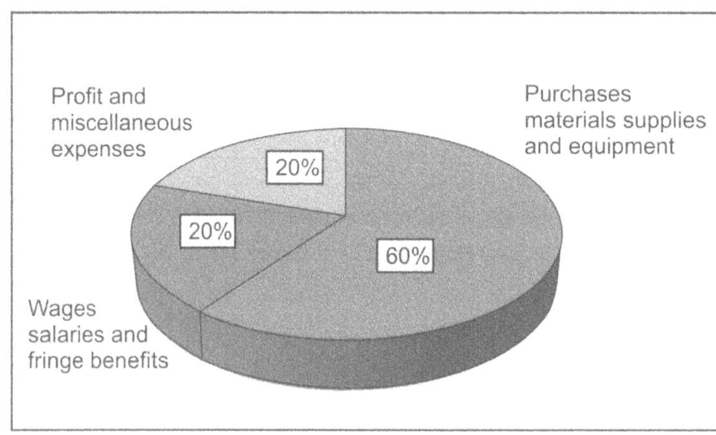

Figure 4.1 How Rupee one revenue is spent by an average hospital

To sum up, **the principle objective of purchasing is not mere procurement of materials or services at lowest price but also to reduce cost of final services to patients,** by reducing cost of materials, finding out substitute materials that are more economical and eliminating elements of costs in purchasing that do not contribute value.

Development of Purchasing Functions in Hospitals

In USA, during 1940's, a typical hospital employed purchasing agents to maintain stores inventory, reorder stock, and keep inventory records. The administrators placed major orders and negotiated large orders. Department heads placed orders directly with salesmen. Thus decentralized purchasing was prevalent in most healthcare institutions. Prices for the same products varied within an area. There was little cooperative or group purchasing. Around the same time, however, hospitals

 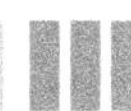

also began to employ purchasing agents comparable to those in industry. Hospital buyers applied the principles of centralized purchasing, negotiation, bidding, inventory control, traffic and transportation, testing, value analysis, and standardization. Initially they were not accepted gracefully by other departmental heads in the institutional hierarchy, and many vendor representatives attempted to go around them to the department heads or administrators. By 1950, there was growing acceptance of the purchasing manager's roles and responsibilities. The first association of hospital purchasing managers was chartered, under the leadership of **Frank Rhatigan** of the Surgical Trade Association and **Dr. Charles Letourneau,** hospital consultant and editor of Hospital Management, as the **National Association of Hospital Purchasing Agents (NAHPA).** One of the first presidents elected in 1957 was **Joseph A. Heeb,** the group purchasing director for the Sisters of St. Joseph Hospitals, Wichita, Kansas. At that time, he was implementing for the first time the concept of group purchasing in programmes nationally. In 1980, the president was another group purchaser **John Vernet,** director of materials management, Yavapai Community Hospital, Prescott, Arizona. The Society for Hospital Purchasing Agents, an affiliate of the American Hospital Association, was chartered in 1963. It is now called the **American Society for Hospital Purchasing and Materials Management (ASHPMM).** The ASHPMM was founded in 1962 in response to numerous requests from hospital administrators and purchasing agents for a professional organization for hospital purchasers. The society had a charter membership of about one hundred; it now has several thousand members worldwide, with affiliated chapters nationwide. The society is one of the fifteen personal membership groups sponsored by the American Hospital Association. Both NAHPA and ASHPMM are active in the professional status and certification of the healthcare material managers, and both sponsor professional training programmes. In India, the corporate hospitals felt the importance of the role played by purchasing during the later half of `1980's but much more needs to be accomplished.

MODERN CONCEPT OF PURCHASING

John H Hill, president, Air Reduction Company, Inc., speaking before National Association of Purchasing Agents, explained the development of purchasing function in the following terms. **"Purchasing was traditionally considered as a service function, a place where money is spent, not made.** Recent developments have shaken this point of view. Good purchasing is essential to good profits. The difference between good purchasing and poor purchasing can be the difference between outstanding results and mediocre performance. Modernized purchasing departments have shown that, skillful procurement can cut 5 to 10 percent from total cost of goods purchased. The fiercely competitive conditions in late 1950's in U.S., spotlighted its unique abilities in cost reduction."

DEFINITIONS OF PURCHASING

Purchasing is an activity responsible for getting the right materials from right source in the right quantity at the right time at the right price. Purchasing, more precisely procurement, can be called as a function responsible for all phases of material cycle from requisition until delivery to user. This includes direct responsibility for selection of vendor, negotiation of price, assurance of quality and delivery. It can also include direct or indirect responsibility for transportation, receiving, inspection and inventory control.

National Institute of Governmental Purchasing Inc. Falls Church Virginia defines purchasing as: "The act and the function responsible for the acquisition of materials, supplies, equipment and services. In a narrow sense, the term describes determining the need, selection of supplier; arriving at a fair and reasonable price, and terms, preparing the contract or purchase order and following up to ensure timely delivery."

Peter Bailey and David Farm state in their book entitled "Managing Materials in industry": "Purchasing means procuring goods and services from outside organizations in return for a price." While price paid is important, what is more important is obtaining value for money. What we have to assess is the cost of goods or services taking into account quality, quantity, source, time and price.

SPECIAL FEATURES OF HOSPITAL PURCHASING

Hospital purchasing is highly specialized and refined activity. Modern healthcare institutions on an average spend almost half of their revenue income on materials, goods and services. The procurement of inputs from other organizations is assigned to specialists who have authority to select suppliers and commit company's funds. Purchasing responsibility has direct effect on financial and competitive position. The buyer in addition to investing money prudently must satisfy the demands of operating departments. Thus the best price he constantly seeks, involves much more than the selection of lowest offer.

In selecting the suppliers and negotiating the price, a buyer must also be certain that what he buys will:

- Meet specifications and quality standards
- Ensure all inputs arrive on time to meet schedules
- Stock sufficient quantity to meet demands of doctors and patients and other Paramedical staff without incurring excessive inventory carrying expenses or stock-outs
- Ensure that the supplier gives prompt and adequate service.

Hospital purchases can range from simple to highly complex items. The buying of an intricate electronic subassembly for Magnetic Resonance Imaging (MRI) equipment obviously poses a greater problem than buying of a stethoscope. The electronic unit involves advanced engineering and exotic materials. Nothing like it may have been ever used before in that hospital. Neither the buyer nor the medical specialist has real cost data to rely on in negotiating price. On the other hand, a stethoscope is a standard product.

Every principle of good purchasing applies to purchases made for healthcare institutions. Good purchasing follows the same guidelines for hospitals run by corporations, government, and charitable institutions.

 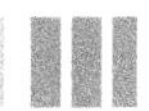

- Hospitals deal with a very broad spectrum of materials and services. Challenging specifications, therefore, is especially important and fruitful.
- A doctor's knowledge of his field does not entail knowledge of economics and market availability of the equipment and supplies needed to conduct teaching and research.
- When it comes to the purchase of unique capital equipment, the situation can be different. Here, the purchase manager, by working with the doctor knowledgeably can save his time and needless worry, as well as save the hospital's money.
- Ethics in medical purchasing is probably more critical than in industry. This is especially true because of increasing interrelationships, among businesses, government and healthcare institutions.
- Controlling salesmen and their attempts at back door selling is frequently more difficult in healthcare institutions than it is in manufacturing or retailing.
- In theory, reciprocity should be easier to control in hospitals than it is in industry. In practice, however, this is often not the case.
- Trustees, donors on occasions, bring great pressure on healthcare institutions for purchases of their companies' products. Normally, such purchases, if made on any basis other than quality, service, and price should be resisted as being an expense, rather than a benefit.
- Healthcare Institutions frequently place their purchasing departments too low in the management structure. This is one of the primary reasons why hospitals have lagged in attracting top purchasing talent.
- It is also a paramount reason why their purchasing accomplishments to this point have lagged behind industry, government, and other non healthcare institutions.
- A purchasing manager is constrained in carrying out top management's desire for good purchasing principles if he himself is not a member of top management.
- Effective centralization of the purchasing function is virtually impossible when the purchasing department is not high in the management hierarchical structure.
- Hospitals have tended to lag behind industry and government in recruiting the most competent purchasing personnel.
- Healthcare institutional salaries historically have been lower than industrial salaries. Fortunately, this situation is now changing and some purchasing professionals are beginning to migrate from industry to healthcare institutions.
- The purchasing operations of a large healthcare institution call for highly competent materials managers. What is required here is the proper perspective based on review of the classification of procurements found in typical large hospitals.

- Healthcare Institutions have the same two reasons for carrying items in stores as industry i.e., economy and service.
- To prevent loss of life, hospitals must have immediate access to reserves of certain materials. These reserves, however, do not have to be stored in the hospital itself. They can be stored in the vendor's storeroom. This concept treats the vendor as being an extension of the hospital's stores system.
- Many healthcare institutions do not have a traffic specialist and this can be a mistake. The salary for a traffic specialist is only slightly more than that for a traffic clerk, which all institutions must have.
- Many institutions tend to run an unreasonably expensive delivery system, with daily delivery service being provided.

It is estimated that in the next few years, the nation's medical bill will exceed Rs. 5000 billion. The purchasing budget for materials and services, hospitals will then probably exceed Rs. 2000 billion. To help restrain rising hospital bills and to get the optimum results, it is desirable, if not imperative, that this large sum of money be spent competently.

OBJECTIVES AND SCOPE OF PURCHASING

The standard objectives of purchasing department can be summarized as acquisition of materials or supplies of the right quality in right quantity and at a right time from a right source for a right price. **These five rights have connotation and implication far beyond their dictionary meanings.** (These five R's are discussed in detail in chapter no.7)

To state it more generally, the main objectives of purchasing are:

- Maintaining continuity, in respect of supply of materials to support hospital's operations and schedules of the planned activities.
- Accomplishing the above objective with minimum investment consistent with safety and economic advantage.
- Avoiding duplication, waste and obsolescence with respect to materials.
- Maintaining standards in quality of materials based on suitability for use.
- Developing good and reliable suppliers and ensuring satisfactory vendor relationships.
- Procuring materials at the lowest cost consistent with quality and timeliness. Benefits of efficient purchasing can accrue to an organization in terms of economical sourcing and greater value for money spent.
- Maintaining the hospital's competitive position by controlling costs relating to materials and thereby maximizing profits. A non profit organization like government or charitable hospital

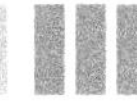

cannot of course maximize profits but saving in purchasing can help to increase service level for the same budgetary provision.

In all the above mentioned activities, reduction of costs becomes the foremost goal of purchasing.

FUNCTIONS OF PURCHASING

Today's purchase manager has to acquire both professional knowledge and professional skills. Purchasing involves the activity directed towards securing materials, supplies, equipment and services required in the operation of a hospital. **The activity has to be performed with optimum efficiency, economy and effectiveness.** These three key factors are for obtaining excellence in material performance. Purchasing is a much broader concept than buying and covers a wide range of managerial functions right from participation in corporate planning and policy to product improvement, working capital management and profit improvement. The functions of purchasing are broadly classified into primary and secondary functions and they are discussed in the following paragraphs.

Primary Functions of Purchasing

Effective hospital purchasing organization eliminates friction, duplication of effort, and non-coverage by clearly demarcating responsibilities and authority.

The following are some of primary functions of purchasing.

Procurement: The identification and quantification of all hospital related purchases is the first step required in the process to determine purchasing duties and to assess the overall department workload.

Procedures and job analysis : The development of understandable and workable procedures that identify job responsibilities and duties by commodity and function is necessary to avoid duplication and possible gaps in coverage. Formal procedures covering purchasing performed by individuals outside the formal purchasing department provide for standardizing the efforts and activities.

Cost management Cost management includes the following activities:

- Establishment of programme that regularly analyzes purchase requirements, and suppliers to identify lowest total cost and maximize total value to the hospital. The development of a savings forecast is necessary to define budget parameters.
- Establishment of the purchasing cost concept. All materials' costs going into a complete patient care are tracked and managed by one purchasing professional, as opposed to having several buyers responsible for different items.
- Establishment of overall and individual cost saving targets and goals.
- Measurement and documentation of the results and progress of cost reduction and containment.

Supply Management

In supply management, purchasing department must:

- Conduct periodic purchase item reviews to assess and identify any item considered to be a risk or vulnerable in relationship to supply or cost.
- Identify single source or sole source supply conditions that may require a secondary source supplier development programme.

Planning

Materials manager of a hospital needs to sell his programme to administration, nursing, pharmacy, laboratories and other departments. This requires a plan. The planning function requires purchasing to:

- Plan near and long term programmes compatible with major hospital objectives and policies seeking advice and counsel of immediate superiors as necessary.
- Keep immediate superiors informed of major plans and programmes and of the progress and the problems of operations for which they are responsible.
- Develop a portfolio of cost saving projects that generate a constant source of activity to contribute to the profitability.

Organization

Organizational duties include the following:

- Maintaining a sound plan of organization, which matches the purchasing business plan, and overall patient care objectives and values.
- Maintaining and updating the purchasing succession plan, which identifies key critical backup personnel and organizational gaps.
- Ensuring that competent employees are available at all times and training programmes are available to support continuous development of new skills.

Personnel

Personnel management requires that the purchasing department:

- Establish qualitative and quantitative performance goals and targets in the area of cost, quality, and service.
- Regularly appraise the performance of immediate subordinates, measuring such performance against established goals and objectives.

Operations

Operations related tasks include the following responsibilities:

- Through proper collaboration, direction, control, coordination, and delegation, implement approved department and hospital policies, plans and programmes.

 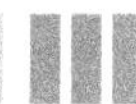

- Establish linkages with appropriate internal functions that must provide support to achieve purchasing goals and targets.
- Review progress against approved programmes and provide constant feedback to departments and individuals against current performance.

Secondary Functions of Purchasing

In addition to primary functions, a purchasing department in a hospital would have several harmonizing activities to share with other departments. **Some of the important ones are as follows:**

- Establishing and maintaining a good professional rapport with the medical staff, administration, nurses, employees of patient care areas, and staff of all other hospital departments.
- Establishing departmental policies and procedures in accordance with hospital policies.
- Assisting the director materials in the annual departmental budget preparation and assuring adherence on a monthly basis.
- Establishing in conjunction with the director realistic and obtainable goals for purchase department on an annual basis.
- Submitting monthly reports to the chief of materials management concerning the functional, budgetary, and administrative phases of the department.
- Performing the appropriate committee functions as assigned, from time to time.
- Developing and distributing information on supplies, drugs, and equipment to all members of the medical staff and all other related hospital personnel.
- Evaluating the effectiveness of services available to various supply consumers from materials management.
- Performing other related tasks as may be deemed necessary for an effective and efficient function of the department.
- Working with engineering standards and cost improvement groups.
- Establishing and developing specification for materials. (The main objective is to ensure just the right quality, neither too high nor too low, both of which increase costs and reduce profitability).
- Accounting of materials purchased including payment to suppliers.
- Inventory control.
- Construction contracts or service contracts and agreements.
- Disposals of surplus obsolete and scrap materials.

- To determine whether to make in one's own hospital or buy them from outside.
- Advising concerned departments of any changes in price or procedure and of restrictions imposed on materials, which would prohibit purchase. Keeping interested departments advised with respect to lead time required for critical materials.

RESPONSIBILITIES OF PURCHASING

Following is list of responsibilities of purchasing department in healthcare institutions, some of which are entirely its own and some of which share with other departments.

Exclusive responsibilities of purchase department

- Maintain good image of the hospital and supplier relations through daily business contacts with patients.
- Supervision of the supply, process, and distribution functions.
- Specifying mode of transport and delivery. Transportation of materials including clearing of goods from transporters and customs authorities in case of imports.
- Conducting daily purchasing rounds of the nursing units to check with head nurses regarding concerns involving the cart and supply systems.
- Reviewing daily special requisitions with appropriate management representative.
- Assuming responsibility for the quarterly physical inventories of all official and unofficial supply areas.
- Interviewing sales representatives promptly and courteously and keeping current on supply publications and price changes.
- Establishing and maintaining the proper and appropriate professional and ethical relationships with all sales representatives.
- Evaluating supply, process, and distribution supervisor and the receiving clerk annually.
- Negotiating prime supplier contracts with major suppliers and distributors of the hospital.
- Conducting the business affairs of the purchasing department prudently.
- Supporting and participating in group purchasing and shared services efforts with other hospitals and related healthcare facilities.
- Searching continuously for improved and/or less costly materials and supplies within the classification assigned.
- Selecting and maintaining sources of supply, using progressive purchasing techniques and methods.

 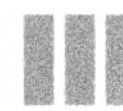

- Visiting supplier plants to analyze facilities and capabilities before enlisting them as approved vendors.
- Completing each requisition by selecting the supplier, setting the proper price, and studying the terms, free on board (FOB) point, and other buying considerations and advice when and in what quantities materials should be purchased to meet market conditions in healthcare industry.
- Expediting deliveries and, where necessary, getting the required approvals for alternative materials if delivery is not available when required.
- Scheduling orders on suppliers and fixing delivery dates.
- Corresponding tactfully with sources or potential sources of supply to overcome misunderstandings, complaints, etc., or to secure further pertinent information regarding purchased material.
- Reviewing invoices as required referred for approval by the invoice audit department, particularly where price or other items do not tally with the purchase order.
- Negotiating supplier rejections and advising suppliers of reasons for rejections and costs incurred as a result of defective material.
- Approving expense orders charged to defective purchased materials and negotiating settlements with suppliers.
- Issue debit notes to suppliers on charges resulting form returned materials and labour performed.
- Issuing credit notes under circumstances that require cancellation of debits or wherever adjustments are necessary to settle disputes.
- Supervising the maintenance of current and potential sources of information in connection with materials under their jurisdiction.
- Using good judgement in consulting with superiors about all materials in which the proper application of organizational hospital policy is uncertain.
- Performing miscellaneous assignments as required from time to time.

Responsibilities Shared with other Departments

- Obtaining technical information and advice on supplies.
- Establishing and developing specifications for materials. The main objective is to ensure that quality is just right not too high or not too low, both of which will have an impact on costs and profitability.
- Scheduling orders for materials on suppliers and setting up delivery dates for supply of materials.
- Specifying modes of delivery and transportation.

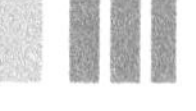

- Receive and inspect materials received and ensure that the specifications laid down have been compiled with.
- Accounting of materials purchased, including coordination with bills payment department for settlement of payments to suppliers.
- Control of inventory both physical and controls
- Receiving, store keeping and warehousing
- Coordinating construction contracts or service contracts and agreements
- Disposal of scrap and surplus materials and salvaging
- Transportation of materials including clearing of goods
- Determining whether to make or buy (i.e., make the item in one's own hospital or buy them from outside)

ROLE OF PURCHASING VIS-À-VIS CUSTOMERS AND SUPPLIERS

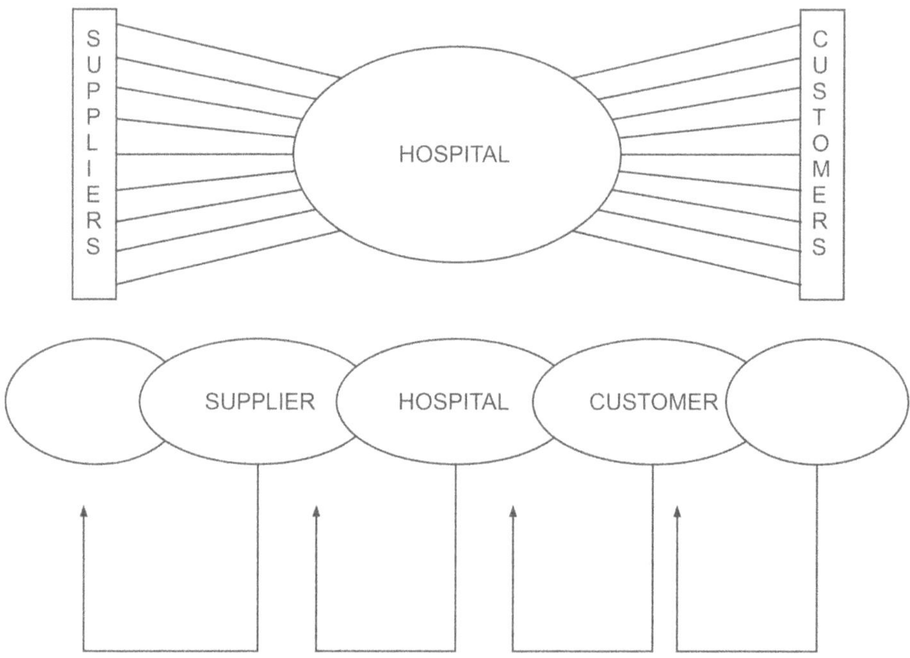

Figure 4.2 The Supplier-Customer Perspective of Supply

Source: The figure is modified version from the book "Value Driven Purchasing" of NAPM

Customer goodwill is a major organizational asset for a hospital. The supply chain can also be seen as equivalent to a typical input-transformation-output system. The inputs influence both the transformation process and the output and vice versa. Many healthcare institutions are starting to

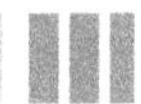

recognize that supplier goodwill is also a key asset. In order to achieve international accomplishment and competitiveness, hospitals must deal with their customers, their own employees, and their suppliers in a congruent and effective way. **By definition, every organization plays three major roles in the supply chain. The first is as a customer to some supplying organization. The second is as a transformer of the input; and the third is as a supplier to a customer.** This normally involves more than just three organizational entities because each organization in the chain continues to have customers and suppliers. For hospital services, the patient is identified as the "end customer," implying an end to the supply chain. If one views any hospital as located between customers on the one hand and suppliers on the other (see Figure 4.2), it is not difficult to see that this is a continuous change of organizations. Each hospital places demands on its suppliers that are appropriate to meet its or his aspirations in terms of customer satisfaction i.e., patients' care (see Figure 4.3).

Within each hospital, a similar pattern may exist as information, materials, products, or services are passed from one department to another. The term internal customer is often used to distinguish them from external customers. The additional notion has been that the supply function provides for the needs of such internal customers too. However, there is a growing concern that focusing exclusively on internal customers may not be in the best interest of external customers.

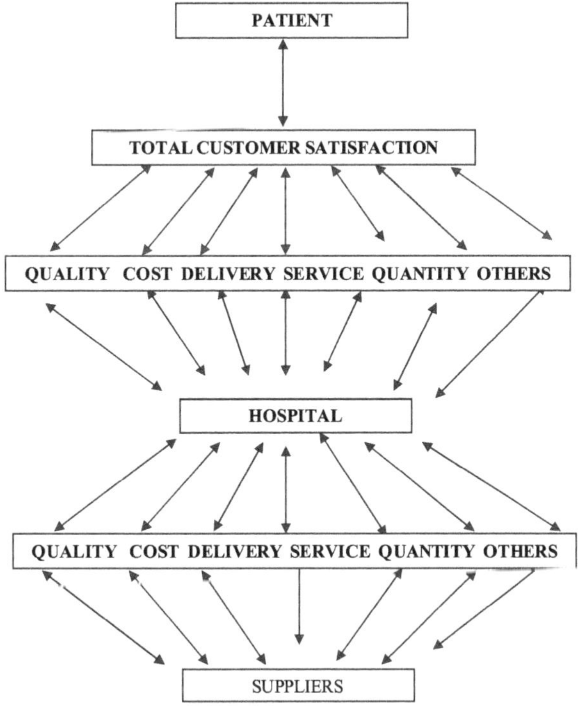

Figure 4.3 Total Patient Care Satisfaction Depends on Supplier Performance

Source: The figure is modified version from the book "Value driven Purchasing" of NAPM

COST SAVINGS IN PURCHASING

It is important that purchasers recognize the difference between cost savings and cost avoidance in order to understand and explain the results of any given cost study. Failure to recognize these important points can result in poor information input into the decision-making process and could, ultimately, cause increased, unnecessary expenditures. Cost avoidance results when available, underutilized resources are used instead of new or additional resources acquired. A cost avoidance also results when the wants and needs for a product are clarified and the wants (nice to have) features are eliminated. For instance, assigning expediting duties to an existing employee rather than hiring another individual to accomplish the expediting function is cost avoidance. A cost saving, results when the monies that would normally be spent are reduced. A saving in labour costs occurs only when a position is eliminated from the budget. Improved efficiency resulting from a technological change without a budget reduction is not a saving. There must be an actual reduction in available budgeted hours to achieve labour savings. It is also important that any labour saving achieved be just that, a saving. There are also many ways to contain costs through effective purchase management. Purchase function can be a major contributor to the cost containment efforts of today's hospitals. It has a large human resources component, enormous paper trail, complex systems, inventories, and sometimes duplications. **The methods for cost containment are as follows:**

- Reducing official and unofficial inventory.
- Amalgamating supply process and distribution functions.
- Eliminating excess staff.
- Stockless purchasing.
- Product standardization.
- Buying items locally as for as possible.
- Indirect or wholesale purchasing.
- Obtaining materials at lower prices through developing new competent sources of supply.
- Market research (It indicates when to buy in a situation of uncertainty, where to buy and how much to buy etc.)
- Price negotiations with vendors.
- Using modern techniques like: cost and price analysis, to determine reasonable price for a material.
- Managing taxes payable: This area has a large scope and is unfortunately a much neglected subject.
- Reducing cost of packaging: Many hospitals incur unnecessary expenditure because they do not have proper idea of what kind of packaging is necessary. The first question that may be asked is whether packaging is necessary at all.

- Optimizing the transportation costs. This calls for proper study of market conditions and selecting the best means of transport.
- Determining whether quality of materials is right (if not, a large quantum of wastes can arise because of scrap).
- Value analysis.

SUMMARY

In any commercial transaction however primitive, there is always a buyer and a seller. Every economic process consists of converting materials into goods that have a higher commercial value or greater utility for consumer. The cost of materials in final price ranges between 50 to 60 percent. This means that added value is between 40-50 percent. The difference between costs of material inputs and the final price is called value addition. Purchased materials consume over half of the average manufacturing firm's sales revenue. Consequently, the profit potential of effective management of purchasing and supply activities is enormous when compounded with other practical management alternatives. An objective analysis of potential importance of hospital purchasing function in management functions shows that purchasing is an essential business function, which should make the same level of contribution to a hospital's success as other major business functions. Suppliers are essentially an extension of buyer's operations. As such it is the responsibility of purchasing to ensure that the innovativeness and quality of materials and services provided by these external organizations are fully compatible with the requirements of the purchasing firm. Purchasing also occupies a pivotal function in a hospital's information and decision making systems. It is a key linkage, along with marketing between service providers and ultimate customers. Over the years, the purchasing function has become more complex, more professional and more encompassing evolving into procurement and now into supply management. The focus is shifting from tactical to strategic.

It is necessary for the purchaser to exercise utmost prudence in ensuring that best ultimate value is obtained for every rupee spent on materials. Value for money has to be the objective of purchasing department.

As the organizations grew larger, the buying jobs were delegated to engineering and manufacturing managers on the premise that those who specified and used materials know how best to buy them.

Hospital purchasing is highly specialized and refined activity. Modern healthcare institutions on an average spend almost half of their revenue income on materials, goods and services. Hospital purchases can range from simple to highly complex items. Say stethoscope to Magnetic Resonance Imaging (MRI) equipment. The electronic unit involves advanced engineering and exotic materials. Neither the buyer nor the medical specialist has real cost data to rely on in negotiating price. On the other hand, a stethoscope is a simple standard product.

The principle objective of purchasing is not mere procurement of materials at lowest price but also to reduce cost of patient service, by reducing cost of materials. Good purchasing is essential to good profits. The difference from good purchasing and poor purchasing can be difference between outstanding results and mediocre performance. Skillful procurement can cut 5 to 10 percent from total cost of goods purchased. Purchasing is an activity responsible for getting the right materials from right source in the right quantity at the right time at the right price. Purchasing has direct effect on financial and competitive position.

The best price that one constantly seeks involves much more than the selection of lowest offer. While selecting the supplier and negotiating the price, a buyer must ensure that what he buys meets specifications, arrives in the hospital in time, sufficient quantity is stocked and that the supplier renders prompt and adequate service.

Effective organization eliminates friction, duplication of effort, and non-coverage by demarcating responsibilities and authority. Purchasing performs several line and staff functions. Every hospital is part of a value chain in which it procures products and services from vendors, transforms the same into patient service and markets that service. Cost savings in purchasing are possible by developing alternative sources, conducting market researches, price negotiations with vendors, managing taxes payable, etc.

The functions of purchasing department in hospital are either entirely its own, or shared with other departments. Purchasing activities cut across all departmental lines and consequently the function is a hub of much of hospital's business activity.

Customer goodwill is a major organizational asset for a hospital. The hospital operations can also be seen as equivalent to a typical input transformation output system. The inputs influence both the transformation process and the output and vice versa. In order to achieve international accomplishment and competitiveness, hospitals must deal with their customers, their own employees, and their suppliers in a congruent and effective way.

It is important that purchasers recognize the difference between cost savings and cost avoidance. Failure to recognize these important points, ultimately cause increased, unnecessary expenditures. Cost avoidance results when available, underutilized resources are used instead of new or additional resources acquired.

REVIEW QUESTIONS

1. Discuss special features of hospital purchasing.
2. Explain objectives and scope of purchasing in healthcare industry.
3. Every principle of good purchasing in manufacturing industry applies to healthcare institutions also - discuss.

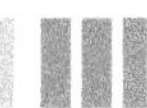

4. What is the role of purchasing in hospital customer satisfaction? Elaborate your answer with suitable examples.
5. What are the objectives and functions of purchase management?
6. What are the responsibilities of purchasing department and why should one maintain good relationships with other departments?
7. Write short notes on
   a) Modern concept of purchasing
   b) Cost management
   c) Primary responsibilities of purchase department
   d) Secondary responsibilities of purchase department
   e) Customer satisfaction the role of buyer in healthcare industry
   f) Supply management
   g) Cost control and cost avoidance

PART - II

Organization for Purchasing Function

Contents

- *Introduction*
- *Basic Concept of Organization*
- *Organization Structure*
- *Responsibilities, Authority and Accountability*
- *Centralized Versus Decentralized Purchasing*
- *Centralization Versus Decentralization in Terms of Supply Management*
- *Part Centralization and Part Decentralization*
- *Summary*
- *Review Questions*

CHAPTER - 5

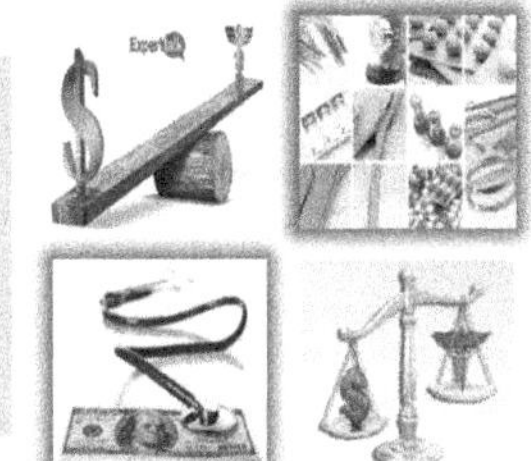

Organization for Purchasing Function

INTRODUCTION

Purchasing department is normally considered a service or staff department. As a service department, purchasing must demonstrate that it is a value adding contributor to hospital profitability. If purchasing does not add value in executing its responsibilities, the department would be a liability and not an asset. Value adding purchasing is accomplished by acquiring the highest quality materials, at the lowest possible total cost, delivered to the ultimate consumer (internal or external), when needed. If this is achieved, the organization can be said to be competitive. The basic objective in the organization of purchasing should be a structure that facilities the motivation of purchasing personnel and coordinates their professional efforts towards the goals of the business. The structure should not get in the way of the various other departmental heads' approaches to their strategies but rather should integrate purchasing into their strategies harmoniously. Very few hospitals have adopted identical organizational structures for purchasing. The purchasing structure usually represents a compromise designed to accommodate the hospital environment and the various operating problems. The purchasing organization usually is tailored to a particular situation, and the imprint of the personalities within the business is evident in organization design. Market environment is one of the greatest single influences in shaping the final organizational design. Organizational structure must adapt to the changing business needs and the market place environment. The organizational design process is dynamic, and management must make numerous trade offs. The choice of an organizational structure should evolve from a thoughtful study of the various factors within and outside the hospital that must be addressed in the application of purchasing management skills. **Organization of purchasing departments refers to its structure and allocation to various officers, inter relationship with other departments, delegation of powers and the process of coordination between various functionaries.**

BASIC CONCEPT OF ORGANIZATION

The basic concepts of organizing include the following:

- Organization principles are guidelines that make organizational structure workable.
- Organizational structure is a framework of relationships between various parts of the organization.

- A Healthcare is a group of people working together, under the direction of a leader, to enact certain plans.
- Organizing is the work of providing, in advance, those things needed to carry out a plan. It is the process of assessing the requisite organizational activities, designing tasks, grouping tasks in manageable units and establishing the relationships between tasks and groups of tasks.

ORGANIZATION STRUCTURE

When the job to be done is known and the factors in the environment have been identified, the purchasing organization should be fitted to the job to be done. Thus,

- Functionally, a healthcare organization, if it is to be flexible, quick to react to change, and competitive, it must be dynamic with emphasis on the job to be done.
- Simplicity should be the goal in setting up the organization, in writing procedures for its operation, and in making contract with others within and outside the company.
- Regardless of the size of the purchasing department, its work force, or the value of its purchases, the corporate results are required to be achieved.
- The goal of optimum purchase is the same, although the manner of achievement will vary depending upon the size of the department and the type of products purchased.
- The buying job is so basic that the procedures and policies developed at great expense by large organizations are usually available and adaptable at least in part, to the smallest company.

Purchasing departments in larger hospitals may be partially self sustaining for many services, such as maintenance, inspection, and records, whereas smaller purchasing departments must secure those services from other departments or individuals. Naturally, the smaller the hospital, the more versatile its personnel must be to successfully combine functions that are the responsibilities of individual specialists, or in some cases even of sections or departments, in the larger hospitals.

Single location hospital

Purchasing department in the basic single location hospital is the foundation of practically all purchasing departments, regardless of the type and size of the hospital, the types of services offered, or the geographical spread of the hospital facilities.

An organization chart for this type of department is shown in Figure 5.1.

- Primary responsibility of the purchasing department is to fill the company's requirements for materials, supplies, and services.
- Red tape and procedural complexity should be kept to the minimum required for orderly buying procedures and adequate control of money spent by the function.
- The responsibilities and duties of the various members of the department will remain essentially the same as it grows. With diversification and/or expansion, organizational modification,

enlarged expertise, and specifications that evolve in a dynamic organization may become necessary.

Expansion and contraction should be possible without disrupting the basic structure of the organization. There should be a capability to withstand boom or depression.

- A good basic purchasing organization has a measure of flexibility, but even with forward planning, there may come a time when the department should be reorganized to meet changing conditions.
- Evolutionary changes occurring frequently in the department are preferable to radical change long due.

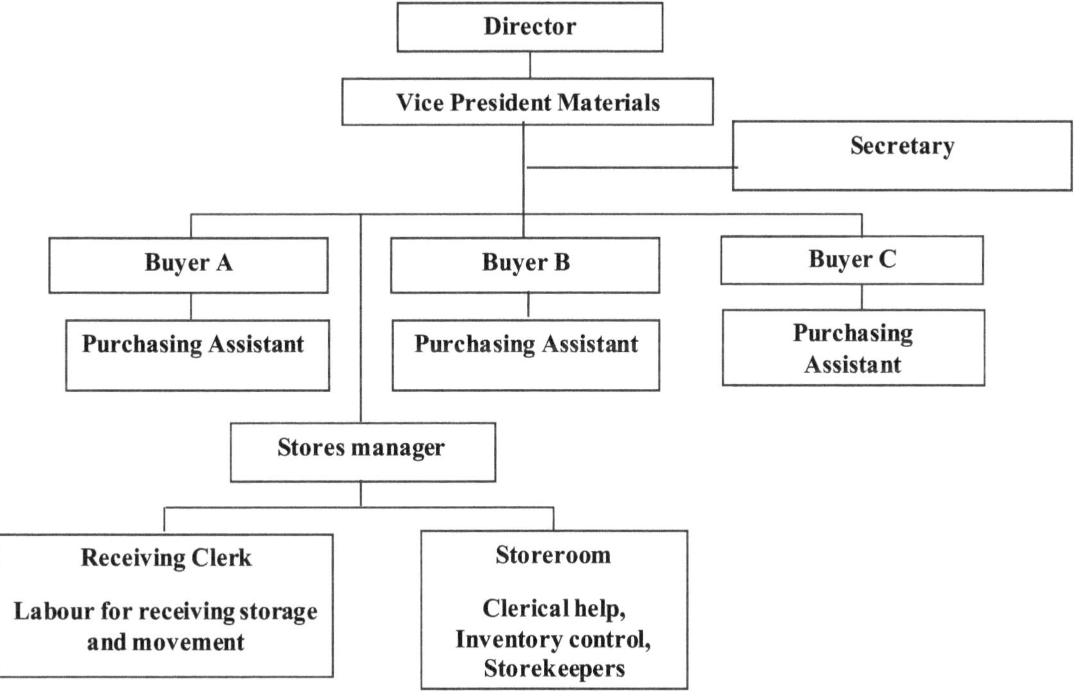

Figure 5.1 Purchasing department for a single location hospital

Small hospital typically will require significant flexibility among all members of the organization. Often the owner of hospital/ chief executive will handle the major expenditures and assign the remaining purchasing responsibilities to a single individual. This individual, whom we may call the purchasing manager, may have a secretary or an all purpose assistant to perform clerical duties as well as place orders for repetitive purchases or for orders where the sourcing may be further sub delegated.

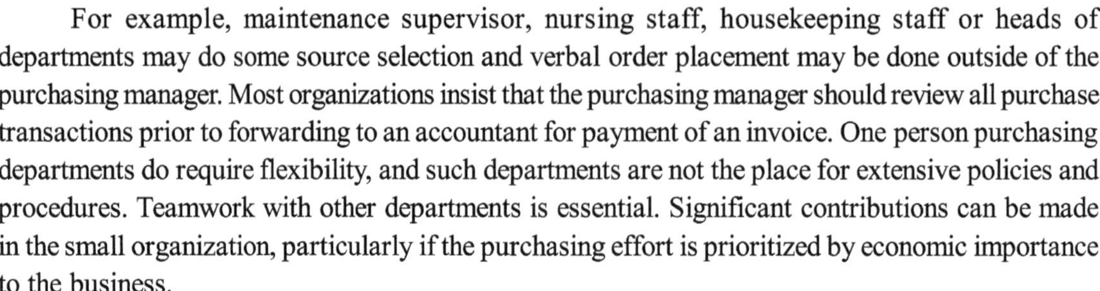

For example, maintenance supervisor, nursing staff, housekeeping staff or heads of departments may do some source selection and verbal order placement may be done outside of the purchasing manager. Most organizations insist that the purchasing manager should review all purchase transactions prior to forwarding to an accountant for payment of an invoice. One person purchasing departments do require flexibility, and such departments are not the place for extensive policies and procedures. Teamwork with other departments is essential. Significant contributions can be made in the small organization, particularly if the purchasing effort is prioritized by economic importance to the business.

RESPONSIBILITIES, AUTHORITY AND ACCOUNTABILITY

Authority for the purchasing function is delegated to purchasing department. Purchasing encompasses those disciplines, which purchase or otherwise obligate the company to a fiduciary responsibility.

Authority is the formal right to require action of others or to act oneself on behalf of the company.

Responsibility means the accountability for the performance of duties.

Functional authority is the explicit right to require the necessary action of others or to act oneself to ensure that the function will be performed.

The purchasing department must be given functional authority; this responsibility and authority is normally part of the company's official policies and procedures governing the purchase of materials.

Major purchasing objective is to keep the operations going. Key to accomplishing this objective is to ensure there are enough materials on hand, without too many inventories to drain the cash flow and working leverage of the hospital's assets.

- A careful balancing is needed between the right mix of materials at the right level of inventory to minimize the carrying cost of inventory.
- All inventory costs money to carry. Too much inventory, or wrong mix of materials, is costly.
- Purchasing should not be viewed as spending the hospital's monetary resources but rather as an investor of the hospital's resources. Purchasing mission is to invest the hospital's resources for maximum returns.
- The key to successful investment of the hospital's resources is the combining of disciplines into a cohesive, decision making group commodity management.
- Purchasing management is the managing of the acquisition and strategic direction of materials and services, globally, to achieve the best quality and delivery at the lowest total cost.

CENTRALIZED VERSUS DECENTRALIZED PURCHASING

Centralized Structure

Completely centralized purchases are best suitable for a single location hospital e.g., Nizam's Institute of Medical Sciences, Hyderabad. Certain multi-location hospitals also practice the same concept of centralized purchasing to economize on the cost of materials and inventory cost e.g., one corporate hospital, located at three different places in Hyderabad; however purchases are centralized at one of the three units.

- A centralized management structure adheres to the example set in the military. Decision making is centralized under a single authority.
- The structure forms a hierarchical, multi-layered chain of command, and decisions tend to be made at higher levels in the organization.
- Centralization necessarily implies that similar functions are handled in one location.

Highly centralized organizations usually have a number of levels of management between top management and the line buyers.

Some of the advantages and disadvantages of a centralized management structure are listed below.

Advantages

1. Decisions are made by purchasing managers who have a broad view of the whole organization.
2. Decision makers at higher levels are usually better educated and better trained than lower management.
3. Eliminates duplication of efforts in cost saving measures.
4. There is a greater chance for specialization, leading to better skills.
5. Decisions are more consistent throughout the organization.

Disadvantages

1. Decisions are made by managers who have a narrow focus.
2. Decision makers at the top rarely deal directly with the buyers who must carry out the decision.
3. Long lines of communication cause long delays.
4. Lower level managers are often frustrated because they are far removed from the decision-making process.
5. Since more people are involved in communication, there is greater chance for error, additionally; personal bias and politics enter the picture.

Decentralized Structure

Decentralized operations are necessary for hospitals geographically located in different parts of the country e.g., Apollo group of Hospitals. Each hospital is responsible for its own purchases in a decentralized manner.

- In a decentralized organization, decision-making power is assigned to individual operating units.
- Decentralized organizations usually have fewer levels of management hierarchy. The decentralization of a centralized organization is accomplished first by removing some levels of management and then by delegating increased authority and responsibility to the remaining managers.
- In general, decentralization stems from the management philosophy that decisions should be made at the lowest level possible.

Choice of a centralized or decentralized purchasing organization, or combination of the two types, should be based on ultimate rather than temporary benefits, and should consider all relevant facts and unusual conditions.

Major functions to be considered are:

- Organizational pattern of the hospital, i.e., multiple units or profit centres, functionally organized or highly centralized.
- Similarity of services provided in the hospitals.
- Impact of profit leverage of purchases on corporate hospital performance.
- Managerial attention required or desired for the purchasing function.
- Geographical distribution of the hospitals.
- Overall size of the organization and the volume of purchases in total and by major commodity or product categories.

Advantages of Decentralization

1. Decisions are faster.
2. The decisions are made by a manager who has the most information about the situation.
3. Higher morale and motivation among first line and middle managers results from their increased involvement in decision making processes.
4. This structure provides good hands on training for first line and middle managers.

Disadvantages of Decentralization

1. There could be lack of information and coordination between departments.
2. Cost per manager is greater because better trained, better educated, & higher paid managers are required at lower levels.
3. Managers tend to have a narrow viewpoint and might be more interested in success of their own departments than of the hospital.
4. Policies and procedures vary widely throughout the organization.

In the final analysis, the best organizational structure synthesizes the benefits of both centralization and decentralization by combining the advantages of having some form of purchasing decisions made at the location of the requirements, with the advantages of volume buying which come from handling common requirements, on a centralized, aggregate basis. The structure that a hospital actually chooses may depend on top management philosophy, the caliber of lower management, the nature of the business, or other factors.

In a study conducted by, **Centre for Advance Purchasing Studies (CAPS)** in USA it was found that

- 59 percent of the responding organizations used some combination of a centralized-decentralized organization.
- 28 percent had adopted a centralized purchasing structure.
- Only 13 percent were oriented in a decentralized fashion.

CENTRALIZATION VERSUS DECENTRALIZATION IN TERMS OF SUPPLY MANAGEMENT

Totally decentralized purchasing would entirely eliminate the purchasing department. All departments would do their own buying. In a totally centralized purchasing department, everything is bought at one location by one purchasing department. Neither of these represents the usual case though many small organizations have no purchasing department. Centralization versus decentralization is concerned with the degree to which attempts are made to consolidate activities at higher levels of the organization. In particular, this is the extent to which the procurement activities are organized to consolidate requirements and combine orders. In the scheduling of work, Japanese hospitals often stress local responsibility. The traditional western approach requires centralized procurement. Frequently, an effort to centralize all procurement, in order to leverage economies of scale in the marketplace and short term schedules, typifies western procurement. At the other end of the spectrum, integrated product teams make centralization versus decentralization decisions based on Total Systems Cost. In practice, virtually every organization answers this question differently. Some centralize the activity almost completely, doing the buying for all sites at a central headquarters office. Others decentralize the function entirely, giving each hospital full authority to conduct all its purchasing activities. Majority of organizations, however, operate somewhere between these two extremes. Each approach offers significant benefits, which are discussed in the following sections.

Centralization is often used for one or all of the following reasons:

- Budget allocation for materials is a very high percentage of total product cost or budget.
- Centralized items are used by the majority of the operating units.
- Management feels the need for tight control on purchases and choose
- To place the authority and responsibility into one central group, which often also assumes the responsibility for developing purchasing policies and control measures too.

Centralization of purchasing in a multi location hospital that does all or most of its buying in one location has the advantages described below.

Communication with suppliers: A central buying group becomes the spokesperson for the organization with its suppliers, thereby making it easier for both buyer and seller to make known their objectives and work together efficiently.

Buying clout: Centralized purchasing permits consolidation of requirements for all operating units. It usually leads to lower prices for goods and services. Sellers generally control costs more effectively when they sell to one department or buyer and know that they are reaching the entire organization.

Greater knowledge: Centralization generally affords more specialization among the staff about specifications and characteristics of the goods that they buy. This focus permits buyers to be more effective in obtaining value, as they understand what they buy.

Job contentment: The centralized purchasing set up contributes to increased job contentment among buyers as they are able to make a more significant and quantifiable contribution to the organization.

More time to manage: Planning, organizing, professional development, and personnel issues require time, and it is easier to allocate resources to these areas if the centralized department is adequately staffed.

Lower operating costs: Consolidation occurs in a centralized organization in terms of purchase orders, requisitions, telephonic, electronic and written communications, sales interviews, and the coordination and scheduling of meetings.

These combined efforts usually lead to lower operating costs. By consolidating like requirements of all the units of the hospital, it improves purchasing strength in negotiation and facilitating suppliers' relationships. It avoids price anomalies between group units and of competition between them for materials in short supply.

In addition to above, the other advantages are:

- A hospital is best able to meet its corporate objectives. Functions can be managed as if the hospital is a single entity, and the materials programme can be well coordinated. Thereby, economies of scale can be achieved.

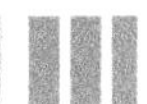

- Centralization avoids duplication of effort and/or working at cross purposes between divisions on items of common concern.
- Centralization allows consolidation of orders for materials commonly used by more than one department or unit, greater buying power, and more favourable national contracts and trade agreements.
- Centralization permits and enhances establishment of unified purchasing policies, practices, procedures, and product standards.
- Purchasing and materials management are recognized as major functions.
- Correlation of each division's resource acquisition cycle improves companywide material flows.
- Greater knowledge and concentrated skills are developed by materials managers specializing in Materials Management for all divisions.
- Effective relations with suppliers are facilitated.
- Supplier certification programmes can be implemented and coordinated.
- Volume buying through national agreements reduces ultimate material, energy, and equipment costs.

Advantages of Decentralized Purchasing

Decentralization means sub delegating purchasing to the local or unit levels. It does not imply total decentralization. An example of decentralized purchasing in a multi location hospital with centralized corporate functional supervision at the overall level is shown in figure below.

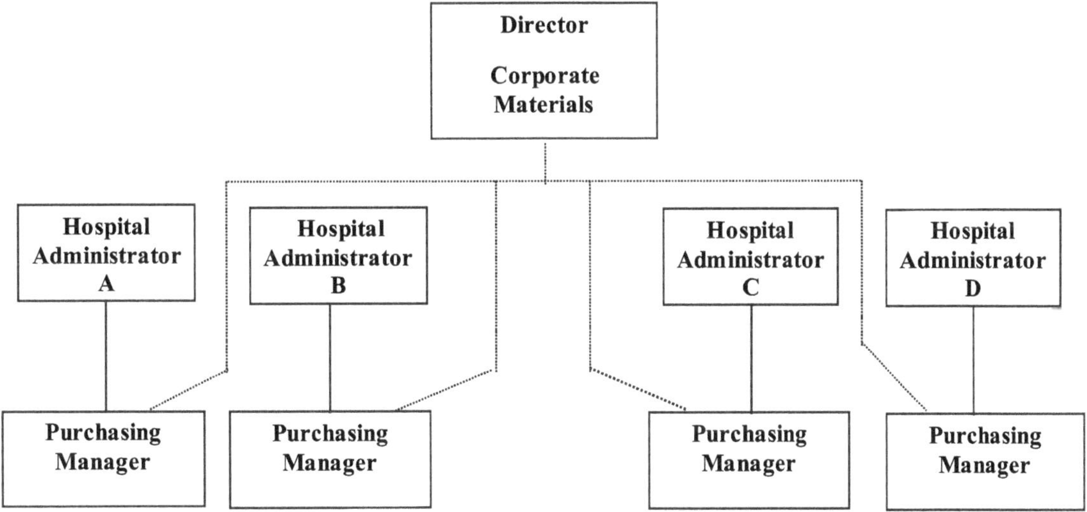

Figure 5.2 Decentralized Purchasing (Multi location Hospitals)

Advantages of decentralized purchasing are:

- Communications with internal customers.
- Better Knowledge of needs.
- More authority.
- Broader responsibilities.

Communications with internal customers: The closer buyers are to their internal customers, the better they understand their needs and respond effectively.

Better knowledge of needs: The local buyer will have better knowledge of the needs of his particular unit and local suppliers. He will respond more quickly to emergency requirements partly because of shorter line of communication and partly because of greater awareness of local circumstances than someone sitting at a distant place.

More authority: The decentralized buyer often has more decision-making authority due to the lack of a reporting hierarchy.

Broader responsibilities: The decentralized buyer must necessarily accept a wider range of responsibilities, quite often involving tasks that are not traditionally associated with purchasing e.g., customer contact or operations liaison function.

Functional Authority of Decentralized Purchasing

Functional authority gives a purchase manager the right to make decisions affecting employees and/or operations that are under the direct control of another manager. It is not uncommon for large hospitals with multi location units to decentralize corporate purchasing but to centralize local purchasing at each plant. The purchasing manager at the local level usually reports to the hospital administrator. Often, but not always, the hospitals also have a corporate purchasing function. Sometimes this corporate entity is only one person, such as a corporate vice president of purchasing, while at other times, it could be a small group of people.

Corporate purchasing departments also provide other services such as:

- Establishing corporate policies and procedures.
- Auditing local purchasing departments to ensure that they are following corporate purchasing policies and procedures.
- Helping to hire, train, and promote purchasing people at the local level.
- Functioning as a resource for those seeking advice.
- Acting as an advocate at the corporate level for local purchasing while similarly serving as the corporate voice at the local level.

PART CENTRALIZATION AND PART DECENTRALIZATION

The typical example of third type of organization is described as follows.

Generally, the advantages of one approach are disadvantages of the other. For example, complete centralization in purchasing is neither always possible nor always desirable, so too, with decentralization. Thus a combination of both these approaches is often used to obtain benefits from the best features of each, while avoiding disadvantages of both approaches. **Part centralization and part decentralization wherein the head office will be responsible for the following:**

- Determining policies, standards, procedures, and group specializations.
- Negotiations of contracts for commonly used, large volume of materials of the group.
- Major plant equipment and capital project contracts.
- Imports
- Legal aspects of purchase contracts, coordination of group inventory and overall control of inventory.
- Training and development of purchasing personnel within the group and providing advice on staff and related requirement etc.

SUMMARY

The fundamental function of a hospital purchase organization is to provide a structure that facilitates motivation of people and the coordination of their efforts towards common goals of the firm. A well designed structure can facilitate, just as poorly designed structure can inhibit such accomplishments. Location of purchasing department within a hospital's organizational hierarchy is determined very simply by one factor management perception of the importance of the function. In a majority of hospitals, the Materials Management function reports to top management executive but in some, it usually reports to a lower level executive. In addition to the complexity of markets and the value and the complexity of materials purchased, the type and amount of specialized expertise in purchasing also influence its profit potential as well as its importance. Hence over a long term, the position of purchasing in the hierarchy can be influenced heavily by department's internal pattern of organization. How purchasing chooses to specialize is important. It can specialize in buying activities by materials categories, or it can specialize by operating functions (e.g., buying, expediting, purchasing research, value analysis, and so on). In practice, all but smallest departments do some of the both. However, with limited staff, each staffing decision represents a trade-off. The managers must decide which type of expertise (material or functional) is most useful to the hospital at a given time and develop the organization accordingly. These needs however change from time to time. Very few hospitals have organizational structures that are exactly alike. Each design represents a trade-off between different criteria. It is for this reason that in U.S.A. many multi-unit hospitals decentralized their purchasing in the 1960s; then with changing conditions of late 1970s moved

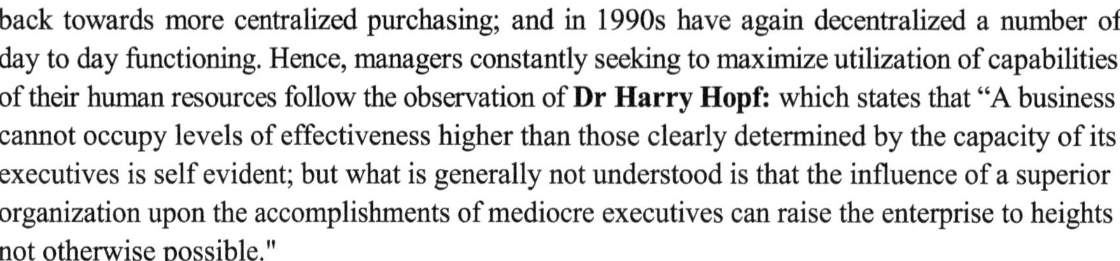

back towards more centralized purchasing; and in 1990s have again decentralized a number of day to day functioning. Hence, managers constantly seeking to maximize utilization of capabilities of their human resources follow the observation of **Dr Harry Hopf:** which states that "A business cannot occupy levels of effectiveness higher than those clearly determined by the capacity of its executives is self evident; but what is generally not understood is that the influence of a superior organization upon the accomplishments of mediocre executives can raise the enterprise to heights not otherwise possible."

A centralized organization structure offers the advantages of broader view for decision making, eliminates duplication of efforts, saves costs, permits specialization and leads to more consistent decisions. The disadvantages are that managers suffer from a narrow focus, long lines of communication cause delays, and lower level managers are often frustrated as they are far removed from the top level decision making.

In a decentralized organization structure, decisions are faster, morale and motivation is higher and this structure provides hands on training to first line and middle level managers. However, there could be lack of information and coordination between departments and policies and procedures vary throughout the organization.

Part centralization and part decentralization purchasing try to obtain the benefits of both the approaches, while avoiding pitfalls of both. The head office is responsible for determining policies, standards, procedures, group specializations and negotiations of contracts for commonly used, large volume of materials of the group. Other activities remain decentralized.

REVIEW QUESTIONS

1. Organization of purchasing function in a large hospital may be
   a) Decentralized by different functional units,
   b) Centralized by commodity group - Discuss
2. What are the responsibilities of hospital materials manager?
   a) Wholly belongs to purchase department.
   b) Shares with other departments.
3. Your Managing Director feels that purchase department in your hospital requires thorough overhauling and needs to be met in a scientific manner. The hospitals are located at Hyderabad, Chennai, Delhi, and Kolkata.
   a) What purchasing organization you would recommend? Give illustrative examples.
   b) What are the results for which the purchase department should be made accountable?
4. Discuss pros and cons of centralized and decentralized purchasing.

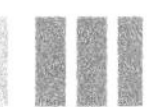

5. In what situation you would suggest part centralized, part decentralized set up for healthcare organization give suitable examples.

6. Write short notes on

   a) Single location hospital

   b) Basic concept of organization

   c) Disadvantages of Centralized purchasing

   d) Advantages of Decentralized purchasing

   e) Advantages of Decentralized purchasing

   f) Disadvantages of decentralised purchasing

PART - II

Purchasing Cycle

Contents

CHAPTER - 6

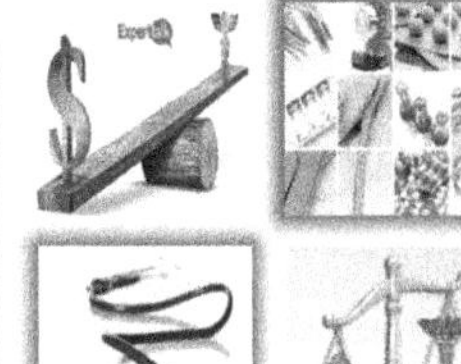

Purchasing Cycle

INTRODUCTION

Organization of a purchasing department and the procedures followed will vary considerably, from industry to industry and also from hospital to hospital. Nature of the items purchased, their volume and variety, the degree of specialization needed to make the purchases, especially the items which have stringent specifications all add up to determine the organization for purchases. Similarly, the procedures adopted in the purchase departments may vary from hospital to hospital in accordance with the policies of the hospital. In some cases, there might be considerable sub delegation of powers to the purchase manager and his subordinates. In other, decisions might be taken in most cases by the top management. In some hospitals, though the delegation might exist on paper, in practice, there might not be much trust and confidence reposed in purchase department and in actual practice, matters might be decided mostly by the hospital top executives. A system best suited for a hospital might not suit an engineering company or the procedures followed by a government hospital may not suit a private hospital. Despite the differences in the sizes of organizations, characteristics of buying units and the sources from which they are obtained.

PURCHASING CYCLE

K.S. Menon, former Director Education Indian institute of Material management had identified eleven elements common to purchasing systems for manufacturing industries which also applies in case of hospitals. In summary, these elements can be divided into eleven general categories of activity.

They are as follows:

1. Need for the material is recognized by user departments and their requirements are determined.
2. Detailed specifications for materials are spelt out.
3. Need is communicated to the purchase department, which in turn will make out a purchase plan and float enquiries.
4. A suitable source is selected for the supply. Sometimes a source may have to be developed.
5. Rates and terms and conditions of purchase are finalized after negotiation.
6. A purchase order is released spelling out the specifications, quantity, price, delivery and terms and conditions of the purchase.

7. The supplier's order acceptance is obtained.
8. Supplier is followed up to ensure prompt delivery.
9. Receiving and inspection - Sometimes the goods are inspected at the vendor's premises.
10. Checking and payment of suppliers bills/invoices.
11. A check is issued to the supplier towards payment for accepted supplies.

Above activities are often refereed to as purchasing cycle.

The purchasing cycle is depicted in Figure 6.1

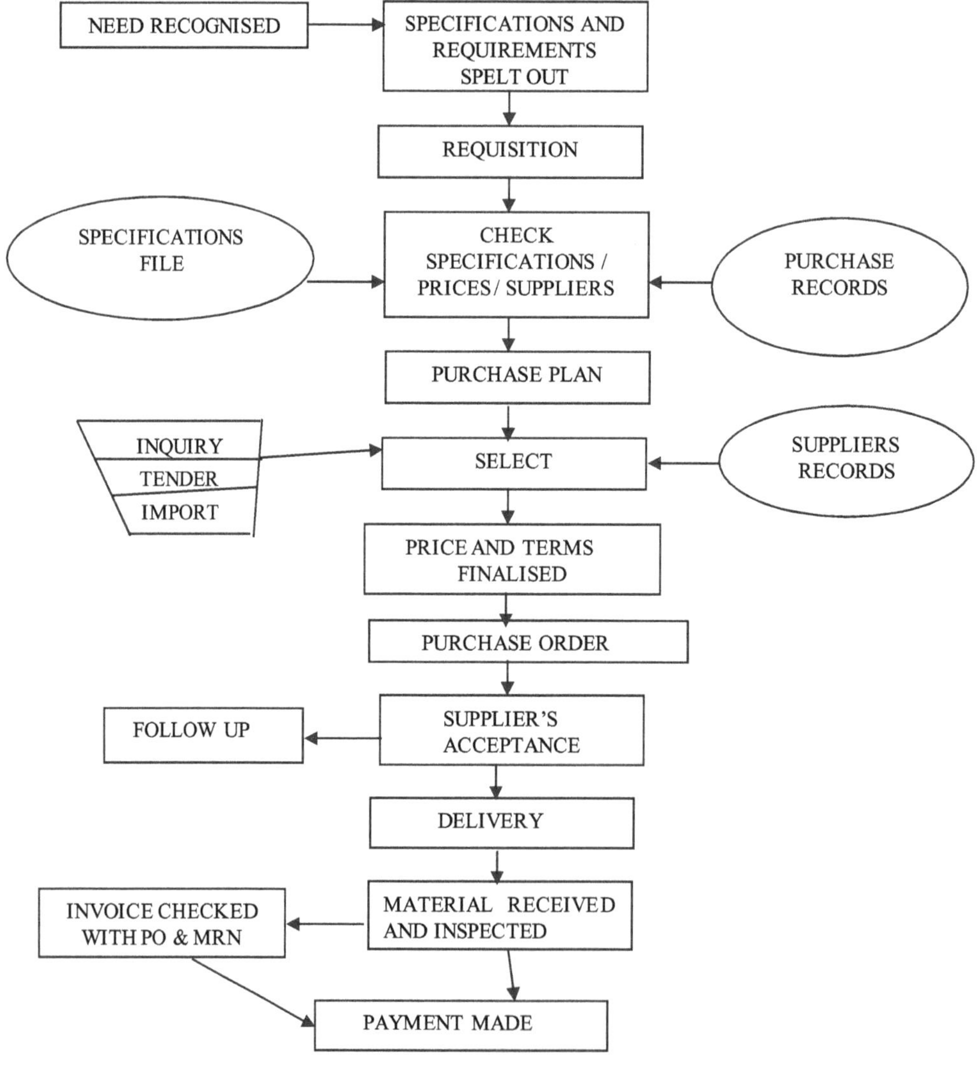

Figure 6.1 The Purchasing Cycle

(Source: Purchasing and Inventory Control by KS Menon)

RECOGNITION OF NEED

Efficient purchasing is a key element of Materials Management. It requires a great amount of detailed information to be handled accurately, promptly, and smoothly. Much of this information is routine and repetitive. The key to efficient purchasing is to organize the routine smoothly so that primary attention can be concentrated on dealing with vendors to obtain necessary items for timely delivery at a best price, or in situations or circumstances that are truly extraordinary and require personal attention outside the routine.

The process has the following steps:

1. Requisition must be stamped with date and time of receipt as soon as it is received at the purchasing department. This is a good control measure. It clearly delineates the time at which purchasing accepts processing responsibility.

2. As soon as possible after being received, the requisition should be checked by a knowledgeable person for completeness and accuracy. If it does not contain sufficient information to complete purchasing action, the situation should be resolved with the official who requisitioned.

3. Purchasing action should be initiated as soon as possible, consistent with effective buying practices.

4. Indenter should be notified, as soon as purchasing action is taken, by sending a copy of the purchase order or by other means. The information which is sent should indicate that the purchase order has been placed and mention the expected delivery date.

5. Purchasing must have a system for prompt follow up of promised deliveries. Expediting is a purchasing service that the indenter has a right to expect. Vigorous expediting combined with regular vendor evaluation also serves to discipline suppliers to adhere to promised dates.

6. Purchasing needs to know when the ordered item has been received and when it was delivered to the user department as specified. Receiving may not be strictly a purchasing function but it is of great concern to purchasing.

Usually, stores or warehouse are responsible for stocking materials and when the stocks reach a particular predetermined level, they raise an indent for purchase. These are for regular stock items. For other items which are one time purchases, the user department raises the indent.

Normally the purchase requisitions originate from three sources and they are:

1. Purchase requisition raised by the user department.

2. Permanent order card or travelling requisition.

3. Bill of materials made in conjunction with the user department.

Purchase Requisition

Professional buyer commits his hospital's funds for items to be used by someone else in the hospital. He must therefore insist upon:

- Adequate and accurate description of what is needed as well as clear identification of those requesting the purchase and authorizing expenditure.
- When a particular department needs some specific materials or equipment etc., it prepares a material purchase requisition. This is sometimes called materials indent form.
- Only officers so authorized by management can sign purchase requisitions. Very often this authority is in terms of value.
- Purchase department should ensure that all purchase requisitions received by it, have been signed by an authorized person. Otherwise, they should return to the originator of the indent with a request for authorization by an appropriate authority.

Purchase requisition should provide following essential information:

1. **Qualitative specifications:** An accurate and full description of the materials required with part numbers or material code numbers, if applicable. This description should in no case be vague or capable of being misunderstood. For unfamiliar or new items, complete details should be given. For a repeated item with which the purchase department is familiar, such details need not be very elaborate.
2. Quantity required: Usually it should be in multiples of a unit.
3. When required: Date by which the materials are required.
4. Work order details: The account, job, department, project or work to which the expenditure is to be charged.
5. Requisition will usually have space for the purchase department to make entries regarding the purchase order number, the company on whom the order has been placed, etc.
6. Date and signature of the indenter and authorization, where necessary.

Formats for materials requisitions for non stock and regular stock items can be had from Tables 6.1 and 6.2

 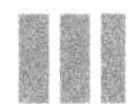

Table 6.1 Materials Requisitions for Non stock Items

PURCHASE REQUISITION NORMAL/URGENT/RUSH			DEPARTMENT Account Code		WORK ORDER REF Date:	
SL. NO	Quantity	Units	Description	Code No	Date when Required	Balance on hand
Indenture Signature Date			Approved by: Signature Date		Distribution Original: Purchase Dept. Duplicate: Office Copy	

(Note: to be used for items not regularly used)

Class of Materials

Table 6.2 Materials Purchase Requisition

Material Code No	Description	Quantity Required	Unit	Balance Stock	Quantity on Order	Last PO No. & Date	Average Consumption in 6 Months	Remarks

Delivery Date:

To

PURCHASE DEPARTMENT Inventory Controller Stores Officer

Note: To be Used by Stores Department for regular stock items

Streamlining the Purchasing Process: Basic Functions and Tasks

Purchasing office must perform the basic purchasing functions well. The total operation is built around these basics viz:

1. Requirements Determination

2. Requisition Processing
3. Forecasting for Regular Use Consumable Item
4. Assisting Users to Prepare Requisitions
5. The Bidding Process
6. Competition Yes and No

Requirements Determination

In theory, user departments determine needs and requirements. Purchasing also can play an important role in such decisions. For repetitively used items, based on anticipated usage, purchasing usually buys inventory. Even for non repetitive items, purchasing can often provide valuable assistance to the user department in determining the actual demand and the requirements for equipment or supplies to meet that need. Every purchasing action should be supported by an authorized requirements determination. For special orders or capital item orders, this normally is in the form of a requisition or some other similar authorization. For repetitively used items purchased into inventory, there should be a procedure that delineates responsibility, authority, and control guidelines for determining stock levels and for ensuring that these are adhered to in line with the corporate policies. These replenishment decisions are based on the authorized requirements determination to support purchase into inventory. Normally, Materials Manager (MM) will be authorized to replenish stock items based on authorized stock levels and actual usage.

Requisition Processing

Requisitions come in several different formats to meet specific needs of a particular organization. Format should be as clear and uncluttered as possible. Especially in a hospital setting, in the interest of expedience, requisitions should be allowed to be filled out by hand rather than required to be typewritten. This of course must not be at the cost of clarity.

Whatever the format, requisitions need at least five elements of information:

1. Who is the indenter?
2. Account which is to be charged for the purchase or issue.
3. Description and specifications of the item which is needed.
4. When is it needed?
5. Location at which the items are to be delivered.

Requisition should follow a definite flow process that should be controlled so that both its status and the overall performance of the purchasing office in processing it will be known at all times.

Role of purchasing includes the following:

- Identifying potential vendors or sourcing of equipment to obtain competition and search out the best value in the market.

- Evaluating competitive pricing and helping to ensure that quotations are compared on an equivalent basis "oranges to oranges".
- Assisting, along with technical personnel, to evaluate particular items, including obtaining samples or demonstration equipment for evaluation.
- Developing financial justification to support the acquisition.

Forecasting for Regular Use Consumable Items

Regular use consumable items are purchased for inclusion into inventory according to an estimate of future need, based on past usage or some other criterion. This is more an inventory control function rather than a purchasing function. However, it is of great interest to purchasing. The more accurately requirements are forecast, the more precisely purchasing commitments can be made. In turn, purchasing commitments that are highly accurate in terms of quantity and delivery date are welcomed by vendors. These also provide leverage for lower prices or for other favourable terms. The more precisely Materials Management accounts for issuance of items, the better will be the usage information upon which to forecast future requirements.

Assisting Users to Prepare Requisitions

Determination of requirements and preparation of requisitions is essentially a responsibility of the user department. However, purchasing often can be helpful to them in this activity. Typical ways in which purchasing can assist users might include identifying and defining particular items or options, accessories, sizing, capacity of equipment. Objective of all purchasing is to buy for value. Value is the optimal combination of quality, service, and price. Unless quality is adequate, the purchase is useless, but if quality is excessive, it is wasteful. There must be adequate service support for such factors as delivery, training, parts, and maintenance. Otherwise, the items may not be ready for use when needed. Subject to adequate quality and service, purchasing at lowest price provides the greatest value. To measure quality accurately, the requirement must be well defined. Unless purchasing knows clearly what is needed, it is difficult to buy effectively. It often is useful for purchasing to become involved in assisting the indenter to determine requirements so that buying action may be more efficient.

BIDDING PROCESS

Bidding process begins with a clear **request for proposal (RFP) or request for bid (RFB).** The materials or services required must be described in sufficient detail so that the vendor knows what is needed. If the request for bid is not clear, the vendor will tend to cushion the price to protect against uncertainty. Bidding process may be formal or informal, public or not public. Unless there are regulatory requirements, the question is a matter of hospital policy. Formal bids sent out in writing, are usually very detailed, and require an equally formal answer. Informal bidding may even be done over the telephone. Public bidding involves the submission of sealed bids that are opened at a public session with all vendors invited to attend. That way,

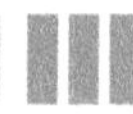

everyone hears details of all the bids and knows exactly where they stand in the bidding. Private openings are done by the purchasing department and only the successful bidder may be announced. Unless there are regulatory requirements, there is no obligation to publicize bid prices or subsequent negotiations with particular vendors.

It is often appropriate to negotiate with one or more vendors before making the final award. If this is to be done, it should be stated in the RFP or RFB. If such negotiations are used, they should be for the purpose of clarifying and sharpening each vendor's proposal. The specific bid price of one vendor should not be used to force down another's bid. To do so is unethical. Furthermore, eventually it causes vendors to pad up their prices in preparation for the price squeeze that they learn to anticipate. It could also raise concerns about legal violations particularly in non profit hospitals.

However, the process is structured. Bidding must always be handled with a high degree of integrity. This means essentially that every vendor must be given an equal opportunity for the business. Buyer cannot disclose information to any bidder that will give the seller an unfair advantage over another bidder. Such information might include prices or terms of competing vendors or special information concerning the purchase that is not generally available to all suppliers. The hospital obviously should seek to obtain the best value for money. Once the proposals are assembled, they must be analyzed carefully, including not only price but terms, conditions, the vendor's past performance and ability in short, the total of all factors of quality, service, and price that make up the value. As soon as possible, after the choice is made and approved, the successful vendor should be notified formally and the actual purchase order issued and accepted by the supplier. The purchase order must contain the complete understanding of the transaction, including all terms and conditions. A little extra time spent in preparing the purchase order, and ensuring that it is complete and comprehensive, usually saves a great deal of time later in correcting mistakes and resolving misunderstandings. Final step in the bidding process is to inform the unsuccessful vendors. This should be done with the same degree of formality or informality as the bidding. It should always be done, out of courtesy to the vendor for the time and effort spent in preparing a proposal.

Competition Yes and No

Competition should be sought and encouraged in all purchasing actions to obtain the lowest price and achieve the best value for money spent. However, purchasing must be cost effective in seeking competition. In procurements of low monetary value, the potential saving simply may not be worth the time and effort involved in obtaining and ensuring maximum competition. In other cases, limited purchasing resources will dictate that they be applied where it is likely to be most effective in saving money for the organization.

Authority to Indent

Needs for procurement originate from user departments. Purchase department, basically a service department, caters to the requirements of the various departments by making purchases of materials, equipment, etc., which those departments may need.

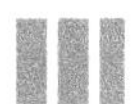

PURCHASE REQUISITION

Most hospitals employ some type of budgeting procedure whereby department heads are held accountable for the supplies and equipments charged to their departmental budgets. Wherever such a budgeting system is employed, the purchasing staff must have some type of supporting documentation to authorize purchases charged to any given department's budget. Purchasing should never be allowed to process purchase orders, except for supplies for their own department itself, without such authorization. **Two most popular methods for departments to initiate an order are the travelling requisition and the direct purchase requisition.**

In general, a travelling requisition is used for items with a high recurrence of reorder. Central stores, central services, laboratory, maintenance, radiology, and surgery are typical examples of departments that could make good use of the travelling requisition.

Travelling requisition is normally exchanged between the ordering department and purchasing and thus its name. Central stores' use of the travelling requisition will naturally correspond to items maintained in their inventory. Each travelling requisition must be marked with the corresponding catalogue or item stock number.

Permanent Order Card Or Travelling Requisition (T.R.)

Permanent order card or travelling requisition form is often used when materials are requested on a repeat basis or for standard stock items, i.e., items which are stocked on a regular basis in the warehouse. In such cases, it helps to:

- Save paper work for such items that are ordered quite often.
- Avoid possible errors like transcribing the information on regular purchase requisition.
- Serve as a continuous record of transactions for a particular item.

A T.R. would normally include the following information i.e.,

- Full description of the material required. (Specifications)
- Stock code number or part number wherever applicable.
- Purchases code or part number, if applicable.
- List of names and addresses of existing or potential suppliers.
- Cumulative record of quantities purchased from various suppliers with prices paid.
- Re order level. When the stock reduces to a particular level, action has to be initiated to purchase fresh quantities of the item. This will depend upon the lead time of the material and also on the quantity required. This level of stocks is called the re order level.

Usually the T.R form is used by the stock control section and the clerk also uses it as a day to day stock card showing receipts and issues. The T.R carries all relevant information required to enable purchase department to place order for fresh supplies. When the stock levels reach re order level the stock control clerk sends the T.R to purchase department. On receipt of card, the purchase department swings into action. It decides up on the sources from which purchases have to be made and also the quantity that is to be ordered and passes the card for typing the order. The number and date of purchase order is then entered on the T.R. and returned to stores clerk, who places it in the appropriate file. Stores then know that the order has been placed. It then awaits receipt of goods.

Table 6.3 A Typical Travelling Requisition (TR)

TRAVELLING REQUISITION CARD

Classification: _________ Description _______________ Stock Number: _________

Minimum Stock: _________

Vendor Code No: Contract Average Monthly Consumption: _________

Approved Suppliers: ____________________________ Inquires Issued: __________

Date	Present Stock	Quantity Required	Unit	Delivery Wanted	Required for	Approved	Date Recd. Purchasing Department	Purchase Order Number	Supp-lier	Price	Transp ort	Settlement

(Note: To be Used for Standard Stock Items.)

BILL OF MATERIAL OR PART LIST

When bio engineering department designs any equipment for captive use, a list of the various components and materials which are required to make that equipment is also made out. This is called a bill of materials or part list. When the bio engineering production schedule is prepared, it is usually converted into a more detailed bill of materials, which will show what materials are required and when and in what number.

On receipt of the bill of materials either directly from the user department or through the stock control, the purchase department then takes out the remaining requirements from the bill of materials and places the purchase orders as deemed necessary. Before issue of purchase order, the purchase department has to ensure that:

- All the information required for making the correct purchases has been received.
- The specifications and description are unambiguous.

- Internal control reference must be very correctly stated. For example, head of account under which the expenditure is to be charged.
- That the specifications are not unreasonably restrictive as this might have an adverse effect on the choice of sources.

It may, therefore, be better to specify the requirements leaving the choice of the suppliers to the purchase department. If user wants to use a specific make, then it is up to him to make a case for doing so by providing adequate justification. Ultimate responsibility of reducing costs rests with both, the purchase department and user department and no action, which is likely to increase such costs, should normally be taken. Purchase department would also have a duty to provide such relevant information as possible to user, so that he may in a position to decide exactly, what the specifications should be in order to meet his functional requirements.

Bill of Materials (BOM)

Table 6.4 Bill of Materials for a Product

Sl no	Name of the Material	Part Number / Code Number	Qty per one Unit of Production	Units	When Required
Indentor	Approved by :		Distribution		
Signature	Signature		Original : Purchase		
Duplicate : Stores					
Triplicate : Office Copy					

BUDGET

When materials are purchased on semi annual or annual basis, the budget often constitutes authorization to purchase. In such cases, the budget usually includes projections of the number of units required by the end user during the budgeted period. **A budget is a plan translated into financial terms.** The basis of budget is to balance expenditure with income. It is one of the functions of budgetary planning to ensure that suitable answers are given to these and many other questions. Budgeting is a management tool used for short term planning and control. Budgets have been typically used as a management tool to monitor expenditure. It should also be noted that Budgets are further useful to treat the budgeting process as a resources allocation for obtaining the most rewarding and profitable use of the company's funds through planning and control. Budget usually includes the projections of the number of units of each service that the hospital plans to provide during the budget period.

Purpose of a budget is to provide:

- Forecast of amount of money a hospital will have to set aside for the operations during a stated period of time.
- Budget is a basis for measurement of performance and control of operations, usually referred to as budgetary control.

Following questions are answered by a budget.

- What sort of service is proposed to be provided?
- What equipments and facilities are required?
- What types of inputs are required, and where can they be obtained?
- What rate of expansion is aimed for?
- What future development is intended?
- What level of staffing is required for patient care?
- What level of overhead expenditure is to be incurred?

PURCHASE BUDGET

A purchase budget is prepared giving estimates of the costs to be incurred on purchase during the year. This represents the spending plan. The purchase plan, which involves the physical quantities, is prepared after taking into consideration the materials requirement spread on a time chart. This estimate materials requirement is often called as Material Budget. One would then know what materials are required and when. Procurement action would then be planned on a systematic basis.

It is usual to prepare a **Performance Evaluation Research and Testing (PERT)** chart to determine when the various steps in purchasing should begin and end. Purchase budget differs from materials budget in two respects:

- Materials budget is limited to quantity only while purchase budget involves both quantities and money value.
- Purchase budget is concerned with actual receipt of material on purchase order or commitments. Materials budget details only the gross requirements.

PURCHASE PLAN

Purchase department must prepare a plan for carrying out its purchasing activities. Without a plan, purchasing will tend to be carried out in "fits and starts" and the department may be very much overloaded during some months and relatively without work for the rest of the year.

- A plan is a predetermined course of action regarding what is to be done to achieve an objective.

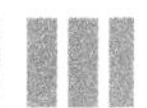

- At the beginning of the year, the purchase department would determine what to buy, when to buy and how much to buy.
- It prepares time schedules and a programme for purchases. **In purchasing, "Time is the essence".**

SELECTING THE ALTERNATIVES

After evaluating the pros and cons of make or buy, if the organization decides to purchase rather than manufacture or to negotiate than call bids, the buyer must select a vendor to receive the order or a group of vendors among whom the order will be divided. Although the complexity of selection process varies with nature of the purchase, it is determined by the buyer's perception of what constitutes a good supplier and the usefulness of available information on suppliers.

APPRAISING ALTERNATIVES: VENDOR SELECTION AND EVALUATION OF COMPETITIVE BIDS

When need for material has been established and specifications of material detailed, the purchase department proceeds to select the source of supply. While deciding a suitable supplier, it is necessary to evaluate the capacities of suppliers to make the supplies in time without fail, and then decide upon placing contracts with him. Negotiations have to be carried out with regard to prices and other terms and conditions, for example, mode of transport, delivery dates, packaging etc. Provisions would have to be made for penalties for breach of contract by either party and so on.

- As a general rule, the buyers use the bid system primarily as a means of exploring or identifying price factor.
- No market price exists for many non standard, materials, complex fabricated products for which design and manufacturing methods vary and items might be made to buyer's specification. In these circumstances, asking for competitive bids is the simplest way of exploring prices and evaluating the reasonableness of quoted prices.
- Having received competitive bids from a group of reliable suppliers, the buyer can select the lowest price offered or the lowest price could be weighted alongside other considerations.
- While evaluating the bids, it should be noted if there is a wide range of quotations, both excessively high and extremely low, the bids may be open to question, "Do the bidders understand the requircments?"
- On the other hand, insignificant variation or identity of quotations leads to suspicion of collusion or cartel formation.

NEGOTIATIONS

Negotiation is not haggling over price. Nor is it an attempt by the buyer to play one vendor against another to force prices down. Negotiation is an art and technique and a process of arriving at a common understanding through discussing the essentials of a purchase, such as specifications, delivery, price, and terms. Price negotiation is typical in hospital purchasing, particularly in complex buying situations, where buyers and sellers make a number of proposals and counter proposals before price is agreed upon. Most major purchases by institutions, government agencies and commercial businesses are negotiated; not only price, but service, delivery, technical assistance, product characteristics and quality are commonly negotiated. Every purchaser needs good negotiation skills and must begin to learn proper techniques early on in his career. Lack of sound negotiation skills by buyers is the primary reason why many departmental heads act as quasi-purchasing agents. They feel as skilled as the purchasing agent who has little, if any, formal training in this critical discipline.

Successful negotiation of a contract requires skills, experience and preparation on the part of seller. Like a good lawyer, the industrial marketer must analyze the firms' strengths and weaknesses compared to potential competition. Factors most important to the buying firm, future growth opportunity and projected profitability must be considered. A buyer who becomes locked into a set style becomes an ineffective negotiator. He cannot remain open to new options and cannot break out of this pattern of inflexibility. Negotiation is a dynamic activity. Each event is unique as it brings together a new combination of persons and situations.

Keys to effective negotiation are as follows:

- Allowing sufficient time to plan for and carry out important negotiations.
- Developing a detailed plan.
- Rehearsing the key elements.
- Adjusting the performance according to what works.

By adopting the above mentioned steps, buyers are able to increase the effectiveness of their negotiations. (This sub topic is dealt in detail in chapter 8 on negotiations).

MAKE OR BUY DECISIONS

Costs as related to manufacturing decisions, whether an organization should "make or buy" materials, parts or completed products is a common type of business decision. Theory underlying make or buy decisions is neither ambiguous nor controversial. Making often entails a capital investment. A decision to make should take place whenever the expected cost savings provide a higher return on the required capital investment than can be obtained from employing these funds in an alternative investment, bearing the same risk. Major as well as minor make or buy decisions are determined primarily by two basic criteria: relative cost and quality. In make or buy decision involving, say, printing, the buying institution might well question whether the quality will be as good as that of a professional printer. In all other decisions, institution is usually concerned about whether the outsider will do as good a job as it does itself. Evaluation of the quality of goods or services involved in make or buy decisions could be subjective when adequate test equipment or testing methods are unavailable. There is usually a wide scope for error. Hence, make or buy decisions should focus initially on cost, where the data is obviously more objective. Subjective evaluations cannot be overlooked. However, there is no point in making them until objective data suggests that it may pay to change. While cost and price considerations are usually paramount, there are varieties of other factors like suppliers' reliability, collusion among suppliers, monopolistic supply situation, uneven production of end product, lack of capital, space requirements etc. that must be considered in "make or buy" decision.

Typical Make versus Buy decisions in hospitals are as follows:

1. Printing and laundry is the most frequent make or buy decisions in Hospital Materials Management. Most hospitals operate small plants in which they print simple/small forms, stationery, and sometimes even hospital publications. Smaller hospitals rely exclusively on outside printers for any work that cannot be done on a Xerox copier. For washing, ironing and disinfecting etc., many hospitals operate their own laundries. Others either have the work done by commercial laundries or rely on cooperative laundries, as in American hospital, which is usually operated by a branch of the local hospital association or purchasing group.
2. Food service is sometimes delegated completely or partly to caterers, as is housekeeping and maintenance.
3. The ultimate in make or buy decision is when a hospital's trustees contract with an outsider (BPO agency) for Materials Management or even for complete operation of the institution.

It is much easier for a hospital to decide to buy rather than make, something which it may be presently buying. Suppose a hospital presently operates its own laundry. A new co operative laundry operated by the local hospital association might offer to do the job for substantial saving per kilogram of clothes. Quick comparison of the two figures might suggest that it is economic for the hospital to close its own laundry and to rely on the co operative for its needs. This decision might be the right one at least eight times out of ten. However, a hospital can improve its chances of making the right decision in this case by taking these four additional factors into account:

1. Co operative laundry's record on linen losses and damage.
2. Likely increase in supplier's costs than those of the hospital itself.
3. Possible saving in internal costs of the existing operation.
4. Is it possible to adapt facilities required by the make activity to some more-lucrative service?

Full costs must always account for when the hospital is considering making something that is presently being purchased. Non cash costs must also be deducted from the saving. The major non-cash cost is depreciation of equipment that must be purchased for the laundry. If the hospital finances the capital expenditure by borrowing from a lending financial institution, it may find that its savings are offset by interest and amortization of the loan. In addition, most hospitals are so strapped

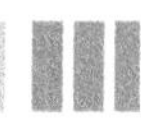

for cash that they prefer to use their limited borrowing limits only for expansion or diversification projects that are critical to survival and growth. In fact, the typical hospital is generally so hard pressed for cash that it would probably not make any additional investment if the only objective was cost reduction. If the hospital also believed that it could do a better job with its own facilities, it would have to weigh the presumed benefits of higher quality against the true cost, after taking all cash and non cash costs into account, including opportunity cost of capital employed.

ORDER PLACEMENT

After the supplier has been selected and terms of supply agreed upon, a purchase order is issued to the supplier. A purchase order is the commitment by a buyer to pay for goods ordered and the supplier's authority to ship the goods and charge the buyer for them. A purchase order is a legal contract and all precautions have therefore, to be taken by the buyer to safeguard his interests. In a purchase order issued, various terms and conditions pertinent to the contract are spelt out. Acceptance of that order by the supplier assures the buyer of acceptance of all terms and conditions stated therein.

FOLLOW UP AND EXPEDITING

After purchase order has been issued and supplier has accepted the same, a regular watch has to be kept by the purchase department to ensure that the deliveries are made in time. There are various follow up procedures. Besides the normal function of following up with supplier to ensure prompt deliveries as per schedule indicated in the purchase order, the purchase section will also have the following duties and responsibilities.

- Advancement or postponement of deliveries, if and when so required.
- Liaison with logistic service providers for transport, off loading etc.
- Liaison with clearing and forwarding agencies.
- Liaison with works of the supplier to maintain schedules and for pre-dispatch inspection at supplier's plants whenever called for. Expediters are often vested with considerable responsibility and spend much of their time visiting supplier's plants to investigate deliveries and to keep shipments moving.

RECEIVING AND INSPECTION

When materials ordered for have been received, they are to be checked for quantity and quality with reference to the purchase order. Receiving of materials should not be treated as a routine clerical function. In fact, it is of considerable importance. Unloading and counting provides an additional internal control to ensure that orders are actually counted. Receiving clerks must have an understanding of the importance of their role in controlling the flow of materials into the hospital. They must pay close attention to detail in verifying descriptions, quantities, and correct units of measure. Ideally, all shipments should be completely counted and inspected before the delivery

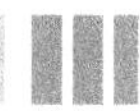

truck is allowed to leave. This usually is found to be unrealistic. normal practice is to inspect for obvious external damage and to ensure that the facility's bulk piece count agrees with that on the vendor's packing slip before signing for the shipment. Shipment should be completely counted and inspected as soon as possible after unloading. Any discrepancies must be documented immediately and communicated to the receiving supervisor. The supervisor must notify purchasing agent to coordinate for resolution of the problem. Receiving is an important control point in the purchase system. Properly maintained receiving records will show up the suppliers who are consistently late in their deliveries. These vendors add to the problems of the hospital. A close coordination is therefore necessary between stores receipts section and the purchase department. Inspection for quality is another important work. An inspection programme must be in place to examine the product periodically for desired quality. Regardless of how quality is described, a regular programme should be established to ensure that the quality specified is being maintained by the manufacturer and/or vendor. At times, product manufacturing methods or specifications are modified without the hospital's knowledge. After inspection for quality, the receiving clerk prepares a report called the materials receipt note or goods inward note. Sometimes goods are rejected, in which case, he also prepares a rejection memo. Sometimes, there is a short receipt or excess supply. All these have to be recorded in various forms.

CHECKING AND PAYMENT OF SUPPLIER'S BILLS (INVOICE HANDLING)

Next step is the payment of the supplier's bills. Bills are sometimes received along with the goods or sometimes later, along with the copy of delivery challan. The bill is checked for payment. Purchase department may do this or may get it done directly by the accounts department, which has to be provided with a copy of purchase order and the material receipt note, forwarded by the receiving section. After bill has been audited, amount is paid to the supplier on the due date, by cheque or through electronic clearing service/e-payment mechanism. After the purchase order has been completely executed, the purchase department retains all papers in one file, which is termed, as **"closed file".**

SUMMARY

Organization of purchasing department and procedures followed will vary considerably depending upon the company's policies, delegation of powers, confidence reposed on the purchase department. A system best suited for a hospital might not suit an engineering company or the procedures followed by a government hospital may not suit a corporate hospital.

Despite differences in size, characteristics in industrial buying, there are eleven elements, which are common to purchasing systems. They are 1. Need recognition 2. Description of specifications 3. Floating of enquires 4. Selection and development of suitable vendor 5. Finalization of rates and terms and conditions 6. Placement of purchase order 7. Obtaining order acceptance 8. Follow up with suppliers for prompt delivery 9. Arranging receiving and inspection 10. Invoice handling 11. Arranging payment for accepted supplies.

Recognition of need in the form of indent may come to purchase department through (a) purchase requisition or (b) permanent order card or travelling requisition (TR) or (c) the bill of material or part list.

When materials are purchased on semi-annual or annual basis, the budget often constitutes authority to purchase. Budgets usually include the projection of, number of units of each and every product or service. Purchase budget is prepared giving estimates of costs to be incurred on purchasing during the year. This represents spending plan.

Purchase plan, which involve physical quantities, would be prepared taking into consideration the material requirement spread over a time period. This estimation is called materials budget. Basic difference between purchase budget and materials budget is that purchase budget involves both estimation of quantities and money value, whereas materials budget is limited to quantity only.

Next step is to arrive at cost related decisions: whether a company should "make or buy" materials, parts, or completed products which are common to business decisions. The basis is techno-commercial evaluation.

While deciding a suitable supplier, the buyer has to evaluate the capacity of suppliers, keeping in mind price, quality, timely delivery and capacity. Before finalization of orders, sometimes the buyer may resort to negotiations. Price negotiation is typical in corporate purchasing, particularly in complex buying situations. Cardinal principle in negotiation is "win-win strategy," established on the basis of careful examination of company's needs and alternatives as well as the recognition that suppliers must make profit too. After the supplier has been selected and terms of supply agreed upon, a purchase order is placed on the supplier. A purchase order is a commitment by buyer to pay for goods ordered and supplier's authority to ship the goods and charge the buyer for the same.

After purchase order has been issued and supplier has accepted the same, a regular watch has to be kept by the purchase department to ensure that the deliveries are made in time. There are various follow up procedures. Besides the normal function of following up with supplier to ensure prompt deliveries as per schedule indicated in the purchase order, the purchase section will also have to perform the following duties and responsibilities.

- Advancement or postponement of deliveries, if and when required.
- Liaison with logistic service providers for transport, off loading etc.
- Liaison with clearing and forwarding agencies.
- Liaison with works of the supplier to maintain schedules and for pre dispatch inspection at supplier's plants whenever called for. Expediters are often vested with considerable responsibility and spend much of their time visiting supplier's plants to investigate deliveries and to keep shipments moving.

When materials ordered have been received, they are to be checked for quantity and quality with reference to purchase order.

Last but one step in purchasing cycle is checking of supplier's bills. Bills are checked for quantities, rates and terms of payments. Last step in purchasing cycle is arranging payment for the material accepted.

After the order has been completed, purchase department keeps all the papers in one file, which is termed, as "closed file".

REVIEW QUESTIONS

1. What do you understand by the term purchasing cycle? Explain in detail various stages of the purchasing cycle.
2. How need arises for materials, how the need is processed?
3. What is purchase requisition? How will you handle the requisition received by the purchase department?
4. What role does the materials manager play in purchasing cycle of Materials Management?
5. Write short notes on
   a) Travelling requisition
   b) Purchasing cycle
   c) Requirements determination
   d) Requisition processing
   e) Purchase budget
   f) Checking for payment of suppliers bills
   g) Assisting users to prepare requisitions

PART - II

Purchasing Parameters

Contents

CHAPTER - 7

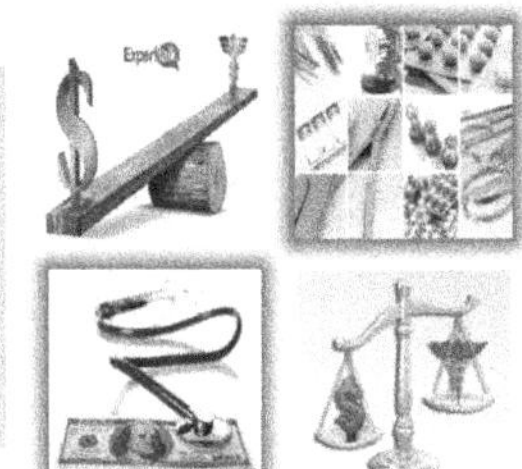

Purchasing Parameters

INTRODUCTION

Purchasing is now considered the most important function of Materials Management. When a buyer places a purchase order, he commits a substantial portion of the finance of the hospital which affects the working capital and cash flow position. A buyer is a highly responsible person who interacts with various salespersons and can be considered to have been contributing to the public relations efforts of the hospital. Thus a buyer can make or mar hospital's image by his excellent or poor interactions with vendors. Basic objective of purchasing function is to ensure continuity of supplies of material inputs, sub contract items and spare parts and, at the same time, reduce ultimate cost of patient service. In other words, the objective is not so much to procure materials at the lowest possible price, but to reduce the cost to the ultimate customer, the patient. For ensuring this, there are many well known parameters such as right price, right quality, right contractual terms, right source, right materials, right time, right place, right mode of transport and right attitude. All these "rights" have to be considered jointly and severally. Just as inefficient marketing techniques and outmoded healthcare practices can lead to a decrease in profit, similarly, an inefficient purchase management system often can lead to reduced profits. Professional competence is therefore the essence in managing the purchasing function. Purchasing is a professional job. Purchase manager must acquire professional knowledge and skills. Purchasing involves activities directed towards securing the materials and supplies of equipment and services required in operations of an enterprise. This activity has to be performed with optimum efficiency, economy and effectiveness. These three factors are the key to obtaining excellence in managerial performance. Since materials constitute the largest chunk of the cost in the creation of value for which the customer alone pays the price, it is necessary for the purchaser to exercise utmost prudence in ensuring that the best ultimate value is obtained for every rupee spent on materials. These five rights have meaning and significance far beyond their respective dictionary meanings.

Prof. P. Gopala Krishnan, former Professor, Administrative Staff College of India, Hyderabad, suggests that some more R's should be considered along with the above mentioned five R's viz., right material, right transport, right contracts, right place of delivery and a right attitude. These rights, as described by Prof. Gopalakrishnan, are graphically presented in Figure 7.1.

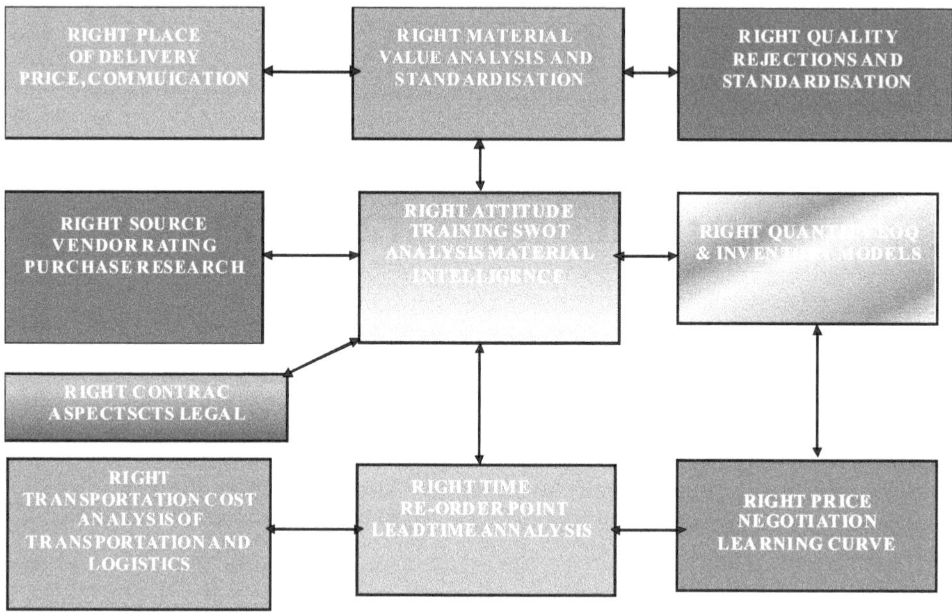

Figure 7.1 Purchasing Parameters

(Source : Materials Management - An Integrated Approach by Prof. P. Gopala Krishnan and Sundaresan

Developing the right attitude, too, is necessary as one often comes across such statements as:

- "Purchasing knows the price of everything and the value of nothing."
- "They buy price and not cost."
- "When will the order placers become purchase managers?"
- "Purchasing acts like a post box."
- "Purchasing should, therefore, keep 'progress' as its key activity and should be future-oriented."

The materials manager should not follow the safe and well trodden path; he should be innovative and his long term objective should be to minimize the cost of ultimate product. He will be able to achieve this if he arms himself with techniques such as

- Value analysis
- Materials intelligence
- Purchase research
- SWOT analysis
- Purchase budget
- Lead time analysis etc.

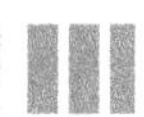

Buyer must adopt separate policies and procedures for capital and consumable items. He should be able to differentiate between indigenous and international purchasing practices. He should be aware of the legal and contractual obligations in global contracts. However the discussions in this chapter are limited to 5 R's only as mentioned earlier.

RIGHT QUALITY

Where an item is purchased to be used in the hospital patient care and if the product has qualities which are really not required, then we are unnecessarily paying the money for something which is not needed. It is like "using a field gun to kill a centipede." (K.S. Menon) If quality is less than what we require, the patient care suffers. Quality assurance is therefore essential for user satisfaction. Quality should be just right; neither more than what is required for a given purpose nor less. Before purchase is made, it is necessary to determine and define quality that we want. Once this is done, purchase department's task is to ensure that the quality of materials purchased conforms strictly to the specified quality.

SPECIFYING QUALITY

Quality of an item is its power to accomplish a function, its compatibility or ability to do certain things. The starting point for determining quality is end use. We have to establish specifications without any ambiguity. A full and complete specification is an essential part of purchase contract. Quality can be specified by several parameters such as dimensions, weight, chemical composition, physical properties, tensile strength, hardness, surface finish, colour, resistance, conductivity, elasticity, capacitance, inductance, life characteristics, appearance, design etc. For machinery or equipment, quality can be defined by factors such as productivity, versatility, dependability, economy, etc. Emergency stock outs are sometimes caused by quality failures. Material may be on hand but, when package opened, it may turn out to be bad quality material.

Hospitals are especially vulnerable to quality failures. Such failures may be literally matters of life and death. It has no facilities for objective measurement of quality. Large industrial purchasers determine their own quality standards and then develop procedures to assure adherence to them. On the other hand, healthcare institutions, often accept vendors' assurances on quality. On drugs and related items, vendor must have proven to the satisfaction of the Drug Controller that its product and process by which it is made, meet minimum specified standards. Other purchases legally or customarily must meet standards imposed by various other quasi or real regulatory agencies. Milk and other food products must usually meet the standards of a local food inspector. Plumbing and other maintenance supplies must be compatible with building codes. Various healthcare groups set standards for other supplies. Hospitals should also develop simple tests that are within their technological capabilities.

WRITING A SPECIFICATION

After all the elements of acceptable quality have been specified, the next step is to establish product specifications. Quality specifications are generally utilized in competitive bidding procedures to determine which product or group of products meet the hospital's exact requirements. In the hospital industry, quality specifications are generally expressed by the use of one or more of the following: hospital-developed purchase specification, brand name, catalogue designation, and market grade.

PURCHASE SPECIFICATION

Specifications developed in a hospital are perhaps least used of all methods for expressing the quality requirements of hospital. The principal reason for this lack of use is that the medical practitioner assumes responsibility to describe the hospital's requirements in complete, positive terms. Many buyers feel that they are unable to perform this function adequately and rightfully so. **Development of a purchase specification is the responsibility of user, not purchaser.** Users who intend to generate their own specifications for quality determination require a few words of caution. Writing purchase specifications for every purchased item may not be economical because of the cost involved. For example, for small, non repetitive purchases, of which there are many, it must be recognized that the user assumes the responsibility for the performance of a product, since user has determined its composition, and possibly its method of manufacture too. User should be very familiar with the product or service being specified, not only as a basis for preparing clear, concise specifications, but also to prevent hospital from incurring avoidable additional expenses as a result of poor performance. Therefore, it is more important that user adopt the various methods of quality specifications wisely than to be able to prepare purchase specifications for every purchased item for use within the hospital.

For users who will utilize purchase specifications as one method of expressing the quality requirements of the hospital, the following methodology and explanations should be useful. Purchase specifications must not be written so restrictively that the number of potential vendors is limited and thereby competition is reduced. Specifications should be broad enough to provide an equal opportunity to all qualified vendors. They must also be stringent enough to ensure maintaining of high quality standards while excluding products that may be undesirable from quality perspective. **A well written specification should inform the vendors clearly and concisely of all the characteristics that must be included in the product or service to produce the results desired by the hospital.** Well written specifications will also serve as evidence that careful thought has been given to the intended use, need and specific characteristics of the items that are procured. Most purchase specifications employ some of the key elements on at least a limited scale. Requirements for polished stainless steel provide the element of composition. The size definition provides the element of physical dimension. A drawing to scale, if included, would more clearly define the physical dimensions. Concept of manufacture is specified as "welded by spot welding method."The element of expected performance should also be included. Hospitals buy most of products in supposedly sterile containers. Clinical laboratory should occasionally examine a package to see if it can grow a culture. Non sterile products probably should also be reviewed by the laboratory sometimes to determine just how much non sterile they are.

 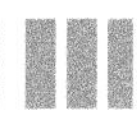

Purchase specifications are expensive to prepare and should be used wisely. Detailed specifications for capital equipment and repetitive high cost items are probably worth the effort involved.

Any system of purchase specification tends to accomplish three things:

1. Providing for specialized clinical review and comment prior to presentation to the standards committee.
2. Poor or unworkable recommendations should be deleted.
3. It tends to promote finalization of function and specification.

An individual who initiated the request or the concerned department head, who recommended some products to the standards committee, should be invited to participate in the committee discussion. This participation by requesting department tends to create a positive environment.

Use of an agenda is necessary. Agenda should be sent out along with copies of complete relevant documentation pertaining to the agenda items. Chairperson of the standardization sub committee must keep meetings running smoothly. One of the problems generally associated with committees is that the members prefer to be somewhere else. The by words here are punctuality, productivity and a sense of accomplishment.

Final aim is to be able to quantify the effectiveness of the committee. Committee's effectiveness can be measured quantitatively in terms of money saved. However, real effectiveness lies in prudent use of hospital's resources and improvement of the quality of patient care. Quality of patient care is the overall objective of a hospital.

Any system of purchase specifications requires updating from time to time. The process should reflect combined efforts of purchasing and the user. User involvement should be encouraged. The resourceful and imaginative purchaser will discover that the time spent on preparation and user involvement results in weaning the user away from brand name purchasing.

BRAND NAME

Use of a recognized brand name is an alternative to the detailed purchase specification.

Brand name specification is simple. Its advantages over purchase specifications include:

- Vendors readily understand the hospital's requirements.
- Users readily accept the product.
- Purchasers can be sure of obtaining the desired product or services.

Most important disadvantage of using brand names is that it eliminates competition at the manufacturer's level. In order to overcome this disadvantage, "acceptable brand names" list, which names manufacturers whose products have been accepted as meeting the required quality or performance standards of the hospital can be used. Use of a brand names list is particularly

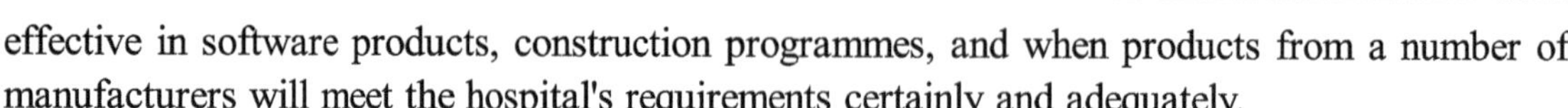

effective in software products, construction programmes, and when products from a number of manufacturers will meet the hospital's requirements certainly and adequately.

SPECIFYING BY CATALOGUE NUMBERS

Use of catalogue numbers or descriptions is quite similar to brand name specification. The desired quality is easily recognizable to the vendor whose catalogue is used; however it prohibits competition by other vendors. Catalogue descriptions can be effectively utilized provided the purchaser converts the description from the specific to the generic, by eliminating or modifying descriptions of features or parts/components that are relevant to only one manufacturer. Such conversions are facilitated by comparing all of the catalogue descriptions for the various manufacturers and extracting the most common and necessary features or specifications. Preparation of this type of specifications is time consuming. Hence, many of the purchasers may prefer this method to brand names

Some caution is to be exercised in the use of catalogue descriptions and brand name specification. **Addition of the phrase or "equivalent" to a catalogue number or brand name for bidding purposes is generally not advisable.** The term or "equivalent" is not clear or concise, and leaves the quality determination to the vendor. Listing all of the acceptable manufacturers and their associated product numbers is a much better way to communicate desired specification.

Quality specification by way of market grade is highly accepted and is most often used in the purchase of food commodity items. Market grades are established by either government agencies, or trade associations, or some independent commodity authorities. Use of market grades for such commodities is one method of establishing quality standards. However market grades, at best, are generalizations that may allow for some fluctuation in quality.

REAL VERSUS APPARENT QUALITY

Product quality needs to be defined within the general framework of cost, inventory, storage, deployment, disposal, processing, user training, and patient charges, and specific clinical needs. Selection of quality cost effective products obviously is related to the growing cost per patient care or prospective payment environment. In this economic environment, purchasing disposable supplies on a cost per unit basis, as opposed to a cost per use or cost per case basis is sometimes self defeating. While, at first glance, it may be difficult to distinguish between unit cost and cost per case, there often is a close and adverse connection. It is critical to distinguish between true and apparent costs. Supplies with a high defect rate, results in use of greater quantity, with excessive consumption perceived as a pilferage problem rather than one of quality. For example, a relatively high quality scalp vein needle had long been in use in a particular hospital. The materials management department, without consulting users, arbitrarily changed products. It obtained another manufacturer's needle at a unit cost 35 percent lower. Obviously they believed that needles were needles and a 35 percent saving was highly desirable. However, the most cursory observation of house staff and intravenous (IV) teams demonstrated that the less expensive unit was harder to

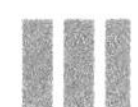

use and needle sharpness was decidedly inferior. Physicians and IV team members had to make three and four times as many attempts to place needles, causing great pain and tissue damage especially in infants and debilitated adults. They also used two to three times the number of scalp vein sets and even threw them away as an act of frustration as well as an effort to preserve sterile technique, when they failed to enter veins successfully. Many more of these needles were used per case than with the superior brand ignoring the cost of their time and lowered productivity. While the unit cost was 35 percent lower, the usage and throwaway rate climbed so rapidly that the actual cost of needles consumed to achieve successful placement increased by more than 55 percent. In another hospital which charged for administration of intravenous fluids, but did not charge the patients specifically for the number of scalp vein needles used, this clearly was a losing proposition. Had the patients been charged for each needle used, this increased expense would have been recovered in a cost reimbursement environment. There still would have been a net loss because of the increased time of placement, the greater investment in inventory, and the higher cost of storage and deployment besides causing more discomfort to the patients. In a **diagnosis related group** (DRG) cost per case environment, the hospital would have lost even more from the change. The lesson is clear in this case. Higher quality meant lower true cost in this case. Purchase price is not always the best index of cost. In this case, the concept of life cycle cost analysis should be applied to single-use items as well as to capital equipment in order to understand true cost. This requires full understanding of how a product is used, by whom, and under what conditions. Understanding true cost needs analytical thinking. It requires sharing of information and perspectives on a continuing basis among all participants, including purchasing, Materials Management and central supply departments besides clinical users. Communication about quality should not stop with the purchase but continue well after the new product has been placed in service. The impact of purchasing decisions is not always obvious to material managers. It is essential that follow up analyses be undertaken when vendors, models, or types of supplies are changed. Detailed analysis before decision making is common in some institutions. However evaluation of the long-term consequences of those changes is equally necessary. Selecting the optimal product involves much more than simply comparing prices. Purchasers choose between products based on their needs and budgets. Materials manager must similarly match the hospital's needs for performance, safety, and reliability with cost considerations against the available products. Equipped with such techniques and tools, the material manager can provide the hospital with the optimal product with less investment in time and with a far greater level of confidence that the best choice has been made.

PURCHASE DEPARTMENT'S ROLE IN QUALITY

- Purchase department must know exactly what is needed and pass on the required information to the vendors.
- Department must ensure that the vendor supplies the material strictly as per the specification.

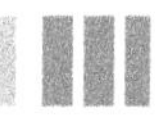

- Department must take such steps as are necessary to protect its hospital against financial loss from materials or parts, which do not meet the quality specifications.

In order to accomplish, the above responsibilities, buyer may have to seek the assistance of others. Quite often, it may seek the assistance of others outside the company, such as test houses for testing the quality of materials being developed or received.

The following points are important and deserve special mention:

- Buyer must ensure that information on quality is complete and unambiguous. This is part of his joint responsibility with the user.
- Internal control reference should be completely stated. For example, the work order or job order references would be necessary in many cases. Code numbers of parts or materials are important information required to be stated correctly.

VENDOR'S ROLE IN QUALITY

- He must know precisely the quality that the buyer wants.
- He must know exactly how to meet the quality specifications prescribed by the hospital.

DETERMINATION OF RIGHT QUANTITY

If a hospital requires 2000 bottles of IV fluid every week, it is necessary for the buyer to make available that much quantity every week. He might buy this once a week or once a month or once in a quarter or once in six months or even once a year provided shelf life is good. For each of these methods of buying, the costs incurred by the hospital will vary. Buying once in a year will result in excessive inventory, higher costs, obsolescence, need for additional storage facilities and investment blockage. On the other hand, if one week requirement is purchased, the unit cost may be high, shortages are likely to increase, more expediting will be necessitated, and relationship between buyer and supplier will need to be excellent. While determining the quantity, a large number of factors influence the decision making of the buyer. **The factors that influence right quantity can be broadly classified into two categories. i.e., internal and external factors**

Internal factors:

- Is the item needed at all, and at any rate is it really needed now?
- How much quantity is needed?
- What is the requirement profile? Is it regular, consistent or sporadic depending upon special requirement of customers?
- How much storage space is available?
- Financial considerations.

 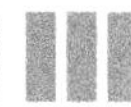

- Administrative effort to place an order. Ordering in small lots is ideal for inventory management but has any one taken care to see that adequate personnel and other facilities are available to under take this task of buying a large number of times?
- Shelf life of the item.
- Problems associated with obsolescence.

Above are factors just illustrative and not exhaustive. Each hospital will have its own peculiarities.

External factors:

- Availability
- Seasonality
- Market conditions
- Packing sizes: Quite often this is an important factor. The item may be packed in standard gross or a barrel and buying loose may be costlier.
- Export Import (Exim) policy
- Fluctuations in lead time i.e., the times taken by the suppliers to deliver the item after orders have been placed might vary.
- Price discounts for larger volumes.

In view of the foregoing, the quantity determination has a very large number of factors influencing a decision and the buyer necessarily has to consider all these aspects before determining the quantity to be purchased. **To have a clear understanding of how quantities come to be determined for purchase, one must start with demand forecasting.**

DEMAND FORECASTING

Forecasts of customer demand are fundamental to the operation of a business. Demand forecast is a link between the evaluation of external factors in the economy, which influences the business and management of company's internal affairs. Forecasts are also a basis for production, inventory control and purchasing. A forecast is by nature, an evaluation of incomplete evidence indicating what the future may look like. Thus no forecast can be expected to be entirely accurate. In production, planning and inventory control, the basic function of inventories and production flexibility is to absorb unexpected fluctuations in demand or departures from forecast. From past experience, one can estimate the degree of forecasting error and make provision for this.

There are many techniques of forecasting some of which are:

- Collective opinion
- Statistical extrapolation

- Economic forecasting
- Market research

Demand forecasts have to be drawn up in great detail. Essential details required to aid the material planning are product, packaging, quantity and the time when it is required. Time factor is particularly important and the requirement must preferably be broken up into months. One major factor to consider is the seasonality of production or availability of the item.

It is therefore, necessary to forecast how much of each product one would need during each month of the year. Once this exercise is completed, one has to make the material forecast. In order to meet the demand efficiently, it is necessary to establish the quantities of materials, the direct and indirect human resources, plant, machinery and facilities required in order to achieve desired output. Planning sets the framework, within which detailed schedules and inventory control schemes operate. The framework of planning should be designed to meet recognized hospital goals.

BILL OF MATERIALS (BOM)

After plans have been drawn up, a bill of material is prepared. Bill of materials is a list of materials required to produce one unit of a particular product or service. It may also be called a part list. As stated earlier, demand forecast is translated into materials schedule and the same is broken down into its constituent materials. By coupling bill of materials with services schedule, purchase manager can establish total requirements and the exact times when various materials will be actually required. **Essential information of a bill of material is as follows:**

Table 7.1 Format of Bill of Materials

S.No.	Name of material	Part no. or code no.	Quality (specifications)	Quantity	Time when required.

It should be noted that the last column of time is most important. It forms the basis of purchase planning and inventory controls.

ECONOMIC ORDER QUANTITY (EOQ)

It would be appreciated, the time wise quantities needed by production need not necessarily be the same as the time-wise quantities purchased. Several other considerations, other than production needs, would determine the quantities to be purchased. The objective is to keep the over all costs to a minimum. One of the most effective techniques for determination of quantities is "economic order quantity (EOQ)".

There are two major costs involved in purchasing viz.

1. Purchasing costs or acquisition cost
2. Inventory carrying cost

Ordering costs and carrying costs are two opposing costs. By balancing these two costs, the economic ordering quantity can be arrived at.

MATERIALS REQUIREMENT PLANNING (MRP)

With the advent of computers, it has become possible to use sophisticated techniques for determining how much quantity to buy or stock one of them is called, **"Materials Requirement Planning (MRP)."** It is a time phased priority planning method. The system calculates the requirement of materials and schedules of supply to meet the demand pattern.

RIGHT PRICE

Price knowledge for a buyer is based on experience and so familiarity with general price conditions. This does not necessarily imply quoted price on enquiries, nor does it imply that prices printed on catalogues are always right.

To determine the right price, it is essential for a buyer to be conversant with:

- Business trends
- Trade cycles
- Supply and demand
- How price advances and declines may be anticipated.
- Quantity discounts
- Many other factors making up the price.

On deciding the right price, a purchaser must take a broad and objective view. For example, lowest price quoted by a supplier whose deliveries are erratic or post sales services are poor, the lowest price is not a right price. As discussed earlier all the five rights must be seen as one composite whole. Each part must fit into the others like a **jig-saw puzzle.** A purchaser must, therefore, examine the prices quoted by different suppliers and attempt to determine which price in combination with the quality features of the product and the service aspects plus the relationship with the suppliers, will afford greatest value for money.

PRICE TERMS

Before we can fully appreciate the concept of a right price, it would be desirable to have a fairly good knowledge as to how price is made up and what are the kinds or type of prices one is

 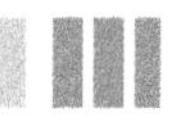

offered when one is making purchases. Price offered may take various forms. Some of the most common terms are described below:

1. **Firm Price**

   Price quoted by vendor will be valid for the period of the contract, which may be 3, 6, 9 or 12 months and may be extended by mutual consent.

2. **Price in effect at the time of dispatch**

   The price is not firm but will be the market price quoted on the day of dispatch. Commodities like foods, vegetables, meat and beverages are items whose prices fluctuate almost daily. In many cases, the price is fixed by government, for example, petroleum products or drugs.

3. **Cost Plus**

   This type of agreement is entered into for construction or service contracts, or in sub-contracting for specialized items. The contractor is given a fixed percentage as compensation or profit over his costs (material, labour, overheads, taxes, tooling etc.). It pre supposes that the buyer will have full access to the supplier's accounts.

4. **Guaranteed Maximum Price**

   It is a cost plus contract but the final price will not exceed a guaranteed maximum.

5. **Price Adjustments**

   Various types of price adjustments can be agreed upon in a purchase contract. Some of these are discussed below:

   a. **Escalation Clause**

      Economic conditions vary considerably and price fluctuations are literally the order of the day. An escalation clause is intended to protect the seller and buyer against the risks of such changes in price. An escalation clause provides for a price variation in accordance with an agreed formula or agreed condition based on materials and labour pricc indiccs.

   b. **Price Decline Protection Clause**

      This is opposite of the escalation clause and it is intended to protect the buyer when prices of materials, or labour decline.

PAYMENT TERMS

These might also vary from case to case and thereby affect the ultimate cost to an organization:

1. **Cash on delivery:** No credit is allowed in this case.
2. **Pre payment discounts:** Discounts would be available if advance payment is made for the purchase, say discount @1percent for 30 days advance payment.

3. **Cash discounts, or prompt payment terms,** result in a lower net cost to the hospital. The accounting department is responsible for meeting payment terms, but purchasers should be sure to include the terms on the purchase order and to advise accounts section. This can be simply accomplished by using a rubber stamp stating "discount terms" on accounting's copy of the purchase order. Purchasers should also clearly define when the discount period begins. The notation of "2.50 percent 15 days; net 30" is less than adequate. A more appropriate statement would be "a 2.50 percent discount will be taken for invoice payment within 15 days of receipt of merchandise. Net amount will however be paid within 30 days." As a general rule, purchasing practitioners should include this type of statement on the hospital quotation form and allow the vendor to modify it if desired. It never hurts to ask!

4. **Consignment terms:** This is frequently used in retailing. Buyer in this case is a usually a trader and he pays the price of the goods to the seller after he has sold the goods. A pharmaceutical company may, for example, agree on consignment terms of payment to a firm of druggists and chemists. Payment may be made, in this case, after the goods have been sold.

5. **Progressive payment terms:** In this case, payment is made in instalments. For example, a company may sell a refrigerator to a customer who pays the price in 12 equal instalments (Equated Monthly Instalments) or (EMI's). In such cases, the company may charge a higher price in order to cover the cost of financing the credit.

6. **Price schedules:** Price may vary with quantity purchased, size of shipment, quality or grade specified, container size, level of distribution and the season (for seasonal products).

7. **Price variation with order size:** This is commonly referred to as quantity discounts. Because of larger orders, the seller is able to obtain economies in production, packaging, billing, selling expenses, etc. He is prepared to transfer a part of these economies to the buyer.

8. **Discounts:** In the healthcare marketplace, usually two types of discounts are available quantity and cash. Quantity discounts are of two types:

   a. Specific quantities in connection with a single purchase. Quantity discounts on a particular purchase refer to the fact that the larger the quantity ordered, the lower the price per unit. One must also consider possible impact of a large quantity on inventory costs in evaluating this type of discount. An increased quantity discount will lower the unit cost, but it may increase holding costs, thus resulting in an uneconomical purchase over the long term.

   b. Discounts involving quantities estimated to cover the hospital's requirements for a specific period of time. Quantity discounts covering a specified period of time are advantageous for both the hospital and the vendor. The vendor is sure of the hospital's business for a specific period of time, say 6 or 12 months and for an estimated quantity. The hospital has some assurance of a reliable source of supply at a good price for the same specified time period.

9. **Price variation with savings in loading and transportation costs:** For example, a full wagon load or full truck load will be cheaper than transportation as smalls. Similarly, transportation in bulk is cheaper than transportation in packages. For example transporting oil in steel or synthetic drums would be far costlier than transporting it in a rail tank wagon or road tanker.
10. **Price variation with container size and type:** Quantities obtained in 205 litre steel drums would be cheaper than five litre cans. Packing in gross would be cheaper than packs of a dozen. Delivery in returnable containers would be cheaper than otherwise, etc.
11. **Price variation with level of distributive function e.g.,** A company may offer different prices to original equipment manufacturers:

    For example, a tyre company may offer a special discounted rate to a car manufacturer.

    - A wholesaler
    - A distributor
    - A broker
    - A dealer or
    - A direct consumer: For example, a pharmaceutical firm may offer a special discounted price to hospitals who consume regularly in bulk.
12. **Other elements in Price are:**
    - Transportation cost: This will vary according to mode of transport.
    - Taxes: Customs and excise duties, municipal taxes (entry tax or octroi duty), goods and services tax (GST), value added tax (VAT), etc., all add to the price. An excellent knowledge of tax laws is necessary for every purchasing executive.
    - Insurance: This again will vary depending upon the material, the packaging, the mode of transport etc.
    - Packaging and materials handling costs: Packaging has a direct bearing on the mode of transport and, of course, on the material being packed.
    - Incidental purchasing costs: There are many kinds of such costs e.g., follow up costs, pre delivery inspection etc.

Determining Right Price

Three basic methods of determining the right price are:

1. Published price lists (with various types of discounts): many manufacturers publish periodically the price lists of the various goods produced by them. Most of these show the prices for

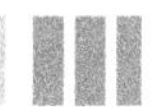

various types of packing sizes or discounts for varying terms of payment and also discounts
2. for various types of purchasers i.e., wholesalers, retailers, consumers etc.,

3. Obtaining competitive bids or quotations for individual specifications.

Negotiated price for specific jobs or for specific materials.

In the case of last two cases cited, it is assumed that there exists a competitive market for the materials that are required. Very often it may not be the case and the specifications may require specialized manufacture, the ability for which rests with only one or few suppliers. Ab-initio negotiations will have to take place in deciding the price of such materials.

Many factors influence price and these have to be properly evaluated. Some of them are:

Economic conditions: Have a great effect on price, the buyer should, therefore, equip himself with information on such conditions. For examples: inflation, recession, business cycles etc.

Price paid by competitors: It will, often be prudent to find out the prices paid by the other buyers of the supplier's products. A comparison of these prices would enable the buyer to determine whether he is paying a fair price.

Quantity: Purchase of larger quantity generally represented a saving compared to smaller purchases. However, the inventory carrying costs would increase with higher quantities.

PREMIUM PRICES FOR NON PREMIUM PRODUCTS

Purchase department for objective evaluation has to surmise ways measure within their own available resources. Sometimes they have to rely on the suppliers.

General tendency among hospital suppliers always prefer to supply premium products as against standard identical products. Generally premium products or branded products command higher share of market. In this context, it is worth remembering **Dean Ammer's** observations on Premium Prices for Non premium Products in his book on Purchasing and Materials for Healthcare institutions. **Dean Ammer observed** that "only the price differs and the highest priced product usually commands the largest market share there are abundant examples of this type. One hospital discovered that it paid $25.42 per 100, 500 mg capsules for Wyeth's brand of ampicillin. But if it simply bought ampicillin made Wyeth without specifying the particular brand, its price was as low as $8.27 for the same product. Interestingly, while **Wyeth and Ayerst** are both divisions of American Home Products and presumably share manufacturing facilities and research capability, the Ayerst brand of the same product was priced at $25.42."

Another example of **Dean Ammer** was "A hospital made a study of ECG probes. It discovered that at least ten allegedly different brands were all made by Texas Instruments Company. These competing products were sold at widely varying prices even though quality was

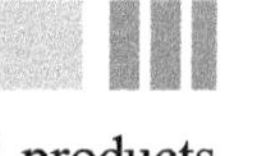

almost identical. Interestingly, prices charged by competing manufacturers of identical products are often inversely related to market share. The highest priced product enjoys the largest share of the market even though it may be identical with a lower priced product that has a much smaller market share." **Thus, the buyer who wants quality need not really pay a premium for it.**

RIGHT TIME

Importance of purchasing timing depends to a great extent upon type of market in which purchases are proposed to be made. Timing becomes more critical as markets become less stable as risks associated with fluctuating price increase. If materials are purchased in stable markets, the choice of timing policies is based primarily on operating factors within the firm, such as administrative costs, indirect material costs, and operating costs.

Right time has the following aspects:

1. Firstly it determines when exactly the delivery is required.
2. Purchasing procedure is to be initiated so as to obtain the requirements about the right time within the short safety margin.
3. Arranging delivery much earlier than the required delivery time or after stock out is not efficient procurement. Former means overstocking and avoidable blocking up of working capital, while the latter implies loss of production and is known as stock out cost.
   - In case of requirements of materials needed for special jobs, purchase section should be given reasonable time.
   - In case of project buying, various materials including capital equipment may be required at different times during the project. In such cases, PERT/CPM networks are extremely useful.

Following basic timing policies can be employed:

1. Purchase according to current requirements (one to three months supply in most cases).
2. Purchase according to market conditions, which includes:
   - Hand to mouth buying, normally covering up to three to six days operating requirements.
   - Forward buying, covering approximately three to twelve month's requirements.
   - Speculative buying, defined as buying in quantities exceeding foreseeable operating requirements. This may also be for hedging.

In unstable markets, selection of timing policies for materials purchased is based largely on the potential costs which can arise from external fluctuations in market price and material availability. In fluctuating markets, a buyer may attempt to use market price fluctuations to his advantage, or he may attempt to reduce the financial risk resulting from price fluctuations. In the former case, major techniques employed are the deliberate volume timing of purchases and the financial budget of purchases. In the latter case, while attempting to reduce market risk, a buyer can use the time budgeting technique, or he can hedge his purchase if a futures market exists for the material. In order to make an intelligent decision concerning the use of specific policies and techniques, the buyer must identify and carefully study the economic factors which influence the market in which he deals. This involves an estimate and forecast of the specific and general economic conditions and a subsequent prediction of resultant activity in the market under study. The purchaser's final decision is generally based on the analysis of both qualitative and statistical data. A purchasing department cannot attain full management status or make its full contribution to the hospital unless it correctly determines the right time to buy. This can be accomplished only when the purchasing department uses the tools of the economist and the forecaster along with his other resources. Inventory control measures such as MRP-1, MRP-II, and JIT concepts can be made use of to arrive at the determination of the right time.

RIGHT SOURCE

The five rights of purchasing are to a significant extent independent of each other. However, selection of the right source can have great influence on the attainment of the other four rights. In purchasing process, the single most important step is choosing right supplier. Hospital purchasing managers often find themselves confronted with no opportunity for any decision to be made. User brand preferences make it impossible for the purchase department to invite bids from competing manufacturers or vendors. The choice of supplier can be made only at distributor or wholesaler level for many purchases of both drugs and medical, surgical supplies. This in fact greatly simplifies the problem of selecting a supplier. Quality is determined by the manufacturer and the purchase is often not made if the item is not in stock for immediate delivery. Hence price becomes the only factor the buyer can take into account when making a purchase decision. Thus, the purchasing process is ultimately reduced to soliciting a reasonable number of suppliers in the area; asking each of them two questions: what is the price and do you have the merchandise on hand? The supplier quotes the lowest price and also has the item in stock automatically gets the order. In more complicated cases, there is a recurring need for the item. While the buyer could theoretically canvas the market each time he makes a purchase, it is not a considered a good practice. The bidding process is costly in itself. In addition, more advantageous terms may be obtained if the supplier knows he is not quoting on a one shot purchase but on a requirement that might sustain his business for a period of several months or even years. With other purchases, the supplier can really influence either quality or availability of the product or service that is sought. For example, the supplier of a seemingly simple purchase like the laying a pipeline at wash area may or may not skip on quality or fail to complete the job on the date that it is promised. In such cases, prices of competing suppliers cannot really be compared until the purchaser is able to assess supplier quality and delivery capabilities in a reasonably rational manner.

Customer goodwill has long been recognized as a valuable asset. Supplier goodwill is an equally valuable asset. However, its importance is still to be fully recognized in healthcare industry

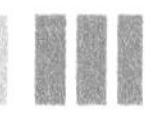

especially in India. Unforeseen emergencies inevitably occur in business. As a result of this, materials must be expedited; quantities increased or decreased, or returned if profit margins are to be protected. The goodwill of vendors is essential if these and similar adjustments are to be made with minimum expense and hassle.

There are many factors, which must be properly evaluated before the right vendor can be selected. When selection starts from scratch, information can be gained about prospective vendors from trade registers, directories, trade journals, the yellow pages of the telephone book, a file of mailing list, salesmen, trade exhibits, purchasing associations, and other purchasing departments.

INVESTIGATION

Most purchasing managers prefer a known evil to an unknown one. All other factors being reasonably equal, they rightly prefer to award business to suppliers with whom they have had favourable experiences rather than to take a chance on any new ones. However, loyalty is a misplaced virtue in purchasing when there is no rational basis for it. In fact, excessive vendor loyalty leads automatically to suspicion of corruption. If past experience with an existing supplier has not been very satisfactory, or if other suppliers quote lower prices, then purchasing manager should seriously consider awarding business to a newcomer. If the purchase is a relatively unimportant one, the purchasing manager might simply give the new supplier a trial order and hope for the best. In such cases, little may be lost if the supplier fails to deliver merchandise of the desired quality on schedule. If the purchase is more important, some investigation of the supplier's antecedents and capabilities should be made. There are limits to how much time and money should go into this process.

However purchasing manager should consider the following:

1. Supplier's reputation with his customers.
2. Supplier resources and management.
3. Supplier's financial soundness.
4. Plant visits can disclose such facts as adequacy and care of equipment, systems used to control quality and care of equipment, systems used to control quality and cost, morale of personnel, and competence of technical staff, the operating staff, and general management. From these facts, the buyer can form a realistic judgement concerning the ability of the vendor to supply his company.
5. Knowledge of a vendor's financial condition can often save time and efforts of further investigation. It is not unusual for small business to aspire unwisely to large orders. Financing such orders often exceeds the capacity of the firm's working capital and borrowing ability. Financial soundness can be judged by calling for the audited financial statements mainly, the balance sheet and profit and loss accounts for the past 2 or 3 years. Reliance can also be placed on banker's opinion

6. Service is often an abstract value; nevertheless, it is an important consideration in vendor selection. Service is usually measured by the vendor's compliance with the quantity and quality conditions of the order, whether he delivers on time, and whether competent technical assistance is provided as and when needed. Price can be easily measured. Quality and service are harder to quantify. Industrial purchasers frequently measure them by recording each shipment from a supplier in their computers and calculating vendor ratings that objectively measure performance. The purchasing manager can do almost as well by keeping data on each supplier concerning each failure in quality or delivery that is important enough to be called to his attention. In every case, he must warn the supplier that such failures are being watched and recorded. Such records can not only be a guide to a more rational decision-making on a future purchase but can also be used to encourage improvement, even by suppliers whose overall records continue to be satisfactory. Vendors who facilitate stockless purchasing provide additional service to the buying organization. In such cases, their products could be obtained under weekly or semimonthly shelf replacements.

7. Company size of the supplier is also an important consideration in selecting vendors. Large companies usually have better infrastructure but their customer relationships sometimes suffer from lack of personal attention.

8. A buyer must always aim to have multiple suppliers for all vital inputs. The fewer the number of vendors, the greater will be the risk of losing continuity of supply.

9. Reciprocity and trade relations continue to play an important part in vendor selection. In fact, increased national and international competition, increased product diversification, the decentralization of management and the complexity of management decision making are causing an increased use of reciprocity and trade relations. In evaluating the effects of reciprocity, management should be aware of two important considerations.

   - First, is a kind concerning materials and components used in the firm's products?
   - Second, firms selling standardized, highly competitive products are more susceptible to the pressures of reciprocity than firms selling nonstandard, non competitive items.

10. Buying locally is sometimes an important factor in vendor selection. Most buyers prefer to patronize local sources whenever possible. Local buying normally results in quicker deliveries, better service, and greater ease in resolving misunderstandings.

11. The choice between dealing directly with manufacturers and dealing through a distributor is often a difficult one. The critical factor in this choice is not the distributor's location. Rather it is the function he performs. If the buying company can perform the functions of distribution at a lower cost than the distributor, then purchase should usually be made directly from the manufacturer, if possible.

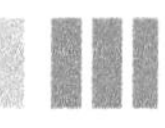

12. Ethics are most important when it comes to vendor selection. Expensive gifts, kickbacks, nepotism, bribery and personal friendships have no place in a properly administered purchasing department. Board of trustee conflict of interest is sometimes witnessed in case of local suppliers used for dairy products, meat products, pharmaceuticals, office supplies, and equipment. Vendor evaluation must take care of these contention aspects. Many healthcare purchasers inherit suppliers from their predecessors or from built in relationships with management. There may be good reasons to continue with these sources.
13. Foreign buying is increasing. The world is shrinking, time-communication wise. As the underdeveloped countries progressively industrialize, increased world trade is inevitable.

SUMMARY

Principle objectives of a purchase department can be summarized as the procurement of materials or supplies of the right quality, in the right quantity and at the right time, from the right supplier, at the right price. These five Rights have meanings and significance far beyond their dictionary meanings.

Quality has been defined as the "power to accomplish or the compatibility or ability to do certain things." The starting point for determining quality is end use. Quality of materials has a direct relationship with quality of services rendered by the hospital. In other words, if materials of inappropriate quality were used, it would mean:

- That, if quality is higher than what is needed, patient service might have features which are unnecessary for management of a disease and as a consequence of it, the cost of patient care might be more than what they should be. As a result, competitiveness in the market might be diminished!
- That, if quality is lower than what is needed, patient service would be too poor and though it might be cheaper, it might entail customer dissatisfaction and also not stand up to competition!

Both these situations are harmful to the interest of the hospital. Specifications are required for providing to the vendors a clear understanding of what the hospital is looking for, as well as a basis for inspection following delivery. Although a quality specification cannot be written out in detail on every purchase order or agreement, it is an absolute necessary part of every purchase agreement.

We can define right quality as totality of features and characteristics (technical and economic) of a product that bear upon its ability to satisfy a given need.

Certain basic facts about quality which are worth remembering are 1. Judgement on quality cannot be delegated to the supplier, 2. Defining quality by words like "good quality", "reliable", etc., are meaningless. What is good for the supplier might be totally unacceptable to the buyer, 3. Inviting three or more quotations does not guarantee quality, 4. Quality is not measured by price. A material or equipment costing more does not mean that it has better quality or assured quality, 5. Right quality means "for the purpose" i.e., the minimum

 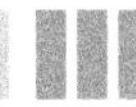

acceptable quality, 6. Availability is a practical requirement, and 7. The buyer constantly seeks alternatives and substitutes.

Determination of right quantity is one of the major tasks faced by the buyer. Right quantity is arrived at taking into consideration the demand forecasting. The factors that influence right quantity can be broadly classified into two categories i.e., internal and external. The various techniques that are used to arrive at the right quantity are: 1. economic order quantity, 2. Materials requirement planning, 3. manufacturing resources planning, etc.

Price may be defined as the sum of money at which a thing is valued or the value which a seller sets on his goods in the market. Price knowledge for a buyer is based on experience and familiarity with general price conditions. This does not necessarily imply quoted price on enquiries, or price printed on catalogues.

Right price is most important from buyer's point of view. Very often, the word price is qualified by terms like best price, lowest price, most economical price etc., which makes the subject more complicated for a buyer who is seeking the "right price". Theoretically, right price is a suggested figure at which seller can deliver his goods at a profit and which the buyer pays, expecting to receive full value in use or manufacture.

Broadly speaking there are three basic methods of determining the right price: 1. Published price lists (with various types of discounts); many manufacturers publish periodically the price-lists of the various goods produced by them, 2. Quotations or bids on individual specifications, 3. Negotiated price for specific jobs or for specific materials. Various factors influence price and these have to be properly evaluated. Some of them are: 1. Economic conditions, 2. Price paid by competitors, 3. Quantity, and 4. Transportation costs.

Right time has two aspects, firstly it determines, when exactly the delivery is required and when the purchasing procedure should be initiated so as to obtain the requirements about the right time with the short margin of safety. The importance of purchase timing depends to a great extent upon the type of market in which the purchase is made.

Right timing depends to a great extent upon type of market in which purchases are proposed to be made. Timing is more critical in markets wherein price is fluctuating. Right time has the following aspects,

1. When exactly the delivery is required?
2. When the purchasing procedure is to be initiated so as to obtain the requirements about the right time within the short safety margin.

Arranging delivery much earlier than the required delivery time or after stock-out is not efficient procurement.

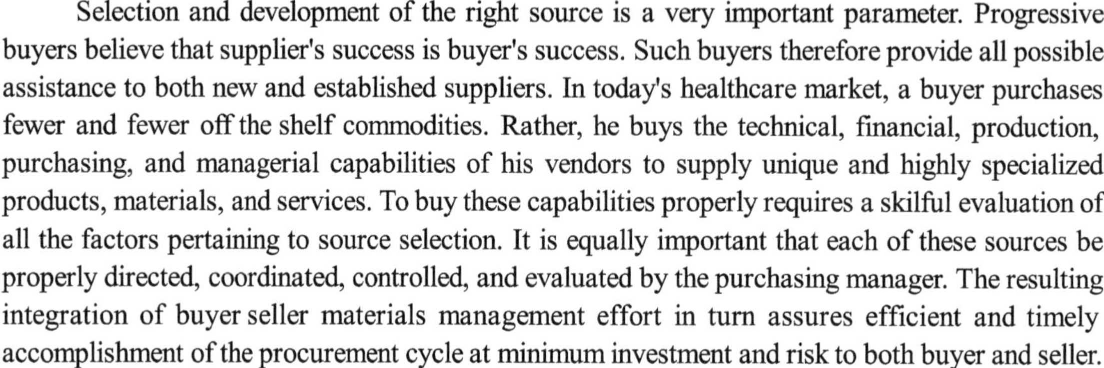

Selection and development of the right source is a very important parameter. Progressive buyers believe that supplier's success is buyer's success. Such buyers therefore provide all possible assistance to both new and established suppliers. In today's healthcare market, a buyer purchases fewer and fewer off the shelf commodities. Rather, he buys the technical, financial, production, purchasing, and managerial capabilities of his vendors to supply unique and highly specialized products, materials, and services. To buy these capabilities properly requires a skilful evaluation of all the factors pertaining to source selection. It is equally important that each of these sources be properly directed, coordinated, controlled, and evaluated by the purchasing manager. The resulting integration of buyer seller materials management effort in turn assures efficient and timely accomplishment of the procurement cycle at minimum investment and risk to both buyer and seller.

For ensuring excellent patient care, all known parameters such as right price, right quality, right contractual terms, right source, right materials, right time, right place, right mode of transport and right attitude have to be considered jointly and severally.

REVIEW QUESTIONS

1. The 'Panchsheel' of purchasing **comprises** of 5R's - explain.
2. The 'Panchsheel' of purchasing **compromise** of 5R's - explain.
3. Does lowest price imply right price or does highest price imply right quality? Discuss
4. What are usual price terms, price adjustments and payment terms practiced in hospital purchasing?
5. Describe the technique of cost and price analysis and state how such an analysis helps in arriving at right price?
6. The importance of purchasing timing to a great extent depends upon type of market in which purchases are proposed to be made. Discuss
7. What is the role of purchase department in quality explain the terms, reals and apparent quality in health care institutions.
8. Write short notes on
   a) Right quality
   b) Right price
   c) Right source
   d) Right time
   e) Price terms
   f) Premium price for non premium products
   g) price ajdustments

PART - II

8

Chapter

Negotiations in Purchasing

Contents

CHAPTER - 8

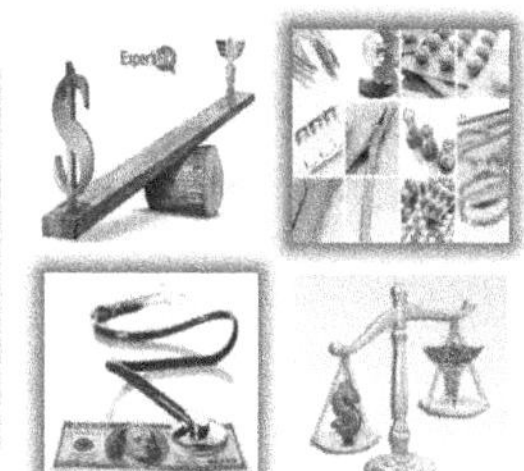

Negotiations in Purchasing

To Get To The Promised Land You Have To Negotiate Your Way Through The Wilderness.

- Herb Cohen

INTRODUCTION

Life is full of negotiations. In fact, the world we live in is one giant negotiating table where nobody can be a bystander. An individual negotiates with several others: family members, colleagues, competitors, entities with big names like the establishment or the power structure. We may like it or not but our participation is inevitable. **Negotiating is a field of knowledge and endeavour that focuses on gaining the favour of people from whom, we want things like money, love, prestige, status, security, freedom, justice, and recognition.** Some of us know better than others, how to get what we want. In industry or commercial establishments, negotiation is one of the most important as well as one of the most interesting parts of purchasing. In industry and at most levels of government, the term negotiation frequently, causes misunderstandings. In industry, negotiation is sometimes confused with haggling and price chiseling. In government, negotiation is frequently visualized as a nefarious means of avoiding competitive bidding and awarding large contracts surreptitiously to favoured vendors or organizations. Negotiation is a very personal art and skill. We must develop our own style: the one that suits our personality and situation at hand. Good preparation and proper technique can make negotiation a pleasant experience from which both parties gain what they want. In fact, negotiation is a delicate art of give and take. Indian industry is gradually switching over to the concepts of MRP II with an ultimate goal of achieving just-in-time management etc. In such a situation, buyers have to interact with the vendors more frequently and devote more time to negotiations.

Suppliers sometimes not only get sloppy on quality and delivery but also try to boost prices and profit margins. The price that is paid can be influenced by the purchasing manager within limits. The competitive bidding process may reduce prices. Negotiation may reduce them further. Competitive bidding can be handled impersonally with written bids. Negotiation inevitably involves face-to-face or at least telephone to telephone or E-mail confrontation between buyer and seller. It is thus a time consuming, expensive process and should be used selectively.

Typical buyer's day in MRP environment is depicted in the following Figure 8.1.

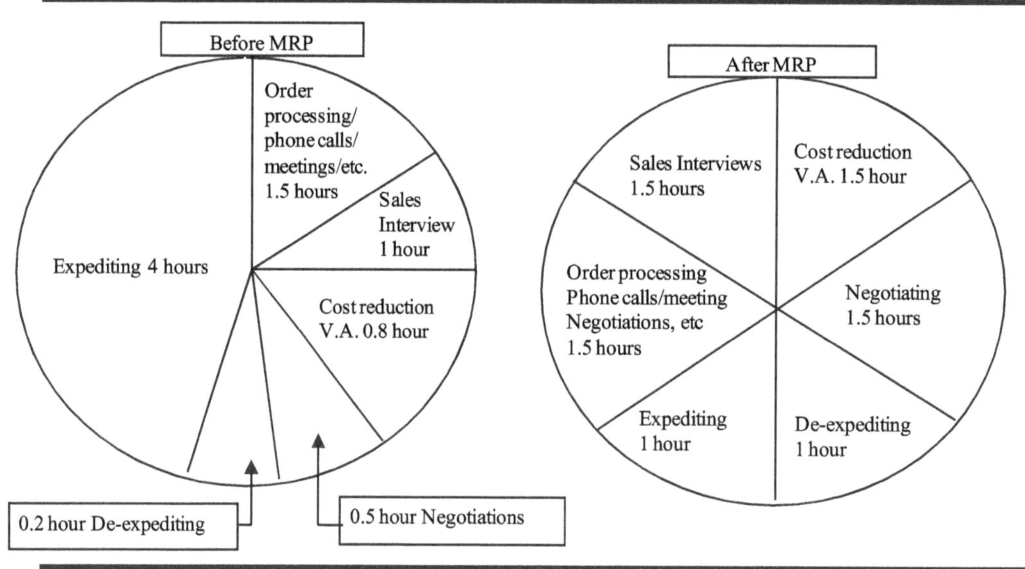

Figure 8.1 Typical Buyer's Day in MRP-II Environment

(Source: G. Bevis, Closed-Loop MRP at the Tennant Company George Bevis Co., Wayzata, Minnesota, U.S.A)

DEFINITIONS OF NEGOTIATION

The word negotiation is derived from Latin and civil laws, and means trading or deliberation leading to an agreement.

Dean Ammer states that the buyer and seller carry on an animated conversation exchanging either insults or compliments.

According to **Walte E Willets,** negotiation in purchasing terminology, is the technique or art of arriving at an understanding with a vendor on the essentials of a contract including specifications, terms, prices and delivery; it requires, a great deal of skill, judgement, and tact to be a good negotiator.

US Air Force defines negotiation in the following manner: Procurement by negotiation is an art of arriving at a common understanding, through bargaining on the essentials of contract; such as delivery, specifications, price, and payment terms, etc. Because of interrelation of these factors with many others, it is a difficult art and requires the exercise of executive judgement, tact and common sense. Negotiator should know where to be firm and where he may make permissive concessions in price or other terms.

Negotiation can also be defined as proposing terms of accommodation with respect to purchase or sale of goods or services. Negotiation should not be considered as haggling over the

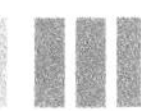

price, as is common in many open air markets. Nor it is an attempt by the buyer to play one vendor against another. Negotiation is an art and technique, a process, of arriving at a common understanding through bargaining on the essentials of a purchase, such as specifications, delivery, price, and terms. Every purchaser needs good negotiation skills and should begin to learn proper techniques early. The lack of sound negotiation skill by practitioners is the primary reason why many department heads act as quasi purchasing agents, since they feel as skilled as the purchasing agent who has little, if any, formal training in this critical discipline. **The negotiation process should be used selectively because it is often lengthy and very costly.**

PURPOSE OF NEGOTIATION

The mode of purchase determines vendor selection and price fixation in a competitive bidding environment. Negotiation is another important approach to price determination.

Apart from price, the buyer resorts to negotiation when:

- Requirement is so urgent that there is no time for competitive bidding.
- The number of bidders is few and the value of purchase is high.
- Willingness to compete is lacking.
- High buyer and seller uncertainty.
- Buying production or service capabilities.
- Product or service is neither standard nor a commercial one.
- Prices are fixed (because of patent, collusion etc.); it is possible to wangle only fringe concessions from the suppliers.
- For finalizing various terms and conditions of contact such as delivery, packing, insurance and so on.
- It is impractical to draft exact specifications or detailed descriptions of certain supplies or services.
- Price escalation or de escalation clause is to be incorporated.
- Supplies and services are from only one source.
- Variations in quantities being purchased are expected.
- Additional amount of extra work on a project is relatively small and may not be of interest to contractors other than those already at work.
- Price as it relates to the terms and conditions of a competitive bid or proposal.
- Changes in delivery points (FOB), method of delivery, or packaging.
- Termination of a previously agreed contract is desired or considered necessary.

- Overhead rates for cost plus contracts are to be finalized.
- Validity of prices is in question.
- No acceptable quotations are received from competent vendors.
- Production is interrupted frequently because of numerous changes in orders.
- Business risk and costs cannot be accurately predetermined. It is expected that if buyers seek competitive bids under these circumstances, excessively high prices are likely to result.
- As a matter of abundant caution, suppliers factor every conceivable contingency into their bids. In reality, all those contingencies are not likely to occur. Hence, the buyer is likely to pay for something which may not be received.
- Tooling and set up costs represent a large percentage of supplier's total costs. These tools are useful only for specific job and have limited use.
- Buyer is contracting for a portion of seller's production capacity rather than for a product. In buying production capacity, the buyer's objective is not only to attain production capability, but also to acquire such control over it as may be needed to improve the product and production processes. This type of control can achieved only after negotiation and the voluntary cooperation of suppliers.

In all the above cases, negotiations are essential; and in each case, quality and service are as important as price.

ERRONEOUS BELIEFS ASSOCIATED WITH NEGOTIATIONS

There are number of erroneous beliefs associated with negotiations. Among them the most common are:

- **Negotiation is a win-lose confrontation**

  Negotiations differ, from ball game or war where only one side wins and the other loses. In a successful negotiation, both sides win something, seldom equally divided. Invariably, one side wins more than the other side, as it would be in business. Skill merits rewards.

- **The idea of negotiation is to overpower the other party.**

  The objective of negotiation is not to win an argument, but to reach an agreement. It should not be considered as a series of skirmishes over isolated issues. Who wins an individual point, is unimportant.

- **Each negotiation is an independent isolated transaction.**

  Purchasing executive must optimize not only today's purchase but also should not jeopardize his tomorrow's negotiating power. A cardinal principle is that both buyer and seller have got to benefit from transactions. Only one sided gains impair overall purchasing efficiency.

OBJECTIVES OF NEGOTIATION

There are five major objectives common to all purchasing negotiations:

1. To obtain fair and reasonable price for the quality specified.
2. To get the supplier to perform the contract on time.
3. To exert some control over the contract performance.
4. To obtain supplier's maximum co-operation to buyer's company.
5. To develop and maintain sound and continuing relationships with competent suppliers.

The above objectives necessitate negotiations, before the deal is struck for purchase of material. The primary function of each negotiation is to discuss the terms and conditions of purchase so that both parties are clear in their obligations.

Factors Influencing Objectives of Negotiations

Major factors that influence the objectives of negotiation are:

- **Fair and reasonable price:** Many factors have to be considered to establish fair and reasonable price. If it is a standard item and is readily available ex-stock, there may not be any need for price negotiation. Usually, the terms and conditions of supply of such items are well defined and negotiations may be centred on quantity discounts, staggered deliveries and payment terms etc.

- **Fixed price:** If a vendor reduces his price for one customer, he might have to reduce it for all his other customers too. This makes price cut extremely expensive and very difficult to negotiate. In some cases the price of an item is legally fixed by a regulatory agency. It may even be illegal for the seller to reduce price under those conditions.

When dealing with a monopoly source in seller's market under scarce availability conditions, the buyer may be forced to agree to whatever terms and conditions are imposed by the seller, especially if he adopts take it or leave it attitude. Sellers run the risk of competition in the long run as the buyers always try to develop new sources, who can deliver materials at better prices. In negotiations, short term or immediate advantages gained almost certainly end up with disappointments and retaliation at the earliest opportunity.

PROCESS AND TECHNIQUES OF NEGOTIATION

Process and techniques of negotiation involve the following steps.

1. Planning
2. Understanding buyer's needs
3. Understanding suppliers' needs

4. Understanding suppliers' systems

5. Recalling what had happened during earlier negotiations

1. Planning

Sufficient time must be allowed for planning. That is to ensure effectiveness in any activity, but particularly in negotiation. It does take time to do proper planning. A wise approach is to identify issues or items directly related to managers' primary operating objectives or, in case of purchasing, items that have the greatest dollar impact, and concentrate their efforts on them.

A materials manager might decide to handle key negotiations personally, delegate others to the director of purchasing, some others to specific buyers, and also some to the concerned user department heads such as the pharmacy or **stores, processing, and distribution (SPD).** The materials manager can also provide overall coordination of total effort without having to conduct all negotiations personally.

Negotiation process starts with the preparation or pre negotiation planning stage. Before that, it is important to set specific goals of what is to be achieved. Specific needs should be expressed, such as terms and conditions, delivery time, and FOB. Without defining needs in specific terms, the buyer's ability to prepare for and conduct negotiations will be seriously impaired. Once the needs are defined, one should establish a level of expectation to achieve during the actual negotiations. Negotiators who set high levels of expectation e.g., lower prices; better delivery, higher quality etc. tend to be more successful than negotiators with lower levels of expectation. One must aim high, and once the level of expectation is set, make all possible efforts to stay with it. The goal of planning for a negotiation is to document both short and long term objectives.

The following outline will assist a negotiator in pulling together the information necessary to be prepared for the negotiation.

2. Understanding buyer's needs

- What are you buying and why (custom product or a commodity)?
- What is the time frame for delivery (soon or next year)?
- What is the length of time the contract will cover?
- What is the technology level of the item you are buying (low or high)?
- What is the driving force behind your position?
- What, if any, external forces affect your position?
- What equals success?
- What is acceptable?

 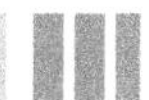

3. **Understanding suppliers' needs**

- Where do they rank in their industry?
- What are your counterparts needs (market share or profit)?
- Are they interested in booking orders or shipping product?
- Is your business the key to their businesses?
- Do they make products for your competitors too?
- Do you know what equaled success for them in the past?

4. **Understanding suppliers' systems**

- How is their pricing decided?
- Are you buying their main product or a secondary one?
- How sensitive are their costs to changes in volume, labour costs, material costs, or process yields? Are any of these changing?
- How is the product manufactured?

5. **Recalling what had happened during earlier negotiations**

- What were the results?
- Will you be negotiating with the same people? If not, what do you need to know about the new players?
- What issues did you agree on?
- What issues did you disagree on?
- What have been the rules of the game?
- What rules would you like to change this time around?

In answering these questions, a buyer would have generated a great deal of information on what you are negotiating, your goals for the negotiation, and what you are likely to encounter during the negotiation. Depending on the rupee value of procurement and the importance of this purchase to your company, it may be worthwhile to analyze several items. Prices are subject to many influences and are determined by competition among buyers and sellers of each item as well as external factors such as business cycles, seasonality of availability or manufacture or competitive strengths and bargaining capabilities.

After specific needs and expectations are defined, one can begin to define clearly the specific goals to be achieved. Two important criteria should be remembered in setting goals. Goals must be realistic and supportable. Even goals set with a high expectation level can be supported but they may not be as supportable as lower goals. Once goals have been established, they may have to be

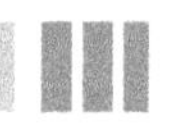

reviewed and approved by hospital administration and, sometimes, by the board. This is because of budget limitations or levels of commitment imposed by administration. Typical examples include Rs. 1,00,000 value or only items specifically expressed in the operating or capital budgets. Armed with the necessary authority to proceed, the goals become foundation around which ranges of settlement can be determined. This range refers to the maximum and minimum positions that are acceptable to the hospital. As a purchaser, the minimum position represents the initial position upon entering the negotiations.

For example, if upon entering a negotiation session for catering services, one were to state something to the effect that this proposal has no value to the hospital; one would clearly state the minimum position. Any concessions should be made upward towards the highest level of expectation or maximum position. It is important that both the maximum and minimum positions be supportable by fact and logic.

ANALYSIS OF SUPPLIER POSITION

One must start by gathering relevant information and defining needs. Conceptually, the framework for gathering relevant information is rather simple. Short and long-term information needs to be gathered for our side, and also about the other side. Furthermore, information needs to be gathered about the strategic and operational implications at an economic and psychological level.

The psychological level requires answers to questions like:

- What kind of person, am I going to be negotiating with?
- What are their short or long term needs?
- How can I recognize them in planning this negotiation?

The short term information can be reasonably easy to gather. Information for the long-term perspective is more difficult to gather, but it is vital nevertheless. One of purchasing responsibilities is forecast of future organizational requirements and future market conditions for key requirements.

Analyzing positions of strength: The desire for agreement, the perceived certainty of getting an agreement, and commitment or intention to perform after agreement depends on relative strengths and weaknesses of each side. One critical element in preparing for a negotiation is assessing the positions of strengths of both or all parties. Performing this task helps to establish future negotiation points. It also avoids setting unrealistic expectations, and may reveal ideas about possible strategies. Analyzing the factors that give either party a position of strength should be done in light of the key objectives of the negotiation. Key objective of one party may not be the key objective of the other.

Michiel R. Leenders and Anna E. Flynn have identified 40 potential points of strength, each for purchasers and supplier.

Some of the most important among them are listed in the following Tables 8.1 and 8.2

Table 8.1 Potential Points of Strength for a Purchaser

1. Pays on time	14. Stands behind commitments
2. Financially strong	15. Ability to make the requirement in-house
3. Excellent reputation	16. Other suitable suppliers are available
4. Significant market share	17. Substitutes are available
5. Large volume requirement	18. Buyer's market
6. Substantially growing future requirements	19. Willing to go long term
7. Steady use or counter seasonal requirement	20. Can and will help suppliers to improve.
8. Strong technical expertise	21. Ethical, honest, and trustworthy
9. Can add additional products or services to the requirement	22. Strong brands or patents; has a sustainable competitive advantage
10. Can influence other purchasers	23. Tolerant of mistakes if repetition will be avoided.
11. Long history of successful supplier relations	
12. Global strength	
13. Accurate forecasts	

Table 8.2 Potential Points of Strength for a Supplier

1. Superior service	10. Future growth assured
2. Superior price	11. Strong brands or patents
3. Superior terms and conditions	12. Reputation as innovative
4. Superior warranties	13. Reputation as environmentally superior
5. Superior flexibility as to specifications, delivery, quantity, timing, terms and conditions, packaging, and special requirements	14. Global strength
	15. Only supplier available
	16. Larger organization than the buyer
	17. Stands behind commitments
6. Superior research and development facilities.	18. Seller's market or market shortage
	19. JIT and EDI capability
7. Financially strong	20. Good public image
8. Excellent reputation	21. Other purchasers anxious to buy
9. Significant market share	

It is also useful to ask, which points are the stronger ones for each side? This allows the negotiators to stress and elaborate their key strong points and be prepared for the arguments from the other side. In most purchasing negotiations, these points of strengths are essential.

Relative Bargaining Powers

Real negotiation pays no lip service to the last price but, instead, focuses on ways in which the supplier either gets something that is desirable in exchange for a price concession or something undesirable is withheld by the buyer. Negotiation is a trade off. Most obvious first undesirable that may be withheld is that of not giving the supplier the contract. This strategy can be effective only if the buyer does not bluff. Otherwise, it is simply an extension of a ritual whereby buyer wins a final price concession that might have only been held in reserve by supplier all along. The buyer must have an alternative available if the supplier calls bluff and refuses to make a concession. With equipment, this might mean managing to make do for another year or so with old equipment rather than trading it in on a brand new model. In other cases, it may consist of making rather than buying. However, the only alternative available when a supplier refuses to reduce a price is to purchase the same item from another supplier. Suppliers soon catch on to this game regardless of how it is played. They discover two obvious ways in which they can prevent the buyer from winning. They either refuse to reduce a quotation or deliberately quote high and then let the buyer negotiate a reduction. Thus, the buyer's threat not to buy is an empty one unless he can get along without it or can produce it himself. In order to be effective, a buyer must have credibility with the seller. **Bluffs and lies are unethical as well as ineffective.** There should be no advantage for the seller who is last to bid. Sellers want to work things out informally with a buyer to negotiate and wrap up the deal in a face to face meeting. When there is real competition among sellers, this is poor strategy for the buyer. One on one relationship effectively blunts the competitive process. If the buyer negotiates individually, he should be willing to do so with every promising bidder and not conclude the deal until he is certain that he has each bidder's best offer.

Negotiations with strong suppliers may be difficult, but this situation is preferable to negotiating with weak, unreliable, incompetent suppliers. That is why purchasing may be defined as fight for good suppliers. The reputation of the purchaser can be assessed by the quality of the suppliers a purchaser can attract. When you have an established position, it is also important to understand the vendor's position. Normally, the vendor's stated goals are contained in their proposal. Through a careful comparison of hospital's goals and vendor's proposal, one should be able to discern areas of disagreement.

Value analysis can yield much more cost reduction than negotiations. A value analysis checklist that can be used by healthcare purchasers is as follows:

1. Value of the item to be purchased.
2. Are all features needed? It should be ensured that the item is essentially needed; that it is without unnecessary features if it is an equipment item; and that it is of good quality, if it is a supply item such as surgical gloves or tape.
3. Is the cost porportionate to end use?

4. Consideration of a less expensive product which could serve the same purpose.
5. Cost analysis to reasonably account for materials, labour, overhead, and profit.
6. At what price are others buying the product?

Complete cost analysis should be conducted to determine what attitude vendor may have in cost reduction. Value analysis and cost analysis can be most beneficial to buyer's position and supportive of his expectations. For example, if you are dealing with a custom made artificial limb for an orthopedic patient, it would be wise to ask the vendor to provide a complete cost analysis of how the unit cost was arrived at. Vendors may not be willing or even able to provide you with this information, but it never hurts to ask. Terms and conditions of the vendor proposal should be closely examined. In almost every instance, despite claims to the contrary from the vendor representative, all terms and conditions are subject to negotiation. For example, many vendors prefer to submit proposals on their standard bid forms. Close examination of terms and conditions printed on the reverse will reveal that they protect the vendor and effectively negate the terms and conditions on buyer's hospital's purchase order.

During negotiations with a large company for purchase of major capital equipment, negotiating team can successfully negotiate terms and conditions that were mutually beneficial to both sides. The company maintained many of its original terms and conditions and the hospital terms and conditions added to the standard sales contract that provided the protection which the hospital desired. Not only was the hospital successful, but as a result of this experience, the company, which had targeted healthcare industry as a new market revised its terms and conditions on its standard bid formats in an effort to reduce future negotiating costs and to improve the company's marketing edge. Realistically, these results are not an everyday occurrence but they do prove that vendors' terms and conditions can be negotiated and high levels of expectations can be attained if you are determined and persistent.

When dealing with contracts for items with alternative or substitutes, every effort should be made to become familiar with those substitutes and their associated costs. This can be accomplished by referring trade/technical literature, by visiting other hospitals, and through interactions with technical experts. The more your knowledge, the more you can support your position. It is equally advisable to learn as much as possible about the vendor's negotiators. During the bidding process, your dealings are normally with the sales representatives. **During a negotiation, you can expect the representative to appear with their general manager, or even a Director. We must make sure that our opponent has the necessary authority to negotiate and commit to the contract.**

PRICE VERSUS COST ANALYSIS

Ability to distinguish between price and cost and to analyze prices and costs are necessary skills for buyers. Most hospitals have accountants who can perform this function. However every purchaser should also be familiar with the fundamental processes involved. Price analysis is aimed at subjecting two or more comparable items to an analysis of their respective direct costs. This can be as simple as comparing the purchase costs of **Kendall versus Johnson & Johnson** surgical gloves, or as complex as for scanner, printer, copier cum fax machines.

On the other hand, cost analysis encompasses all of the factors involved in the procurement, use, and disposal of any given product. Price analysis is included as one of the factors in the cost analysis formula. Cost analysis quantifies all the expenses, such as transportation, receiving, handling, recording, and storage, which must be added to the price to determine the ultimate costs (landed). Cost analysis provides a more complete picture of true expense. A cost savings results when the monies that would normally be spent are reduced. For example, if a hospital spends Rs. 2,00,000 per year on aprons and a reduction of 10 percent in the unit cost results in a reduction of total costs to Rs. 1,80,000/, then a Rs. 20,000/ cost savings has been achieved.

A cost avoidance results when available, underutilized resources are used instead of new or additional resources acquired or when the wants and needs for a product are clarified and the wants (nice to have) features are eliminated for example, assigning expediting duties to an existing person rather than hiring another individual to accomplish the expediting function. A saving in labour costs occurs only when a position is eliminated from the budget. Improved efficiency resulting from a technological change without a budget reduction is not a savings. There must be an actual reduction in available budgeted hours to achieve a labour savings. It is important that the difference between a cost savings and a cost avoidance is understood in order to explain the results of any given cost study. It is also important that any labour savings achieved be real. Failure to recognize these important points can result in poor information input into the decision-making process. These could cause the hospital increased, unnecessary expenditures.

The first step in the cost analysis process requires that the objective or purpose for the cost analysis be stated clearly and concisely. For example:

- To provide a cost comparison for a decision on using disposable diapers versus a diaper service.
- To determine the cost of a Xerox copier versus Modi copier.
- To determine if the current charges for operating room disposables are reasonable and accurate.

The second step is to determine what factors must be included to make an objective analysis.

Typical factors influencing cost analysis include:

- Potential revenue
- Capital investment

- Supplies
- Labour
- Maintenance costs
- Depreciation costs
- Disposal problems
- Investment on inventories
- Alternative investment costs
- Replacement costs

Each cost analysis may require a different set of factors, i.e., what is applicable for one analysis may not be applicable for another analysis. One must identify the source of information for each of the factors involved and the method of determination or computation. Such detailed work is necessary to provide documentation or "proof" of how the results were determined. In most cases, the cost analysis will be reviewed by the administrator, or another department head, or the product utilization committee as part of the decision making process. It is important that everyone involved in the decision understand how the results were arrived at. No matter what the outcome of the analysis is, someone might challenge the final results. Buyer should be prepared to substantiate the methodology used. Finally, as a matter of routine, buyer should be prepared to follow up the process to ensure that a cost savings, cost avoidance, or increased revenue is realized. This analysis should be reviewed with the appropriate department heads to determine whether the objective of the analysis has been accomplished.

Cost/price analysis is a powerful tool used in the negotiations. It means analysis of all factors that enter into price computation and is an attempt to ensure that the final price is reasonable and right one. **Cost represents the actual cost;** it is a fact which could be determined and verified by classifying, recording, and appropriate allocation of expenditure. **Price is the sum of money at which a thing is valued or the value a seller sets on his goods.** Price is the suggested figure at which seller can deliver his goods at a profit and for which the buyer pays; this is obviously more than cost and includes profit.

Cost/Price and Value

The illustration given alongside demonstrates manner in which price can respond to the economic power of parties in negotiation

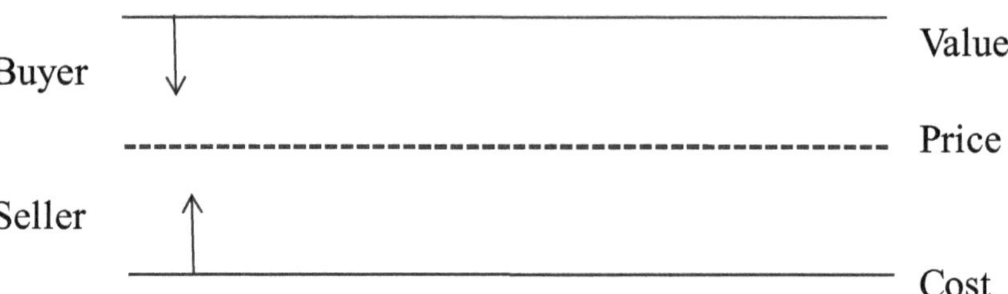

Value represents the utility (in economic sense) of the item to the buyer. Costs furnish a floor for price but they do not determine the price. The price lies between value and cost. The seller is trying to push the price as close to the value as possible while the buyer does the opposite. In order to succeed in this exercise, the buyer must acquire knowledge of seller's productive capacity, the degree to which that capacity is being utilized and his own company's plans and needs. Based on this information, the buyer can secure bids from potential suppliers. The buyer may also attempt to ascertain from the potential suppliers, the various components of their respective costs that are included in their prices.

TYPES OF RELATIONSHIPS BETWEEN BUYERS AND SELLERS

The two basic approaches to negotiating an agreement are win/lose and win/win. Prior to defining the characteristics and pitfalls of each of these negotiating approaches, we need to review various types of buyer seller relationships.

Relationships between buyers and sellers can be of three types and are as follows:

1. Antagonistic relationship

In this relationship, buyers and sellers are enemies, always contriving ways to demoralize each other. A sign of an antagonistic relationship is what is called externalization.

Characteristics of this relationship are as below:

- Each party considers the other as enemy and tries to demoralize the other.
- Faults are always externalized - i.e., always the faults of the other party are highlighted.
- Neither party takes responsibility for what takes place in relationship. Each party disowns responsibility for a bad outcome.
- There is no compassion.

2. Adversary relationship

This relationship is the most common type of buyer and seller relationship. It is an extension of our competitive culture.

Characteristics of adversary relationship are:

- Adversary relationship relies on external stimulation. Each claims that his behaviour depends on how well the other person is behaving.
- Buyer/seller adversaries often believe that they are behaving in a cooperative way, e.g., we provide QC training and they provide cent percent defect free supplies.
- Cooperation in this contest means that everything is in balance; each party is getting equal share and neither is getting ahead of the other.

Win-win negotiation is generally not possible in this type of relationship.

3. Cooperative relationships

In this kind of relationship, there is a mutual acceptance without preconditions.

The buyer and seller accept each other and do not predicate that acceptance on any conditions.

- Both parties accept the fact that human beings and human organizations are imperfect and that the differences of opinion, discrepancies, and inconsistencies in people and their organizations always exist.
- Limitations of both buyer and seller are expected. Acceptable difficulties can be understood and resolved by talking them over.
- In reality, they spend little time or energy determining which party is right or wrong.
- The parties involved do not always haggle over justice, reward or punishment.
- Cooperative buyer and seller relate to each other as a team without merging their separate identities.
- They assist the counterpart by raising their self-esteem.
- Win - win negotiation is possible. **Results in self help made effective through mutual help.**

POSSIBLE APPROACHES TO NEGOTIATIONS

There are three possible approaches to negotiations.

1. Lose-Lose Negotiation

In this case, both parties lose. There is no meeting point and there is no agreement. The contract cannot be signed. Both buyer and seller have to seek other avenues. There is no continuing relationship, no remorse afterwards. Each feels I am drowning, he should drown with me. Let us both sink together. **Lose-lose strategy is embodied in the expression we all bleed together and perish.**

2. Win-Lose Negotiations

The only objective in the win/lose approach is to win by capturing as much value as possible. In this type of negotiation, more is always better. This approach is also known as a competitive positional negotiation or a zero-sum game (in order for buyer to gain rupee 1, seller has to lose rupee 1 and 1-1=0). Value is viewed as being fixed and unchangeable. Goals are viewed as single points and not ranges. The focus is on minimizing losses. Your counterpart is your enemy and cannot be trusted to give you the best price.

Your major thrust is to understand the lowest price that the other party will agree to and still deliver quality goods. It is a static situation. **I defend my position while I attack yours.**

3. Win-Win Negotiations

The objective of a win/win negotiation is that one party is unable to win unless the other wins. The focus is on assisting one's counterpart with achieving their needs, and this is a mutual goal. This approach is collaborative, issue oriented, and a non-zero-sum game. Value is created through the process of negotiation. Goals are viewed in terms of ranges of outcomes.

The focus is on maximizing gains.

- The counterpart is viewed as a partner. (Partners contribute to the success of a business while fulfilling their own interests. Partnerships where one partner does all the work do not last long.)
- The objective is to create as much value as possible. There is openness regarding the goals and support for achieving them.
- During the negotiating process, creativity is present, as interpersonal contact is spontaneous, responsive, and flexible.
- All moves are open and honest.

The last step in any negotiation is to distribute the value that has been created. Again the focus is on satisfying the needs of both parties.

The negotiators first decision involves whether to plan to adopt a win-lose or a win-win approach. The latter provides best long term results. When both sides can come away feeling that their key objectives have been met, and that neither has been taken advantage of, the stage is set for a long lasting, mutually beneficial relationship. However, it is vital to be able to detect a deceitful situation in which the other party is stating a win-win philosophy while trying to take undue advantages from the buyer. If this occurs, the buyer will have to decide whether to counter it with a win-lose approach or simply to avoid doing business with that party.

Identification of Buyer and Seller Objectives

In order to increase the frequency with which they achieve objectives, managers must have a clear understanding of what their objectives are. It is not sufficient to seek just a better price for

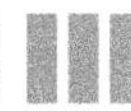

intravenous fluids; it is necessary to decide what price the hospital will be willing to pay as well as what other items are needed. These might include frequent delivery, price protection, local warehousing, and so on. Managers should also identify how important each of these items is to their overall plan. In addition, they should determine what they have to offer for these in return.

It is also equally important to determine the other party's objectives. This is usually more difficult. Obviously, the other party's primary objective is to obtain all of the hospital's business at the vendor's most favourable price. There usually are also additional elements that are important to the sales representative and to the current circumstances in the seller's company. Having some idea of these is helpful in setting up a strategy. The best way to determine these is to establish a positive and open relationship with the other party well before formal negotiation. Additional sources of this information are other managers who have earlier dealt with the vendor, company documents such as annual reports, and general information from newspapers, trade journals, and so on. The idea is to establish a clear picture of the total event in establishing a consistent and effective strategy.

DEVELOPING STRATEGY

Developing a suitable strategy is the final step in the preparation stage for negotiation.

There are three major tasks involved in this.

1. The first is to develop arguments and counter arguments by using the data collected. Not only should you support your position, but also try to anticipate the vendor's defense against your position and in support of theirs. A useful technique for preparation is to have other members of the purchasing department or the requesting department head rehearse with you.

2. The second task is to anticipate the vendor's range of settlement. Remember, the original proposal contains the vendor's high expectation. The vendor's lowest/ minimum position has not been stated. One easy method is to talk to other hospitals or local businesses that the vendor serves in order to find out what they are paying for similar products or services.

3. The final task is to prepare an agenda of the topics to be discussed. That agenda should be sequenced with our most powerful arguments presented first, our weakest arguments next, and our best arguments last. Psychologically this is based on the primacy immediacy effect.

The primacy effect relates the fact that people tend to retain information presented first in the discussion. The immediacy effect relates to the fact that whatever is said last will be best remembered. Our weakest arguments should be placed in the middle because they are most often forgotten first. The vendor is also aware of the primacy immediacy effect and will use it on you.

Next, the managers should think up the details of how to conduct the actual negotiation sessions. This includes matters like when and where the negotiation meetings will take place, whether to meet one on one or to use a team approach etc. The managers also must organize the points to be discussed and decide what items of lesser importance to their overall objectives they might be willing to concede, if necessary, for achieving those of relatively higher importance. Various

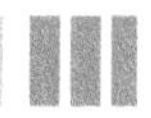

books have been written on this subject. It will be helpful, in developing strategies, to select the suggestions most relevant to the buyer's individual style and circumstances.

Following list of steps may serve as a starter for managers on what they should do:

- Establish a sense of power and legitimacy. They must believe that they have something which the other side needs and that they have every right to negotiate assertively.
- Make the other persons feel important. Then they will be more likely to respond to the buyer's needs.
- Establish a positive relationship in which each side invests time and energy.
- It is not always necessary to tightly control the interaction. Let the other person feel free to try and meet their objectives too.
- Always offer multiple alternatives and be persistent in trying options until points of agreement are covered.
- The buyers must neither rush nor allow themselves to be rushed.
- They must always try to meet the other person's needs without losing sight of the obligation to make sure that the hospital's needs are being met, as well.
- During the meeting someone must take notes on behalf of the buyer's team and follow up the meetings with a letter of agreement.

DO'S AND DON'TS OF NEGOTIATION

One important rule in negotiation is never to over emphasize the price to the detriment of other avenues for cost reductions. The materials manager should conduct tough negotiation sessions on an annual basis for all supply categories, and all major agreements on price and service should be effective for at least a year. Since the hospital suppliers have been in control so long, the materials manager must be creative and innovative in his approach at the negotiation table. It must, however, be remembered that concern about prices can over shadow the more important actions such as inventory reduction. We must understand the supply price in proper perspective. The maximum reduction obtainable from the toughest, most stringent type of negotiations is only about two percent if the hospital is getting good prices to begin with. At this rate, the hospital could possibly pick up another Rs. 20, 000 per each million rupees worth of purchases, so the money saved through purchasing is miniscule compared to that which can be possibly saved through internal material practices. In fact, hospitals practicing prudent purchasing are at a point beyond which a supplier cannot give.

Do's

- **Negotiate at home when possible.** Isolate members of the selling team by seating arrangement with buying team members between them to break up their attack.

- **Negotiate with those who can make concessions.**
- **Remain silent** at times; often greater concessions result from a seller's fear of losing business. Vendors may talk themselves into a better settlement than expected.
- **Know what you can expect to gain by negotiating** and keep your target in mind. Analyze the amount of concessions the vendor can reasonably be expected to have.
- **Plan ahead** and prepare the agenda to your advantage.
- **Brief your team members** before hand to be sure that none of them ignorantly give in on a point before you do.
- **Negotiate for a major advantage** not merely a short sighted one which may backfire at the first turn of economic conditions.
- **Be confident of facts presented.** Don't use information that you may have to acknowledge it as wrong.
- **Use new techniques** such as the learning curve concept and price cost analysis.
- **Divert their attention if the negotiation hits your weak point.** Shift the strategy of attack to minor points which you may later concede.
- **If talks hit a snag,** it is advisable to call for a recess, or arrange for a lunch break. It is advisable to set the meeting at a time that will allow the vendor to relax at lunch with company people (at buyer's expenses, of course).
- **Enlist the aid of specialists in the organization** in manufacturing, operations and methods (O&M), finance, and engineering to help to evaluate tooling and other special costs. Purchasing research will help supply basic data for negotiating.
- **A good suggestion is to give away relatively, minor concession** generously in return for a compromise which is still satisfactory.
- Always be fair.

Don'ts

- **Browbeat suppliers** to submit lower quotations.
- **Reveal your strong points too early;** withhold something for later concession in return for a point.
- **Get so bogged down in details that the overall objectives are lost.**
- **Act as a price chiseler.** In most cases, the price reduction they negotiate is illusory. Suppliers who know them simply quote higher than normal and then make concessions.
- **Try to prove that the vendor is wrong.** You may win an argument point, but he would not reduce price and may leave the negotiating room to back off gracefully from stated position.

All the above indicates clearly that no other skill or responsibility is more basic to the universal description of the purchasing manager's function than the requirement that he negotiate in the interest of his company.

NEGOTIATION PROCESS

Basic Rules

Some of the principles applied by successful negotiators include:

- Think from the supplier's perspectives.
- Let the supplier talk - The best thoughts sometimes come from others.
- Let the supplier save face.
- Satisfy the supplier's needs too.
- Always talk to the proper person.
- Build up confidence early in the meeting. Anything well begin is half done.
- Discuss one point at a time.
- Always be honest, dispassionate and impersonal.

Less experienced purchasing managers simply ask the supplier, "Can you reduce further?" after he has presumably made his last offer. Such negotiations do seem to produce tangible results sometimes. It often turns out that the supplier can do better and makes one more last price cut. The sophisticated buyer is more cynical. He knows fully well that he has probably wound up with a price that is exactly what the supplier intended to charge, neither more nor less. No buyer is so powerful that he can force a supplier to reduce prices. Suppliers cut prices only because they believe this is in their selfish interest. They may feel that the buyer may purchase from a competitor. The intelligent buyer goes on playing the game of asking a supplier if he can do better, before reaching final agreement. This is an accepted ritual between suppliers and buyers in particular areas. However, this is not really negotiation but simply a long drawn-out bidding process in which the supplier makes his final price known just before the contract is actually awarded.

NEGOTIATION TECHNIQUES

There is no need for negotiation if all competing suppliers put forth their lowest possible offers. Buyers too do not have time for negotiation of anything but their largest contracts. However, in certain instances, negotiation process permits buyer and seller to identify a relationship that is more or less unique to that contract. In some cases, the buyer may negotiate individually with several competing sellers. A final decision involves weighing the value of each offer. In other instances, the negotiation would be only with the lowest bidder, who is going to get the contract anyway. In this instance, the discussion would focus on ways in which the contract could be designed to yield a greater net benefit to both parties.

Negotiation techniques vary depending upon the situation and the party's levels of expectation. Early in the negotiation session, every effort should be made to establish mutual interest.

Reinforcement of this position is necessary from time to time to remind the vendor that the objective of the discussion is to obtain an agreement in the best interests of both the vendor as well as the buyer The buyer must convey the feeling that the hospital welcomes the vendor as a member of the team which is supposed to achieve the objectives. This provides them a sense of participation and makes them willing to help. Listening is one of the most important techniques a skilled negotiator can use. The vendor will often feel the need to respond to your silence by talking. The more you get the vendor to talk, greater the possibility of gaining information relative to vendor's range of settlement and overall position.

There are number of techniques to gain information on vendor's range of expectations. Important among them are:

1. **Asking questions aids in soliciting information:**

   The use of questions is valuable in diverting attention from an area you are not fully prepared to discuss, to the area the vendor will be on the defensive. It is also useful for eliciting support for the buyer's position, and, finally, to help the vendor to accept your position.

2. **Exploring alternatives:** Another technique that can provide a measure of success is that of exploring alternatives. Use of this technique can serve three purposes:

   a. **Obtaining information by sending a trial offer.** By offering an extreme position, one may be able to learn the vendor's actual level of expectation.

   b. **Problem solving:** When you offer an alternative solution, you may find an area of compromise. However, you should offer only those alternatives that are totally acceptable to you.

   c. **Making concessions:** It is common for some type of impasse to occur during negotiation and it should be anticipated. Making concessions during negotiations requires careful timing and consideration. Concessions can be used to break an impasse, to win a corresponding concession from the vendor, and to conclude an agreement. Making a concession is like making a trade off. Always trade upward. Concede on a minor point to win a major point. Concessions should not be made early in the session, lest you give the impression that you are an easy negotiator. This technique is best saved for the middle or end of the session to show your sincerity regarding mutual interest.

3. **Role playing:** In team negotiation situations, the use of role playing, known as **"tough guy/ soft gal,"** may sometimes be an effective technique. The "tough guy" assumes an extreme position that might impose a serious threat to the vendor. The "soft gal" assumes a more reasonable position, one that team is actually striving for. By disagreeing with the "tough guy" and, perhaps, even supporting the vendor, the "soft gal" should attempt to win the

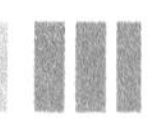

confidence of the vendor and increase the chances of attaining the team's objective. When this technique is utilized against you, ignore "tough guy" and concentrate on effectively responding to "soft gal's" position and arguments. If the "tough guy" becomes too disruptive to the session, suggest that "tough guy" leave or negotiations be suspended temporarily.

4. **Use of a deadline date:** This technique uses a deadline date by which an agreement must be reached. This is probably the one technique that vendors utilize effectively. They may say, "If you order today, you can save 5 percent because tomorrow, there will be a price increase." The vendor is trying to arrive at a quick agreement that is probably unfavourable for you. In most cases, such a deadline date is more imaginary than real. When a vendor really wants your business, whether the deadline date is real or not, and the vendor can often hold the price for "a few days". When negotiating from the buyer's position, deadline dates should be used only if they are real. It is unwise to try a deadline date as a bluff. Unless you are a skilled negotiator, you may put yourself into a corner and may later have to make concessions you had never planned to. The use of empty threats has no place in purchasing negotiations. Threats are risky and incur a high cost in the long run. Threats should be replaced with good solid data and logic to support your position.

5. **Offering a deal to the vendor:** In the course of negotiation, buyer explores ways to exchange something that is of less value to the buyer's organization than it is to the vendor, in return for something that is valued more highly by the hospital than by the vendor. With this form of exchange, both parties win. The win for the buyer may be some sort of direct price concession. For the vendor, the win is something that is worth more than the price or other economic concession.

Here are some of the deals a buyer may offer:

a. **Assurance of future business:** Such an offer may be incorporated into a formal contract in which buyer agrees to purchase all or part of his needs from the seller for some particular period of time. In other cases, the agreement may be entirely oral. In either case, the buyer should faithfully carry out any promises he makes as otherwise, he loses credibility on future deals he may wish to negotiate.

b. **Assurance of other business:** This involves combining purchases of items that are not monopoly priced with those that are. Supplier and his competitors cannot usually offer attractive discounts on proprietary items. Manufacturer has complete control over the price structure and can cut off dealers who deviate from his monopolistic rules. But there is no limit on offering low prices for other items. Thus, it is sometimes possible for a buyer to get prices on certain items that are even below the seller's costs as long as he also agrees to purchase the high-profit, proprietary products from the same supplier.

c. **Helping to reduce supplier's costs:** This form of cooperation is in the buyer's interest if it reduces prices. For example, frequent supplier sales calls are viewed as service by many

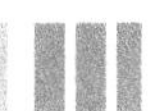

purchasers. For sellers these are costs. A salesman who works strictly on commission may occasionally be willing to pass on at least part of his earnings in the form of lower prices provided he is assured of getting the business with less frequent calls. The same approach is even more likely to be successful when the supplier has salaried salesmen and also makes deliveries. Distribution costs can almost always be reduced and may result in reduced prices.

d. **Concealed price cuts or non price benefits:** Suppliers are often in an awkward position when they believe that it is in their selfish interest to make a price concession to a particular customer. They fear that they may be forced to offer a comparable price to other customers and this may make the total loss much greater than the benefit gained from pleasing a particular customer. Suppliers are more inhibited in price cutting by the fear that news of it is bound to leak out either to competitors or other customers. If the competitors meet the new prices, only the buyers will gain. If other customers demand the same price, the cost of the price concession is just too high. For these reasons, sellers resist overt price concessions that are otherwise in their selfish interests. In such cases, the buyer can seek and often obtain other concessions that have value while the official price ostensibly remains unchanged. In some cases, the supplier's concession is a concealed price cut. For example, **buyers occasionally get suppliers to offer unusually favourable payment terms. This is a thinly camouflaged price cut.** In other cases, the supplier guarantees to the buyer that some minimum inventory will always be on hand, reserved for the buyer's exclusive use. The cost of carrying this inventory is obviously the equivalent of a price cut. Such non price fringe benefits become progressively less useful to the buyer as their relationship to price becomes more remote. It should be noted that it is poor strategy for a buyer to press a vendor to deliver a benefit that really does not fall under his control e.g., price caps offered by a distributor of medical-surgical supplies that allegedly protect them against price hikes beyond some predetermined ceilings. Actually, the distributor has no control whatsoever over the prices it pays the manufacturer. Such caps are masterpieces of slippery wording by the distributor's lawyers. These permit the distributor to charge whatever it pleases, or they are possible only because the original price is so high that there is plenty of padding for possible escalation. In either case, the buyer loses. Naturally, each supplier tries to make its particular package of non price fringe benefits look as attractive as possible to its customers at minimum cost. From supplier's point of view, object of the game is to appear to offer a lot while still spending nothing or little.

PRICE NEGOTIATIONS

Negotiation process involves use of logic, persuasion and sometimes economic pressure to arrive at a reasonable agreement in areas in which two parties have divergent interests.

Successful buyers have a more sophisticated approach to negotiation. **They know that they can negotiate nothing but what suppliers are willing to concede.** So they concentrate on creating an environment conducive to voluntary concessions by the suppliers.

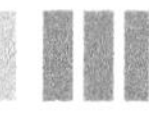

Here is an illustration of how to start from the most favoured price (MFP) and inch towards an acceptable price.

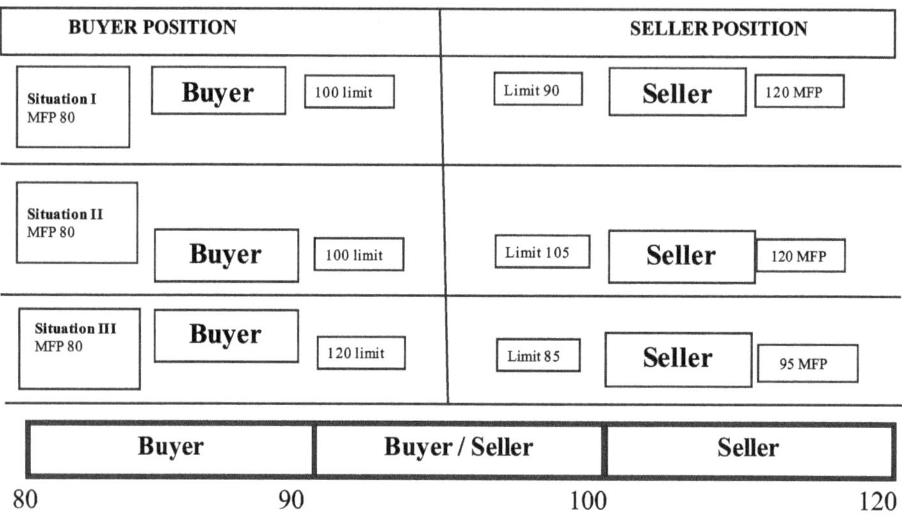

Figure 8.2 Possible situation in price negotiation

In situation I and III, there is an area of common acceptance. Both the parties start from their extreme on MFP and move towards a compromise or mutually acceptable position. It will be seen from the above that in situations I and III, there is a common acceptance. When the parties move into that area of agreement, probably they will become harder and harder in their approach. The movement is slow and each party moves slowly, step by step. One does not agree to what the other party demands all of a sudden. One must remember that one does not know what is in the other party's mind. **Supplier's first offer might be acceptable to him. Never accept the initial proposal, because the other party will have psychological feeling that he has not won his case and has been taken for a ride.** If the movement is slow and bargaining is stiff on both sides, then both parties come out of negotiating room with a feeling that they really argued and won the case, on the basis of their strengths or their negotiating skills. This psychological impact is very vital to the success of a contract.

In the second situation, there is no meeting ground for the two parties. The buyer does not have authority to go beyond certain monitory limits. The negotiations may involve a movement but will abruptly end at the terminal point beyond which the parties cannot proceed. In such a situation the negotiations may break down or both the parties seek time to discuss with their superiors and may come to the negotiation table once again if further concessions are made.

OTHER FACTORS THAT MAY INFLUENCE PRICE NEGOTIATIONS

Delivery Schedules

Inability to meet delivery schedules for quality and quantity specified is the single greatest instance of suppliers' failures encountered in purchasing operations. Buyers should attempt to investigate whether a defaulting supplier's plant is genuinely overloaded to the point that his production is running behind schedule. Despite having gained such knowledge, some buyers continue to place orders with suppliers, who constantly fall behind on their scheduled production dates. The reasons could be either a very attractive price or dependence on a single source or reciprocity etc.

Control over the Execution of the Order

Deficiencies of supplier's performance can seriously affect and in some cases completely disrupt the operations of the buyer's organization. For this reason, the buyer should exercise controls, which will help to ensure compliance with quality, quantity, delivery and several terms of contract.

Supplier's Cooperation

Supplier's cooperation is best obtained by the policy of rewarding with additional orders those suppliers who perform well. Good suppliers also expect courteous treatment, pleasant working relationships, timely payments and cooperation from their customers Cooperation begets Cooperation.

Sound and Continuing Suppliers Relationships

Negotiating conditions which permit buyers to take unfair advantage of sellers invariably change with time to conditions, which allow sellers to hold up buyers. For this reason, a buyer must realize that any advantage dishonestly won will in all likelihood, be recovered by the supplier at a later date probably with interest.

WHO SHOULD NEGOTIATE?

Who negotiates, buyer acting alone or buyer as a leader of a team? While negotiating a buyer have two options. First option is to as a sole negotiator on behalf of the company, while the second alternative is to act as a team leader of specialists drawn from various heads of departments concerned with the item to be procured. The team as a whole collectively negotiates.

Buyer Acts Alone

For recurring and or standard purchased items, regardless of their value, the buyer invariably acts alone. A buyer's sole negotiations are not limited to formal negotiations sessions. Rather, such negotiations continue on a daily basis with both current and prospective suppliers.

Buyer Acting as a Team Leader

This is done especially in purchase of high technology capital goods, complex contracts or high technology products. The team traditionally consists of a combination of specialists drawn from fields such as design, production, or user departments, engineering, industrial engineering, cost analysis and estimation, finance, price panelists, traffic, purchasing and law. The heterogeneous group of different specialists will view similar matters differently. As head of the team, the negotiator must make it into an integrated whole. A special mention may be made here of the necessity for an industrial engineer on the team. Even if the hospital cannot afford a staff industrial engineer, it

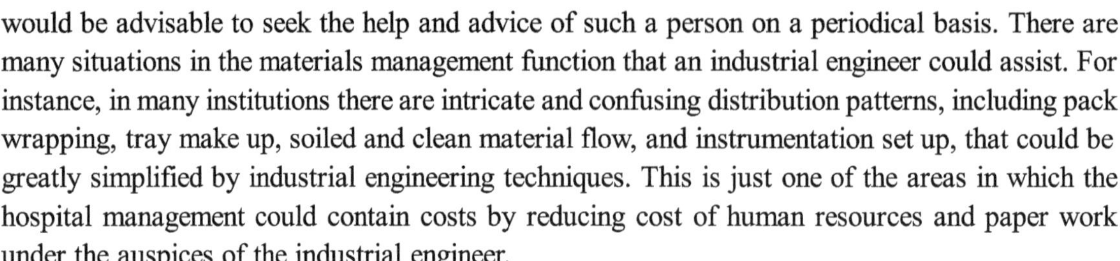

would be advisable to seek the help and advice of such a person on a periodical basis. There are many situations in the materials management function that an industrial engineer could assist. For instance, in many institutions there are intricate and confusing distribution patterns, including pack wrapping, tray make up, soiled and clean material flow, and instrumentation set up, that could be greatly simplified by industrial engineering techniques. This is just one of the areas in which the hospital management could contain costs by reducing cost of human resources and paper work under the auspices of the industrial engineer.

Individual versus Team Comparison

Mostly, hospital purchasers function as individual negotiators. However, there are occasions when the team concept is more practical and worthwhile. Purchase of services is a good example. The user usually has greater knowledge of the technological processes involved than the purchaser does. In a situation such as this, team concept comes into play. A team leader should be the one with the best negotiation skills; this should always be the purchaser. The team leader plays a vital role in the negotiations. He is the spokesperson for the team and also acts as mediator, unifier, and consolidator. Team leader must consider various individual opinions of the team and create a solid, unified position.

Moreover, each team member must recognize and support the leader's role as spokesperson for the group. For this reason, team members should also be chosen with care, on the basis of what each can specifically contribute to the actual negotiations. All team members must be involved in the preparation process from the outset and be totally familiar with goals and strategy. The most disastrous effect of a poorly prepared team can be the lack of proper presentation of information or position to the vendor's representatives. Each team member should be responsible for specific areas or sections to be negotiated. For instance, if negotiating for catering services, the dietician may be responsible for nutrition requirements, while the finance expert may handle taxes and duties. By having designated areas of responsibility, the team members present the psychological impression of a solid, unified front representing all areas affected by the contract to the vendor. In team negotiations, a caucus can be used to evaluate new information presented by the vendor, evaluate concessions by the vendor, restore calm if an emotional situation presents itself , divert attention away from an area that one is unprepared for or that may require a concession or to gain additional information in support of an important point. The caucus is a useful technique and should be employed as necessary. No matter how careful and complete your preparation, something new that was never anticipated will probably be presented during the actual negotiations.

PERSONAL ABILITIES, QUALITIES AND ATTITUDE OF A GOOD BUYER

1. Knowledge

He must be completely familiar with products specifications, with relevant standards and with acceptable quality levels. An effective negotiator must also understand the environment in which the procurement takes place. Knowledge needed to negotiate effectively takes several forms. **Important among them are:**

- Knowledge of the product itself
- Market knowledge
- Knowledge about suppliers facilities
- Where and how is the products used?
- How is it manufactured?
- What are its alternative methods of manufacturing?
- What substitutes are possible for the products itself as well as materials used in the manufacture of the product?
- Knowledge about suppliers work load.
- Complete knowledge of various types of contracting agreements, law of contracts, accounting and pricing.
- Familiarity with engineering, basic psychology and human behaviour.
- Knowledge of business management and business.
- Knowledge about cost, price analysis.
- Knowledge about learning curve.
- Knowledge about different types of discounts.

2. Attitude

This involves knowledge of self, the psychology of individuals and the interactions of groups. The buyer's attitude should be positive one, a resoluteness to reach an agreement and not to win a battle irrespective of what happens to other party.

3. Skills

The negotiator must have skill in identifying the issues during a negotiation and in planning the strategy and tactics required to resolve the issues satisfactorily, by effective communication and persuasion.

4. Other Attributes

- Ability to think in midst of complex negotiation.
- Ability to analyze alternatives emanating from the opposite camp and to determine their effect on his own negotiating position.

- **Ease of expression:** This is derived from the knowledge of the problem and experience in negotiating.
- **Leadership qualities:** He should lead his team and take initiative in understanding the strategy of the opposing side and negotiating his own position to his best advantage.
- **Emotional stability:** He must remain calm and composed in the midst of heated arguments. Statements made in anger may affect the buyer and seller relationship in the long run.
- **Patience:** It often pays to allow other side to talk themselves out and then try to resolve the issue without heated arguments.
- **A sense of humour:** A good humour can create goodwill. Humour has a utility in negotiation. It can divert direct confrontation and relax tensions. As a negotiation technique, humour can divert the vendor when he is concentrating on an argument that you may not be prepared to deal with except, perhaps, when some concession is involved.

The buyer's total professional knowledge must be brought to bear at the negotiation table. Only then he will be able to negotiate effectively.

PRACTICE FOR NEGOTIATIONS

Practice comes in three forms.

1. Rehearsal
2. Actual experience
3. Reading on the subject

Rehearsal: For major negotiations, managers should plan their strategy in detail, and then rehearse key elements either alone or with a team member. Practicing behaviour in a non-threatening or reduced stress environment makes it easier to carry out the conduct successfully under increased pressure. For extremely important negotiations, this step is definitely worthwhile.

Actual experience: The more often managers negotiate, the better negotiators they will become. This is particularly true if they take the time to analyze their performance, build upon their strengths, and take steps to correct their weaknesses. Finally, practice comes from searching for and seeking out new information and incorporating it into our own knowledge bank for improved performance. This can come from finding a particularly effective negotiator and observing such an individual in action.

Reading on the subject: It can also come from reading on the subject, selecting the ideas that work, and building them into their behavioural repertoire. It sometimes is difficult to admit that negotiating skill can be learnt and stand improvement. However, this is true for even the most experienced negotiator.

An ineffective negotiator is one who becomes locked into a set style and does not remain open to new options. In order to break out of this pattern of inflexibility, learning is essential. Each unique event brings together a new combination of people and circumstances. The keys to effective negotiation are to allow sufficient time to plan for and carry out important negotiations, develop a detailed plan, rehearse the key elements and then, to adjust performance according to what works. By adopting these steps, managers are able to increase the effectiveness of their negotiations.

CONCLUDING THE AGREEMENT

A suggestion to wrap up should be made when a satisfactory agreement appears imminent. When the vendor makes this recommendation, the buyer should consider whether they are prepared to accept the agreement. The final agreement should ensure that all agreements reached during the negotiations are understood by both parties. Often an area or issue, on which one of the parties thought agreement had been reached, but it actually had not been, might surface. When this happens, the problem needs be resolved immediately. It is beneficial to have purchase orders pre typed, setting forth agreements that are expected to be concluded. However, the purchasing secretary should be on stand by to type the final agreement. Once completed, the final agreement draft should be reviewed by both the parties and signed as a token of acceptance. If the agreement is to be prepared by the vendor, it should be reviewed carefully by the buying team to ensure that the contract reflects the totality of all understandings agreed upon. If an agreement cannot be signed immediately, a memorandum of understanding may be prepared that shows the exact wording of any agreements reached, and that should be signed by both parties. **When the final contract is presented, it should be compared carefully with the memorandum of understanding earlier signed by both the parties. If the contract is found to be in order, they must again sign it and conclude the negotiations.**

HOW TO NEGOTIATE FIXED PRICE?

Even rigid pricing, leaves buyer plenty of room to negotiate for lower prices. The buyer often has opportunity to:

1. **Become a unique buyer:** Sometimes, it is possible to become a unique buyer of materials with nominal changes in specifications. In such a case, the buyer and seller can negotiate any price they please. Then if the supplier reduces his price, he need not reduce prices of similar items sold to other customers.

2. **Negotiating for more favourable payment terms:** Although the price is fixed, individual sellers of material often have different payment terms. Some organizations have been known to offer thinly disguised reductions on fixed price items by offering unusually generous payment terms. Some vendors who are hard pressed for cash are willing to pay cash discounts equal to or more than bank lending rate of interest.

3. **Using concealed discounts:** When a company buys both fixed price and non fixed price items from the same vendor as often happens in the case of procuring from distributors, it is

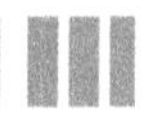

possible to negotiate discounts on the non-fixed price items. The buyer simply lists both fixed price and non fixed price items on the purchase order. By previous agreement, he deducts his negotiated discount on the price fixed from the non-fixed price items.

4. **Using vendor's inventory:** Inventories are expensive to maintain. If a buyer can get a supplier to carry a part of his inventories for him, he is getting equivalent of a reduction in purchase price.

5. **Obtain quantity discounts:** Sometimes a buyer can persuade a supplier to give quantity discounts even though he is not actually buying the quantities required for such a concession. His gimmick is something like a purchase order is placed for 10,000 units, but it does not call for immediate delivery. It permits the buyer to draw the required quantities as and when he needs them. The buyer may draw 1000 units each month and still get discount for a quantity of 10,000 units. This amounts to taking advantage of bulk purchase orders with staggered deliveries.

6. **Centralized purchases:** When centralized purchases are made, it improves the bargaining power of the purchasers of all plants which buy directly from the same manufacturer on a national accounts basis and they can get higher percentages of discounts directly from same manufacturers.

7. **Adjusting packing and shipping costs:** There is almost no limit to the number of ways this can be done. An imaginative buyer can find myriad ways to reduce costs even when prices of items which he buys are theoretically fixed. Various packing and shipping arrangements offer numerous possibilities. **The simple act of buying FOB destination instead of FOB shipping point can itself bring a substantial savings.** Packing and palletizing arrangements can cut costs. For example, one company persuaded its vendors to ship in cartons that can be reused for shipment to its own customers.

8. **Getting Extra Services:** Sometimes, suppliers can be persuaded to render free extra services. Suppliers may be asked to train buyer's personnel in use or maintenance of equipment. In smaller hospitals, suppliers sometimes take over much of the materials function; they periodically check buyer's stocks and automatically replenish them if they find that stocks have depleted to levels lower than those specified by the buyer. In most cases, vendors are over generous in keeping their products well stocked. (The points at 2 to 5 above are dealt in detail under the sub topic negotiation techniques.)

NEGOTIATING A PRICE INCREASE

Before the buyer should even bother analyzing the supplier's cost break down, he should ask himself these questions.

- Is the supplier's proposed new price still competitive with that of other qualified producers?

- Do purchase order terms and conditions permit price escalation?
- Are other producers in the supplier's industry also confronted with these higher costs, and are they succeeding in passing them on to their customers?
- Has the supplier passed on, in the form of price reductions, the benefits of increased productivity or other changes that have escalated his costs?

If the answer to any one or more than one of these questions is no, then the buyer has a basis for negotiation with supplier other than cost of production. In such a case, he might possibly be able to convince the supplier that he should forego his price increase.

CENTRAL VIGILANCE GUIDELINES FOR PUBLIC BUYING IN HOSPITALS

A) Post-Tender Negotiations

As per Central Vigilance Commission (CVC) Guidelines vide letter No. 8(1)(h)/ 98 (1) dated 18 November 1998, it was brought out that the tenders are generally a major source of corruption. In order to avoid corruption, a more transparent and effective system must be introduced. Post-tender negotiations are banned with immediate effect except in case of negotiations with L1 (i.e., lowest tenderer). Among other issues, the CVC had directed that when the quantity to be ordered is much more than what L1 alone can supply, in such cases, the quantity ordered may be distributed in such a manner that the purchase is done in a fair and transparent and equitable manner.

However the government of India, Central Vigilance Commission, New Delhi vide Circular No. 4/3/07, dated 3 March, 2007, in supersession of the earlier instructions, issued the following consolidated instructions with immediate effect

i. As post tender negotiations could often be a source of corruption, it is directed that there should be no post tender negotiations with L-1, except in certain exceptional situations. Such exceptional situations would include procurement of proprietary items, items with limited sources of supply and items where there is suspicion of a cartel formation. The justification and details of such negotiations should be duly recorded and documented without any loss of time.

ii. In cases where a decision is taken to go for re tendering due to the unreasonableness of the quoted rates, but the requirements are urgent and a re-tender for the entire requirement would delay the availability of the item, thus jeopardizing the essential operations, maintenance and safety, negotiations would be permitted with L-1 bidder(s) for the supply of a bare minimum quantity. The balance quantity should, however, be procured expeditiously through a re tender, following the normal tendering process.

iii. Negotiations should not be allowed to be misused as a tool for bargaining with L-1 with dubious intentions or lead to delays in decision-making. Convincing reasons must be recorded by the authority recommending negotiations. Competent authority should exercise due diligence while accepting a tender or ordering negotiations or calling for a re-tender and a definite timeframe should be indicated so that the time taken for according requisite approvals for the entire process of award of tenders does not exceed one month from the date of submission of recommendations. In cases where the proposal is to be approved at higher levels, a maximum of 15 days should be assigned for clearance at each level. In no case should the overall timeframe exceed the validity period of the tender and it should be ensured that tenders are invariably finalised within their validity period.

iv. As regards the splitting of quantities, some organisations have expressed apprehension that pre disclosing the distribution of quantities in the bid document may not be feasible, as the capacity of the L-1 firm may not be known in advance. It may be stated that if, after due processing, it is discovered that the quantity to be ordered is far more than what L-1 alone is capable of supplying and there was no prior decision to split the quantities, then the quantity being finally ordered should be distributed among the other bidders in a manner that is fair, transparent and equitable. It is essentially in cases where the organisations decide in advance to have more than one source of supply (due to critical or vital nature of the item) that the Commission insists on pre-disclosing the ratio of splitting the supply in the tender itself. This must be followed scrupulously.

v. Counter offers to L-1, in order to arrive at an acceptable price, shall amount to negotiations. However, any counter-offer thereafter to L-2, L-3, etc., (at the rates accepted by L-1) in case of splitting of quantities, as pre-disclosed in the tender, shall not be deemed to be a negotiation.

It is reiterated that in case L-1 backs-out, there should be a re-tender.

B) Reasonableness of Prices

It was noticed by Central Vigilance Commission (CVC) that purchases were being made in some of the organizations in an ad hoc and arbitrary manner without satisfying some prime requirement of establishing the reasonableness of the rates in relation to the estimated rates, last purchase price or the prevailing market rates. It is very important to establish reasonableness of prices on the basis of estimated rates, prevailing market rates, last purchase prices, economic indices of raw materials/ labour, other input costs and intrinsic value etc. before the award of the contract.

SUMMARY

Negotiation is one of the most important as well as one of the most interesting parts of purchasing. In industry, negotiation is sometimes confused with "haggling" and "price chiseling". In government, negotiation is frequently visualized as a nefarious means of avoiding competitive bidding and awarding large contracts surreptitiously to favoured vendors or organizations. Lowest bid may not necessarily mean best bid. Negotiation is important either after bidding or after requests for quotations. The essential technique of negotiation is communication of ideas. Negotiation involves convincing the other party of your point of view and reaching an agreement. An effective negotiator must be a real shopper alive to the possibilities of bargaining with the seller only through the awareness of relative bargaining strengths.

In a competitive bidding, the mode of purchase results in selection of a vendor, and price determination. Negotiation is another important approach to price determination. Apart from price, the buyer resorts to negotiation on various other parameters of purchasing.

There are five major objectives common to all purchasing negotiations:

1) To obtain fair and reasonable price for the quality specified.
2) To get the supplier to perform the contract on time.
3) To exert some control over the manner in which the contract is performed.
4) To persuade the supplier to give maximum cooperation to buyer's company. 5) To develop a sound and continuing relationship with competent suppliers.

A buyer plays one of two distinct roles in negotiation either as a sole negotiator or as head of a negotiating team. Personal abilities and qualities of good buyer are knowledge, aptitude, skills, ability to think, ability to analyze, ease of expression, leadership, emotional stability, patience and a sense of humour.

Conceptually, preparation for negotiation involves gathering relevant information. Furthermore, information needs to be gathered about the strategic and operational implications at an economic and psychological level. Obtaining information is a time-consuming process. Analyzing the factors that give either party a position of strength should be done in light of the key objectives of the negotiation. Purchasers must have more strengths than the vendor and plan the negotiations accordingly. Negotiations with strong suppliers may be difficult, but this situation is preferable to negotiating with weak, unreliable, incompetent suppliers. Purchasing is a quest for good suppliers.

Relationships between buyers and sellers can be of 3 types. They are: 1. Antagonistic relationship, 2. Adversary relationship, and 3. Cooperative relationship. The last type is the most preferable.

Negotiation requires a skilled interviewing technique, direct and indirect, which is carefully planned to gain purchasing objectives. Negotiating is an art. In order for negotiation to be successful there should be a free, honest, open interaction between bargainers of both the sides. In order to interview vendor effectively, the buyer should be prepared to negotiate from a position of strength.

A good negotiator carefully develops his strategy for each negotiation and uses it to the best advantage of his hospital. Hospital purchaser should conduct tough negotiation sessions on an annual basis for all supply categories. All major agreements on price and service should be effectively negotiated. Buyers must not be overly concerned about prices as compared to inventory reduction. Finally, negotiation is a personal process whose objective is to safe-guard the capital investment of the hospital, an increasingly important consideration in a cost-conscious, inflationary, consumer market.

The government of India, Central Vigilance Commission, New Delhi Guidelines vide letter no. 8(1)(h)/ 98 (1) dated 18 November 1998 brought out that in order to avoid corruption, a more transparent and effective system must be introduced. Post tender negotiations were banned except in case of negotiations with L1 (i.e., lowest renderer). Among other issues, the CVC had directed that when the quantity to be ordered is much more than what L1 alone can supply, in such cases, the quantity ordered may be distributed in such a manner that the purchase is done in a fair, transparent and equitable manner. However later, CVC vide circular no. 4/3/07, dated 3 March, 2007, in supersession of the earlier instructions, issued the following consolidated instructions with immediate effect.

There should be no post-tender negotiations with L-1, except in certain exceptional situations which would include procurement of proprietary items, items with limited sources of supply and items where there is suspicion of a cartel formation. The justification and details of such negotiations should be duly recorded and documented without any loss of time.

In cases where a decision is taken to go for re-tendering due to the unreasonableness of the quoted rates, but the requirements are urgent and a re-tender for the entire requirement would delay the availability of the item, thus jeopardizing the essential operations, maintenance and safety, negotiations would be permitted with L-1 bidder(s) for the supply of a bare minimum quantity. The balance quantity should, however, be procured expeditiously through a re-tender, following the normal tendering process.

Negotiations should not be allowed to be misused as a tool for bargaining with L-1 with dubious intentions or lead to delays in decision-making. Convincing reasons must be recorded by the authority recommending negotiations. Counter-offers to L-1, in order to arrive at an acceptable price, amount to negotiations. However, any counter-offer thereafter to L-2, L-3, etc., (at the rates accepted by L-1) in case of splitting of quantities, as pre-disclosed in the tender, shall not be deemed to be a negotiation.

It was reiterated that in case L-1 backs-out, there should be a re-tender.

Regarding reasonableness of prices, it was directed by CVC that it is very important to establish reasonableness of prices on the basis of estimated rates, prevailing market rates, last purchase prices, economic indices of raw materials/labour, other input costs and intrinsic value etc. before the award of the contract.

Splitting of orders: It is essential in cases where the organizations decide in advance to have more than one source of supply (due to critical or vital nature of the item). The Commission insists on pre-disclosing the ratio of splitting the supply in the tender itself.

REVIEW QUESTIONS

1. Define the term "negotiations" and explain when negotiations are resorted in purchasing?
2. "Negotiation is not to be used as a tool by powerful buyers to bully the weaker vendors - Elucidate.
3. "Objective of negotiation is to persuade and convince the other side to agree with one's view point. Elaborate this objective as applicable to Hospital Purchasing.
4. Who is a negotiator? What should be his qualities? How does one go about planning for negotiations?
5. What are the guidelines of Central Vigilance Commission with regard to public buying?
6. What are Do's and Dont's of purchase negotiations.
7. Enumerate purposes of negotiations in purchasing.
8. Write short notes on
   a) Antagonistic relations
   b) Understanding suppliers needs
   c) Win-win negotiation
   d) Unique buyer
   e) CVC guidelines for post-tender negotiations
   f) Erroneous beliefs associated with negotiations
   g) Cost, price and value

PART - II

Hospital Purchasing and Industrial Purchasing - A Comparison

Contents

CHAPTER - 9

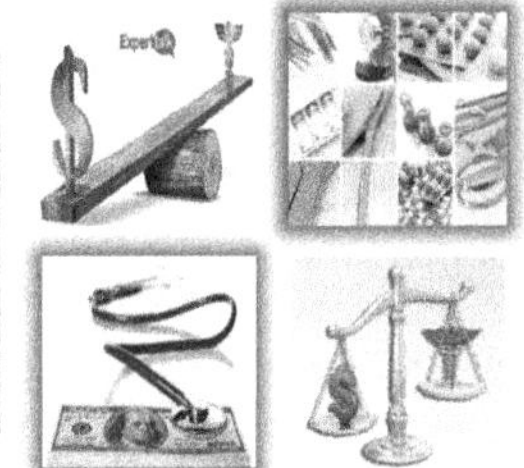

Hospital Purchasing and Industrial Purchasing - A Comparison

INTRODUCTION

Health care industry continues to be in news as business and society struggle to contain unsustainably escalating healthcare delivery costs. Developments in US economy have seen its change from a production economy to a service one. Hospitals have become an important and rapidly growing segment of the economy. With the growth of hospitals and healthcare institutions, both profit and non profit institutions have benefited with the infusion of sound management concepts and strategies. This trend is well set in USA which was the first nation in the world to have a service oriented economy. American Management Association Bulletin 33 states that every dollar invested wisely in purchasing should return $3 to $5. Hospitals must understand what industry understood years ago; money spent on good purchasing is not an expense, but an investment. India is in the midst of a major revolution in healthcare services. With liberalization, privatization and globalization, the management concepts and techniques are beginning to have impact now on healthcare and medical institutions.

One important factor viz., Health Insurance schemes will bring in lot of innovative and competitive schemes to be offered. The present monopoly of public sector has come to an end giving room for more corporate bodies entering healthcare sector further. Indian economy has also witnessed gradual transition from production economy to a service oriented economy in recent years. Such an economic change is the hallmark of advancing society which, calls for a new emphasis on purchasing and what it can contribute to nation's economy.

Healthcare in India is basically urban oriented. The urban population is estimated as 32 percent of the total population of 122.0 crores (2011 census). They live in 7925 towns each town having population over 10,000 people. There are 23,303 hospitals in the country with a bed strength of 10, 98,180 of which 68 percent are located in urban areas and of total 7,46,762 beds covering these hospitals. Healthcare is predominantly available in urban areas. (Source: National Health profile 2010).

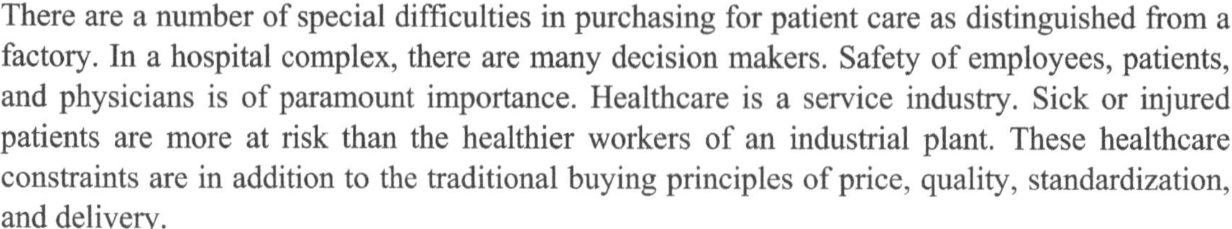

There are a number of special difficulties in purchasing for patient care as distinguished from a factory. In a hospital complex, there are many decision makers. Safety of employees, patients, and physicians is of paramount importance. Healthcare is a service industry. Sick or injured patients are more at risk than the healthier workers of an industrial plant. These healthcare constraints are in addition to the traditional buying principles of price, quality, standardization, and delivery.

DEFINITION OF HOSPITAL AND HEALTHCARE INSTITUTION

Webster defines HOSPITAL as an institution where the ill or injured may receive medical, surgical, or psychiatric treatment, nursing care, food and lodging.

HEALTHCARE means protection of physical and mental well being. In this chapter, the words hospital and healthcare institutions are used as synonyms.

Thus, a hospital as healthcare organization has been defined in varied terms as an institution involved in preventive, curative/ameliorative, palliative or rehabilitative services.

However, the definition given by W.H.O is quite exhaustive and exclusive, in which it is defined as an integral part of medical and social organization, which is to provide for the population complete healthcare, both curative and preventive and whose outpatient services reach out into the family in its home environment. The hospital is also a centre for training of health workers and for bio-social research.

Hospitals also provide bio social research; teaching, training for all members of hospital and a health team, which include not only doctors and nurses, but also professionals, paramedics, pharmacists, etc. Operationally, a hospital could be viewed as consisting of service faculties for outpatients, inpatients, general wards, emergency special wards, intensive care units, operation theatres, delivery suites and support services such as pharmacy, radiology and imaging, blood bank, laboratory, **Central Sterilization System Department (CSSD)** and stores, etc.

DIFFERENCES IN HOSPITAL AND INDUSTRIAL PURCHASING

Discussions here focus on purchasing for hospitals and healthcare institutions. Most of it will also be applicable for other types of service organizations such as colleges, universities, hospitality industry, etc.

- Every principle of good purchasing in purchasing management applies to purchases made for healthcare institutions.
- All buying activities, whether industrial or governmental or healthcare institutions have one cardinal objective: **"Obtaining maximum value for each rupee spent."**
- There is no separate group of principles for hospital purchasing when compared to industrial buying. However, hospital purchasing places different emphasis on certain areas of healthcare institutional purchasing. **The important differences are as follows:**

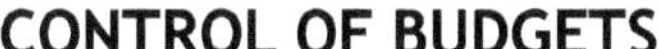

CONTROL OF BUDGETS

Parkinson's Law on budgets states expenditure will always rise to exceed income. This law is applicable to all business operations. It is more so with service organizations like hospitals. The will and determination to control expenditures in healthcare organizations is not as strong as it is in industry. Thus, it has proved easier for hospitals to raise room rents and treatment charges than it has been for industrial companies to raise the selling prices of their output. Consequently, hospitals have not been motivated to control purchasing costs as much as the competitive industry. However, this situation is now gradually changing. The government and individual tax payers alike are increasingly concerned about high cost of Medicare. A resistance by consumer to higher medical bills is changing this attitude. Prices as costs continue to rise for healthcare. Of late, employees and retirees are taking medical insurance policies. These insurance companies fix ceilings on rates for different procedures. **Thus, the concept of arbitrarily enhancing costs of treatments may not be possible in future.**

SCOPE FOR SAVINGS

Savings in hospital purchasing are as valuable as they are to the industry. In industry, profits increase a firm's capability to survive in the competitive environment. In healthcare, savings permit the hospitals to further accomplish its goals of better patient care, better physical facilities, better salaries etc. Most purchasing savings recur year after year thus creating a snowballing effect. For example, if a corporate hospital with return on investment at 5 percent achieves purchasing savings of Rs. 50 lakhs, the recurring saving is equal to an additional investment of Rs. 10 crores. Stated another way each rupee saved by prudent purchasing has same budgetary effect as Rs. 20 additions to hospitals invested funds.

Cost reduction in hospital purchasing is possible in two ways:

1. Identifying items that may not be needed
2. Paying lower prices for items that are needed

Standardization and value analysis programmes focus primarily on identifying items or features of those items which may not be really required.

Standardization

Cost reduction efforts begin with a standardization programme. The objective is to reduce the variety of items that are purchased. Effort is focused both on reducing the number of different brands of essentially identical products that are bought and also on eliminating genuinely different products. For example, that a purchasing manager and the pharmacist review purchases of tetracycline and discover that three different types of 250 mg capsules are being purchased: a generic variety from company X for Rs. 1050 per thousand and two branded versions from company Y, an Indian MNC, and company Z, a foreign MNC priced at Rs. 4275 per thousand and Rs. 5910 per

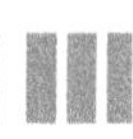

thousand numbers respectively. These drugs might be purchased and classified under three names: tetracycline, panmycin, and achromycin. First step in standardization programme would be to determine if these three drugs were really identical in every respect. If both medical staff and the pharmacist agree that they are, then pharmacy could simply stop buying Panmycin and Achromycin and purchase 250 mg of generic tetracycline exclusively. In this case, all requirements could be purchased for not more than Rs. 1050 per thousand, eliminating purchases made at Rs. 4275 and Rs. 5910. In some cases, the cost of the cheapest item could also be further reduced because it would be bought in larger quantities. In addition, standardization always reduces investment in inventory. If one item is made to do the jobs of three, then two separate inventory items are eliminated. For example, if the hospital carries a stock of Rs. 2,25,000 for each of these three similar drugs and carrying cost is @20 percent per year, each item inventory costs Rs. 45,000 per year to maintain elimination of inventories of two items, therefore, saves Rs. 90,000 per year even if there are no savings in price either by consolidating purchases or by buying the cheapest item that will do the job. Standardization yields dividends especially on two types of items Viz. the items which are used in extremely small quantities and the items where it is possible to adopt some other standard.

Preventive Cost Reduction Measures

Equipment standardization not only simplifies repairs and maintenance but also reduces both purchase and inventory carrying costs. A standard conscious purchasing organization will also discourage users who tend to introduce new brands and, possibly new stocking and repair problems. For example, if a hospital has one Maruthi Suzuki ambulance, its second ambulance should also be Maruthi Suzuki, unless there is compelling reason to change. Similarly, if most computers are HP's, then the organization should think twice before it buys IBM PC's. If a hospital can standardize its pillows, it can also standardize pillow covers. Similarly, standardization of printers promotes standardization of cartridges.

CHALLENGING SPECIFICATIONS

Specifications are detailed descriptions of the materials, parts, and components used in making the product. Proper specifications and standardization can materially improve the profitability of a hospital's operations. Purchasing department is responsible for economic considerations and hence, has the responsibility of challenging the restrictive specifications by requesting for reconsideration of technical parameters for economic reasons.

Major factors that call for reconsideration are:

- Material availability
- Potential substitutes
- Suggestions made by vendors
- Standardization
- Total value considerations (TVC)

Healthcare institutions deal with broad spectrum of materials and services than an average industrial organization. Further medical professions tend to become more specialized than their industrial counterparts. **Doctors are very knowledgeable in their professional fields, that does not entail knowledge of economics and market availability.** However, the ultimate responsibility for quality decisions rightfully rests with doctor or user department. For example, assume that a radiologist wishes to acquire a new portable X-ray machine. Purchasing department can help him by arranging a demonstration of competing X-ray machines from several manufacturers. This is something that a radiologist cannot always accomplish by himself for lack of economic leverage. Because of this economic capability, the purchasing department is in a logically stronger position to challenge restrictive specifications. Buyer in the purchasing department perforce, learns much about many varieties of items which he buys because he continuously deals with them. He knows what models are available, who sells them, and which company has the best facilities for servicing and who prices them most economically. He discusses technical and marketing changes and improvements with the manufacturers' salesmen on a continuous basis. On the other hand, even the largest users make only infrequent purchases; therefore, they cannot possibly keep up with many advancements and changes of all major manufacturers. But the purchasing department buys many things in addition to X-ray machines from the distributors of scientific equipment; it can get from distributor a superior response in terms of sales efforts, timing and price. When it comes to purchase of unique or seldom purchased capital equipment, the situation can be different. Here, the technical competence of the doctor/user must fully be relied upon when making this type of purchase. Purchasing staff helps by working with doctors/users upstream. In planning and procurement, purchasing can help with economic problems of capacity, prices and obtaining favourable terms and conditions in general and especially in the purchasing of higher cost machines like **Magnetic Resonance Imaging (MRI) equipment.**

A competent materials manager can effectively combine his skills with the technical knowhow of electronics engineers and with the professional needs of doctors. Ultimately, the contract can be awarded based on manufacturer's product quality along with the consideration of his responsiveness to non technical aspects of funding and other desired contractual provisions.

INSPECTIONS OF MATERIALS AND SERVICES

Ensuring quality has its own unique difficulties and challenges. Emergency stock outs are many a time, by products of quality failures. A package of material is on hand but, when opened, turns out to be of poor quality. **Hospitals are extremely vulnerable to quality failures. At times, such failures may be literally matters of life and death.** Problem is further compounded due to lack of facilities for objective measurements of quality specifications. Hospitals have more difficult problems in inspecting purchased items than industrial organizations. Hospitals are required to purchase wide range of materials, services, and products. The very range of incoming materials, therefore, makes centralized inspection practically impossible. This calls for many kinds of quality control inspectors and wide range of inspection equipment. In most hospitals and Medicare institutions, receiving departments inspect

 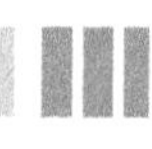

for bulk quantity and outward damages. Unit quantity, quality, and compliance with specifications is done by doctors, who originated the request for materials. If desired, the receiving department can of course, inspect for general stores types, or common use items. Large industrial purchasers determine their own quality standards, and then develop procedures to ensure compliance with the same. Healthcare institutions, in contrast, often must accept vendors' assurances on quality. On drugs and related items, the vendor has to prove to the satisfaction of the Drug Controller that its product and the process by which it is made, meets minimum standards. Other purchases by law or by custom must meet standards imposed by various other quasi or real regulatory agencies. Milk and food products must usually meet the standards of a local medical and health department. Plumbing, electrical, and maintenance supplies must be compatible with building codes; and various healthcare groups may set standards for other supplies. Hospital should also develop simple tests that lie within their technological capabilities.

Here are some examples:

a. **Count:** While the contents of every container need not be counted, random checks must be made. Suppliers' employees sometimes get lazy or careless and it is obviously less effort to ship a carton that is less than full. In addition, under shipment is a common form of dishonesty. Either a hospital employee or a supplier's employee steals a part of the shipment and no one knows as long as no attempt is made to verify what was received.

b. **Weight and measure:** For many purchases, quality is largely or partly measured by how much you get. A high-quality product uses more or better materials; a poor quality product uses less and/or inferior materials. To cite a simple example: quality of a trash can liner is usually directly proportionate to the quantity of plastic (PVC) material used. An easy quality check involves simply weighing a carton of the liners. If the weight falls below some previously established standard, it is likely that either the hospital got a short count or less plastic was used in making each bag. Carton can then be opened and a more detailed investigation can be made. Similarly, the contents of one quart or litre containers can occasionally be measured to make certain that they contain as much fluid as the hospital paid for. If price is linked to a key ingredient, destructive testing may be needed to determine if a standard is being met. Another simple example in food items is of opening a can of fruit juice to determine the proportion of food and syrup and to evaluate the quality of the fruit juice.

c. **Sterility:** Hospitals buy many products in supposedly sterile containers. Occasionally, incoming inspection staff should examine a package to see if it can grow a culture. Non-sterile products probably should also be reviewed by the lab in certain instances to determine just how non sterile they are.

BACK DOOR SELLING

Purchasing manager may be prone to sabotage by his suppliers in his effort to strengthen user relations. While there may not be conflict between user and purchaser, the relationship between

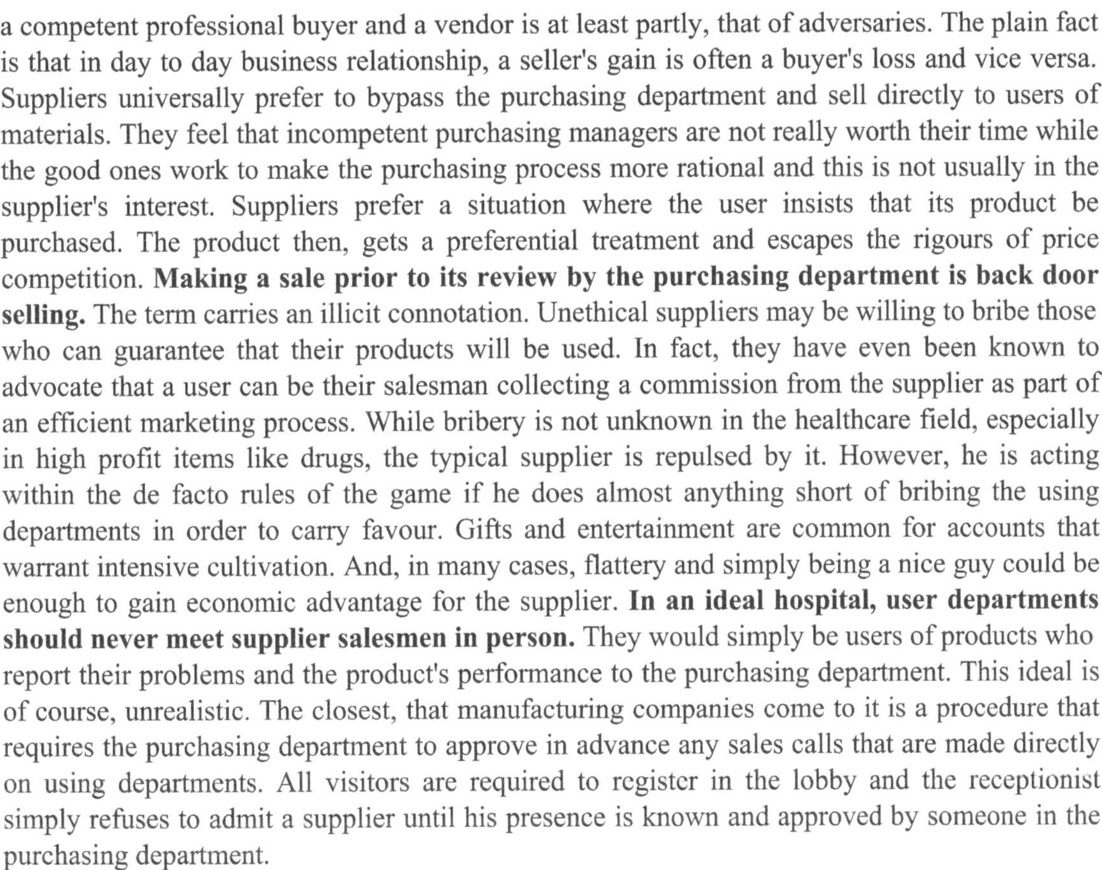

a competent professional buyer and a vendor is at least partly, that of adversaries. The plain fact is that in day to day business relationship, a seller's gain is often a buyer's loss and vice versa. Suppliers universally prefer to bypass the purchasing department and sell directly to users of materials. They feel that incompetent purchasing managers are not really worth their time while the good ones work to make the purchasing process more rational and this is not usually in the supplier's interest. Suppliers prefer a situation where the user insists that its product be purchased. The product then, gets a preferential treatment and escapes the rigours of price competition. **Making a sale prior to its review by the purchasing department is back door selling.** The term carries an illicit connotation. Unethical suppliers may be willing to bribe those who can guarantee that their products will be used. In fact, they have even been known to advocate that a user can be their salesman collecting a commission from the supplier as part of an efficient marketing process. While bribery is not unknown in the healthcare field, especially in high profit items like drugs, the typical supplier is repulsed by it. However, he is acting within the de facto rules of the game if he does almost anything short of bribing the using departments in order to carry favour. Gifts and entertainment are common for accounts that warrant intensive cultivation. And, in many cases, flattery and simply being a nice guy could be enough to gain economic advantage for the supplier. **In an ideal hospital, user departments should never meet supplier salesmen in person.** They would simply be users of products who report their problems and the product's performance to the purchasing department. This ideal is of course, unrealistic. The closest, that manufacturing companies come to it is a procedure that requires the purchasing department to approve in advance any sales calls that are made directly on using departments. All visitors are required to register in the lobby and the receptionist simply refuses to admit a supplier until his presence is known and approved by someone in the purchasing department.

In some hospital purchasing managers may be able to wield so much control over suppliers' movements within their institutions but the objective is certainly a worthy one. The purchasing managers should make it clear both to suppliers and to users that any agreements reached between suppliers and users are not binding on the institution unless they have the concurrence of the purchasing department. In most cases, if one makes an effort, it is possible to find an alternate source of supply which offers terms that may be slightly more favourable. An action of one purchasing manager was consistent with hospital objectives, even though he did not announce the basis of his decision at large. **Dean Ammer** cites an example, that a large supplier first convinced nursing department that it was not possible to operate without a particular proprietary product. Then, the purchasing manager bought the product. Six months later, supplier hiked the price by 40 percent. Nursing department refused to drop the product and the supplier, secure in the knowledge that it could not be displaced. The supplier insisted that the hospital pay a higher price or discontinue the use of that product. Purchasing manager took it, but he made the supplier regret its greed. Every other item which he had earlier bought from that supplier went out on bid and, after some months of work, he managed to place every item with other suppliers for prices no higher than he had been paying to the delinquent supplier. He believed that by proving his resourcefulness, even

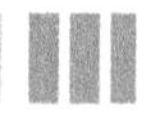

when powerless on a single product, the supplier will alter his policies in the future. **A competent purchasing manager is friend of no supplier but neither their enemy.**

Controlling Back Door Selling

Controlling visits of sales personnel is considerably more difficult in hospitals than it is in manufacturing industry. Most of the doctors are extremely individualistic. This fact at times creates problems in establishing and enforcing effective business procedures. Added to this, the physical layout in most hospitals does not provide separate areas for meeting vendors as in industrial organizations, where separate reception rooms for vendors are provided. Visitors cannot get reception without clearance. **In hospitals, vendors are free to roam about. In such situations, controls can seldom be accomplished by fiat.** There may be situations where the subject matter is highly unique or complex and users may have genuine and urgent need to talk to sales representatives. In such situations, the purchase department should do everything possible to bring competent sales personnel and the doctors or users together.

Controlling salesmen involves scheduling their visits in accordance with the following commonsense alternatives.

1. Salesmen, who from organization point of view, can be utilized most effectively in purchasing department can be handled by purchasing staff.
2. Salesmen who can best be handled most effectively by appropriate technical personnel, as for new surgical products development or improving performance of existing ones as per doctor's ideas, should not be obstructed from achieving this relationship by unduly restrictive purchasing procedures.

In USA, surgical sales executives visit every one of the 5,000 hospitals where surgeries are performed at least once in every ten days. They gown up and accompany surgeons into operating rooms to provide technical assistance in the use of U.S. surgical products. Importantly, they also listen to what doctors like, and don't like, need, and don't need. hospital's close connection has resulted in many innovative products. (Philip Kotler and Gary Armstrong)

RECIPROCITY

In theory, reciprocity should be easier to control in hospitals than it is in industry; in practice, exactly reverse is often the case. Trustees, donors, and alumni of teaching hospitals on occasion, bring great pressures on healthcare institutions for the purchases of their favourite company's products. Normally, such pressures are difficult to resist. A hospital has nothing to sell back to its vendors. This obviously is quite a different situation than can exist in industrial reciprocity. There, the objective of reciprocity is, in theory at least, for the buyer and seller to reach an agreement on an exchange of business that is mutually beneficial. Suppose a vendor gave a donation of Rs. 5,00,000, to the hospital, and now demands business which will yield for his firm a profit in excess of Rs. 5,00,000 then he is actually asking the institution to give him a gift. Healthcare institutional buyers should always be alert to this widespread unfair practice of exchange.

The preceding discussion on reciprocity should not be implied to mean that donors cannot be good suppliers as well. They certainly can be. In fact, if they are willing to compete on quality, service, and price; they can be the best suppliers. It is only when they are unwilling to compete openly that their motives become suspicious. The answer to the vendors' proposals of reciprocity in healthcare institutions could be appreciation of their generosity. However, beyond that, the hospital has many supporters and benefactors, and obligations towards patients. Hence, it must give impartial treatment to all stakeholders if it is to maintain a reputation for integrity, fair dealing, and progressiveness. Consequently, it has no alternative to selecting its vendors on any basis other than the best combination of quality, service, and price.

PERSONNEL

Despite their rapid growth, hospitals have so far lagged behind industry in recruiting most competent Materials Management personnel. Hospitals frequently place their purchasing personnel too low in their management hierarchy. This is one of the reasons why hospitals could not attract talent. Fortunately, these institutions are now trying to attract personnel with top flight qualifications and skills. **Good purchasing results from professional competence.** Determining the best combination of quality, service, and price is the result of effective negotiations, value analysis, price analysis, vendor analysis, cost analysis etc. All these activities require high levels of competence. Purchasing personnel, who lack such competence, work as order placers, not as competent buyers. Low salaries still remain as the greatest single obstacle to good healthcare institutions buying.

ORGANIZATION

The location of purchasing department in the organization structure can have a single significant influence on the department's ability to function optimally. Healthcare institutions routinely place their purchasing departments too low in the management hierarchy. Despite the fact that procurement is a major area of potential cost saving in most hospitals, hospitals have not fully capitalized on this source of cutting costs. Most materials managers in industry report either directly to the chief executive officer or to a senior vice president. It should be emphasized that organization is merely a logical group of tasks. Motivation and integrating of people gets the work done. This comes from coordination and communication. These are most important responsibilities of any manager. A purchasing manager who must work with every department head in a hospital cannot effectively carry good purchasing principles if he or she is not member of top management itself.

PROFESSIONAL LOYALTIES

A doctor with MD qualification working in a super speciality hospital or DM in a teaching hospital or a corporate hospital, may be motivated more by his professional accomplishments than by the performance of the institution which he is supposed to serve. This is not to cast an aspersion on his loyalty. Typically, Doctor's loyalty to his profession comes first, and to the organization where he works, stands second.

This is the anti thesis of a business manager's loyalty. A business manager's loyalty is to his firm first and then to his profession. For a business firm to operate successfully, the managers of various functions, such as marketing, materials, operations, finance, personnel, and engineering must subordinate their desire for individual achievement. Their paramount motivation must be directed towards their firm's achievement as a whole. If marketing or engineering fail, it will result in failure of other functions and of the firm as a whole. For individual gains, business managers must cooperate and become integral parts of the team. Business managers, like vital organs of human body, are parts of a body that will die or operate at a reduced efficiency, unless all the vital parts function properly. A business executive's loyalty must first be to his organization then to his profession, otherwise neither the firm nor the executive can be fully successful. If any basic business function in a firm fails or weakens, the firm as a whole suffers similar consequences. This is the reason that business managers cannot achieve optimum individual success unless they cooperate and become team players.

An industrial organization sustains on the principle of **self help made effective through mutual help.** This is not the situation that exists in healthcare organization. Doctors more often than not, feel that they are entities unto themselves. They can succeed or fail individually, without regard to the success or failure of the organization in which they are employed. The managers, working in hospitals consequently deal with unique people; people who, frequently are in great demand and short supply. Working with them successfully requires different appeals and techniques from those used successfully in industry.

CENTRALIZATION OF PURCHASING

In a large hospital or research oriented healthcare institution, the broad scope of its technical effort and the complete lack of departmental routine usually make it difficult to centralize purchasing. To complicate matters further, hospitals tend to spread themselves over large geographical areas. "A wit once defined a university as a collection of colleges and schools connected with more or less inadequate plumbing. It is difficult to coordinate widely separated units under any circumstances; in an atmosphere of academic freedom, it is especially difficult in academic environment, very few things can be accomplished by edict; consequently total centralization of purchasing is often very difficult." (**Lammer Lee and Donald Dobler**) This aptly applies to large multi speciality healthcare institutions. The problem is further aggravated because the recognizable strength of a hospital flows from a general policy of independence and autonomy of medical experts. Procurement is a justifiable exception. Competent institutional management strives for purchasing centralization in the highest practical degree. It is costly for a hospital if different departments carry out their own purchasing in an unprofessional manner without consolidating purchase orders and delivery schedules. There would be confusion in unloading, checking, routing, processing, recording, and generally keeping on top of hundreds of daily deliveries made to hundreds of delivery points instead of to a centralized receiving and processing area. Expenses on such a system would be prohibitive due to high internal cost of close control which is needed for such activities without even taking into

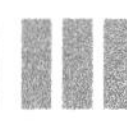

account the high prices that would inevitably be paid for the materials ordered under such a system. If all using departments attempted to get lower prices from higher volumes, this would add additional costs for inventory control of stocks, storage space, usage records, and the like. It has been estimated that centralized purchasing in hospitals yields savings of at least 10 to 15 percent over a decentralized system. Additionally, centralized purchasing allows vendors to render better services as well as offer better prices because their expenses in servicing the institution which they serve are reduced. For example, their salesmen have fewer persons to call on, fewer orders have to be serviced, fewer invoices have to be prepared, fewer shipments have to be made, and finally, fewer financial records have to be kept. Centralized purchasing and Materials Management in healthcare institutions will eventually develop sufficient bargaining power to deal directly with manufacturers and possibly eliminate one entire level of distribution for higher healthcare products such as X-ray films. The savings would accrue if the centres are collectively strong enough to act as countervailing forces to manufacturers themselves, rather than their fragmented dealers and distributors.

DIFFERENCES BETWEEN PUBLIC AND PRIVATE HEALTHCARE INSTITUTIONS

There are notable differences between public and private hospitals in respect of responsibilities of executives, and organization of Hospital Materials Management (HMM). A few public hospitals may be free of political purchasing constraints but most of them are highly constrained in their operations by governmental regulations. Private hospitals on the other hand, are usually free to use their economic clout in the ways best suited to them. The considerations for good purchasing in all hospitals should be the same as found in industry. Procedures in either public or private hospitals should be directed towards creating goodwill for the hospitals. Goodwill is achieved when patients feel assured that a hospital treats all customers impartially. To satisfy such diverse groups as trustees, donors, business firms, and governmental agencies, a private hospital has no rational alternative but to buy without favouritism just as public hospitals are required to do by law. **Difference between purchasing for public and private hospitals is not a matter of concept; rather it is a matter of how to implement the concept of buying without favouritism**. Political pressures can cause public institutions to ridiculously extend otherwise sound concepts. For example, they may be often forced into using competitive bidding in situations where effective negotiations would give better price and service.

In India, government hospitals, dispensaries, and in medical institutions and organizations attached to the **Director General of Health Services (DGHS)** under Ministry of Health and Family Welfare procures a variety of medical equipment and drugs under various national programmes. A separate procurement cell is constituted for procurement of medical equipment exclusively where the value of equipment exceeds Rs. 10 lakhs. Where equipment costs below this limit, procurement is undertaken by respective healthcare institution/ organization. The procurement of capital equipment by DGHS is based on predetermined specifications. specifications are drawn by the approved committee of technical experts. Generally, the procurement is done by open tender method. Tender enquires are published in Indian Trade Journal or Indian Trade Bulletin and newspapers to attract good manufactures as well as bring in

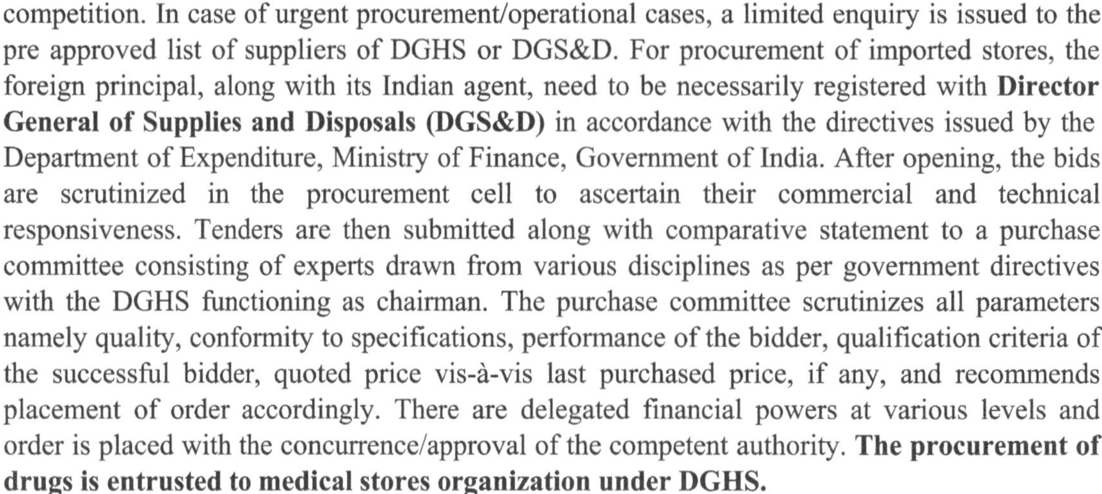

competition. In case of urgent procurement/operational cases, a limited enquiry is issued to the pre approved list of suppliers of DGHS or DGS&D. For procurement of imported stores, the foreign principal, along with its Indian agent, need to be necessarily registered with **Director General of Supplies and Disposals (DGS&D)** in accordance with the directives issued by the Department of Expenditure, Ministry of Finance, Government of India. After opening, the bids are scrutinized in the procurement cell to ascertain their commercial and technical responsiveness. Tenders are then submitted along with comparative statement to a purchase committee consisting of experts drawn from various disciplines as per government directives with the DGHS functioning as chairman. The purchase committee scrutinizes all parameters namely quality, conformity to specifications, performance of the bidder, qualification criteria of the successful bidder, quoted price vis-à-vis last purchased price, if any, and recommends placement of order accordingly. There are delegated financial powers at various levels and order is placed with the concurrence/approval of the competent authority. **The procurement of drugs is entrusted to medical stores organization under DGHS.**

COOPERATIVE BUYING

Cooperative purchasing among hospital groups can be most beneficial, when properly implemented. Cooperative purchasing involves establishment of cooperative buying organizations that negotiate prices with suppliers based on the estimated total demand based on individual needs of cooperative members. Cooperative buying is most commonly used by state and local government hospitals in U.S.A. around 50 to 70 voluntary hospitals belong to one or more such cooperatives. In India, quite a few of government hospitals are adopting a concept similar to cooperative purchasing, to overcome some of their purchasing problems.

Such purchasing takes place in one of three following forms.

1. **Full purchasing services:** Under this, local government hospitals purchase from a common warehouse which is operated by another government agency. Almost every state has an organization for state stores purchasing.

2. **Open end contracts:** Under cooperative open end contracts, the central agency (i.e. city, state or central government agency) awards contracts which permit other local, state, and central government hospitals to order directly from the contractor at the same price quoted to central agency. Rate and Running contracts by DGS&D and DGHS fall in this category. Hospitals gain the advantages of superior prices and services as a result of large volume contracts. They also benefit from the convenience and economies of placing their orders to get quantity discounts. Every state government entrusts to a nodal agency, the responsibility to pool the requirements of all state government hospitals and procure requirements on behalf of them. Medical equipments and drugs required by government healthcare institutions under Ministry of Health and Family Welfare are procured through DGHS.

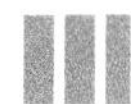

3. **Joint bid procedures:** Under this method, a number of government hospitals consolidate their requirements for large joint bids after standardization of items and their descriptions; a collection and collation of each individual hospitals requirements and a joint call for competitive bids. Thus, an extra administrative work load is imposed on the central activity coordinating the joint bid procedure but the resultant reductions in price more than compensate for added expense. Joint bidding is most effective in procurement of large items of equipments and largely used common medical items.

In the United States of America, cooperative purchasing is mostly among private hospitals. Hospital Bureau, Pleasantville, New York, is an outstanding national cooperative serving hospital. A number of hospitals have also formed local purchasing cooperatives, which also sometimes engage in local service ventures such as laundries. Successes of these local ventures have been proportional to the skills with which the cooperatives have been conceived and managed.

There is no doubt that savings can result from the proper harnessing of economic power and professional talent. **However, many cooperatives fail because they are ill conceived, poorly managed, and too small to reap the rewards resulting from larger volume of business.**

PRICE FACTOR

Earlier, hospital market segment was small. Suppliers felt that it was their philanthropic duty to help these institutions financially. Today, it is not the case. The market has undergone a change; now suppliers view hospital market as large and highly profitable and worthy of their sales efforts. Many large corporations, which earlier ignored this segment, are now eagerly entering into it. Pricing is always a problem when entering into any long term contract with a distributor. The distributors are unable to control prices paid to manufacturers. A distributor may buy at Rs. 450 and be willing to sell at Rs. 495. If the manufacturer raises its price to Rs. 495, the distributor will want to boost its retail price by at least Rs. 45. In practice, he will probably boost it by Rs. 49.50, so that it preserves the 10 percent mark up. For this reason, most distributors are willing to enter into fixed price contracts with their hospital customers only when they have some assurance of predictable prices from the manufacturers. When they do not have this assurance, the hospital usually has little option but to agree to an alternative pricing system. In most cases, this involves negotiation with the distributor for a discount from manufacturer's list. In other instances, the hospital will prefer to buy at predetermined mark up over cost.

Suppose hospital X pays Rs. 150 for an item, that hospital Y buys the same item for Rs. 200. If this fact becomes known to hospital Y, and it persuades the vendor for the price reduction, there is little likelihood that it will get it. Instead, the vendor will equalize the prices; he will either start charging hospital X Rs. 200 or he will charge both Rs. 175. In either case, the hospital that is buying well loses. This is a basic reason for not revealing price information.

AUXILIARY FUNCTIONS

Many hospitals have found it organizationally desirable to group their auxiliary purchasing functions such as traffic, receiving, delivery and surplus and salvage together, in what can perhaps be called the "Purchasing Auxiliary Services Division".

Traffic: As contrasted to industry and government, many healthcare institutions do not have a traffic specialist. All hospitals should consider the advantages of having one. Outgoing shipments in hospitals are small in number and incoming shipments are usually consigned F.O.B. destination. Nonetheless, there still can be a need for a traffic specialist. A healthcare institution cannot avoid paying a reasonable salary to an experienced clerk, for clearing its freight bills, for payment, and for initiating settlements of its freight claims. For a little additional salary, a skilled traffic specialist can be hired. In all likelihood, this individual can generate cash savings that will recover his salary several times over. In addition, improved traffic and claims service will be a gain for the institution. A good traffic specialist can help in many transportation situations, when there are minimum rates but no maximum rates. He can advise buyers on the best and most economic routings to use. He can follow through on lost and delayed shipments. He can also be of great assistance in getting materials cleared through customs and other governmental agencies.

Receiving: Hospitals, sometimes underestimate the importance of receiving function because they do not have production schedules. Poor receiving can produce costly consequences for hospitals as in manufacturing industry. **Receiving is a critical control point in Hospital Materials Management (HMM)** system. The receiving dock directs the flow of purchased materials and relevant documents. Discrepancies, if any, are uncovered. Errors are easily corrected. Cost of correcting them later is higher. receiving clerk can also easily identify suppliers who do not meet the minimum standards of quality and services for his hospital. Hence, importance of receiving function should never be underestimated by a hospital.

Delivery: All materials received both by purchase from vendors and by requisition from stores must be delivered to the user department. To the extent possible, these two categories of materials should be combined into a single, integrated delivery system. Such an action prevents duplication of effort. Failing to plan ahead for their material requirements is a common shortcoming of many healthcare institution departments. To compensate for this shortcoming, they request immediate deliveries of all materials which they requisition. Ignoring all other aspects of the problem, institutions simply cannot afford the cost of making continuous deliveries. Hospitals especially can support only a reasonable delivery system, not an express one. Each hospital must determine for itself what is reasonable.

Surplus and Salvage: In a healthcare institution, surplus and salvage sales are not usually handled, either with same efficiency or with same interest, which industry directs to these profitable areas. Healthcare institutions are however generating larger and larger surpluses of increasing values. In absence of a formalized surplus and salvage programme, department heads tend to

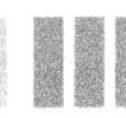

dispose off surplus materials on subjective basis rather than in a businesslike manner. In disposing of surplus, the first consideration should be whether the surplus can be used elsewhere in the hospital or in other hospital operations. This is normally the most profitable form of disposal. If the material cannot be used within the hospital, possibility of returning it to the original supplier should be investigated. **Many suppliers accept the return of salable materials at original price or current price, whichever is lower after reducing the stocking charge.** If it appears that surplus items will have an eventual use within the hospital, then the decision on whether to sell straight away or later depends on the expected time required for utilization of materials, the hospital's cost of capital, rate of income tax, and the shelf-lives of the item(s).

MATERIALS MANAGEMENT PROBLEMS IN HEALTHCARE INSTITUTIONS

HR problems of healthcare institutions are undoubtedly important. But they have been given so much attention that another major and growing problem has been overlooked; i.e., the materials problem in healthcare.

Some of the issues involved are:

- Hospitals are not only labour intensive but also materials intensive.
- According to American Hospitals Association data on reporting the trend on hospital salaries per patient's day and that of non salary costs per day, non-labour (primarily purchased materials and services) costs of hospital care have been increasing faster than labour costs. **Every 10 percent increase in hospital salary and fringe benefits cost, is accompanied by an approximately 15 percent increase in non personnel costs (purchased materials and services). Dean S. Ammer**
- Hospitals are not only paying higher prices for purchases but are also using more of them.

Some of the reasons for the problems are:

- Usage of purchased materials has increased of late, partly because of advancement in technology. This becomes most obvious when present day hospitals are compared with the earliest hospitals.
- Earlier, the hospitals offered nursing care along with room and boarding but not much else, while progress in healthcare techniques has created brand new paramedical skills; its effect on materials has been even greater.
- In addition, continued progress is primarily a matter of development of new materials, drugs, equipment, and a host of other items. New skills will undoubtedly be developed in order to use these new materials more effectively.

However, **aggregate healthcare man hours per patient will not increase as much as materials usage.** In short, the suppliers to the healthcare institutions will almost certainly continue to enjoy a higher growth rate than that of the institutions themselves.

MAGNITUDE OF PURCHASES

Purchasing costs per hospital bed per year varies widely depending upon the number in type of specialities and how they account for unofficial inventories. Hospitals are paying more for purchases each year, not only because of higher prices, but also more materials are required directly or indirectly for each patient. For example, most important categories of drug purchases like antibiotics and tranquilizers did not exist in India, a generation ago. These drugs perform functions that simply were not fulfilled in the past. Large sums of monies are also being spent on products that perform the same old functions better or cheaply. In some cases, these products are a response to soaring hospital labour costs. It has often become economical to substitute supplier labour and capital for hospital labour (i.e., subcontracting). Food, beverages and drugs are often purchased in unit packages, thus saving preparation and handling time in kitchen, and the pharmacy syringes and other disposables not only improve quality of care but also substitute purchased materials for hospital labour, which would otherwise require sterilization operations.

Institution Passive Role

Hospitals undoubtedly benefit from a flow of new products; they are not able to develop them on their own. Their role is strictly that of passive purchasers of whatever their suppliers have to offer. In fact, it has been implicitly assumed that the supplier's interests parallel those of their customer institutions. User wants and needs the product offered by the supplier. Thus it appears that, what is good for seller may also be good for buyer. Although the buyer and seller are mutually dependent, purchasers are gradually becoming more sophisticated. What is good for seller now is often but not always good for the buyer. Supplier's goal of profit maximization is certainly not in consonance with the buyer's interest.

DEVELOPMENT OF PURCHASING IN HEALTHCARE INSTITUTIONS

User buyer in the past, the healthcare institutional user of material dealt directly with healthcare suppliers. Each department head in the healthcare institution was responsible for his or her own purchases. He was the expert. If he did not know what he wanted, his friendly supplier helped him to make decisions. In this environment, there was no recognition of the existence of buying skills. There were only user expertise and supplier marketing prowess. Lack of buying skill need not be crippling as long as the institution is small one, its needs are limited, and the buyers of institution's services are not price conscious.

Applying New Skills

It is obvious that marketer's selfish objectives do not always further those of its institutional customers. Further, institutions are gradually squeezed by steadily rising costs and resistance to increases in its charges to patients. At this point, there is recognition, that a third party, the professional buyer can influence the user seller interaction in the best overall interests of the hospital. This situation calls for some rethinking on some aspects of hospital purchasing function. Buying skill is

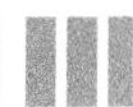

quite different from using and specifying skills. User knows how to apply or administer what is sold to him. Professional buyer in contrast, may have only a superficial knowledge about the function of the product purchased. But he is able to identify the institutional objectives, which are not always completely in consonance with those of the user, let alone the vendors. Professional buyer is now in a position to influence the seller to behave in a manner that is more consistent with overall objectives of the buying healthcare institution. To a user, price of material is simply what the supplier charges. In such a case, the price that is paid will reflect almost entirely the seller's selfish interest in profit maximization. In contrast, for a professional buyer, price is a result of negotiation between buyer and seller; it reflects a compromise between the conflicting selfish interests of both the parties. User of purchased material is generally interested only in possessing enough of material on hand and in ensuring that it will always remain available. Professional materials manager sees the stock of materials in the stores as representing a compromise between two conflicting objectives i.e., the desire to have it available as opposed to the goal of minimizing costs that are always associated with the existence of any stock pile of inventory. It is barely visible physically hospital inventory ranges from Rs. 3.75 lakhs to Rs. 15 lakhs per bed. The reason for this large scale variation is that different hospitals adopt different measures of performance for example the stock values at one hospital in present only official inventory. Where as, at another it include both official and unofficial inventories. Next reason for variation may represent total bed strength or occupancy rate. "This measure is most useful when it is used for comparing progress over a period of time with in a facility adjusting of course of changes in scope of service and utilization". **(Willam Sheyer)**

SUMMARY

One of the important developments in the United States economy during of 1960's has been its change from a production economy to service economy. Hospitals have become an important and rapidly growing segment of the American economy. India is also going through a major revolution in healthcare services. The economic liberalization, and the management concepts and techniques are beginning to have impact now on health and medical institutions. Healthcare in India is basically urban-oriented.

There is a wide spread impression that purchasing for healthcare organizations is totally different from industrial purchasing. There is no separate group of principles for hospital buying; however, it involves certain special considerations, which are not usually applicable to purchasing in industry.

Advances in healthcare technology not only create demand for specialized skills, but also probably work to increase rather than decrease employment in healthcare institutions, making them more labour intensive than ever. Purchased materials usage of late has increased partly because of advancements in technology. Progress in healthcare techniques has created new paramedical skills; its effect on materials has been even greater.

Aggregate healthcare man hours per patient will not increase nearly as much as materials usage. The suppliers to the healthcare institutions will almost certainly continue to enjoy a higher growth rate than that of the institutions themselves. Though hospitals undoubtedly benefit from a flow of new products, they are not able to develop them on their own; their role is strictly that of passive purchasers of whatever their suppliers have to offer.

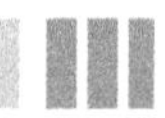

Large sums of monies are being spent on products that perform the same old functions better or cheaply. In some cases, these products are a response to increasing hospital labour costs. To the professional buyer, the price is a result of negotiation between buyer and seller.

Negotiated price reflects a compromise between the conflicting selfish interests of the parties concerned. For most items, the aggregate cost of carrying distribution inventories probably exceeds the actual manufacturing cost of drugs.

Every principle of good purchasing in purchasing management applies to purchases made for healthcare institutions. All buying activities whether, industrial or governmental or healthcare institutions, have one cardinal objective: "Obtaining maximum value for each rupee spent."

Hospital purchasing however places different emphasis on certain areas of considerations of healthcare institutional purchasing. Important among them are: 1. Control of budgets, 2. Scope for savings, 3. Challenging specifications, 4. Inspection of materials and services, 5. Back door selling, 6. Reciprocity, 7. Personnel, 8. Organization, 9. Professional loyalties, 10. Centralization of purchasing, 11. Cooperative purchasing, 12. Differences in public and private health care institutions, 13. Prices, 14. Materials Management, 15. Stores, 16. Auxiliary functions such as traffic, receiving, delivery and surplus and salvage.

Parkinson's Law on budgets aptly applies to all service organization more so for hospitals. The will and determination to control expenditures in service organizations is not as strong as it is in industry.

It has proved easier to revise room rents and service charges than it has for industrial companies to raise the selling prices of their products. Hospitals have not been motivated to control the purchasing costs in the same way that competitive industry has.

Hospitals deal with a much broader spectrum of materials and services than does the average industrial company. Challenging specifications, therefore, is especially important and fruitful. The purchasing department that is responsible for the economic considerations has the responsibility of challenging the restrictive specifications - this means to request reconsideration of technical decisions for economic reasons. In most hospitals and medical centres, receiving departments will inspect for bulk quantity and outward damages; quality and compliance with specifications is checked by doctors, who originated the request for materials. When desired, the receiving department can of course, inspect for general store types, or common use items.

Doctors are highly knowledgeable concerning what they want to do professionally in their fields. However, this does not entail knowledge of economics, and market availability.

A doctor working in a large hospital or learning institution may be more concerned with his professional accomplishments than with the institution for which he is working. Typically his first loyalty is to his profession and second to the organization where he works. This is anti-thesis of what a business executive's loyalty should be. It should be to his firm first and to his profession second, for a business firm to operate successfully.

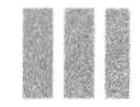

Hospitals should develop simple tests that can be performed within their technical capabilities. Some examples are count, weigh, measure and check.

Process of making a sale prior to its review by the purchasing department is called back door selling. Controlling visits of sales personnel is considerably more difficult in medical centres than it is in industry. Controlling salesmen properly involves, scheduling them in accordance with two alternatives: 1. Salesmen, who from organization point of view, can be utilized most effectively in purchasing department, can be handled by purchasing staff; and, 2. Salesmen who can best be handled most effectively by appropriate technical personnel should not be obstructed from achieving this relationship by unduly restrictive purchasing procedures.

Good purchasing results primarily from professional competence. Determining the best combination of quality, service, and price, is the result of actions such as effective negotiation, value analysis, price analysis, vendor analysis, cost analysis etc. All these activities require high level of competence.

A purchasing manager, who must work with every department head in a hospital, cannot effectively carry good purchasing principles if he or she is not a member of top management itself. Managers, working in hospitals, deal with unique people, people who are frequently in great demand and short supply. Working with them successfully requires different appeals and techniques from those used successfully in the industry.

Properly guided cooperative purchasing among the institutional groups can be most beneficial. In India, quite a few of the government hospitals are trying to overcome some of their purchasing problems through concepts similar to cooperative purchasing. Cooperative purchasing takes one of three forms: 1. Full purchasing services, 2. Open end contracts, and 3. Joint bid procedures.

Medical equipment and drugs required by government healthcare institutions under Ministry of Health and Family Welfare are procured through Directorate General of Health Services.

Pricing is always a problem, when existing into long-term contract with a distributor. The roof of the problem lies with the distributor's inability to control prices paid to manufacturers. From buyer's point of view, low prices are major motivation for a system or prime vendor contract. This is hardly supplier's motivation; in fact, many so called prime vendor contracts lead to higher not lower prices. Healthcare institutions continuously try to compare their prices with those of other institutions. In most cases, such price comparison is really meaningless and such action is unethical.

Materials Management process begins with the supplier and does not end until materials are consumed. Many healthcare institutions have found it organizationally desirable to group their auxiliary purchasing function traffic, receiving, delivery and surplus together, in what can approximately called the "Purchasing Service Division". A good traffic specialist can help in many transportation situations when there are minimum rates but not maximum rates. He can advise buyers on the best and most economic routings to use. Receiving is a critical control point in hospital materials system. It is at the receiving dock that the papers directing the flow of purchased materials and physical materials themselves meet for the first time.

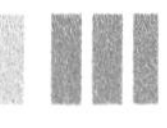

All materials received both by purchasers from outside vendors and by requisition from stores must be delivered to the user department. To the extent possible, these two categories of materials should be combined into single, integrated delivery system. Thus, such an action will prevent duplication of effort.

Healthcare institutions are generating larger and larger surpluses of increasing values. Without a formalized surplus and salvage programme, department heads tend to sell surplus materials on subjective basis rather than on business basis.

Trustees/donors bring great pressure on institutions for the purchase of a particular company's products. Normally, such purchases (if made on any basis other than quality, service, and price) should be resisted.

Hospitals frequently place their purchasing departments too low in the management organizations structure. This is one of the primary reasons why hospitals have lagged in attracting top purchasing talent. It is also a paramount reason why their purchasing accomplishments to this point have lagged behind industry, government, and other institutions. A purchasing manager is constrained in carrying out top management's desire for good purchasing principles if he is not a member of top management himself. Effective centralization of the purchasing function is virtually impossible when the purchasing department is not high in the management structure.

Hospitals have tended to lag behind industry and government in recruiting the most competent purchasing personnel. Institutional salaries historically have been lower than industrial salaries. Fortunately, this situation is now changing and some purchasing professionals are beginning to migrate from industry to institutions. The purchasing operations of a large institution call for highly competent managers.

Healthcare institutions have the same reasons for carrying items in stores, as industry i.e., economy and service. To prevent loss of life, hospitals must have access to immediate reserves of certain materials. These reserves, however, do not have to be stored in the hospital itself. They can be stored in the vendor's storeroom. This is based on the concept of the vendor being an extension of the institution's stores system.

REVIEW QUESTIONS

1. a. Making a sale prior to its review by purchasing department is back door selling? What steps are to be taken to control back door selling?

   b. What are the peculiar problems that hospital purchase manager faces?

2. What do you understand by the term "reciprocity"? How difficult it is to control reciprocity in healthcare institutions than in industry?

3. Describe major differences between public and private healthcare institutions purchasing.

4. What do you understand by the term backdoor selling and how it has be controlled in hospitals?

5. Savings in hospital purchase are as valuable as they are in industry - elaborate the statement with suitable examples.

6. How are hospital materials and service inspected as compared to industry?

7. Write short notes on

   a. Preventive cost reduction techniques

   b. Challenging specifications

   c. Role of DGHS in hospital purchasing

   d. Reciprocity

   e. Professional loyalties

   f. Auxiliary functions of purchasing in hospitals

   g. Back door selling

PART - II

Special Features of Hospital Purchasing

Contents

CHAPTER - 10

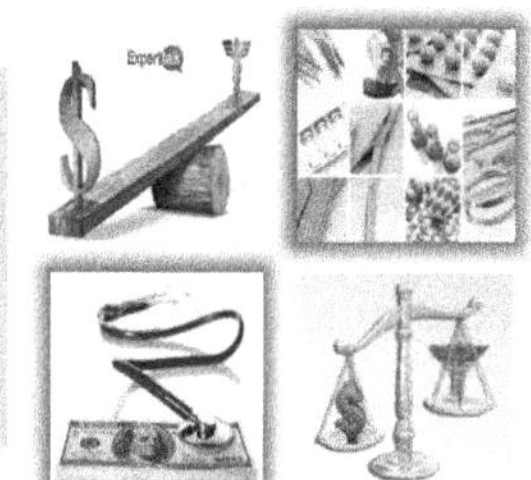

Special Features of Hospital Purchasing

INTRODUCTION

Efficiency and effectiveness are twin objectives of Materials Management. There are several distinctly, different difficulties associated with purchasing for patient care when compared to buying for a manufacturing company. Decisions in healthcare purchasing can be attributed to many individuals like hospital administrators, doctors, nurses, and other paramedical staff; in addition, service features of patient care. These constraints are over and above to traditional buying for manufacturing companies. **Hospital inventories are broadly classified as expendables and unexpendables. These expendables are further classified as reusable or disposable.**

Based on the author's interactions with hospital professionals in the capacity of a Professor, Hospital Operations Management and as chief executive of manufacturing companies, he had identified some special categories of products in hospital buying processes viz. digital medical electronic monitors, stretchers, linens, disposables and reusables to highlight in this chapter on special features of hospital purchasing.

Electronic equipments are purchased to monitor ventricular fibrillation, a fairly common cardiac emergency requiring immediate diagnosis. Hooking up the electrodes and obtaining a quick reading of the patient's condition from a monitor is very important because "irreversible brain damage occurs in three to four minutes". After operational switch on, some time is required for attaching electrodes.

Stretchers are used in all patient care areas. Each area requires a variation on what was, historically, just a frame on four castor wheels with a metal top covered by a pad, all designed to carry a patient from one place to another. Today's hospital has stretcher transports for emergency rooms, surgery, intensive care and coronary critical care units, **post anaesthesia recovery rooms (PAR),** radiology, and general transportation.

Less technical than digital medical electronic monitoring equipment and stretchers is linen, classified as either a reusable or disposable. Hospital linens require careful evaluation and testing, as costs for linens are rising. Hence the need for economy measures such as more patching of torn linen, making hand towels out of bath towels that are torn, and prolonging the life of linen by increasing inventory (so that linens are not used immediately after each laundering).

Oil shortage and energy crisis are matters of international concern. For the past several years, the use of disposables and non woven items has been steadily increasing in healthcare institutions. Hospitals, nursing homes, clinics, and doctors' offices have relied on disposable syringes and needles for at least past twenty five years. **Anything used in patient care that must be cleaned, sterilized, washed, or otherwise converted to its original aseptic condition, can be considered either a disposable or a reusable.**

Although hospital purchasing managers differ in their approaches to acquisitions of these items, some considerations are generally common. These considerations apply in fact to all health facility equipment or multi use products. Guidelines for hospital purchasing and strategies for group purchasing must give special attention to these items.

DIGITAL MEDICAL ELECTRONIC MONITORS

These monitoring equipments consist of LED (light emitting diode) display, solid-state circuitry, modular systems, and interchangeable circuit cards and are found in specialized medical surgical areas including intensive care, coronary care, paediatric and neonatal nursing, surgery, and emergency. These are also used for heart catheterization in critical and non critical patient areas and for stress testing in cardiovascular complications. These machines are most valuable only because of their accuracy, reliability, safety and functionality. Their bidding specifications generation needs assistance of bio medical engineers or research and testing laboratories. The purchasing manager arranges for demonstrations of multiple brands/models of equipments for the consideration by bio-medical experts, who ultimately recommend the selection criteria.

1. **Safety, accuracy and reliability:** Accidents are totally undesirable in patient care.
2. **Supplying company technical competence:** This is an important aspect which requires to be gone into in greater details and thoroughly especially where quality and technical competence is of critical importance to buyer.
3. **Promptness of after sale service:** Firms marketing capital equipment face the problem whether to go in for their own costly modern service centres or ensure that the dealers invest in a service set up after considering aspects such as overhead expenses, pilferage, working capital for slow moving spare parts inventory, wage bill, labour indiscipline, technical quality of service etc. In such a situation, a purchase manager has to obtain first hand information to assess the capabilities of the original equipment manufacturer (OEM) or his authorized service centres
4. **Testing cost:** This may not be playing a major role in selection, as higher cost might sometimes represent better equipment.

5. **Pre standardization and standardization programmes:** The objective is to reduce the number of different items that are purchased. Preventive measure in a standardization purchasing will discourage purchases that tend to introduce new brands and possibly new stocking spares and maintenance problems. Standardization leads to cost containment.

6. **Compatibility with the hospital's existing equipment:** Computers and other electronic equipments as well as with expected new technological developments that in the near future has also to be borne in mind

While drawing up specifications, there is a need to answer such questions as:

- The number of beds to be monitored.
- Recording needs.
- Whether automatic alarms and displays should be only at bedsides or at central station or at both the places.
- Will the equipment involve conventional patient cables or biotelemetry?

One should also determine whether the monitors should be fixed or mobile, size of display, digital or analogue display formats and safety requirements e.g., X-ray emission levels which are important for **occupational health and safety Act (OHSA)** requirements and local electrical codes. Qualified bio-medical engineers can help train medical personnel in the technical aspects of all kinds of electronic equipment as a requirement for safety and proper use. Sometimes, the bio-medical engineers develop their own apparatus or systems, but this can open up problems of hospital liability, and in such cases, hospitals should take up this legal liability. Electronic monitors maintain surveillance over critical care and operating room patients during and after a crisis. These monitors graphically record and report heart rates or other vital signs on a continuous basis; newer monitors record, store, and retrieve a patient's medical symptoms every twelve or twenty-four hours while in the hospital's coronary care or intensive care areas. Several factors have been clearly identified as influencing the investment for such equipment.

The following factors are to be examined before actual purchase takes place and should include comparative figures on:

1. Original purchase price.
2. Probable downtime, which depends on reliability, service, and ease of maintenance.
3. Savings in nursing time by making use of monitoring and warning devices (including alarms, buzzers).
4. Depreciation and cost of obsolescence.
5. Cost benefit issues i.e., the total cost of the equipment over its expected lifetime by weighing for service and/or installation costs or lease or buy equipment needs to be in good

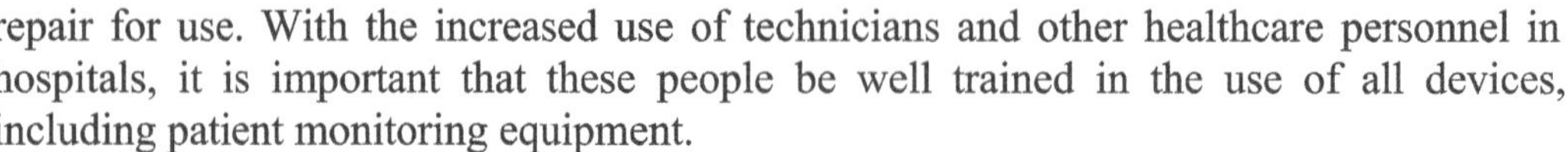

repair for use. With the increased use of technicians and other healthcare personnel in hospitals, it is important that these people be well trained in the use of all devices, including patient monitoring equipment.

For example, if electrocardiograph electrodes are not properly placed on the patient, noise interference can occur. Safety, repair, and maintenance of these equipments are important because of the increased problem of product liability, where the hospital is sued, along with the manufacturer, in cases of injury or illness allegedly caused by healthcare devices. In addition to safety and consumer protection laws, the threat of damage suits is imminent. **Reliability should be built into a machine, but not at the cost of safety.** Conversely, safety can be enhanced without reducing reliability. Possibility of micro shock, equipment reliability, and safety can be evaluated by the seller's representative, a bio technician, an electronics engineer, the physician/user, or maintenance in charge.

Factors important for safety are:

- Age of the equipment, with reference to number of machine hours in use.
- Location of equipment in relation to interfering equipment, if any.
- Availability of standby power.
- Training needs and levels of personnel using the equipment.
- Knowledge and availability of service personnel, and degree of acceptable risk.

Now a days, many hospitals are employing qualified medical electronic engineers who are capable of maintaining electronic equipments of all types, till the need for overhaul is felt. The hospital can also enter into **Annual Maintenance Contract (AMC)** services with manufacturer. Alternatively, hospitals can contract to maintenance service organization employing medical electronics technician, bio medical engineer, clinical engineer, or medical engineer. These technicians/engineers have varying levels of education, ability, status, and salaries. Another problem with purchase of capital equipment is standardization. Purchase of many types of monitoring devices in a single institution complicates repair and maintenance. Further, all emergency medical care programs, whether operated by hospitals, private ambulance service providers, or state governments, need to standardize mobile medical telemetry equipment purchased for remote electrocardiograph transmissions. In absence of such standardization, another manufacturer's equipment cannot always process the signals produced. The problem of **equipment selection is two fold: technical and personal relations.** The purchasing manager is in a key position to enlist the right people in selecting the right electronic equipment for both short and long range uses.

STRETCHERS

Stretchers are one of the basic equipments in use in almost all patient care locations in the hospitals. Several stretchers are modular, with one basic frame to which accessories can be added for different uses, such as side rails, adjustable arm boards, oxygen bottle holders etc. Some modular

 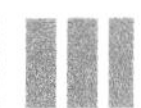

stretchers have an additional fifth wheel in the centre, on the floor, to enable one person to move a patient and maintain the stability of the stretcher. The wheel engages automatically and acts as a steering wheel. Generally, diameter of casters fitted to stretchers would be of 15 to 20 cm. The material specified should be strong gauge tubular steel (class 'C' tubes), and the stretcher fitted with hydraulic lift pedals to facilitate height adjustment.

Stretcher tables that are used as operating or emergency room tables are provided with a braking lock so that all four wheels can be locked by one brake pedal. This braking lowers the four bumper guards to immobilize the wheels. Raising the pedal releases the wheels. Some stretchers have two-wheel brakes, which lock two wheels at one end of the stretcher. These are less convenient for braking, but they are adjustable in case non medical personnel wish to have one end of the stretcher table movable. Trendelenburg position is often needed in stretcher tables. It is achieved by hydraulic height adjustment, which also helps in transferring patients to a bed or a fixed table. The Trendelenburg position adjusts to 15 to 30 degrees. On the Fowler backrests, there are nine positions with three ranges i.e., low, semi and high positions. Stretchers have to be constructed to provide maximum patient comfort, easy and efficient handling for attendant, and three way adjustment.

1. Hydraulic height control.
2. Torsion-balanced Trendelenburg positions pull out control knob allows tilting to desired position in seconds, locks safely in place.
3. Built in Fowler backrest that easily adjusts to nine comfortable positions. It includes built in, self storing, folding chrome plated side rails or metal transfer rails. Stainless steel corner protectors and nylon buttons protect finish. Two built in stainless steel clips are provided to hold rod that carry I.V. fluid.

Criteria for selection of stretchers are:

- The manner in which use relates to the physical characteristics of the rooms and furnishings to which the stretcher is taken.
- Will the stretcher height adapt to the patient height?
- If used in the emergency room, can one wheel it in and out an examining or trauma room?
- What is the turning radius?
- Can the stretcher accommodate rods for holding intravenous solutions for patients, if it is a general transportation stretcher?

Assembly of any stretcher or stretcher table should be done by qualified manufacturer's engineers or under his supervision. An improperly assembled stretcher is prone to collapse and cause injury in a number of ways. Sometimes there may be failure, due to breaking of a castor while a patient is being moved, and then the problem is the manufacturer's product liability. Preventive

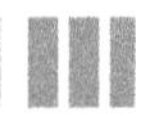

maintenance of stretchers at regular intervals is absolutely essential. The maintenance department should coordinate this with nursing service by labelling unique identification number of each stretcher and date- cards indicating when the stretcher was inspected and its status. There are also cases where some hospitals wait until the equipment comes to grinding halt or state of disrepair and obsolescence before replacing it. Standardization of stretchers by area and purpose is an advantage in terms of price because of volume discount and in terms of service by manufacturer's representative. Because of the distance to be travelled between departments, there is a danger of cardiac arrest for patients with a myocardial infarction or cardiac arrhythmia. Efforts should therefore be made to be prepared for cardiopulmonary arrests en route.

In summary, purchase of stretchers involves product evaluation, standardization, special purpose, and quality. These factors should be taken into account when buying this kind of equipment, as well as cost price considerations and the reputation of the manufacturer.

LINENS

Linen selection is important for patient beds. Non-woven disposables are being increasingly used in many corporate hospitals in areas where linens were formerly used. Patient comfort calls for the need for traditional sheets and blankets. Selection of linens involves man made fibres such as nylon, acrylic, and polyester. A newer synthetic in the market is triacetate. It has renewed the use of nylon because of its durability in repetitive washings. All these are primarily fibres. These new generation fibres are suitable for twinning, where two fibres are combined in varying ways for different uses. Polyester linens have replaced all cotton linens in many hospitals. Through the use of synthetic blends, hospital linen costs have decreased due to greater durability qualities and easier laundering. All modern synthetic products are labelled showing the percentage of product mixes used. Labels indicate fibre content, generic name of all fibres included in the material, name of manufacturer, country of origin if imported, and whether the article is finished. Some hospitals use polyester cotton blend for all linen, except in surgery where static electricity may be hazardous. Annual orders for mixes are usually issued with staggered delivery based on annual demand to facilitate assured deliveries and price is maintained at least for a period of one year.

To purchase linens of any type, hospital may develop or adopt its own versions of **Indian Standard Institution (ISI)** specifications. Specification committees generally comprise of key personnel to evaluate linen usage, misuse, durability, cost, and patient comfort, as well as to assist in ordering speciality woven linens. The committee should include representatives from nursing, laundry, and housekeeping.

Specifications for sheets should cover several aspects. Important among them are:

- **Number of threads per square centimeter:** 30 for polyester cotton or 20 for cotton percale and cotton muslin.
- **Quality:** Percent of cotton or man-made fibres, if blended.

- **Flame:** Retardant/resistant qualities.
- **Weave:** Plain
- **Selvage:** Both sides of sheet shall be 3 cm minimum tape selvage.
- **Size:** Length and width (cut size) with preshrunk quality and not more than 2 cm tolerance, plus or minus.
- **Finish:** Bleached
- **Weight:** Specified in terms of grams per square metre.
- **Tensile strength:** A pull of at least 5 cm.
- **Hems:** 5 cm at each end, turned securely, with stitching at not less than 5 per cm.
- **Shrinkage:** Not more than 2 percent.

Specifications are also relevant for items such as patient pyjamas and gowns.

- For pyjamas, method of closure (snap, zip, tapes, or buttons) should be specified.
- For patient gowns, the important specifications include length of gown and method of closure.
- The concept of equivalence can be applied to specifications for linens by specifying the brand name, number, and type of linens in use, and requesting bids on equivalent basis.

Following is an example of an equivalent specification for surgeon's gowns:

- Colour : White, barrier style.
- Sanforized: i.e., stretched, shrunk and fixed woven cloth before cutting and stitching (Bombay Dyeing fabric).
- Zipper closures
- Overlapping sterile back
- Neckline reinforcement with yoke
- Large size of a particular brand or its equivalent etc.

All cotton cloth is still preferred by hospitals because it is more absorbent, less expensive, and has a higher loss ratio for small items which arc somtimes prone to pilferage by patients and lower level employees. Cotton thermal blankets are difficult to acquire. Substitute materials for all-cotton items are various polyesters. Because of the shortage of cotton products, some hospitals now use anti static cotton polyester with a 2 percent stainless steel wire woven into the fabric for use in surgery. Some hospitals buy disposable sheets, but patients do not normally prefer these because of their papery feel. However, with the improvement in the finish of disposable linens, this difference will reduce. All cotton sheets do not last quite as long as mixes. However before switching over to blended fabrics, there must be close interaction of the laundry in charge with purchasing department to ensure that the laundry equipment can launder the desired linens and that all orders relate to a master linen plan. New types of synthetic materials should be introduced only after testing and validation. The master linen plan is a general guideline establishing quantity of inventory by each classification of linen, by department, by type of material, by number of washings or cleaning processes planned etc. It also provides a basis for selecting and purchasing linens. Selecting linens on the basis of specifications helps in maintaining a master linen plan and a workable inventory system. Some materials require dry cleaning. It is a more expensive process than washing; however a few less expensive dry cleaning chemicals for polyester cottons have now been introduced. Cotton polyester thermal blankets are being increasingly used in hospitals and nursing homes because they are easily laundered. **Flame-retardant linens are more expensive, but they outlast linens that are not flame retardant.** Many hospitals have increased cotton polyesters to 80 percent of their total linen requirement. Polyester cotton lasts a longer number of washes than pure cotton. Generic, standardized names e.g., acetate, acrylic, azlon, fibre glass, metallic, modacrylic (a synthetic copolymer), nylon, mytril, olefin, polyester, rayon, rubber, saran, spandex, vinyl, and vinyon have been defined and established for manufactured fibres. Generally, the larger the quantity, the lower the price, as competitive buying reduces prices wherever there are open manufacturing and marketing channels and no shortages of materials to complicate the open bidding.

Flame retardant fabrics are tested by setting on fire in order to ensure durability, flame-retardant hospital garments for use in the hyperbaric chamber. Such materials include flame-retardant polyesters, phenolics, and polyamides blended cotton. Some of the so called flame retardant fabrics are either flammable or emit lethal noxious fumes when heated to temperatures comparable to a fire situation. As a result of investigative tests, hospitals now use flame retardant pyjamas that resist fire and do not have as great a toxicity. There is a need to check by a simple match test certain factors before buying flame-retardant linens: melting, toxicity and the resultant odour. Washability and cost effectiveness are judged by computing original cost of a garment divided by the number of uses that can reasonably be expected. **Cotton sheets are cheaper and safer than synthetic sheets.** Switching over from polyester cotton to all cotton sheets can save on energy and laundering costs, cause less skin abrasion; need less water to wash, are folded more easily, and not usually prone to pilferage as they are contoured to fit hospital mattresses, which normally are larger than home mattresses.

DISPOSABLES AND REUSABLES

Disposables are generally plastic items and are petroleum derivatives. Hence, the trend towards disposables was not questioned until the availability of petrochemicals became problematic. In 1970's, US hospitals detected two trends: a critical, developing fuel shortage and consequently, anticipated shortage of disposables.

However, if alternatives to petroleum are brought in to use, demand for disposables will continue to rise in healthcare facilities. However, some experts feel that, at some time in future,

 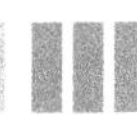

cost increases will certainly force a return to the reusable. At this time, it is a matter of conjecture, but cost is certainly a factor in evaluating disposables as well as their comparison to reusables (Holmgren and Wentz). Both options are important. Early resistance to disposables was caused by their higher prices. For example, the sterilization of needles was less expensive, than buying, using and discarding them, largely because labour cost was less. Later, the acquisition prices of disposables became competitive vis-a-vis reusables, when evaluated objectively. As sales of disposables increased, manufacturing costs fell with higher volumes of manufacture. The prices of disposable needles, syringes, gloves, and drapes decreased on account of economic scales in manufacturing. It became more cost effective to use disposable items.

PROS AND CONS OF DISPOSABLES AND REUSABLES

Advantages of disposable items

- **Cost factor:** In small hospitals and nursing homes, the use of disposables as well as non-woven items may be economical, where volume does not justify cost of manufacturing or reprocessing reusables such as surgical trays, intravenous sets, and pre-assembled disposables.
- **Safety:** Pre packaged, sterile products offer quality control to protect the patient against hospital acquired infections.
- **Convenience:** The product is available of the shelf as soon as need arises.
- **Technology upgradation:** Manufacturers in order to improve their market shares try to invest in techniques to improve patient care disposables; this is a protection against obsolescence.
- **Preferences for disposables:** Preference for disposables is ever increasing as physicians, nurses, technicians, housekeeping staff, and others prefer these items.
- **Legal responsibility:** Manufacturer shares the responsibility in medico legal cases.

Disadvantages

Arguments against using disposables are far less relevant now than they were earlier i.e., at the time when plastic items were first introduced in healthcare industry. Those arguments were based on the belief that disposables would be expensive. Cost comparisons can only validate this assumption. With labour costs are escalating at an unprecedented rate, this argument will certainly not be valid in future.

Make Or Buy Considerations

Cost comparisons are needed to compare costs of reusables and disposables. While buying, the manufacturer absorbs costs of production and material handling. However, for reusables processed in central facility in a hospital reflect all production and overhead costs. Convenience, safety, advanced technology, and demand are the other considerations. Sometimes a small difference

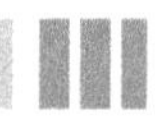

in cost may be outweighed by these intangible characteristics. Data can be obtained from purchasing, finance and user departments, primarily nursing, housekeeping, or dietary, central services and administration. Hospital industrial engineers can develop flowcharts of the processing or acquisition of items as a basis for comparisons of costs of acquisition and delivery for disposable items, with acquisition, processing, and reprocessing costs for reusable items. Verifying the desirability of disposables is a matter of accounting for all costs.

Outside vendors usually try to convince a purchaser to buy their disposables by pointing out that it saves money through elimination of processing costs. The vendor, however, projects only cost of acquisition i.e., the cost incurred up to the time of delivery of an item to hospital. The purchaser should however include in his analysis the ordering and carrying costs too. Disposables are complementaries to, and not always replacements for reusables.

Most healthcare facilities suffer from scarcity of space. Many of these facilities stock 50 to 75 percent more items than they did 2 decades ago. While planning for new facilities, centralization of stores and the increased need for stores expansion must be factored and is the principal reason for the increasing preference for off-site warehousing by hospitals.

It is advisable to pay for a high quality disposable or reusable, in order to obtain maximum benefits, inspite of inexpensive disposable products are available. However considering the fierce competition, increased government surveillance, product liability suits, and rising expectations of patient care, these are not always preferable. Operating room supervisors and consultants insist on disposable dressing trays instead of carts, which can cause cross contamination. The factor stressed here is that of safety, and most plastics are safe.

Environmental Issues

The most potent argument against the use of disposables is pollution and disturbance to ecological balance. Hospitals face the problem of waste disposal daily and have to regularly seek ways and means to control waste and decrease pollution. Methods of solid waste collection in healthcare facilities include bulk collection, automatic pneumatic or drop chute and compaction, pulping, shredding and grinding. Final disposal of infectious solid wastes, away from the site utilizes a community sanitary landfill, on site or off site incineration, or conversion to liquid waste before ultimate disposal. Fewer new convertibles to disposables are now entering the market. Reusables for such high volume items, as surgical packs, instruments, and bed linen and processing them avoid idle time of central processing department personnel. Labour is less expensive when processing, sterilization, and similar activities are generated daily. Also, healthcare facilities function on a twenty four hour basis and hence it may not be advisable to depend on outside sources. Reprocessing of many reusables can be efficient and economical if it ensures proper delivery, low inventory, and adherence to standards, and adjustments in stock levels as needed.

Problems Associated with Disposables

Some vendors now offer both disposables and reusables, and one must consider all factors i.e., labour, storage, convenience, patient safety, and pollution to choose between both the two options. Before the advent of the worldwide oil shortage in 1973, predictions for disposables and plastics in general were optimistic. It was predicted that, by 1976, more than 10 percent of all healthcare supplies and equipment would be disposable, but that did not happen. There are several industrial applications to the make or buy comparison which can be utilized by the healthcare facility purchasing manager. **Dean Ammer's** Material Management and **Lammar Lee and Donald Dobler's** Purchasing and Material Management include separate chapters on make or buy decisions. Georgia Hospital in the US converted to a total system of disposables several years ago and was able to reduce costs without experiencing any increased wastages. St. Johns Mercy Medical Centre in St. Louis, felt that manufacturers of these products need to work closely with hospitals to help eliminate the hazards of throw away needles, syringes, and other sharp pointed disposables because employees sometimes carelessly mix these up with laundry, especially in operating rooms. This problem invariably surfaces during a combined reusable linen disposable medical supplies programme.

When disposables first came in the scene, it was believed that they were most suitable for small hospitals but not in the larger ones which are equipped with extensive central supply departments. This opinion did not survive long and big hospitals too started using disposables because they are easier, better, and more economical to use. In large, impersonal hospitals, processing personnel in central supply tend to become lax. Sterile disposables help eliminate infections; are ready for immediate use, and, for first time, one time use, they are superior to reusables. Anyone who ever received an injection with a re sharpened, reusable needle that had a burr on it, surely believe in disposable needles now. The most important influences on the demand for disposables will continue to be the healthcare wage costs and inflation, as well as the availability of petroleum derivatives. Spiralling labour costs narrow the gap between the costs of disposables and reusables. **The annual disposable growth rate has been 15 percent in recent years.** This is despite the phenomenal increase in cost of petroleum products, some discomfort to patients, and their artificial appearance and texture. Pollution is still a problem. Paper products make up 36 percent of all disposables in the hospital. Recycling (by others) could save on operating supply costs of healthcare institutions. In several hospitals, glass and metal articles have been collected, segregated, packaged, and sold for recycling. Such efforts help reduce pollution. Present trend in hospitals is to use disposable linen as well as packs, pads and garments to save cost towards laundry.

Factors of comparative assessment are as follows:

- Life cycle costing analysis.
- Comparison with neighbouring institutions.
- Estimating both cash and additional costs of handling and processing.
- Adding a notional price for quality.

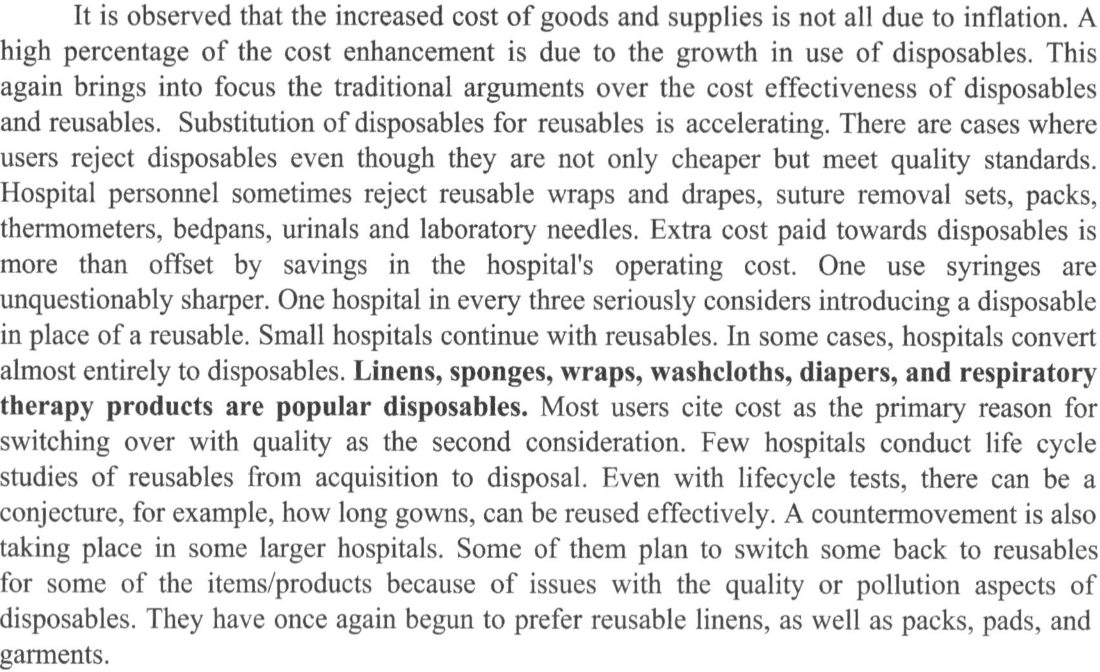

It is observed that the increased cost of goods and supplies is not all due to inflation. A high percentage of the cost enhancement is due to the growth in use of disposables. This again brings into focus the traditional arguments over the cost effectiveness of disposables and reusables. Substitution of disposables for reusables is accelerating. There are cases where users reject disposables even though they are not only cheaper but meet quality standards. Hospital personnel sometimes reject reusable wraps and drapes, suture removal sets, packs, thermometers, bedpans, urinals and laboratory needles. Extra cost paid towards disposables is more than offset by savings in the hospital's operating cost. One use syringes are unquestionably sharper. One hospital in every three seriously considers introducing a disposable in place of a reusable. Small hospitals continue with reusables. In some cases, hospitals convert almost entirely to disposables. **Linens, sponges, wraps, washcloths, diapers, and respiratory therapy products are popular disposables.** Most users cite cost as the primary reason for switching over with quality as the second consideration. Few hospitals conduct life cycle studies of reusables from acquisition to disposal. Even with lifecycle tests, there can be a conjecture, for example, how long gowns, can be reused effectively. A countermovement is also taking place in some larger hospitals. Some of them plan to switch some back to reusables for some of the items/products because of issues with the quality or pollution aspects of disposables. They have once again begun to prefer reusable linens, as well as packs, pads, and garments.

PROBLEMS OF PURCHASING IN INTEGRATED MM ENVIRONMENT

There five major violators of the principle of integrated Materials Management in most hospitals are pharmacy, dietary, radiology, laboratory, and plant maintenance. Foods and beverages and pharmacy are generally under different functional heads because they feel that their needs and products are diverse /singular and only they have the expertise to specify and buy them. Of course, this is an untenable argument. A capable materials manager can purchase them given the proper specifications. Departmental heads should know well enough what they want to instruct the buyer to buy. For the sake of efficiency and cost effectiveness, they should figure out and specify what they really need so that the designated buyers may purchase those goods and services. This policy should be explicit to all heads of pharmacy, laboratory, radiology, dietary, and maintenance to avoid any misunderstandings.

Centralized purchasing sets tone for entire MM programme of the hospital and emphasizes that purchasing is important and should be performed by persons with the requisite training, competency, and authority. Department heads should lay down quality specifications of the products they use. Centralized purchasing must provide the necessary impetus for hospitals to put more emphasis in this area.

BACK DOOR SELLING AND BUYING

Suppliers are often guilty of back door selling. They market, sell, and ship to anyone in the hospital who shows any interest in their product. Most of the times, hospitals are just as guilty of back door buying. As long as decentralized purchasing is overlooked, tolerated, and not explicitly prohibited, it will continue. Integrated MM eliminates back door selling and buying. Integrated MM relieves the various departments of the tasks of interacting with sales representatives. Departmental heads have enough to do without involving themselves into purchasing. When the integrated MM is implemented in the right manner, it sells itself, and the hospital is the ultimate beneficiary. Very few Indian hospitals have switched over to Integrated MM.

HOSPITALS SHOULD SHARE PRICES

Buyers are generally reluctant to share supply prices with their colleagues within and outside the hospital. Unfortunately, in doing so, they play right into the suppliers' hands. Lowest price is not necessarily characteristic of any certain type of hospital. Even group purchasing associations do not always get the best price. No one knows what the best price is because no one knows who is paying what. Prices for the same product can and do vary from hospital to hospital, region to region, and dealer to dealer.

Major reasons for variations are as follows:

- Volume of purchase determines price in some cases.
- Location of vendor: If the supplier is located at far off place, the higher transportation costs results in higher prices.
- Negotiation skills of the buyer.
- Type of supply.
- Size and prestige of the hospital: Large teaching hospitals usually get lower prices because vendors feel that there is likelihood that their products would become de novo standards of practice for future physicians.
- Supplier's need to meet a quota or promotional sale is another motivation for price reduction.

There is need for buyers to share supply prices frequently and regularly. Hospital associations, hospital councils, and purchasing groups must develop, implement, and participate in a supply price comparison survey. This will serve as a purchasing index for individual hospital purchasing professional. Knowledgeable buyers better achieve the objective of purchasing at an advantageous price. The really important issue is not which hospital pays higher prices, but whether that hospital is taking necessary steps to prevent this from happening again. Supply price comparisons are organizational tools to assist buyers to do a more intelligent negotiation. However, there could still sometimes be legitimate reasons for paying more.

Initiative and implementation of a supply price comparison programme can be taken up by any hospital. However, the wider support it has, the more credibility it will receive. **Professional bodies like Indian Institute of Materials Management is an ideal vehicle.** It is imperative that

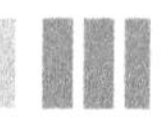

the concept behind the comparison index be communicated to hospital administrators as well as to the buyers. Top management support is a must in such an attempt.

GUIDELINES FOR HOSPITAL PURCHASING

Purchasing should always be simple and result oriented. A simple system must be planned and initiated. Purchase order has long been the basic document of the purchasing process. It represents much work that is both duplicative and expensive. On an average hospital system, the cost of this process is Rs. 300 to Rs. 4,000. Purchase order is a costly artifact but is really essential part to the procurement cycle. No other document can replace it. Act of purchasing should become a repetitive, simple task, and ultimately should not be in the job description of the true materials manager. In the long run, after automating or mechanizing its function for maximum utilization of time and talent, the manager should have to only supervise it. In these days of advanced IT environment, it is easy to lose sight of the basic principles of Materials Management. It must be computerized, centralized, automated, integrated, or amalgamated to get maximum results.

However, all systems and concepts must be built around simple, fundamental principles. Seven fundamental principals are required to be followed for Materials Management concepts to be implemented effectively. **They are:**

1. **Effective management and supervision:** Thrust must be built on the managerial functions of planning, organizing, directing, controlling, and staffing. Good management practices and result oriented supervision must permeate the entire MM effort from the basics to the complexities.

2. **Sound purchasing methods:** To accentuate the art and skill of ethical, hard nosed negotiation. Some rules of negotiation for hospitals have already been discussed in the chapter 8 on Negotiations.

3. **A simple, efficient purchase system:** One which adds to the price of the items being bought, is inappropriate.

4. **Simple inventory control:** Computerization of inventories is basic to advanced inventory models. The hospital must adapt it to suit their requirement and it should be cost effective.

5. A result oriented requisition and distribution system for having the right supply, at the right place and time, in the right quantities.

6. A manual of policies and procedures to provide the foundation for the building of the MM organization structure.

7. A practical receiving programme to fulfill the need for accountability and responsibility. It should have internal controls built into it. For best results, different individuals should handle purchasing, receiving, and payment of invoices because receiving is one of the most important functions in the MM continuum and it should be executed in a professional and ethical manner.

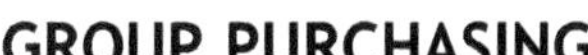

GROUP PURCHASING

William L Scheyer is of the opinion that large volume purchases should result in lower prices. If several hospitals can combine buying from a single vendor, then volumes increase and all other things being equal, prices should be lower. Purchasing practices, value analysis, standardization and other economies occur, thereby reducing total cost. **Group purchasing is a concept based upon the principle that together the member hospitals have greater purchasing power than any individual member.**

Healthcare institutions can strengthen bargaining power and lower the purchase prices by adopting group buying. Value analysis and standardization processes are facilitated when hospitals and other healthcare institutions purchase collectively. The group can carry out more intensive analysis of each item simply because there is a much greater volume of purchases to justify such effort. In due course, the group standard is adopted as a standard of every member of the group. In such a purchasing context, the buyer need not defend his choice of supplier or standard materials; instead he can more or less blame the anonymous group pointing out that everyone is using the same brand or supplier. The individual institution may not always be able to persuade a supplier to reduce prices, because prices paid to healthcare suppliers are determined in part, at least, by bargaining power. Value analysis can disclose why a price should be less. Powerful buyers pay lower prices than weaker ones. Unfortunately, even fairly large hospitals do not really have much bargaining power with suppliers because their total individual purchases usually range between 80 to 100 crores per year and this is distributed among thousands of different suppliers and items. As a result, even large institutions can benefit from group purchasing and for smaller ones, this is the only way in which there is any hope of meeting the supplier in the market place on a reasonably equal footing.

Advantages of Group Purchasing

1. Hospitals can save substantially.
2. A hospital belonging to more than one group can pick and choose among the contracts offered by competing groups.
3. Some groups function as distributors for some products, buying from manufacturers and storing inventory until it is needed by one of the member hospitals.
4. Other groups fulfill a limited warehousing function, usually acting as catalysts for a vendor managed inventory that is available for member use.
5. Most groups limit themselves to a purchasing service. They rarely buy on behalf of members but simply make predetermined purchase terms and conditions available to members, each of whom contract with those approved vendors individually. This is akin to rate contracts adopted in purchases through Directorate General of Supplies & Disposals (DGS&D), Government of India.

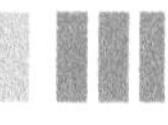

6. Purchasing groups often play a professional development role. Members get to know one another at group meetings by sponsoring seminars and plant visits which keep their members informed.
7. Groups also provide placement services for purchasing managers seeking new or higher positions.
8. A group price can still be further reduced by negotiation after lower competing prices are offered.
9. Because supplier combines the need of many buyers, it is often possible to effect economies of scales.

To summarize, the advantages of group purchasing include reduction in prices, information sharing, standardization, saving on HR costs, and enhancement of purchasing effectiveness. **It has been reported that some of the US hospitals have achieved a saving of 20 to 50 percent through group purchasing.**

Limitations of Group Purchasing

1. System will be ineffective unless the members are well informed and motivated.
2. A group purchasing coordinator is in fact, a sort of elected official. As a politician, he can be as good or as bad as the voters desire.
3. Boards elected from hospital executives run purchasing groups. Sometimes continuity is lost.
4. Group purchasing is ineffective when members are unwilling to standardize or to accept alternative brands.
5. Reduced control might result.
6. Justifying savings in terms of cost benefit of group purchasing is difficult.
7. Commitment of group purchase may not always be acceptable to all hospitals.
8. Diversity within groups reduces effectiveness.
9. Group's internal operations may be inefficient and wasteful unless groups are well managed.
10. Reduced service level of vendors might occur sometimes.
11. Group's selfish interests may sometimes be closer to those of suppliers than of member hospitals.
12. Group coordinator may not be acting in the best interest of members.
13. In a situation, where prices are constantly changing, it is difficult to measure savings, if any.

STRATEGIES FOR GROUP SUCCESS

To be successful, purchasing groups must adopt strategies such as:

- Autonomy to the group: It will be effective, when members of the hospitals are identical in many respects.
- Strategic planning.
- Enhanced vendor relationship management.
- Serve constituent members with common missions.
- Stick to the same group for a substantial period.
- Achieve adequate volume.
- Exchange information regularly and frequently.
- Obtain information inputs from all members.
- Provide liaison with member's pharmacy and therapeutic committees.
- Establish a common formulary.
- Formulate review programmes.
- Deal ethically.
- Enforce exclusivity.

Criteria for making a purchasing group more effective are same as those that make for effective purchasing in the individual hospital. The buyer in both cases must maximize competition by creating conditions under which several firms can win by cutting prices. Unlike professional associations, group purchasing associations have a specific economic goal. This practice is also known as cooperative buying. **Major objective of group and cooperative buying is same.** This phrase of **"group buying"** is mostly applied to private hospitals' procurement, whereas **"cooperative buying"** to government purchases.

SUMMARY

There are several markedly, different difficulties associated with purchasing for healthcare. This can be attributed to several individuals in hospital like administrators, doctors, nurses, and other paramedical staff involved in decision making process, in addition to service features of patient care while making healthcare purchasing.

Purchases special to hospitals include the following items. Digital Electronic Monitoring which is based on a marriage of the physical and life sciences has become very sophisticated due to application of space flight medicine, bio medical engineering, and improvements in digital signal processing. However, some instrument problems result either from poor design or from poor maintenance. Purchasing protocol for monitoring equipments recommends that the using physicians initiate the request and that the purchasing manager in consultation with the evaluation committee, develop a selection procedure.

The criteria to be considered for selection are safety, accuracy, reliability, technical competence of supplying company, promptness of local service, standardization as well as compatibility with the hospital's computer and other equipment.

Modern linens are made of synthetic fibres such as nylon, acrylic, and polyester. Synthetic blended hospital linen costs are lower due to greater wearing qualities and easier laundering. All modern synthetic products must be labelled showing the percentage of synthetic fibres used indicating fibre content, generic name of all fibres etc. Usage, misuse, durability, cost, and patient comfort must be evaluated before selection. Specifications for sheets could cover threads per square cm, percent of cotton or man-made fibres, flame retardant/resistant qualities, weave, selvage, weight in grams per square metre, tensile strength and shrinkage.

Both disposables and reusables have pros and cons. The advantages of disposable items are lower cost, safety, and convenience. The disadvantages include pollution, and ecological considerations. Make or buy cost comparisons have to be used to compare cost of reusables and disposables; convenience, safety, advanced technology and demand are the other factors to be considered.

Selection criteria of stretchers involve: 1. The manner in which use relates to the physical characteristics of the rooms and furnishings to which the stretcher is taken. 2. Will the stretcher height adapt to the patient height? 3. If used in the emergency room, can one wheel it in and out an examining or trauma room? 4. What is the turning radius? 5. Can the stretcher accommodate rods for holding intravenous solutions for patients, if it is a general transportation stretcher?

Generally speaking, there are five major violators for principle of integrated Materials Management for hospital the pharmacy, dietary, and radiology laboratory and plant maintenance department. This is mostly because they feel that their needs and products are different and special and only they have the expertise to buy them. This is untenable. Centralized purchasing sets the tone for entire MM programme of hospitals. It emphasizes that purchasing is important and should be performed by persons with certain training, competency and authority. Suppliers are often found guilty of using backdoor selling techniques and hospitals are also just as guilty due to backdoor buying. Integrated MM of course eliminates both backdoor selling and buying. Buyer should share supply prices frequently and regularly. Hospital associations and purchasing groups must develop, implement, and participate in supply price comparison survey to serve as a purchasing index for individual hospital purchasing professionals.

Act of purchasing should be simple and result oriented. A simple system must be planned and initiated. There are seven fundamental principles that are to be followed for Materials Management concept to be implemented effectively: 1. Effective management and supervision,

2. Sound purchasing methods, 3. A simple and efficient purchasing system, 4. A simple inventory control programme, 5. A result oriented requisition and distribution system, 6. A manual of policies and procedures, 7. A practical receiving programme.

Healthcare institutions can vastly strengthen their bargain power and can lower the purchase prices by adopting group buying. Value analysis and standardization process are facilitated, when hospitals and other healthcare institutions purchase collectively. The group can carry out more intensive analysis of each item because there is a greater volume of purchase to justify that effort. There are several benefits and some limitations of group purchasing. However, the benefits of group purchasing are much more than limitations.

REVIEW QUESTIONS

1. What factors influence purchasing linens for a hospital?
2. Problem of procurement of equipment is twofold: technical and personal relations. Discuss the role of the purchase manager in equipment purchases.
3. What do you understand by the term "disposables"? What are pros and cons of use of disposables in hospitals?
4. Enumerate problems associated with use of disposables.
5. There are five violators associated with integrated Materials Management in hospitals. What are they and as a materials manager, how will you tackle this problem?
6. What is group purchasing? What are advantages and limitations of group purchasing?
7. Write short notes on
   a) Back door selling and buying
   b) Strategies for success of group purchasing
   c) Sharing of prices
   d) Disposal of disposables
   e) Environmental issues in use of disposables
   f) Reprocessing

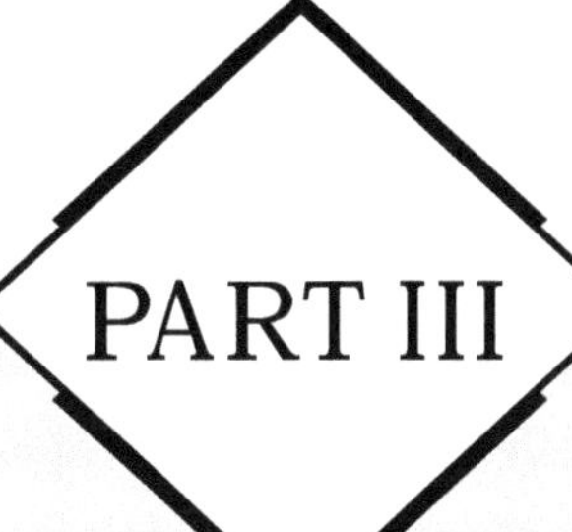
PART III

PART - III

Scope of Inventory Control and its Impact on Profitability

Contents

CHAPTER - 11

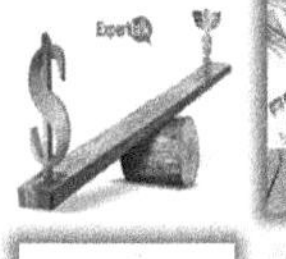
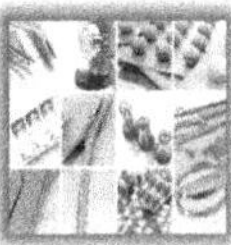
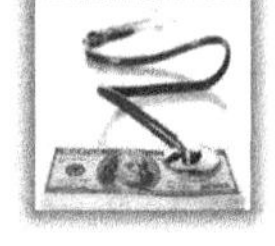
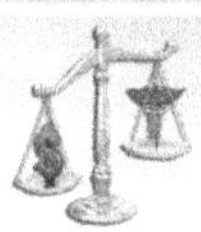

Scope of Inventory Control and its Impact on Profitability

INTRODUCTION

A healthcare institution is said to be successful only when it is able to provide top class patient care and at the same time, remain monetarily viable. For a healthcare organization providing services to patients, the major activity is to make available the required materials at most competitive prices within a reasonable time span. Many constituents of health care industry are involved in setting up this situation. To start with it could be purchasing, and production as in the case of manufacturing orthopaedic implants in a hospital having its own manufacturing facility for making artificial limbs or production of medical gases and other goods incidental to the hospital operations. The main objective is providing continuity of supply for smooth running of the hospital. Inventory control is a planned effort to make the available the required in puts as and when need arises for patient care. It coordinates purchasing, materials management, manufacturing and distribution functions of hospital to meet its' day to day needs. This responsibility includes providing medical care to patients who require a variety of material, new products consumables, spare parts for equipment, and controlling obsolescence. In the event purchase is not able to immediately satisfy demand it may result in customer dissatisfaction. Lack of satisfaction could either be on account to the slow pace of purchasing or due to extended lead time. Thus control is therefore imperative to a hospital. Many hospital activities depend on correct stock being held at correct level; but the definition of 'correct level' varies depending upon who is defining the stock. Stock control is a balancing act between conflicting requirements. **Prime reason for making use of inventory management techniques is to resolve these conflicts in the best interests of hospital and the patients.** In a healthcare organization inventory manager should endeavour to set down procedures enabling programmable problems to as a matter of routine. Areas of activity which lend themselves this treatment other than speciality departments, include production, MM, purchase, Accounts and Finance, quality control, housekeeping contracts and general administration.

ORIGIN OF INVENTORY

"Inventory is as old as man." rather it must have existed even before i.e., before the existence of man. Someone omnipotent that created the universe could not have so successfully evolved the

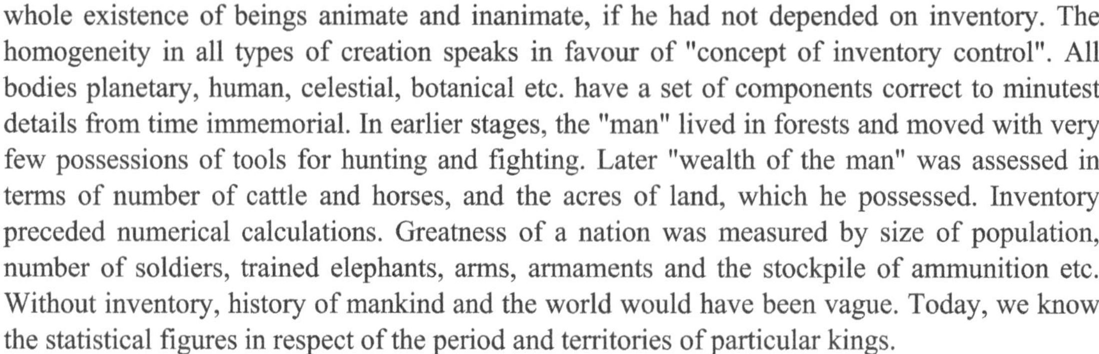

whole existence of beings animate and inanimate, if he had not depended on inventory. The homogeneity in all types of creation speaks in favour of "concept of inventory control". All bodies planetary, human, celestial, botanical etc. have a set of components correct to minutest details from time immemorial. In earlier stages, the "man" lived in forests and moved with very few possessions of tools for hunting and fighting. Later "wealth of the man" was assessed in terms of number of cattle and horses, and the acres of land, which he possessed. Inventory preceded numerical calculations. Greatness of a nation was measured by size of population, number of soldiers, trained elephants, arms, armaments and the stockpile of ammunition etc. Without inventory, history of mankind and the world would have been vague. Today, we know the statistical figures in respect of the period and territories of particular kings.

Inventory gave birth to statistics in every field of our growing civilization. Inventory became unswerving and accurate yardstick to measure the composition of different sciences. Without inventory data and statistical heritage, no scientific progress could be possible. Since numbers fathered statistics, inventory may be termed as mother of all sciences. Inventory control became imperative by virtue of necessity. For welfare of a state, which was considered as largest organization under head of the state, physical marking of cattle, horses, arms, and even trees gave practical shape to inventory control. In order to assess revenues, various kings who made basic regulations for proper inventory controls, measured cultivable land. In modern economy, inventory control evolved itself in every establishment in its accurate form.

INVENTORY DEFINITION

Inventory is defined as materials that have been acquired based upon an anticipated future use, but at the time of review, is awaiting consumption. Accountants use the term inventory to refer to the asset accounts that contain the values of materials held in stocks awaiting usage. Inventories are an integral part of any hospital. Inputs of labour, materials, and technology are combined to provide patient care, which is a service. A variety of influences have had an impact on the way healthcare organizations have accounted for and managed inventories. There have been pressures to reduce inventories, caused by rising costs of capital. These pressures have become particularly intense in hospitals where cash flow became a problem. Increasing cost of space and growing opportunities for alternative uses for existing space has further intensified these pressures to reduce inventories. In contrast, the cost based reimbursement system has promoted expensing of inventories at the time of purchase so that the costs are reportable without any delay. When this has occurred, it often resulted in poorly managed excessive inventories and increased costs. The classic definition of inventory is that, **"it is an idle resource of any kind having an economic value."** Hence, we can identify inventory as those goods, which are procured, stored and used for day to day operations of the hospital.

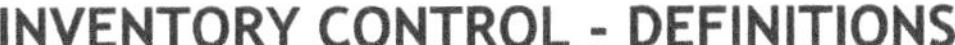

INVENTORY CONTROL - DEFINITIONS

There are seven main terms used in this chapter on inventory management, and are defined below.

1. **Usage:** This refers to the quantity of a given inventory expected to be used based upon past consumption data or projections for a specific time horizon.

2. **Lead time:** Lead time comprises of internal and external lead times. Internal lead time is the time required for a requisition to be processed, a purchase order is issued, resulting in placement of an order with the vendor. External lead time is the time required for vendor to receive the order, enter it, manufacture or buy the goods, pick and ship them, to the time it arrives at the requesting facility for consumption. **"Longer the lead time the more will be inventories."**

3. **Safety factor:** This is the factor by which the expected lead time might be modified to provide a margin of safety to cover potential variations in and/or usage during lead time. Safety factors typically are established through the addition of a percentage of the expected usage during lead time or through use of statistically derived factors.

4. **Re order point:** A pre determined inventory level at which re order of an item is initiated as inventory is consumed. Re order points must be determined scientifically to meet demand during the time it takes to receive the ordered quantity. Fixation of reorder point is discussed in detail in chapter no 17.

5. **Economic order quantity (EOQ):** EOQ includes all costs associated with acquisition of materials, including ordering cost and inventory carrying cost. Ordering and inventory carrying costs are two opposing costs which helps to determine optimum quantity so that overall costs are minimum. Application of EOQ formula is dealt in detail in chapter no. 14.

6. **Re order quantity:** It is desirable to differentiate between EOQ, which is mathematically determined, and re order quantity, which is actual amount that will be re ordered based upon judgement and common sense. For example, EOQ for items known to be used sporadically in large quantities (e.g., burn care supplies and dialysis solutions) should be adjusted. Here, the importance of patient care must override the economic factors that constitute the calculated EOQ. More details are available in chapter 14.

7. **Material requirements planning (MRP)** is a system to determine quantity and timing requirements of demand. MRP normally treats each item of consumption as independent, unaffected by usage rates of other items or by random demand patterns. However MRP has to take into account the interdependence of usage rates between stock and time needed for acquisition of stock.

PURPOSE OF HOLDING INVENTORY

Hospitals may hold inventories of purchased items for many good reasons. Most common reasons are:

- To facilitate patient care operations, inventories are held to act as buffer between different stages of patient care till discharge.
- Inventories are held for consumption during the period between recognition of need and its fulfilment. This period is called "lead time". Consequently, the longer the lead time, the greater will be the level of inventory.
- As a precaution or contingency for increased lead time.
- Speculative element in holding the inventory to meet contingencies like price rise, shortages, etc. This also applies to spare parts inventory to keep machinary and equipment in good repair.

NEED FOR INVENTORY CONTROL

In the post liberalization, privatization and globalization environment of Indian economy, **"seller's market"** is a feature of past and today, inventory control techniques must be used effectively to sustain in competitive environment. Moreover, credit restraints forcing organizations to trim the inventory. In the past, managers of hospitals usually assumed that accumulation of adequate stocks was beneficial to the hospital and they did not therefore feel the need for controlling them. However, large stocks are now often viewed with alarm. This is a complete change in outlook in regard to inventory holdings. In integrated MM, inventory control signifies conversion of idle resources into ideal resource. **If inventories are left to themselves, they have a tendency to expand and go beyond economic limits.** A good inventory control system requires attention only on an exception basis. Starting point in developing a control system is an analysis of the objectives of intended systems. Control should be appropriate for the purpose.

Inventory control system should:

- Reduce financial investment in inventories as the capital invested in inventory costs money and decreases liquidity.
- Provide good customer services.
- Minimize inventory carrying cost.
- Avoid stock outs and over stocking.

INVENTORY CONTROL CLASHING OBJECTIVES

Inventory control is a cross functional activity that has to balance conflicting objectives. Inventory management is always an optimizing function, comparable to a balancing act.

The following goal conflicts have to be resolved:

- High level of customer service vs. low capital and inventory carrying costs.
- Branded material versus generic materials costs.
- Low level of tied up capital accompanied with high liquidity versus continuous customer service.

BASICS OF INVENTORY MANAGEMENT

In the patient care, few things remain the same. Inventory needs have to reflect changing technologies and demands in patient treatment. Management's task is to develop an inventory management system that allows updating, refining and continuous monitoring of inventory needs. The store rooms with too much inventory can never be assessed by mere observation. **Developing responsive systems relies on assessing and understanding existing systems.**

Essential tasks in developing inventory system include:

- Documenting current inventories (in different sub stores and the central stores).
- Eliminating redundant quantity and variety of items kept in inventory.
- Standardizing supplies and instrument and testing equipment.
- Designing realistic inventory levels and models.
- Forecasting demand for existing inventory and also changing needs.
- Organizing inventories in centralized stores locations.
- Motivating all personnel to adapt to new systems.

There is an imperative need to maintain database of supply actually consumed, especially for non-stock items. However, care should be taken in identifying life saving items.

PRE REQUISITES FOR INVENTORY REDUCTION

Inventory reduction should be achieved in a methodical manner based on the following information.

Product information

- Use of the product?
- Criticality of the product in the patient care?
- Possibilities for substitutions for the product?
- Is there a range of similar sizes?
- Product availability
- Normal lead time for procurement of the item

- Predictability (consistency) of lead time?
- Are there other/multiple sources of supply for the product?
- How is the product packaged and shipped?
- Whether the product is available in case of emergency, if need arises?
- Do other hospitals in the area use the same product?

Usage patterns

- Annual usage quantity of the product?
- Is usage seasonal, sporadic or cyclical?
- Variation in usage from month to month?

User information

- Who are the present users?
- Who else are also potential users?
- What type are the users?

Based on above information, a plan should be developed so that process of inventory reduction will become a continuing philosophy, and not just a one time project.

1. **First step is to review existing inventory:** It is useful to calculate turnover for each area for which an inventory account exists.

   To maximize use of resources, it is desirable to identify where greatest rupee values are and/or where the poorest turnover is for incorporation into reduction plan.

2. **Second step involves identification:** The materials manager has to fix cut off point values. This is decided by average value per item. This is obtained by dividing total closing stock value by number of items. Materials manager can focus on items whose closing stock value is twice average value for the inventory reduction programme. By comparing counted quantity on hand with calculated re order point plus economic order quantity, the theoretical maximum is defined. **If physical inventory exceeds the calculated maximum, then there is a potential for cost reduction.**

3. **Third step is review of existing inventory for excess items:** Accuracy of data on usage depends on the inventory system in vogue. For a hospital, the most suitable system would be perpetual inventory model. However, it has its own problems. Items that are grossly overstocked often are apparent but multiple items that are slightly overstocked can be overlooked. It is useful to first review items known to be stored in multiple locations. If those items appear to be excessive, a review of their usage history will permit a determination of whether there is excess or not.

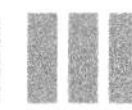

4. **Identification of non moving items:** It is the final step in this process of inventory reduction. This can be achieved by periodic review of movement histories, in relation to number of different users, and types of users.

It is time consuming to detail such information for each product in inventory but it is important that a general understanding exists among those preparing to undertake the task. Many products can be categorized by vendor or by product type and treated similarly, there by simplifying this process. In healthcare industry, generally efforts are put into official inventory for reduction but unofficial inventory is ignored. This is a potential area for inventory reduction.

IMPACT OF INVENTORY CONTROL ON PROFITABILITY

Inventories form an important part of current assets in any organization and also in hospital's. **Return on investment (ROI)** to a great deal depends upon the manner of utilization of materials. Impact of inventory control on profitability can be established from the point of view of return on investment (ROI) on capital.

$$\text{R.O.I} = \frac{\text{Profit}}{\text{Assets}}$$

Assets can be further divided into fixed and current assets.

$$\text{R.O.I} = \frac{\text{Profits}}{\text{Fixed assets + Current asscts}}$$

It can also be represented as:

$$\text{R.O.I} = \frac{\text{Profits}}{\text{Sales}} \times \frac{\text{Sales}}{\text{Fixed assets + Current assets}}$$

Return of investment can be maximized by:

- Increasing the profit keeping capital constant.
- Reducing the capital employed keeping profit constant.
- Simultaneously increasing profit margin and reducing capital employed.

There are limitations to increasing profit as it depends upon many external factors, often beyond management control. The other factor i.e., reduction in capital employed in current assets is well within the control of management. For increasing profitability, first thing that comes into mind is to increase sales. However, there are also constraints to increase sales.

Most important among them are:

- Competition
- Additional investment in facilities and equipment.

- Additional working of capital.
- Aggressive marketing campaign by way of advertisements, developing new or strengthening existing logistics and distribution, production and other support services etc. calls for additional investment.
- Governmental regulations and restrictions

Capital employed refers to fixed assets and current assets.

- Fixed assets are funds employed in land, building and machinery.
- They are permanent in nature and very little can be done to reduce the fixed assets in short time, once expenditure is incurred.
- Current assets mainly comprise of inventories.
- Inventory control carried out on a scientific basis can reduce investment on capital. Generally speaking, inventory should be adequate to achieve maximum reduction and maximum sales.

Consider a 50 bedded private hospital having a turnover of Rs. 200 lakhs

Turnover .... Rs. 200 lakhs

Material cost .... Rs. 120 lakhs

Profit .... Rs. 20 lakhs

Management wants to increase profit by Rs. 6 lakhs.

There are 2 ways to achieve this. By increasing turnover by 30 percent in a given span of time, to achieve overall profit of Rs. 26 lakhs can be achieved. Alternatively reducing materials costs by 5 percent (of Rs.120 lakhs) in the same time, so as to increase the profit by Rs. 6 lakhs. Materials Manager can achieve this either by reducing the materials cost by buying more economically or reduce cost on materials i.e., inventory carrying cost. The second method is based on inventory control.

INVENTORY TURNOVER

In addition to the above, inventory turnover rate is closely connected with profitability.

If a hospital keeps inventories equal to one month's consumption, it means that the inventory turnover in a year is 12 times i.e., entire inventory is used up and replaced 12 times a year. If it maintains 6 months inventories on average, it means that the inventory turnover is 2 times. The inventory turnover rate is a quick guide to the mileage obtained for money tied up in inventories.

Impact of inventory turnover ratio on profitability can be seen from the following Table 11.1.

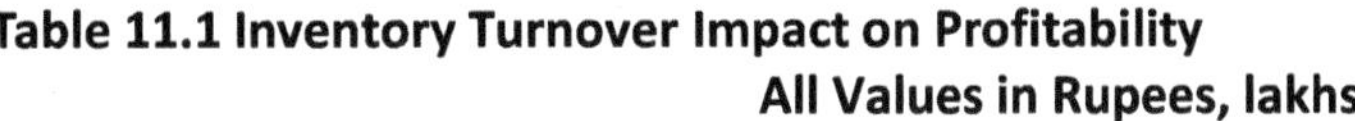

Table 11.1 Inventory Turnover Impact on Profitability

All Values in Rupees, lakhs

	Hospital X	Hospital Y	Hospital Z
1.Revenue	200	200	200
2. Gross profit @ 12.5 percent	25	25	25
3. Materials consumed	100	100	100
4. Inventories held (in number of months consumption)	1	6	12
Turnover rate	12	2	1
Value of inventory held	8.33	50	100
5. Inventory carrying costs @ 25 percent per annum	2.08	12.5	25
6. Net profit	22.92	12.5	NIL

Investment in business is money tied up in assets, including inventories, which are often one of the largest assets, consequently reducing the amount of money tied up in inventories improves return on assets even though profit on sales remains same.

INVENTORY SYSTEM IMPROVEMENT

Each purchase or production situation must be preceded by decision making process. The number of items involved can range from scores to millions. And the number of transactions is far in excess of the number of items. Decision making process may be simple or complex or programmed, intuitive or mathematical, hasty or deliberate. There are many ways that an inventory manager can reduce his costs.

Some of the more noticeable methods are as follows:

- **Reduce lead time:** by selecting local suppliers; substantial reductions in cost can be achieved. Local supply can reduce lead times, which lower re order point and safety stock.
- **Inform suppliers in advance the expected annual demand:** If suppliers are aware of hospital annual in advance, they can plan their production to have sufficient inventory to meet the expected demand.
- **Contract with suppliers for minimum annual purchases:** This approach acts as a hedge against future price increases.
- **Maintain multiple suppliers and at the same time attempt to reduce suppliers base:** If one supplier fails to supply goods, others can meet the demand. Multiple suppliers also permit cost comparisons, which help to maintain a competitive price structure. With supplier competition, unit costs tend to be lower.

- **Buy on consignment:** Arrange with suppliers to pay for their items as and when they are used. This will transfer a large portion of holding cost to supplier.
- **Consider transportation costs:** Failing to consider transportation costs and the most economical mode of transportation can increase unit cost and also inventory holding costs.
- **Order economical quantities:** Over buying in relation to needs result in excessive holding. Under buying results in stock out costs.
- **Control access to storage areas:** Protect against losses from theft, pilferage, unauthorized withdrawals by employees.
- **Obtain improved forecasts:** Substantial reduction in safety stocks can be achieved if the forecasts are reliable and accurate.
- **Standardize stock items:** Standardization helps to reduce variety in inventories. It also helps to reduce the quantities of each item or the number of items used in stock. Carrying one standard item instead of maintaining different items that are used essentially for same end use.
- **Dispose of inactive stock regularly:** All stocks should be reviewed periodically to identify obsolete, surplus, slow moving, and poor quality materials. Disposal alternatives include return to vendor, scrapping, reworking, salvage, and reduced price sales.

IMPACT OF OFFICIAL AND UNOFFICIAL INVENTORY INVESTMENT PER BED

Inventory investment per Bed: Inventories in hospitals are measured in terms of funds invested, usually by category, divided by the number of beds. This is a useful gross measure. Typical aggregate values range from Rs. 25,000 to Rs. 3,00,000 per bed. Obviously such a wide range limits the complete usefulness of the measure. The obvious reason for such a wide range is that different hospitals use different methods. For example, in arriving at value of inventories invested per bed, the value at one facility may represent only official inventory while at another facility, it is a sum total of unofficial and official inventories. Bed figure may represent occupied beds or the total capacity in terms of number of beds available. Inventory measurement is most useful when it is used for comparing progress over time within a facility after adjusting for changes in scope of services and/or their utilization or when comparing similar hospitals i.e., similar, in activity levels and specialities. Simplistic comparisons of inventory value of money invested per bed totally ignore related but critical issues such as inventory service levels and rate of replenishment. To manage an inventory properly, it is necessary to first determine the starting point. This necessitates taking a physical inventory.

Inventories booked as assets are official inventory. This is where most of the reduction efforts have been applied in the past. Materials expensed at the time of purchase comprise of unofficial inventory. These materials were purchased in anticipation of future use but until they are actually used, they represent investment that has been made while expected returns are still

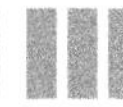

awaited. Efforts to manage and reduce unofficial inventories are rewarded through a drop in materials costs and improved cash flow balance. **Dean Amer** has estimated that unofficial inventory levels may be about 37 percent whereas **Charles Houseley** has suggested that they could be about 58 percent of total inventory. This author estimates that the figures in Indian hospitals could be as high as 80 to 90 percent of total inventory.

Pressure is mounting upon hospitals to reduce both official and unofficial inventories with the advent of prospective payment systems in healthcare. Inventories must be kept to a minimum level but it is critical that as they are reduced, this has to be done in a methodical fashion based on all available information, rather than in a haphazard manner. If these inventories are not scientifically managed, it would result in frequent stock outs or over stocking (i.e., excessive investment in inventory). Management of inventories means to control the resources consumed in anticipation of future use of material. Control of these resources include space allocated to inventories, labour used in their storage and control, capital invested, technology, and equipment used in storage and control (e.g., computers, forklifts, shelving etc.).

TYPICAL PER-BED INVENTORY LEVELS IN INDIAN HEALTHCARE INDUSTRY

Inventories in hospitals and healthcare institutions vary according to type and number of specialities, its teaching programmes, its size and accessibility to suppliers etc. However, in the long run, all these factors tend to average out, and definite projections per bed can be made.

Following rating scale compares inventories per bed to materials management effectiveness.

	Inventory category	Poor	Fair	Good	Excellent
A	Central stores	Above Rs.45,000	Rs. 45,000	Rs. 30,000	Rs. 15,000
B	Pharmaceuticals	AboveRs. 37,500	Rs. 37,500	Rs. 33,750	Rs. 26,250
C	Dietary	Above Rs.6,750	Rs. 6,750	Rs. 4,500	Rs. 3,750

Above comparison scale is based on certain assumptions, first of which is that hospital has definite object oriented inventory reduction programmes.

Charles E. Housley suggests that:

- All hospitals should strive to avoid duplication of supplies in the central stores as well as in the using departments, but should instead adhere to concept of stockless purchasing.
- Furthermore, hospital should not stock unused and used linens and expensive printed forms. The very existence of such high inventory suggests duplication and back up.
- Unofficial inventory this duplication would be tolerable if hospital kept only bare minimum emergency supply of all items in stock. Unfortunately, the fact is that duplication in certain healthcare units is as high as 100 to 500 percent of amount needed.

- In addition, no single person really knows where all this duplication is at any cross section of time. While the official inventory is departmentally controlled, issued to using department as needed, and counted and reviewed at least annually by hospital stock verifiers, the unofficial inventory is subject to practically little control.

METHODOLOGY FOR ARRIVING AT THE INVENTORY PER BED

Table 11.2 Total Estimated Inventory per Bed

Sl.	Categories of inventories	Estimated value of official inventory in rupees
1	Drugs and pharmacy	30,000
2	Medical surgical supplies	22,000
3	Sterile supplies (central supply)	12,000
4	Office supplies stationery	9,000
5	Housekeeping and linen	7,000
6	Food and dietary supplies	7,000
7	Laboratory supplies	5,000
8	X-ray and radiology supplies	5,000
	Total estimated inventory per bed	97,000

Value of Investment per bed

The quantitative method for determining inventory values per bed is to divide closing value of inventory figure by average number of occupied beds during the year. It should be noted that the methodology specifies occupied beds, not total beds. Occupied beds provide a more accurate picture of the inventory activity and need for inventory. For example in the Table 11.2, inventory per bed is calculated as Rs. 97, 000 per bed, which by some standard, would indicate as "good". However, when the calculation is made on the basis of average occupancy, the value of inventory per bed increases to Rs. 1,26,067 as given below, which again by some standards, would be indicative of poor inventory control.

Hospital bed strength		500
Inventory value (500 x 97000)		Rs. 4,85,000,00
Percentage of occupancy	75 of 500 beds	375
A. Calculation by total beds		Rs. 97, 000
B. Calculation by average occupancy		Rs. 1,29,333

Unofficial inventory is expected to be much higher in hospitals ranging from 100 percent to 500 percent on the inventories in central stores as stated earlier.

Question here is, when should an inventory manager begin to recognize that value inventory per bed is too high? Answer goes beyond traditional beliefs of compensating for poor vendor performance and lack of effective systems, and depends upon a large number of additional factors such as:

- Type of hospital
- Length of stay of patient in the hospital
- Types of items maintained within the inventory
- Inventory turnover rates
- Changes in medical staff
- Poor forecasting
- Rate of inflation
- Types of patients treated

This last factor has perhaps the greatest impact. Types of patients treated refers to the general patient population; i.e., medical patients vs. surgical patients. Although patients mix may not have great impact on large hospitals (400 plus beds), it definitely does have an effect in the smaller hospitals. **Dean Ammer** identified that, the root cause for high investment in inventories is due to neglect and inefficiency of the hospital.

INTERDEPARTMENTAL RELATIONSHIPS

In a well managed hospital communication does not remain a means. It represents spirit of the organization working harmoniously and effectively. Basic tenets communication is that it ought to be quick, precise, and consistent. Materials managers have to develop and maintain open communications with medical staff in all departments in the hospital. Materials Management department must endeavour to assist various departments' theoretical goals to accomplish. They should let others know of MM accomplishments in quantitative terms. Again, this is part of creating an image of competency and performance. Interaction with user departments can provide useful feedback through written questionnaires and also involve periodic visits to departments to discuss MM department support, problems, and other concerns. This might some time lead to criticism, at time some of that is uncharitable. Materials manager must be prepared to handle it in a mature way. It is very important that any problems faced by users be followed up and resolved to erase the feeling that MM department does not listen and the positive effect will be reversed.

In any hospital, people who are most apprehensive with inventories are:

- **Finance manager:** To finance manager, inventory connotes the value of inventories, consumables, spares, and scrap in which funds are invested. He is wary of the term because inventory represents to him idle stocks locking the capital.

- Head Departments, nursing and housekeeping, maintenance and other paramedical staff react violently, when there is shortage and start complaining that its lack has been the root cause of dissatisfaction of patients and their attendants.
- Maintenance manager: He is not sure, when he requires a spare part. One thing that is certain in spare parts management is its uncertainty. Maintenance manager's tendency is to hoard as many spare parts as possible.

Each one of above views inventories differently. Under these circumstances, inventory controller has to do a tight rope walking. On one hand, he has to stock various inputs of patient care, so that patient service is uninterrupted. On the other hand, he has to reduce idle capital locked up in the shape of inventory.

IMPLEMENTING CHANGE

Change is unavoidable. There was a situation earlier, when materials managers would not even imagine to discuss something as sensitive as surgeons' gloves. Later, many items became commodity products, and fewer therefore are now Sacrosanct. The healthcare market is shifting rapidly. It has become inevitable take a transitory look at the brass stock of products and demand reasons for the various accompaniments. If less expensive manufactured goods will work from an infection control point and provide proper patient care, then it can be used. The product need not have to be the best or have a major market share. Its' objective it simply needs to work. Cost factor is ever more important.

Conflict to total centralization of inventory control is normally in dietary and pharmacy areas, while laboratory, radiology, and maintenance departments are less responsive. There is no reason why pharmacy and dietary cannot be handled in the same way as other departments. On the other hand, materials managers must be discreet before moving to assume control. Total centralization of receiving is the first stride. They should promote this idea as a way of increasing efficiency, not as loss of control by a department. Receiving departments are best equipped for this activity and provide most efficient utilization of staff time. Objectors will cite physical location problems and security difficulties and will come up with an unending list of pleas for refraining, but managers can be resourceful in building control yet offering them some flexibility. Dietary and pharmacy are more subjective and sensitive because of problems associated with shelf life, spoilage, frozen handling, and so on, but the solution lies in training materials personnel and requiring expertise from other departments in order to help ensure fulfillment with specifications. Many products such as vacuum containers are no different from the type of canned food on any general store's shelves. Distribution can be handled via replenishment against a typical par stock type system similar to that on nursing units. Advent of computers and networking will go a long way in installing controls in these areas since the data collected on site can be downloaded onto computer in MM. Acquisition of drugs through a wholesale or depot method can provide efficiencies that allow pharmacy to project its requirements via local networking system. Accessibility of certain information such as inventory reports and stock analysis from wholesalers, plus rapid delivery that enhances inventory reduction, will allow pharmacy to continue control in this area. Participation with purchasing groups, as well as new approaches with generic and therapeutic drug substitution have reduced the importance of price as an issue at individual healthcare facilities. Foods beverage purchasing was earlier loosely controlled but now requires a formalized system.

From William Schreyer's point of view, it is basically inventory control. For example, pharmacy administrator, as well as other department managers, should know that inventory is the responsibility of MM. If a problem crops up, that is, if statistics indicate lags in inventory turns or controls, MM will assist. Materials managers' ability to implement sourcing strategies professionally must be underscored.

R_X FOR INVENTORY REDUCTION

Reduction process of inventories must include the following steps:

1. **Formulate administrative policies in regard to inventories and define responsibilities.**
   a. Inventory control should be a function of MM, assisted by all related departments involved.
   b. Control of both official and unofficial inventories is the responsibility of Materials Management.
   c. Periodical stock taking must be done at least once every 6 months.
   d. No department should be permitted more than two weeks supply of unofficial inventory. Furthermore, each department head is to requisition from MM 2 weeks supply of operational inventory as stockless purchases. For example, disposal items are requisitioned twice per month, with no stock being kept in central stores. This means that all departmental supplies are to be ordered, expensed, and used in the same month.
   e. All purchases are to be made by Materials Management department only.
   f. Combination of official and unofficial inventories shall not exceed Rs. 35,000 per bed, subject to revision taking in to account, factors like inflation, market conditions, governmental regulations etc.,

2. **Formulate and implement relevant MM policies.**
   a. All nursing stations and related units will be part of a 24 hour total supply cart exchange system.
   b. Stockless purchasing will be practised when and where ever possible.
   c. Prime supplier approach will be practised for all major supply categories and reviewed accordingly.

d. In reference to the prime suppliers, necessary lead times are reviewed and approved periodically by the materials manager to make note of changes in lead times.

e. A multi disciplinary standardization committee has to be constituted to approve all new items prior to induction.

f. Appropriate item substitutes will be made when the supply of the standard item is delayed or becomes difficult/non existent.

g. Certain high rupee value items, such as orthopaedic and cardiac implants, are recommended for purchase on a consignment basis.

3. **Combine all supply, process, and distribution functions under the supervision of MM.**

a. Central sterile supply will be a processing unit, not a source of supply items.

b. Supply quotas are to be reviewed and updated with the user departments periodically.

4. **Develop and use timely administrative reports by materials department such as:**

a. Vendor usage report

b. Vendor performance rating report

c. Departmental purchase report

d. Nursing unit usage reports

e. Shortage reports, by value

f. Inventory standardization report

5. **Undertake timely performance review for all prime suppliers and consumer departments and nursing units.**

There is a need for arriving at level of inventory for smooth functioning of the hospital. Necessary level for most hospitals is many times less than the inventory quantities now maintained. If administrative and managerial attention is paid to this area, monumental costs savings and a more efficient MM programme can be achieved. Holding inventory, which is, more than just enough is wasteful and costly. Materials manager can provide considerable assistance in developing and maintaining an inventory control programme. Materials manager is familiar with various statistical methods used to establish appropriate inventory levels (e.g., economic order quantity determinations, ABC analysis, and material requirements planning). Materials manager, for example, can assist operating room staff in striking most effective balance between surgical suite inventories and those maintained in general store room. Both departments base inventory needs on hard data such as past experience and statistical forecasting. Personnel in both departments who are made responsible to managing inventories must understand the importance of ensuring adequate

 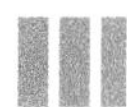

stock levels and their obligation for controlling funds invested in supplies and surgical instruments. Without a clear understanding of the balance between these two facets of inventory management, employees will tend to play safe and overstock or be overly conservative in maintaining stock levels. Frequent and clear communications between the operating room supervisor and the materials manager will avoid credibility gaps and will strengthen the hospital's formal inventory system. This is especially important in hospitals where case carts are assembled by the MM department.

SUMMARY

Inventory is defined as materials that have been acquired based upon an anticipated future use, but at the time of review, is awaiting consumption. Inventory can be defined "as an idle resource of any kind provided that resource has an **economic value**". Hence, we can identify inventory as those goods, which are procured, stored and used for the day to day operations of the hospital. Pre requisites for inventory control are, *Usage, Lead time, Safety factor, Re order point, Economic order quantity (EOQ). Re order quantity, and Material requirements planning (MRP):* To facilitate smooth operations of hospitals, inventories are held to act as buffer between different stages of patient care. Inventories of materials and components are held for consumption during the period between recognition of need and its fulfilment. Inventories are also held as a precaution or contingency for increased lead time. There is special speculative element in holding the inventory to meet the contingencies like price rise, shortages during certain periods of time. An effective inventory control system should be relative, dynamic and true. Relative refers to meeting the needs of organizational functions or departments. Dynamic refers to the time variant nature of inventory needs. Any system must react to expected and unexpected changes. Finally, "true" refers to the ability to report accurately the stock or position of inventory when required. Inventories are troublesome and controversial. In the light of organizational goals, inventory has an impact on functional areas. Globalization and liberalization of Indian economy indicate that seller's market is a feature of past and inventory control techniques can be used effectively. Inventory control is a double edged sword. Excessive control is as undesirable and costly as under control. A new system that saves thousands and costs lakhs of rupees is unhealthy investment. A control system should be installed on the basis of cost benefit analysis and not merely to achieve control as end in itself.

Success of a healthcare institution depends on its ability to provide services to customers or users and remain financially viable. For a hospital, which is providing services to its patients, the major activity is to have suitable products available at an acceptable price within a reasonable timescale. A healthcare institution is said to be successful, when it is able to provide to its patients an efficient and effective services to its customers or users of facilities and remain cost-effective. Inventory manager has to support its customer service, logistics or manufacturing activities in situations where purchase or manufacture of the items is not able to satisfy demand. Inventory control is a planed method of deterring what to indent, when to indent and how much to stock so that ordering and holding cost are lowest possible so as to enable hospital to support its customer service.

In any organization, people who are more concerned with inventories other than materials management department are finance, operations, housekeeping and maintenance departments etc.

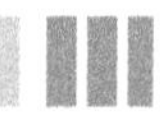

Inventory control is a cross functional area that has to balance conflicting objectives. The primary objective of inventory control is to provide customer service and also maintain return on investment (ROI). The return on investment to a great extent depends on the manner of utilization of materials. Inventory turnover rate is a quick guide to mileage obtained for money tied up in inventories. There are many ways a materials manager can reduce costs. Some of more apparent methods are reducing lead time by selecting local suppliers, informing suppliers of expected annual demand in advance, contracting with suppliers for minimum annual purchases, maintaining multiple sources, standardizing etc.

Healthcare market is changing due to competition. When implementing such a programme, it is important to educate and involve key management and administrative personnel. Without their support, inventory control programme cannot be successfully implemented. Cost savings and system benefits in inventory control function are significant. Final objective of inventory control is to integrate management approach to planning, acquisition, conversion flow and distribution of material. Keys to implementing this process are coordination and communication.

REVIEW QUESTIONS

1. Inventories are idle resources, still we carry - Discuss.
2. Define "Inventory". State the necessity of inventory control and the benefits derived there from.
3. a. Purpose of inventory is "Protection" and "Economy"- Comment.

   b. Today's inventories are for tomorrow's consumption - Comment.
4. How will you arrive at per bed inventory in a hospital? Give your answer with a illustrative examples.
5. Write short notes on
   a) Need for holding inventories
   b) Pre requisition for inventory reduction
   c) Inter departmental relationships
   d) Inventory control
   e) Purpose of inventory
   f) Need for inventory control

Classification of Hospital Inventories

Contents

- *Introduction*
- *Inventory Classification based on Functions*
- *Classification of Hospital Inventories based on Usage and Point of Entry*
- *Expendables*
- *Unexpendables*
- *Spare Parts*
- *Classification of Spares*
- *Spare Parts Planning Pre Requisite*
- *Measures of Reliability*
- *Mean Time Between Failures (MTBF)*
- *Summary*
- *Review Questions*

CHAPTER - 12

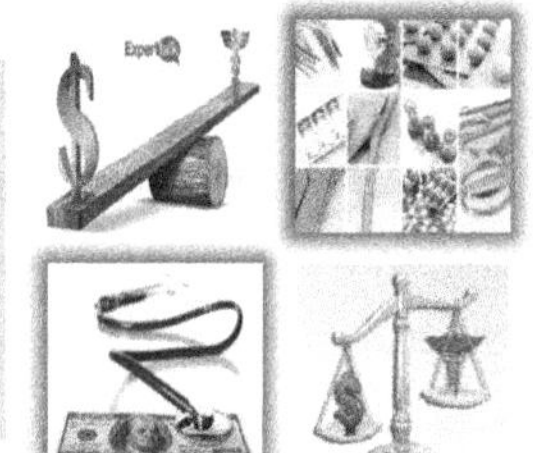

Classification of Hospital Inventories

INTRODUCTION

In every hospital, there are various demands for items for its day to day operations. Everyone in the hospital requires supplies of large quantities of diversified materials like, drugs and pharmaceuticals, instruments, medical surgical, sterile, office equipment, housekeeping, foods and beverages, maintenance, laboratory supplies, radiology supplies, gases and capital equipment etc. These items have to be either procured or produced in the hospital. Infrastructures are to be built and amenities have to be provided. For all these exercises, materials are required in one form or the other, resulting in timely supply of such commodities to meet the needs of a hospital and render satisfactory service to its customers. Users of diagnostic and therapeutic equipments require spare parts in stock to keep the equipment in good working condition.

All inventory items used in healthcare do not necessarily require the same treatment and therefore policy with regard to each item may differ according to their types and need of different healthcare institutions. **Inventories can be classified according to either the functions they perform or their usage and point of entry into the operations of the hospital.**

INVENTORY CLASSIFICATION BASED ON FUNCTIONS

Based on the functions they perform, inventories are classified into four groups as Lot size inventory, Fluctuation inventory, Anticipation inventory and Transportation inventory.

Lot Size Inventory

Most manufacturing companies produce in lots sizes, rather than quantities exactly equal to the supply order. Economic batch production quantity may dictate that production lot sizes larger than demand, are manufactured and held in stock. At times hospitals have to buy excess quantities to fulfill the conditions of minimum order quantities stipulated by supplier or the supplier does not have any other customer other than the buyer.

Fluctuation Inventory

These inventories exist because of demand or supply fluctuations. Safety or reserve stock can be termed as fluctuation inventory. These stocks are held over and above cycle stocks (regular demand quantity) because of uncertainties that occur in demand pattern or variations in lead time. It is an ongoing investment to avoid the costs of out of stock during day to day running of hospital or for sale of medicines by the outpatient pharmacy.

Anticipation Inventory

These inventories are sometimes called as speculative stock and are held in stock often because there have been opportunities to gain advantages of quantity discounts if larger than average orders are placed, Also prudent procurement has been undertaken ahead of forecast shortages or price increases or fluctuations in lead times and rates of consumption, or to meet peak time demand for seasonal products or for holding ahead of holiday season or in anticipation of strikes, lock outs at supplier plants etc. or to provide initial inventories for new product or services.

Transportation Inventory

These inventories are also known as in transit inventories that are being transported from one place to another. Usually, transportation inventories are included while arriving at the inventory carrying costs.

Transportation inventories exist because materials are moved from one place to other. A multi location hospital will have inventories at a centrally located warehouse moved to stock points at other places especially where centralized purchasing is the policy. It should be noted, more distance between production and consumption centres and larger the channel of distribution, the greater will be the level of in transit inventories.

CLASSIFICATION OF HOSPITAL INVENTORIES BASED ON USAGE AND POINT OF ENTRY

Inventories that are used in hospitals are broadly classified based on consumption, criticality, and movement and also on the functions they perform. **All hospital inventories are broadly classified as expendables and un expendables.**

EXPENDABLES

Expendables are used in day to day operations of hospitals and are procured on recurring basis. These include foods and beverages, items like provisions, perishable items like eggs, meat, fish, fruits, vegetables, bread, butter etc., and linen including bed sheets, pillow covers, curtains, gloves etc. In addition to the above, provisioning items for infrastructure e.g., laundry items and maintenance, repair, maintenance and overhaul items also fall under this category. On an average, a total number of approximately more than 15,000 items are held in stock in hospitals. These items can be grouped and classified in a variety of ways as given below.

Drugs and Pharmacy Items

Drugs are classified into different groups according to their common effects and actions on

the mind and body. Depending on the specialities, drugs can be grouped in a variety of ways. One method of classification is according to their use on diseases as:

Antacids, Antibiotics, Analgesics,
Coagulants, Anti-convulsants, Anti-histamines,
Anti-allergy, Anti-dysentery, Anti-malaria,
Anti-spasmodic, Anti-asthma, Anti-tuberculosis,
Anti-diabetic, Anti-nomic, Antibiotic steroids,
Anti-helminthic, Cardiovascular, Bronchodilators,
Diuretics, Anti-carcinoma, Anti-hypertension,
Anti-thematic, Sedatives, Tranquilizers,
Urinary antiseptics, Anti-anaemia,
Depressants, Hallucinogens, Opiates, Stimulants,
Vitamins and Miscellaneous Items.

Drugs are also classified in different forms such as

Tablets	Injections
Drops	Powders
Capsules	Liquids
Over-the-counter items (OTC)	Miscellaneous

A study at a multi speciality PG level teaching hospital has classified its medical stores based on user department and item wise. The same is shown in Tables 12.1 and 12.2.

Table 12.1 Classification of Drugs in a Multi-speciality Hospital

Fluids	IV Fluids	Injections	Sprays
Tablets	Ointments	Insulin	Syrups
Inhalers	Lotions	Others	

Hospital has 15 departments grouped into 13. Department wise distribution of drugs is shown in Table 12.2. The Table 12.3 shows number of drugs in each group and their distribution in terms of numbers and percentages.

Most of the drugs purchased have a finite shelf life beyond which, they cannot and should not be used.

Classification of drugs: user department's help can be sought to decide criticality of the drugs, which is discussed in chapter 15, under application of VED control to medical store items.

Table 12.2 Distribution of Drugs Vis-a-Vis with user Departments of Drugs

	Anaesthesiology		Chest		Cardiology		Dermatology Gynaecology *		Neurology		Endocrinology		General medicine		Medical Gastro-Enterology		Medical Oncology Hematology		Nephrology		Orthopaedic		Rheumatology		Radiation Oncology	
	No.	%	No.	%	No.	%	No.	%	No.	%	No.	%	No.	%	No.	%	No.	%	No.	%	No.	%	No.	%	No.	%
Fluids	29	23													5	6			13							
IV Fluids	31	25																								
Injections	51	40	8	8	64	24			33		27	24	126	36	19	22	121	63	43				15	52	3	60
Sprays																										
Capsules			8	8									30	9	8	9	26	13.5	4		2		1	3		
Tablets			36	35	198	74	15	29			49	61	153	44	38	43	45	23	37		2		13	45	2	40
Ointments							25	49	123																	
Insulin																										
Syrups			18	17									20	6	11	13										
Patches																										
Inhalers			18	17																						
Lotions																										
Others	15	12	15	15	5	2	11	22	6		4	5	20	6	7	8	1	0.5	8							

* Only outpatient services

Table 12.3 Classification of Drugs in Medical Stores

S.no	Category of Drug	No. of Items	Percentage
1	Fluids	47	3
2	IV fluids	31	2
3	Injections	543	33
4	Capsules	79	5
5	Tablets	834	51
6	Ointments	25	2
7	Syrups	49	3
8	Inhalers	18	1
	Total	1626	100

As seen from above Table, 86 percent of items in medical stores are injections and tablets.

Reusables and Disposables

Health care service providers' viz., physicians, nurses, physiotherapist, laboratory technicians and other support services staff are consumers of, reusables and disposables. Disposable items are to be used once in its patient care and discarded or converted it to reusable materials or dispensed with as solid waste. These items are generally inexpensive in nature and are of short term expediency rather than medium to long term resilience. The term occasionally is used for products which are used for more than once e.g., washable air filters. Disposables are made out of paper, cotton and other bio degradable materials. Materials like polystyrene and other plastics, materials are also used

Table 12.4 List of Products that can be considered either Reusable or Disposable

REUSABLES	DISPOSABLES
Aprons Bedpans Blankets Bottles Catheters Clothes Containers Coveralls Covers Examining table Mattress Tray	**Bags:** Blood collection, Laundry, Specimen, Trash, Utility Diapers Dietary Products Gloves, Gowns, Shirts, Handkerchiefs **Kits** : Catheterization, Irrigation, Peritoneal analysis Mops, Needles, Prep sets, Sheets, Syringes, Underpads

(Author is indebted to John Holmgren and Walter J. Went for reproducing above table.)

Anything in patient care that must be cleaned, sterilized, washed, or otherwise converted to its original aseptic condition can be considered either a disposable or a reusable. Table 12.4 lists several examples of healthcare products that can be considered either reusable or disposable.

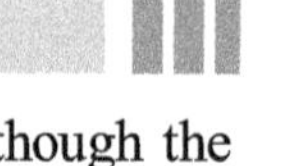

It is often stated, that "disposables cost too much they are too expensive". Although the factor of higher cost is relevant, a cost comparison should be made before this statement can be made with any degree of certainty. With labour costs escalating at an unprecedented rate, this argument may not be supportable. (John H. Holgren and Walter J. Wentz 1982)

Implant and Tissue Makes

Implant is an object or material inserted or grafted into the body for prosthetic, therapeutic, diagnostic or experimental purposes.

Examples of this category includes

S. No.	Item	Function
1	Artificial heart	A pump that replaces the natural heart.
2	Artificial joints	A metal or plastic part that is surgically implanted to replace a natural joint.
3	Dental implant	An implant that replaces a natural tooth.
4	Inter ocular lens	Implant in cataract operations.

Single Use Instruments

During the year 2007 European Union (EU) brought out guide lines to ensure safety and infection control for dental and minor surgeries. **After use, the Single use Instruments are termed as clinical waste** and have to be disposed of in accordance with clinical waste laws in force. If free collection of clinical waste facilities is not available then hospitals are required to remove and destroy the waste under the supervision a specialist. Single use surgical instruments are conventionally made out of special alloy steels. The instruments which are to be recycled can be resterilized to eliminate their clinical waste status and moved to sterile store for future use.

Lab and Chemical Reagents

Reagent is a "substance or mixture for use in a chemical analysis or added to facilitate reaction to takes place." Reactant is a substance that takes part in analysis and undergoes change during a reaction. The terms reactant and reagent are often used as synonym words. However a **reactant** is more specifically a "substance that is consumed in the course of a chemical reaction". Solvents, though they take part in the reaction, are usually not referred to as reactants. Catalysts are not consumed during reaction; they accelerate or retard a reaction and do not undergo a chemical or physical change, hence is not described as reactants.

Medical Gases

Medical gases are manufactured, packaged, to be administered to a patient in anaesthesia, therapy, or diagnosis. In USA, the **Code of Federal Regulations (CFR)** classifies medical gases as drugs. It mandates that the Secretary of the Treasury and/or the Secretary of Health and

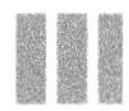

Human Services must promulgate regulations for efficient application and enforcement of Federal **Food, Drug, and Cosmetic Act (FDA).** Other regulatory bodies including the **Department of Transportation (DOT), Compressed Gas Association (CGA)** and the **National Fire Protection Association [NFPA]** establish regulations and standards for compressed gases. Medical gases are to be treated as prescription drugs as their usage is unsafe without supervision of a licensed practitioner or trained emergency personnel.

Medical gases are used for following applications

Oxygen used to support respiratory system; in combination with **nitrous oxide** in dentistry; and also as an emergency standby.

- **Nitrous oxide** used as anaesthetic agent in surgery; supplemented with oxygen it helps patients relax during dental procedures; also used in cryosurgery (which is defined as the use of extreme low temperatures to destroy tissue).
- **Nitrogen** an inert gas meant to provide pneumatic pressure in certain medical equipment; to prevent combustion/ chemical reactions; and as component in several gas mixtures.
- **Carbon dioxide** made use of to inflate body parts for "keyhole" surgery wherein small incisions are made to accommodate **surgical instruments.** Also used in cryosurgery and for testing tooth sensitivity to low temperatures.
- **Medical air** is meant for respiratory treatments; and also as a component for other respiratory cases.
- **Helium** is used in breathing mixtures for treatment of patients whose lung function is impaired.

Medical gases are the most frequently administered drugs in the USA. FDA is attempting to sensitize both consumers and industry about these regulated products.

Medical Sterilization Items

Medical sterilization connotes complete elimination or destruction of all living micro organisms. Some of the agents available for sterilization are steam, hot air, ethylene oxide gas, chemical compounds like hexachlorophene, chlorhexidine etc. Others include: Irradiation, filtration, pasteurization, high velocity electron bombardment, ultraviolet radiation etc. Most of the Sterilization is done either by autoclaving through steam or boiling (where autoclave facilities are inadequate or un available}

Kitchen and Dining Products

Kitchen & Dining Products are dishware drink ware plates bowls cups plastic cutlery, like spoons, knives forks, Cans, bottles, jars, cartons wrappers and other food packaging are generally recyclable, and a few of them are even Bio degradable.

- Cans, bottles, jars, cartons, wrappers and other food packaging are largely recyclable, and some are even compostable.
- Inexpensive Tupperware products are recyclable.
- Cupcake wrappers, coffee filters are compostable.

Food and Beverages

The foods and beverages are generally categorized as

S.No	Type of items	Examples
1	Provisions	Pulses, Wheat flour, Rice, Oil
2	Processed food	Noodles, Oats, Cornflakes, Vegetable and Meat based soups, Sausage
3	Spices	Cinnamon, Cardamom, Cloves, Turmeric, Pepper
4	Dairy items	Milk, Cheese, Butter, Buttermilk, Yoghurt
5	Bakery items	Bread, Biscuits, Tomato Ketchup, Salad
6	Vegetables	Vegetables, Tubers, Leafy vegetables
7	Beverages	Soft drinks, Cool drinks, Mineral water
8	Fruits	Oranges, Apples, Papaya, Watermelon
9	Non-Vegetarian	Meat, Poultry and Fish

Special Diets

Special Diets are of two types, one meeting cultural or spiritual requirements other is personal diets meeting personal preferences "tastes differ from patient to patient. Standard menu adopted by hospitals meets majority of patients' cultural and religious food requirements. When a patient is on therapeutic diet his or her special dietary needs have to be met. Medical tourism sector is one of India's fast growing service sectors with a growth rate of 30 percent per annum by 2015. It expected become a $2 billion industry.

Foreign patients who come to India for treatment belong to different religious and ethnic groups. Their food habits will be distinctly different from each region in the world. This requires, the foods and beverages managers to take note of different food habits, dietary practices of different religious groups. Hospitals, therefore, may need to procure and stock foods and beverages to meet the requirements of people who practice vegetarianism and veganism, Hindu diet, Kosher diet, Halal diet, and Chinese food.

Other Expendables

These include consumables like X-ray films, fixers, developers, surgical cotton, bandage cloth, lab chemicals, gloves, sutures, etc. Another method may be to classify them on the basis of well known selective controls like ABC/VED in particular HML/SDE/GOLF analysis in general.

 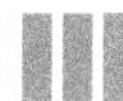

UNEXPENDABLES

Unexpendable items in hospitals are costly equipment, as are used in different departments. Most of these equipments are procured on non recurring basis. These items are not consumed in healthcare activities, and they retain their original identity and characteristics, during their useful life.

The original **Hill Burton** Hospital Planning and Construction Act of 1946, equipment for hospitals and nursing homes has been classified into three groups for planning and ordering purposes as shown in Table 12.5.

Table 12.5 Classifications of Equipment based on Hill-Burton Act, 1946

Type	Group	Description
Fixed	1	Fixed equipment included in construction contract such as pneumatic tubes, elevators, sterilizers, cabinets, and other built-in equipment (coordination by materials manager is important for this group as well).
Major movable	2	Major movable equipment, such as furnishings, X-ray, operating room. "Having a reasonably fixed location in the building," and does not form part in the construction contract, and a "depreciable life of 5 years or more."
Minor movable	3	Includes items having a depreciation life less than that of a major movable, and also not normally purchased through construction contracts; items of small cost, such as stools, silverware, waste baskets, bedpans, and the like.

[Source: U.S. Department of Health, Education and Welfare. Public health service, hospital and nursing home equipment Planning Guide (USPHS)]

Subsequently, the **Department of Public Health Service US** consolidated the above-mentioned three classifications into two major groups, fixed and movable. Fixed equipment includes all equipment normally in the construction contract plus other fixed equipment, such as X-ray machines, normally not in the construction contract. Major and minor movable equipment, formerly classified in groups 2 and 3, have been consolidated. Sophisticated electronic and mechanical hospital equipments are chosen by departments, with the advice of a panel of consultants, engineers, and architects acting as an evaluator or as member of value engineering committee. Ultimate responsibility however lies with the buyer for the final negotiation and order placement. In many instances, the facility administrator is also involved in these matters, and for policy and budgetary reasons, he should be. But he should clearly delegate authority and responsibility for entire construction equipment project to the buyer.

Unexpendable equipments are further classified into three broad categories namely:

1. Diagnostic equipment
2. Therapeutic equipment
3. Support service equipment

1. Diagnostic Equipment

Correct diagnosis leads to correct treatment and helps the doctors to help patients.

Diagnostic equipment is used for diagnosis and prognosis of the inpatients and outpatient clinics or inpatient wards, laboratories, radiology department, specializations like microbiology, biochemistry and bacteriology.

Diagnostic equipment is any type of equipment, whose main purpose is to help doctors detect and diagnose diseases. These items include handy items like stethoscope used by doctors for preliminary diagnosis to costly equipment. The costliest equipments can be found in radiology department (X-ray plants) or in the cardiology department and intensive care units (ICUs).

Some of the most commonly used diagnostic equipment include ultrasound machines, **Positron Emission Tomography (PET)** scanners (which use cameras and tracer fluid to produce images of a patient's internal organs in order to detect signs of cancer or other diseases), **Computerized Tomography (CT)** scanners (which use X-rays and dye to do the same job as PET scanner), **Magnetic Resonance Imaging (MRI)** machines (which use magnetic resonance technology to detect things like tumours, infections and internal injuries), Bio-technology and general analysis equipment. Diagnostic medical equipment may also be used in the homes for certain purposes like for monitoring blood glucose levels.

2. Therapeutic Equipment

Therapeutic is a branch medicine deals with treatment and cure of diseases or disability. Excellence in patient care depends to a large extent proper maintenance of medical equipment, more so with the bio medical. This is one of low priority areas in healthcare management and is a burning problem. In many hospitals medical equipment are lying unserviceable. Without proper maintenance, no equipment can perform satisfactorily. Maintenance and repair of sophisticated bio medical equipment has become more critical necessitating, specialized maintenance crew. **To keep equipment in good repair, calls for right spare part at right time in right quantity at the right place.**

Other Therapeutic Equipments

Other therapeutic medical equipments include devices such as infusion pumps (which infuse the circulatory system of patients under recovery with nutrients and medicines), equipment used in operation theatres, trauma care units, neurosurgery, thoracic surgery, cardiology and psychiatry come under this category. An example of therapeutic equipment is haemodialysis equipment in nephrology department. Equipment in patients' wards of orthopaedics' physiotherapy includes diathermy, ultraviolet, combined treatment, infrared radiant heat, gymnasium equipment and tank for hydrotherapy.

3. Support Service Equipment

Following equipment are classified as support service equipment.

a. Productive Equipment

Productive equipment helps the hospital in manufacture of certain basic requirements of hospital like oxygen, glucose, procurement, and preservation of blood, manufacturing of artificial limbs for physically challenged patients.

b. Service Equipment

Equipment that comes under this category is used in departments of medical store, laundry, dietetics, mortuary, and waste disposal e.g., refrigerators, tools, trolleys, cold storage plants etc.

Central Sterile Supplies Department (CSSD) is responsible for issuing and control of sterile items to various departments in the hospital. Equipment that is used for sterilization is pressure type steel sterilizer operating at a temperature of 121°C.

Laundry: Main function of laundry services is to receive soiled and infected linen and to process it. Important equipment used in the laundry includes washing machines of different capacities, hydro extractors to squeeze water and drain it out, drying tumblers, automatic iron etc.

c. Engineering

The equipment used for regular supply of water and electricity to various departments in the hospital e.g., water coolers, air conditioners, air coolers, elevators, ceiling fans etc. are some of the examples of engineering support service equipment.

d. Ambulatory equipment

Ambulance with necessary equipment is used for bringing patients comfortably during emergency situations. Depending on the type of emergency, the ambulance can be a simple one having only a stretcher to a super speciality one having the following equipment:

- DC shock machine, which is used for cardiac resuscitation.
- Ventilator
- Cardiac monitor
- ECG machine
- Emergency drugs and IV fluids

- Sphygmomanometer
- Single point cane or quad canes

e. **Hospital Beds and Bedroom Aids**

Patients who require instant and/or recurrent changes in body positioning on account of pain, difficulty in breathing or other issues The need for semi electric bed arises. This type of bed is helpful when patients are left alone they can make their own position adjustments head and knee sections using power hand control. However height adjustment is done manually.

Patients who require frequent changes in body position, and allow patient to make positions without adjustments, a full electric bed is desirable Head and knee sections and the height of the bed are adjusted by a power hand control. A beside commode is used by people who have difficulty getting to the bathroom.

f. **Support Surfaces**

A patient who always confined to a wheelchair is at risk for developing pressure sores, or decubitus ulcers. Unless the patient repositions her or himself frequently is prone to decubitus ulcers within a few hours.

Aged bed ridden patients are highly susceptible to pressure sores, whose skin may be sensitive on account of nervous or circulatory conditions and persons for whom paralysis makes change of position impossible.

Examples are bed ridden patients due to any medical condition.

Support Surfaces that may be recommended for use by such patients would be

- An alternating pressure cushion with pump
- Pneumatic pressure mattress
- Gel pressure mattress
- Aqua pressure mattress

g. **Bath Aids**

Bath and shower benches not only give comfort and make bathing easier a **tub transfer chair** is used to relocate patient from a wheelchair to a bathtub.

To get on and off the toilet comfortably an **elevated toilet seat,** with a safety device is provided on the rim of a toilet, making it easier for users, such as seniors.

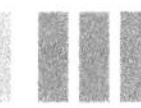

h. Diabetic Supplies

Clients living with diabetes have a convenient, safe way of receiving their diabetic testing equipment and supplies.

i. Office Equipment

Furniture and different kinds of racks, cupboards, and side tables provided for keeping the files and other records in all offices, departments, units and wards come under this category. **Classification of hospital inventories based on usage and point of entry is shown in Figure 12.1**

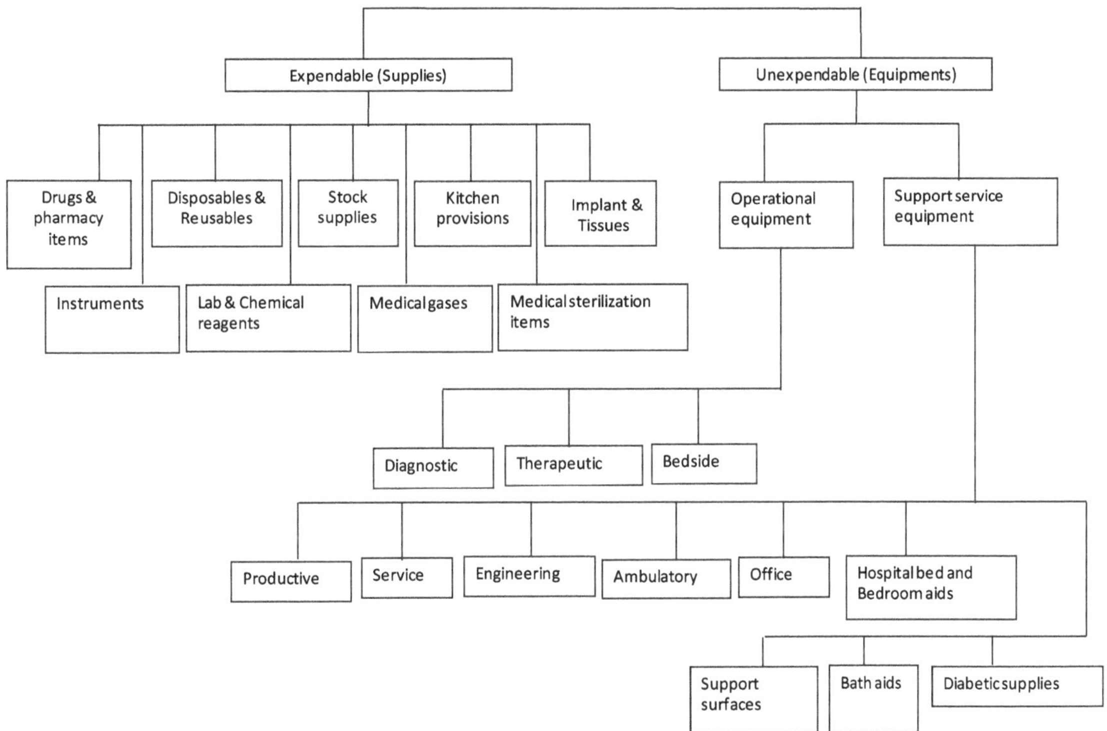

Figure 12.1 Classification of Hospital Inventories based on Usage and Point of Entry

SPARE PARTS

Quality and delivery of healthcare depends to a large extent on proper management of medical equipment more so with the bio medical equipment. This is one of the low priority areas in healthcare management and a burning problem as in many hospitals, medical equipments lying unserviceable without proper maintenance renders unsatisfactory performance and service. As more and more sophisticated bio-medical equipment come to use, requirement of specialized services for maintenance and repair will become more critical. Keeping equipment in good repair, calls for right spare part at right time in right quantity at the right place.

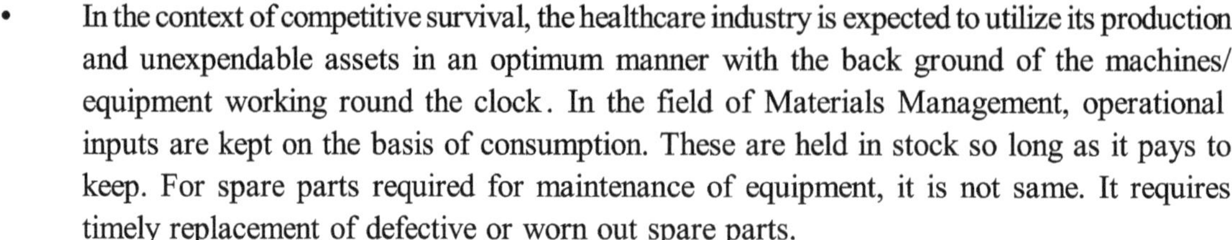

- In the context of competitive survival, the healthcare industry is expected to utilize its production and unexpendable assets in an optimum manner with the back ground of the machines/ equipment working round the clock. In the field of Materials Management, operational inputs are kept on the basis of consumption. These are held in stock so long as it pays to keep. For spare parts required for maintenance of equipment, it is not same. It requires timely replacement of defective or worn out spare parts.

CLASSIFICATION OF SPARES

General Classification

Spares can be broadly classified into three categories on the basis of:

1. Usage
2. Movement analysis
3. Functional characteristics

Based on usage the spares can further be classified into two types:

a. Regularly used spares

b. Irregularly used spares

Classification of Spares based on Movement analysis:

a. Fast moving: Items which have moved at least once in last one or two years are classified as fast moving.

b. Slow moving: Spare parts which have moved at least once in a period of two to four years.

c. Non-moving: Items which have not moved at least once in five years duration are classified as non-moving.

Classification Based on Functional Characteristics

Here, the spare part inventories are classified as:

- Capital and Insurance spares
- Rotable spares
- Maintenance or regular consumption spares
- Over hauling spares

The rate of consumption of spare parts differs from hospital to hospital depending upon type of specialities, bed strength, occupancy rate and age of equipment in use.

Each classification has different behaviour and hence to be controlled differently.

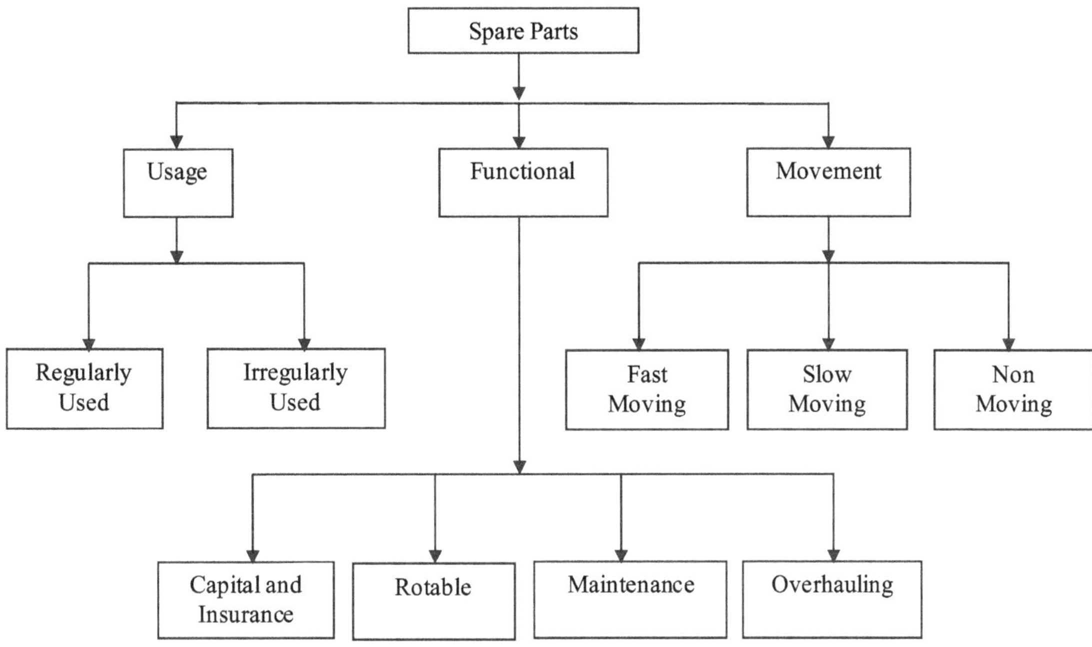

Figure 12.2 Classification of Spare Parts Inventory

Spares are significant set of inventories by themselves. **Consumption pattern of spare parts are distinctly different from inventories that are used for day to day operations of hospitals.** As a result stocking policies of spares are diverse and necessitates special approach to tackle spare parts inventory. One thing certain in spare parts requirement is it's uncertainty. It is usual to define a spare part ironically as **"something, which is available when not required and not available when needed.**

Capital and Insurance Spare Parts

Capital and insurance spares are those critical parts of a machine or equipment which have life nearly equal to the life of machine itself and are held as a contingency against any possible breakdown.

Characteristics of capital and insurance spare parts are as follows:

- These are held as contingency against probable machine breakdowns.
- Their consumption is low during the lifetime of equipment.
- Procurement lead time is high; requires several months or more.
- Normally, these are procured along with original equipment and are carried as standby.

- Reliability of capital and insurance spares is very high and could be 99 percent or more, i.e., almost equal to the life of the equipment. Insurance spares do not become obsolete until parent equipment is retired from service. For insurance spares, one has to decide whether to carry or not. If stocked, they may be retained in stock even if they do not move for many years. Reliability of capital spare is around 95 percent. Number of capital spares to be carried ranges between of 1 to 3.

Rotable Spares

The nomenclature 'Rotable' was first obtained from air force vocabulary. These are expensive spare parts such as pumps, engines and generators, and motors, and are not usually scrapped. Defective rotable parts removed from the machine are repaired and held in stock to be used, when failure of similar equipment occurs. They are easily interchanged on similar machines.

Characteristics of rotable spare parts are:

- These are major functional sub assembles/assemblies of the equipment.
- Procurement lead time is generally high. Some of the spares are to be made to order thus result in long procurement lead time.
- Cost of stock out is high.
- Carrying costs are also high.
- Demand for such spare parts per any single machine is low but for group of similar machines, the demand will be high.

In evolving stocking policies for rotable spares, factors pertaining to 'rotation' of the same part must be considered. In order to reduce downtime of the equipment, the removal should be on replacement basis, which implies that, a reserve of 'rotables' have to be maintained at the store or base workshop. When a rotable spare fails, it is replaced from the **'reserve' (also called as float)** and the failed item is later repaired and brought back to stores. In order to determine the stocking policy of rotable spares, several approaches are available; one of the most commonly used methods is **'Queuing approach'.**

Queues are formed due to lack of just right balance between the pace of arrival of customers and the pace of servicing at the facility. In such cases, a surge of customers towards the 'service facility' is turned into queue as it is not possible to serve all customers immediately on arrival. A typical example include people waiting at the outpatient departments in hospitals, application of queuing approach is to lessen waiting time to a minimum after considering the service cost and waiting cost. In queuing theory, breakdowns are treated as "**customers**"; and those replaced are termed as "**servers**".

Maintenance Spares

Spare parts, which are consumed on a regular basis, are called "maintenance spares". These are required for replacements of old parts due to frequent breakdowns caused by wear and tear. These are generally fast moving and demand for these spares is repetitive in nature compared to other categories of spares. Typical examples include V belts, standard bearings, oil seals, fasteners couplings, gaskets etc.

Characteristics of maintenance spares are as follows:

- Compared to other categories, these spare parts are faster moving and requirement is repetitive in nature.
- It is possible to build adequate database on failures and consumption, according to actual withdrawals from the stores.
- Normally, these do not create problems in planning and procurement or requirement. Usually the design of equipment is such that, parts which need to be frequently replaced are easily accessible for replacement without stripping open the machine.
- Set pattern of consumption facilitates fixing of ordering quantities, frequency of replenishment and safety levels.
- Usually, the spares parts that often fail are also cheaper compared to other categories of spares.
- Part that often fails, the **mean time between failures (MTBF)** will be low.

Influencing Factors

Important among the large number of factors that influence maintenance spare parts inventory controls are:

- Inventory holding cost
- Under stocking/downtime cost
- Importance of the item/equipment
- Criticality of the spare part
- Administrative, procurement and inspection lead times
- Service level
- Movement analysis (FSN)

Selective controls such as ABC, VED analysis also help to arrive at the requirement of spare parts thoroughly. While ABC analysis categorizes the items according to consumption value, VED analysis helps to identify the criticality of the item. ABC/VED analysis matrix will help to identify the service level, which forms the basis for inventory policies. A typical illustration of service level indications is shown below in the ABC-VED combination matrix

Table 12.6 ABC/VED Combination Matrix for Maintenance Spares

	Consumption value as percentage		
Criticality	A	B	C
Vital	90	95	99
Essential	75	85	95
Desirable	60	70	80

Overhauling Spares

Overhauling gives a new lease of life to an equipment or part of it. Organizations undertake periodic overhauling of equipment on a planned basis after pre determined hours of working. In the case of transport industry, it is well known that engines are overhauled after a pre determined number of kilometres run or hours of use. The extent and timing of overhaul are normally predictable with reasonable accuracy. **Main difference between overhaul and ordinary repair is about timing and extent of repair activity scheduled.** Overhaul could also be a preventive action to prevent failure of expensive parts of machines.

Overhaul spares are those replaced at the time of overhauls. Some of these parts like track links are to be adjusted; some parts can be built up. At the time of overhauling of equipment, maintenance engineer has to decide which parts have to be replaced outright and which can be adjusted. Maintenance department then list out only those parts, which, are required to be replaced completely; this list may not be very accurate, unless hospitals maintain equipment record sheets or cards and log tools to arrive at pattern of replacements. Since overhauling is a planned programme timing of overhauling is informed to production and purchase who are primarily concerned. Some activities like overhauling of engines, compressors, and pumps and rewinding of motors can be sub contracted when there is paucity of time. In such situations application of analytical tools like **CPM/Network analysis** techniques comes handy. Overhauling programme has to be planned well in advance say at least 6 months in advance to coordinate with user and purchase departments.

General tendency among maintenance personnel is to overestimate the requirement (i.e. to err on safer side) in such situation ABC/VED analysis will facilitate the maintenance engineer to have second look at the requirements.

Lead times for different spare parts are estimated in advance then, Purchase department can schedule the deliveries depending lead for times of different items so that they arrive only when they are needed to ensure minimum locking up of funds.

SPARE PARTS PLANNING PRE REQUISITE

Prior to installing inventory control policy for spares, a 'diagnostic' study covering following aspects will be useful.

1. List of spare parts required for each machine used in the company should be prepared.
2. A survey of factory to locate all areas of formal and informal storage must be conducted. This survey may reveal that, lockers for workers and cupboards for supervisors and many nooks and corners of maintenance workshop have been converted into informal storage area.
3. List of all the materials salvaged during above mentioned survey must be prepared and should give description of material, place of its storage and its ultimate use.
4. The list must be subjected to thorough scrutiny with the view of scrapping worthless and obsolete items and of identifying the remaining spares for purpose of relating them to the specific machines.
5. Material that needs to be retained should be placed in pre-designed storage spaces after attaching tags or slips to them for identification in future.
6. Salvageable parts should be entrusted to workshop for re-conditioning before taking them on stock.

Usage Rate

Failure rate resulting in the replacement of spare part is known as usage rate and forms the basis for application of scientific management techniques in spare function. From the individual rate of failures, average rate can be estimated. But it will not be possible to predict exact time of when an individual failure will occur. There will be considerable variation in number of spares required in equal amount of time. This variation is very large for low usage rate and low for high usage rate and can be determined with the help of Poisson distribution.

Methodology to Obtain Usage Rate

To obtain usage rate, one has to consider following three stages:

- **First stage:** Initial provisioning will cover a period ranging between 1 to 5 years and are procured at the time of purchase of equipment. The manufacture's (OEM's) recommendation carries an important weight at this stage. It is not uncommon to order the spare parts needed during lifetime of equipments, particularly if there is risk or price increases or non-availability during the later years.

- **Second stage:** This is the easiest stage or phase. The requirement is regular periodic or is as and when needed stage.
- **Third stage:** This is the final stage, when equipment is about to be phased out or the supplier needs that all time requirement should be given to him implying that is the last opportunity to purchase from the original equipment manufacturer. In this stage, the knowledge and experience gained during the operation of equipment could be used to minimize the margin of error in the spares planning.

Reliability

In order to meet increased occurrence of failure of the spare parts, the science of reliability engineering is very helpful. It is obvious that reliability of spare part or rather unreliability and maintainability jointly affect the availability of the equipment to the users.

Reliability of spare part is defined as the probability or proportion of time that, the part will function adequately within specified limits, for at least a specified period of time under operating conditions without failure.

Operating conditions include:

- Impact due to raw materials.
- Environmental conditions such as, humidity, shock, pressure, vibration temperature etc.
- Maintenance policies of the organization etc.

MEASURES OF RELIABILITY

A measure of reliability should be accompanied by the prevailing, physical or operating conditions. The measures of reliability usually adopted in practice are failure rate, probability of survival and mean times between failures. They are explained below.

MEAN TIME BETWEEN FAILURES (MTBF)

Failure rate is commonly expressed as failures per fixed number of hours. Larger the value of meantime between failures, greater is the reliability.

Probability is expressed as a decimal fraction or percent which indicates the number of parts that will function for required time period. Distribution of time of failure of a component is important to arrive at MTBF.

Failure rate curve typical of most of manufactured item is given in Figure 12.3. This is known as **'Bath tub curve'.**

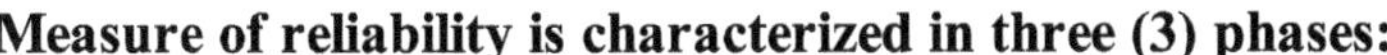

Measure of reliability is characterized in three (3) phases:

- **First Phase:** First phase is characterized by decreasing failure rate; represents the period where poorly manufactured items are weeded out.
- **Second Phase:** The second phase is often characterized by a constant failure rate and here only chance failure occurs.
- **Third Phase:** It is characterized by an increasing failure rate. It is the period during which components fail because of wear and tear of parts.

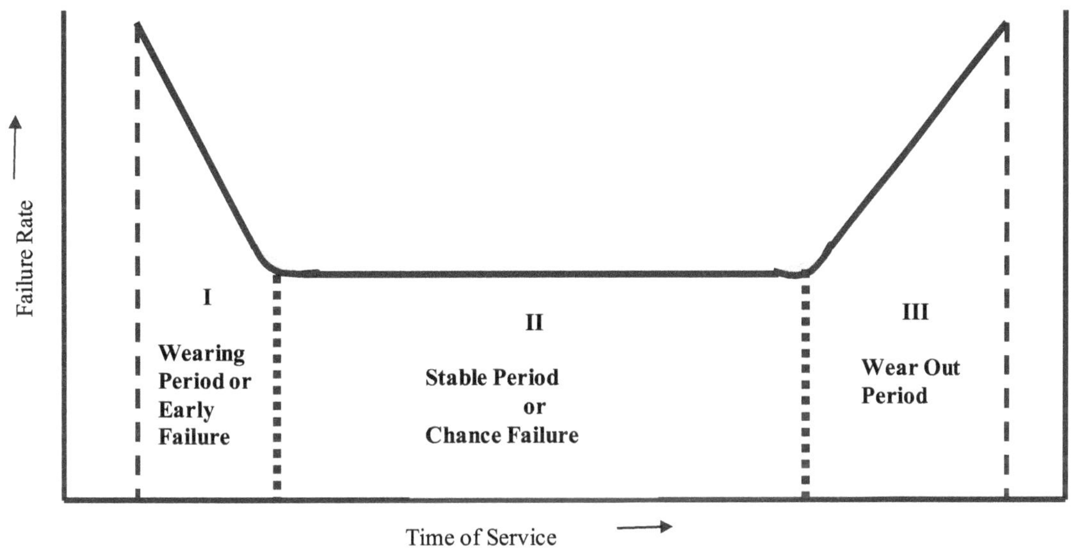

Figure 12.3 Bath Tub Curve

The general bath tub curve is typical of human body, where first phase represents infant mortality, second phase is chance failure and third phase depicts old age mortality.

SUMMARY

Internal and external customers of health care organization requires supplies of plethora of materials like, drugs and pharmaceuticals, instruments, medical, surgical, sterile, office equipment, housekeeping, foods and beverages, MRO items, laboratory and radiology supplies, gases and capital equipment. These materials have to be either procured or produced in the hospital. Users of diagnostic and therapeutic equipments require spare parts in stock to keep the equipment in good repair. Inventories can be broadly classified according to the functions they perform or usage and point of entry into operations of hospital. Based on the function it performs, the inventories are classified into four groups, as lot size inventories, fluctuation inventories, anticipation inventories and transportation inventories. In lot size inventories,

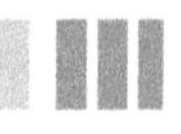

supplier companies manufacture items in lots rather than exactly at the rate at which they are supplied. Fluctuation inventories exist because of demand or supply variations. Anticipation inventories are sometimes called as speculative inventories and are held to take care of fluctuations in lead time and rate of consumption, or to meet peak time demand for seasonal products, Transportation inventories are also known as in transit inventories that are being transported from one place to another.

All hospital inventories based on point of entry into the operations are broadly classified as **expendables and unexpendables.** Expendables are used in day to day operations of hospitals and are procured on recurring basis, which include foods and beverages, and dietary items and linen gloves etc. In addition to above, provisioning items for infrastructure e.g., laundry items and **maintenance, repair and operation (MRO)** items also fall under this category. On an average, in medium size hospital number of stock items will be around 15,000. These items can be grouped and classified in a variety of ways.

Drugs are classified into different groups according to their common effects and actions on the mind and body, depending upon the specialities drugs can be grouped in to variety of ways. One method of classification is grouped according to diseases.

Drugs are also classified under their myriad forms such as tablets, injections, ointments, drops, powders, fluids, capsules, liquids, surgical, over the counter items (OTC) etc. A disposable item is used once during patient care and then thrown away or converted it to reusable materials or dispensed with as solid waste. These items are generally inexpensive in nature and are of short-term expediency rather than medium to long term resilience.

An object or material inserted or grafted into the body for medical procedures is known as implant. During the year 2007 the European Union (EU) brought out guide lines to ensure safety and infection control for dental and minor surgery. After use, the Single use Instruments are called as clinical waste and have to be disposed of in accordance with clinical waste laws in force. The instruments which are to be recycled can be re sterilized to eliminate clinical waste status and moved to sterile store for future use Anything used in patient care must be cleaned, sterilized, washed, or otherwise converted to its original aseptic condition.

Medical gas is intended for administration to a patient in anaesthesia, therapy, or diagnosis. In USA, the Code of Federal Regulations (CFR) classifies medical gases as drugs. Medical gases are to be treated as prescription drugs as their usage is unsafe without supervision of a licensed practitioner or trained emergency personnel. Examples of medical gases are Oxygen, Nitrous oxide, Nitrogen, Carbon dioxide, Medical air and Helium etc.

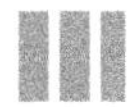

Medical sterilization connotes the complete elimination or destruction of all living micro organisms. There are several agents are available important among them are steam, hot air chemical agents high velocity electron bombardment, heat, or ultraviolet light radiation.

Kitchen & Dining Products include dishware drink ware plates bowls cups plastic cutlery, like spoons, knives forks, Cans, bottles, jars, cartons ,wrappers and other food packaging etc are generally recyclable, and a few of them are even Bio degradable. The foods and beverages generally categorized as provisional items, processed food, spices, diary items, bakery items, vegetables, beverages, fruits, non vegetarian items. Although standard hospital menu meets majority patients, cultural and religious food needs are also required to be considered while planning for procurement of foods and beverages.

Other expendables include consumables like X-ray films, fixers, developers, surgical cotton, bandage cloth, lab chemicals, gloves, sutures, etc. Another method may be to classify them on the basis of well known selective controls like ABC, VED in particular, HML, SDE, GOLF analysis in general.

Unexpendable materials in hospitals are costly equipment, as are used in different departments. Most of these equipments are procured on non recurring basis. These items are not consumed in healthcare activities, and they retain their original identity and characteristics, during their useful life.

Unexpendable equipments are further classified into three broad categories namely diagnostic equipment, therapeutic equipment, support service equipment. Correct diagnosis leads to correct treatment and helps the doctors to help patients. Some of the most commonly used diagnostic equipment include ultrasound machines, position emission tomography (PET) scanners (which use cameras and tracer fluid to produce images of a patient's internal organs in order to detect signs of cancer or other diseases), computerized tomography (CT).

Therapeutic is a branch medicine that deals with treatment and cure of diseases or disability. Excellence in patient care depends upon to a large extent proper maintenance of medical equipment, to keep equipment in good repair, Calls for right spare part at right time in right quantity at the right place.

Other unexpendables include productive equipment, service equipment, engineering, ambulatory equipment, h**ospital beds and bedroom aids, support surfaces, bath aids, diabetic supplies, o**ffice equipment.

Proper management of medical equipment, and Quality and delivery of are entwined in healthcare, more so with bio medical eqipment. Up keep of medical equipment is one of the low priority areas in healthcare management and is a burning problem as in many hospitals, with medical equipment lying unserviceable. Without proper maintenance no equipment can perform satisfactorily. In order to keep equipment in good repair, it calls for right spare part at right time in right quantity at the right place and right attitude of the management. Spares can be broadly classified into three categories on the basis of usage, movement analysis and functional characteristics. Functional spare parts inventories are further classified as capital and insurance spares, rotable spares, maintenance or regular consumption spares, over-hauling spares. Capital and insurance spares are those critical parts of a machine or equipment which have life nearly equal to life of machine itself and are held as a contingency against any possible breakdown. Defective rotable parts removed from the machine are repaired and held in stock to be used, when failure of similar equipment occurs. They are easily interchanged on similar machines. Demand for "Maintenance spares are fairly regular, and are required for replacements due to breakdowns on account of wear and tear of parts. These are generally fast moving and demand is repetitive in nature compared to other categories of spares. Overhauling gives a new lease of life to an equipment or part of it. Overhaul spares are those replaced at the time of overhauls. Prior to installing inventory control policy for spares, a 'diagnostic' study is required to be done. Next stage is to arrive at the failure rate resulting in the replacement of spare part. This is known as usage rate and forms the basis for application of scientific management techniques in spare function.

To arrive at usage rate, one has to consider issues like, initial provisioning, regular periodic replacements and finally when equipment is about to be phased out or the supplier needs that all time requirement should be given to him implying that is the last opportunity to purchase from the original equipment manufacturer. In order to meet increased occurrence of failure of the spare parts, the science of reliability engineering is very helpful.

Other factors that have to be considered in spare parts planning are impact due to raw materials, environmental conditions such as, humidity, shock, pressure, vibration temperature etc., maintenance policies of the organization and measures of reliability, mean time between failures (MTBF) etc. Reliability of system will often depend on the length of time it has been in service and hence the distribution of the time of failure of a component is important. Typical failure rate curve is popularly known as 'Bath tub curve'.

REVIEW QUESTIONS

1. What are the broad classifications of inventories? Explain the classification of inventories based on the functions it performs.
2. Briefly describe how hospital inventories are classified based on usage and point of entry in to the operations of the hospital.
3. How spare parts are usually classified? Describe each of them and state their peculiarities in so far as inventory control is concerned.
4. Describe the general classification of foods and beverages. What are special diets in meeting patient's cultural and religious food needs with the advent of medical tourism?
5. Describe briefly various support services equipment used in hospital for patient care.
6. Write short notes on
   a) Reagent and reactant
   b) Maintenance spares
   c) Support surfaces
   d) Ambulatory equipment
   e) Therapeutic equipment
   f) Medical gases
   g) Special diets

PART - III

Cost Associated with Inventories

Contents

CHAPTER - 13

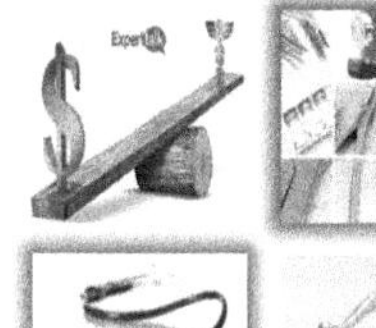

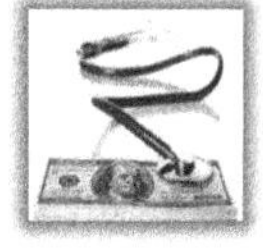

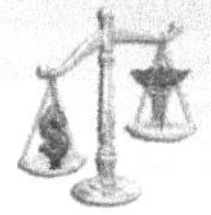

Cost Associated with Inventories

INTRODUCTION

Analysis of inventory problems is fundamentally based on very simple common-sense observation. **Batters Bay** rightly said, "Management of inventory is associated with opposing costs." There are always costs associated with "too much" or "too little" inventory. Optimum decision depends on how often a commodity is ordered and how much quantity is ordered. Ordering too frequently is associated with cost and is referred as "ordering cost". If this was not the case, then the commodity would be ordered, with maximum possible frequency. Perhaps separate orders for each item, when demanded. As a matter of fact, it may be optimal policy for some commodities. If no cost were associated with ordering, then there would be no problem and no analysis is required. But in real life, such costs do exist. Second alternative is not ordering too frequently. In this alternative also, there is cost associated in not ordering frequently enough. It is known as inventory carrying cost or inventory holding cost. If there were no such cost, the commodity would never be ordered at all, or one order might be placed for huge quantity of commodity. **If any one of the two opposing costs i.e. Ordering or holding costs is not in existence, optimal policy would be to go in for one of the two extreme solutions indicated earlier.**

Next question to be answered is how much of a commodity is to be ordered. Once again we can be sure that two opposing costs exist. If there were no costs existing for carrying inventory, then some enormous quantity would be automatically ordered. Correspondingly, if there were no costs associated with ordering too little, then no stock would be kept in the inventory. If these costs do not exist there would be simply no inventory problems. However, such an ideal situation does not exist. Such opposing costs always exist and first step of analysis must be to determine what costs are and, if possible measure them.

- Ordering cost
- Inventory carrying cost
- Over stocking cost
- Under stocking cost

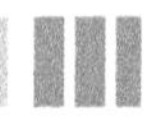

Useful objective of inventory management is minimization of total costs involved and not simply minimization of one or other opposing costs. Total costs include all relevant opposing costs and analytical procedure is to find out an expression for total cost and then discover the course of action, which will minimize the aggregate. Apparent costs are ordering cost incurred prior to arrival and inventory carrying cost incurred after the arrival into the inventory till it is used in the day to day operations of the hospital. Hidden costs are not carrying inventory at all or carrying less than required, called **"under stocking cost"** or **"stock out cost"** and cost of **carrying more than required quantities called "over stocking costs".**

Various internal and external factors influence levels of inventory. Internal conditions start from forecasting a requirement, so that required material is available only at the right time. External conditions include supplier's lead time, environmental conditions, government rules and regulations, credit availability, market conditions etc. All these factors, influence on the inventory management, could be summed up in the following categories.

- Service level
- Obsolescence
- Scrap
- Waste

In addition to above cost factors, lead time plays an important role in management of inventories. Impact of lead time on inventory management is dealt in detail in chapter 16.

ORDERING COST/SET UP COST

Ordering cost is also known as procurement cost. There are at least two possible approaches to calculating this cost of placing an order. All costs associated with placing, receiving, and paying for an order should be included. These ordinarily include the following.

Average order costs are calculated by determining the total annual costs for purchasing, receiving, and accounts payable functions and dividing this amount by number of orders issued per year. The defect in this approach is that it fails to consider variability in costs of placing purchase orders. Number of items ordered per purchase order may vary. In addition, the above mentioned costs comprise of both fixed and variable elements. To facilitate decision making, managers need to know how much it costs to place an additional order or whether anything would be saved if fewer orders are placed. Alternative is to base calculation of ordering cost on incremental order cost. This means that the decision as to whether to order more or less frequently will be based upon, what it will cost to place each additional order and what it will save by reducing number of orders.

To take this step, it is necessary to analyze each of the cost categories in order to determine which are fixed and which are variable. Cost of equipment depreciation is fixed and thus can be ignored until the increasing number of orders would require the purchase of another personal computer (PC). Labour costs behave in a similar fashion. Care needs to be exercised to avoid the assumption that labour costs are fixed when they should be viewed as variable. Time studies help to determine labour costs for each element. In application, it is helpful to determine the average number of line items on each purchase order. The value of total average cost per order is divided by the average number of line items per order to arrive at average cost per item. This information then needs to be incorporated into economic order quantity (EOQ) formula, thus the calculated results will be based upon costs that are as accurate as possible.

Activities, which constitute cost of ordering (Co), ordering cost or set up cost are those involved in processing an order such as handling charges, inspection and testing charges, transportation and receiving costs, postage costs and special expediting costs. The activities pertaining to procurement of materials consume executive and non executive time, stationery and communication charges, which have to be borne by the organization, thus giving rise to the ordering cost.

Activities, which constitute ordering costs, are:

1. Cost of completing the requisition.
2. Cost of reviewing the requisition.
3. Cost of source development i.e., time spent in arranging for material and sharing technical know how and tolerating initial rejections etc.
4. Cost of publication in newspapers, trade journals, supply of tender forms etc.
5. Cost of tender opening formalities.
6. Cost of discussing terms and conditions of supply with potential vendor(s), including pricing.
7. Cost of purchase order forms and other stationery used in purchase department.
8. Cost of distribution and filing the document.
9. Salaries and other statutory payments like gratuity, PF, etc. made to purchase personnel.
10. Salaries paid for the time spent by other departments directly or indirectly connected with purchasing activities.
11. Follow up costs incurred on postage, fax, e-mail, Internet, telephone etc.
12. Cost of follow up for expediting supplies and travel charges.
13. Cost of electronic data processing charges relevant to purchasing.
14. Cost of entertaining the suppliers.
15. Proportionate rent or depreciation on the space utilized by purchase department personnel.

16. Depreciation on equipment and office furniture used in the department, stationery, paper used for typing orders and sending reminders.
17. Cost of inspection of inward materials.
18. Cost of receiving the item(s) ordered, including checking-in, documenting and forwarding the paper work to accounts payable.
19. Cost of moving items from point of receipt to point of storage or use.
20. Cost of matching the invoice to the receiving documentation.
21. Cost of follow up between accounts payable and receiving, if required and cost of follow up between accounts payable and purchasing, in case where pricing does not match.
22. Cost of bills payment.
23. Cost of legal advises.
24. Any other expenses incurred on the activities that are incidental to purchasing activities.

Total costs incurred on the above activities divided by number of orders in a year gives estimate of average ordering cost per order.

$$\text{Cost per Order} = \frac{\text{Total cost incurred on purchasing activity in a year}}{\text{Number of orders issued during corresponding year}}$$

When a commodity is self supplied then ordering cost shall be referred to as "set up cost" (i.e., in the case of production). This takes into account idle cost of labour incurred during change over from one job to other. This is mainly found in jobbing type of activities and has to be taken into account for scheduling production.

Salaries, wages and other statutory payments made to purchasing personnel and follow costs constitute major expense items in the purchasing activities. Hence, the manpower in purchasing should be kept as low as possible. Any increase in total salary already paid should not be allowed, unless there is corresponding increase in number of orders. It will be cheaper to use overtime, when there is marginal increase in number of orders.

In India, cost of ordering ranges from Rs. 300 to 4,000 per order depending upon the size of the hospital and the number of personnel involved directly or indirectly in purchasing activities.

One may be tempted to reduce cost per order by indiscriminate increase in number of orders placed rather than reducing costs involved in ordering. This strategy will lead to reduction of effective time spent on an order thereby resulting in decrease of purchase efficiency. It always pays to carry out O and M study to improve purchase efficiency.

The levels of activities are different for different products. For example, costs incurred on order for import of an item will be much higher, when compared to cost of an order for cash

 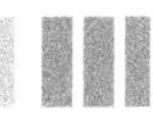

purchases of off the shelf items. **It is assumed that ordering costs are directly proportional to number of orders. This will usually be expressed as cost per order.**

INVENTORY CARRYING COST

Inventory carrying cost is otherwise known as holding cost. The motive factor to control inventory is the cost incurred by carrying it. Inventory holding costs are related to storage and handling of the goods and are calculated by first quantifying as many of the relevant costs as possible. Many will have to be extrapolated from total costs and prorated, based on inventory value and/or space. For example, insurance costs are not likely to be specifically identified with inventory. Rather, the total premium will have to be allocated based on the proportion of total assets that inventory constitutes. This is also true for security and housekeeping costs. Costs related to handling of inventory can be determined by identifying the amount of money spent on labour used to perform these functions. It is much more difficult to define these costs for inventories which are outside the direct control of MM. Costs of material handling equipment consist of the acquisition cost divided by the expected useful life i.e., depreciation. Cost of space is based on historical cost of the building. This figure expressed on a per square metre basis, is available from financial records. Replacement cost should be used when a building addition or an off site warehouse is under consideration. It should be recognized that an opportunity cost is also associated with space occupied by stores holding the inventories. If the option of placing another revenue producing service into the space used for inventories is under consideration, the cost of continuing such use of space is increased to expense of additional space for the service. The remaining costs are related to investment.

Capital always has many alternative uses including the purchase of operating inventories. If the money is not invested in inventory, they could be invested in adding revenue generating services or, at a minimum, with a bank to earn interest. In view of these alternatives, this cost of capital must be assigned to the inventory. The amount to be assigned obviously will depend upon interest rates and alternative uses for the capital. Finance department should be consulted for determination of the present capital cost along with trends. The amount invested so arrived must be divided by the current inventory value to convert them to percentages. The percentages then are added, resulting in the total holding cost percentage. This value is used in calculation of EOQ and economic review periods (ERP). Changes in prime interest rates and inflation will have a severe impact on inventory holding cost.

Major elements of carrying costs (Cc) are:

1. **Cost of capital blocked up due to money invested in inventory** i.e., interest on investment in inventories. This usually is most significant of all. Bank rate of interest (lending rate) is around 12 to 14 percent depending upon credit rating of the organization. If organization's internal reserves are used, then opportunity cost criterion must be applied.

2. **Cost storage space:** This may be on rental basis if the storage space is rented or on opportunity cost basis if the firm owns it. This usually is arrived at on the basis of the number of square metres assigned to the function. Historical costs may be used for existing space but replacement cost is required when considering additions or off site storage.
3. Salaries and other statutory payments like P.F, bonus, gratuity made to stores personnel.
4. Cost of handling: This should account for labour used in moving materials from point of storage to point of use.
5. Cost of material handling equipment: This includes shelving, carts, hand trucks, and forklifts etc.
6. Cost of security services for guarding inventory: This should be isolated for inventory safeguarding from overall security costs.
7. Cost of housekeeping services: This, too, should be spelt out specifically for the space utilized by the stores.
8. Taxes: These should be identified wherever applicable.
9. Costs of periodic physical inventories by stores personnel: Depreciation charges incurred on the storage equipments, handling equipments, bins, racks, and other accessories for storing and handling of inventories.
10. Salaries of stock verifiers and audit staff for time spent by them in the stores at the time of stock verification.
11. Cost due to deterioration of items which have low shelf life.
12. Losses due to evaporation of volatile materials like petrol.
13. Losses due to breakages in stores, while handling.
14. Losses due to pilferage, wastages.
15. Documentation charges for all stationery consumed relating to stores activities.
16. Electronic data processing charges pertaining to stores items. Nowadays it is an important cost element.
17. Cost of insurance to protect against fire and other natural calamities related risks.
18. Overhead costs like electricity, water, maintenance, housekeeping etc. incurred to maintain the stores.
19. Property tax expenses
20. Cost of obsolescence, which could be due to discontinuation of products line, changes in design, changes in machinery/equipment or existence of spare parts when machines are retired from service.
21. Any other costs incurred on stores activities that are incidental to holding inventory.

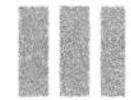

Inventory carrying cost is usually represented as percentage on average value of inventory held.

$$\text{Carrying cost} = \frac{\text{Total expenses incurred on stores activity in a year}}{\text{Value of average inventories held during the corresponding period}} \times 100$$

Since inventory carrying costs are calculated as percentage of average inventory carried. Adding up inventories held at the end of each of twelve calendar months and then dividing the result by 12 gives figure of average inventory. In some cases, stock as on 1st of April and as on 31st March of succeeding year are added and divided by 2. This type of calculation is not accurate and is only approximation.

OVER STOCKING COST

Measurement of this cost is comparatively simple. This cost is basically due to investment in inventory for longer periods than necessary i.e., demand for an item has terminated or becomes excessive. This cost is called "over stocking cost". Interpretation of this cost differs in accordance with the inventory problem, whether it is static or dynamic.

Static Purchase

Some inventory decisions, essentially made only once during its usage time are called static decisions or one shot decisions. A decision concerning hospital bed strength must be made when hospital is first planned. While expansions or further build up of hospital are subsequently taken up, the time lag is sufficiently high to justify such decision as an independent one. Consider an example of static inventory problem, that a retailer who wishes to sell "Christmas trees". His sales season is very sharply limited and any tree left on hand at the end of the season will have very little salvage value. Thus if he has too much stock he will have a cost due to loss he will suffer for each tree he over stocks. Other examples of static situation are printing of diaries or construction of a bridge over river. **In one shot decision, it is not necessary to consider the effect of one decision on subsequent decision.**

Dynamic Purchase

Any inventory decisions of similar nature, which are taken several times for sufficiently long time duration, are termed as dynamic. In a continuing process, the outcome of one decision has an affect on subsequent decisions and it is necessary to take this into account in the analysis.

Dynamic inventory situations are of two kinds

In the first case, there is a standard demand for certain materials for certain reasons found to be procured in excess. In such a case, this item will be ultimately used provided it has got enough shelf life to be used at a later date. This can be equated to "holding cost". Worked out example is given at Table 13.1.

In the second case, for items, which cannot be used after a certain period, this cost will be the difference between the cost of the item and its salvage value. To this amount is added the cost incurred for ordering it and the holding cost till it was salvaged.

Consider, as an example the inventory problem of a textile store with regard to some standard household items such as towels. There is always a demand for towels. So the towels left over after one time period can be sold in subsequent periods and this remains true for an indefinite period in the future. There will never be an over stock as in the case of Christmas trees. Hence no over-stock cost. Only the carrying cost is to be taken into account.

Example of calculation of over stocking cost for items, which can ultimately be used is given below.

Table 13.1 Calculation of Over Stocking Cost for Dynamic Purchases

Inventory norm for carrying a particular item inventory	One month consumption
Average monthly consumption as	100 units per month
Cost of the item	Rs. 1000 per unit
Actual quantity purchased as against 100 units	500 units
The excess quantity purchased (500-100)	400 units
Average inventory 400 × ½	200 units
Assuming inventory carrying cost 30 percent per annum the over stocking can be equated to (200 × 1000 × 30/100)	Rs. 60,000
Thus over stocking for four months period is	Rs. 20,000

Another example, consider women's clothing, for which, there are two selling seasons, in U.S market i.e., fall and spring. If only one order can be placed, we have static inventory problem. If several orders can be placed during a season, then we have a dynamic inventory problem. There will be no over stock cost involved until last order period of the season. At that time, however, any over stock will typically undergo a drastic devaluation and this must be measured as over stock cost. In case of items which cannot be used after a certain period (on account of low shelf life or obsolescence), the cost will be the difference between purchase price of item + cost incurred for ordering it + cost of carrying it till it is salvaged or disposed - salvageable value. Model calculation of over stocking of cost for which demand has been terminated could be seen from Table 13.2.

Example: An insurance spare part costing Rs. 2,00,000 was procured along with the machine. The machine was used for 10 years before it was scrapped. During usage period of the said machine, need for this particular insurance spare part did not arise; estimated holding cost was 30 percent. Then the over stocking cost would be:

Table 13.2 Calculation of Over Stocking Cost for Item which cannot be used Over a Period of Time

	Value in Rs.
Cost of spare part	2,00,000
Add. Inventory carrying cost 10 years (i.e., the period for which the machine is in use) 2,00,000 x 30/100 x 10	6,00,000
Add. Cost incurred for procuring the spare part	1,000
Total costs incurred	8,01,000
Less. Salvaged value realized when sold as scrap	51,000
Total cost of over stocking	**7,50,000**

UNDER STOCKING COST OR OUT OF STOCK COST

The cost of not carrying inventory i.e., a commodity is not in stock at the time when it is required is known as out of stock or under stocking cost. Suppose a fire accident occurs in a factory and extinguisher is out of operation and the whole factory gets gutted by fire, the resulting loss to building and materials, is the consequence of such stock out. In the event if it is happens in a hospital, consequential losses will be much more as life of patients is at danger. In this price of the commodity has no impact on stock out cost. This is usually measured in terms of 'opportunity cost' due to loss of production by keeping the line idle. If a stock out results in expedited orders, the extra charges incurred will be added to this cost.

There are some other intangible elements also, which cannot be measured directly. Some of hem are:

- Inconvenience
- Lay off to labour
- Delay in shipment of sale orders
- Rift among various departments
- Dislocation of entire works
- Loss of goodwill and reduction in future revenue
- Loss of morale and increased laziness of workers
- Because of inertia it will be some time before they pick up their original performance rate after re starting operations.

Computation of this cost is quite tricky. However, many organizations include only profit foregone due to loss of production or revenue.

SERVICE LEVEL

Service level is a measure of stock control effectiveness and it is a function of demand (in terms of quantity or value) routinely met from stock.

Table below lists some commonly used service levels

Table 13.3 Commonly used Service Levels

- Percentage of requisitions/requisitions fulfilled at the first request itself.
- Percentage of items indented in the requisition form/orders satisfied at first request.
- Percentage of items for which requirements are held in stock.
- Percentage of satisfied replenishment period.

$$SL = \frac{\text{No. of units delivered without delay}}{\text{No. of units demanded}}$$

$$\text{It may also be} = \frac{\text{No. of units demanded} - \text{No. of units short}}{\text{No. of units demanded}}$$

Calculation of service level (SL) should preferably cover a time span of a year. It is limited to 0-SL-1. If the service level is zero, it means that complete breakdown of delivery system and if SL=1, it means there were no shortages and that was a perfect hundred percent service.

Service level is usually expressed as a percentage.

$$\text{Percentage of stock-outs} = \frac{\text{No. of order periods when stocks were zero}}{\text{Total no. of order periods}} \times 100$$

Efficiency of inventory control is normally measured against negative scale i.e., by the number of stock outs. On the other hand, achieving zero stock outs requires very high idle investment and even then such service cannot be measured. Solution to this problem is to fix the service level as percentage depending upon the criticality of the items and availability of the material. For critical i.e., life saving drug or spare parts, we can fix 99 percent service level for life saving drugs. This implies that if there are 100 demands, control system will take care of at least 99 occasions of demand. As the importance of the item decreases, service level can be reduced. Required service level can be fixed by arriving at costs involved. **The two opportunity costs related to service level are over stocking cost and under stocking cost.**

$$\text{Service Level} = \frac{Ku}{(Ku + Ko)}$$

Where Ku is cost of under stocking and Ko is cost of over stocking. The service level is generally expressed in terms of percentage.

Example: Let us consider probable requirement for a particular spare part at a given time. Data collected is given in the following table.

Table 13.4 Probability of Demand for a Particular Item in a given Time

Demand	Probability of Demand	Cumulative Probability of Demand
0	0.330	0.330
1	0.369	0.699
2	0.201	0.900
3	0.073	0.973
4	0.021	0.994
5	0.005	0.999

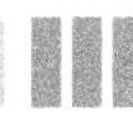

It can be seen from the table above that increasing the stock quantity does not increase the service level in the same proportion. For example, increasing stock level from 2 to 3 improves service level by 7.3 percent; increasing it from 3 to 4 improves the service level by 2.1 percent and increasing it further from 4 to 5 improves the service level by only 0.005 percent. Therefore we can conclude that to achieve a service level of 100 percent, we need large stocks. Level of safety stock to be established must support the definition of service level preferred by a hospital.

NATURE OF SEASONALITY ITS IMPACT ON INVENTORIES

Seasonality is of two types. One is Natural and the other Man-made seasonality. Natural seasonality is very common in agriculture based industry. Man made seasonality mainly occurs because of operations of an organization as reflected in books of accounts. General tendency in manufacturing industries is that purchasing and sales activity will be at its peak as financial year ending is fast approaching. This phenomenon occurs as yearly sales targets have to be achieved and purchase budgets allocations are to be utlised.

Supply and Demand for Natural Seasonality

1. Supply	-	Seasonal	Supply - Uniform
2. Demand	-	Seasonal	Demand - Uniform

1. **Supply Seasonal:** Example, agricultural produce such as food grains, vegetables, cereals and pulses etc.

2. **Demand Seasonal:** Agricultural implements, fertilizers, paints construction material etc., are treated as seasonal demand and their sales are low during monsoon. Normally, the purchase executive is not concerned with seasonal demand and uniform supply.

   - He is faced with a peculiar problem when supply is seasonal and demand is uniform.
   - To assure continuous supply of materials to the company and to make purchases at a reasonable price (since price will fluctuate), the organizations in order to ensure continuous supply resort to forward buying and in the process it is restricted by two major factors.
   - Availability of warehousing facilities.
   - Amount of liquid capital available on hand.

In case of seasonally available materials if a buyer purchases at regular intervals he will pay a high or low price but, by and large cost will be equal to average market price in the long run. Such traditional policy is unavoidable for Organization, in absence adequate storing facility or buyer prefers not to **"buy forward"** On the other hand, if storage space is available, the buyer can, to a limited extent, procure more in anticipation of price increase. To accomplish this effectively requires skill and certain amount of luck equally.

It is essential to strike a balance between likelihood of price declining now and holding costs for later use. Further, agricultural commodities shelf life also should be taken into consideration. Capability to forecast anticipated prices with accuracy is important. But it should be remembered that no forecast can be accurate.

OVER STOCK COST FOR PRODUCTS WHICH HAVE SEASONAL DEMAND

Since some tropical diseases are seasonal, the availability of some products is also seasonal. In the case of agro products, the prices are usually lower at the time of harvest. The inventory manager will have to balance holding costs vs. lower prices in deciding the inventory levels for these classes of items. Apart from that, the shelf life of the item has to be taken into consideration while stocking seasonal products. Prices would fluctuate depending upon demand and supply gap in a free market under perfect conditions.

OBSOLETE INVENTORY

Items which are held physically intact but need terminated are termed as obsolete items. Obsolescence occurs due to one or more of the following reasons.

- Changes in Technology
- Change in the product line of manufacture
- Changes in machines on account of prudent replacement policies
- Changes in surgical procedures
- Over buying of materials in anticipation of demand, which may not take place
- Cannibalization of equipments, when original equipment manufacturers (OEM'S) have already phased out manufacturing
- Faulty planning and forecasting of demand
- Equipment procured but not used during its lifetime
- Improper conservation methods
- When input is rationalized, balance stock of discarded item tends to become obsolete
- Faulty buying of large quantities to take advantage of quantity discounts.

To control obsolescence these loopholes should be plugged. Without proper identification, obsolescence cannot be controlled. A regular movement analysis (FSN) should give an indication of status of inventory.

SURPLUS

Surplus is similar to obsolete inventory. When an item in stock is more than is reasonably necessary to provide an adequate service to an operational activity. If the anticipated operational activity does not take place or there is error on the part of purchase department for required demand, the organization lands up in excess inventory. Excess over the normal is said to be surplus. This has same meaning as redundant. The term surplus material includes obsolete material that will have economic value.

SCRAP

Any manufacturing process will generate scrap, because we do not have 100 percent efficient system which can convert all the input into an output.

Scrap is usually of 3 categories: ferrous, non-ferrous and non metallic.

The following points to be borne in mind with regard to scrap.

- Scrap is unavoidable, in manufacturing activity but should be minimized this calls for continuous effort and vigilance
- Residual value of scrap material is a source of revenue.

  Segregation of scrap as ferrous, non ferrous before it is disposed of will fetch better price

Scrap and surplus material are a contradiction in terms; no organisation would like not to produce them. Yet they are regularly being generated. They are the only resources that are never exhausted

WASTE

Unusable non-metallic items are termed as waste. Examples of it are paper, corrugated boxes, oils, bags, plastics, rubber, timber, etc.

One of the most cogent arguments against the rapid increase in the use of disposables is that it affects ecology.

Hospital wastes are broadly classified as infectious, hazardous and non-nfectious and non hazardous.

LIMITATIONS OF INVENTORY CONTROL

- Efficient inventory control methods can reduce, but not altogether eliminate business risk.
- Risk in healthcare business as elsewhere is essentially a measure of uncertainty concerning the future.
- Inventory planning and control procedures can only help the business assess the risk and plan a strategy as far as hospital operations and purchasing plans are concerned so as to accept the risk on the most favourable terms consistent with the basic policies and objectives of business.
- Power of improved inventory management is limited further by the basic nature of conflict among objectives of a business i.e., better projection of occupancy rate through improved services to customers vs. lower costs through smoother operations.

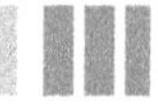

- Lower investment needs through reduced inventories are all legitimate business aims, but they are in fundamental conflict with other objectives.
- Thus, inventory management always is an optimizing function comparable to balancing act on a tight rope.

DETERMINATION OF ORDERING AND CARRYING COSTS

Work sheet for ordering cost

All costs associated with placing order receiving and paying for an order are included to arrive at cost per annum. Average order costs are calculated by determining total annual cost for purchasing, receiving and accounts payable functions and dividing this amount by number of orders issued per year. Various elements involved in ordering cost are discussed in the earlier part of this chapter.

(a) salaries & wages				
S. No.	Description	Work-load as percentage	Salaries/ wages per month in Rs.	Expenditure per annum in Rs.
1.	**(a) Purchase Department**	Percentage		
2.	Materials Manager	75	60,000	5,40,000
3.	Salary of pharmacy Manager	80	50,000	4,80,000
4.	Dy. Materials Manager	20	40,000	96,000
5.	Asst. Manager (PUR) – I	100	25,000	3,00,000
6.	Asst. Manager (PUR) – II	100	22,000	2,64,000
7.	Purchase Office	100	20,000	2,40,000
8.	Purchase Executives (PUR) – 2 persons	100	30,000	3,60,000
9.	Management Trainee	100	10,000	1,20,000
10.	Data Entry Operator & Steno – 2 persons	100	30,000	3,60,000
11.	Purchase Assistance's – 4 in number	100	48,00	5,76,000
12.	Office Boy	100	6,000	72,000
	Total:			**34,08,000**

(b) Finance Section				
1.	Finance Manager	5	50,000	30,000
2.	Accounts Officer	10	30,000	36,000
3.	Bill Passing Clerks – (3)	100	30,000	3,60,000
Sub Total				
	(c) Others			
4.	M.D's Salary	6	2,00,000	1,44,000
Grand Total (b + c)				**5,70,000**

S. No.	Description	Expenditure per annum in Rs.
1.	Salaries & wages paid to purchase personnel	37,08,000
2.	Cost of receiving the item(s) ordered including checking in, documenting and forwarding paper work to accounts payables	7,62,000
3.	Proportionate salaries and wages of finance department connected directly with purchase activity	4,26,000
4.	Proportionate salary of chief executive for time spent in purchase activities	1,44,000
5.	Travelling expenses in connection with purchase, and other follow up expenses	5,50,000
6.	Proportionate depreciation on the area utilized by the purchase department	70,000
7.	Depreciation on the furniture, other office equipment possessed by purchase department	1,50,000
8.	Statutory payments to purchase department staff like gratuity, PF, bonus etc. and other department staff who were involved in purchase activities	8,29,500
9.	Internet and email, postage & stationery expenses	2,50,000
Total cost of ordering per year		**68,89,500**

(B) Categories of Orders released		
S. No	**Category of Purchase Orders**	**No. of orders released**
1.	Drugs and pharmacy materials	186
2.	Medical and surgical supplies	375
3.	Sterile supplies	155
4.	Housekeeping supplies	172
5.	Foods and dietary supplies	160
6.	X-ray, radiology supplies and other consumables	342
7.	Diagnostic lab supplies	150
8.	Maintenance repair and operation materials	136
9.	Spare parts supplies	150
Total number of orders:		**1,826**

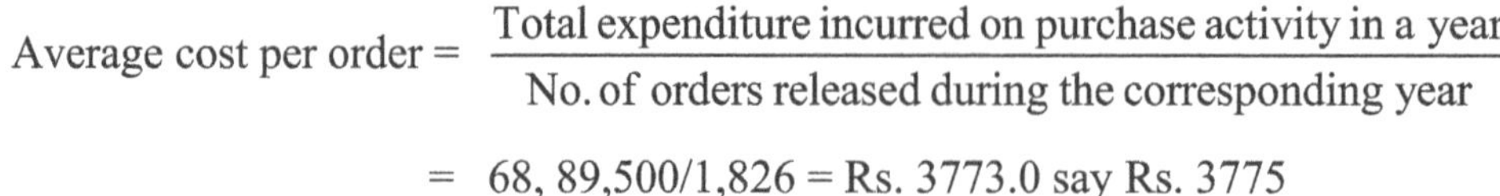

$$\text{Average cost per order} = \frac{\text{Total expenditure incurred on purchase activity in a year}}{\text{No. of orders released during the corresponding year}}$$

$$= 68,89{,}500/1{,}826 = \text{Rs. } 3773.0 \text{ say Rs. } 3775$$

Work Sheet for Calculation of Inventory Carrying Cost

It is difficult to quantify inventory carrying costs precisely. Any cost relating to storage and handling of goods along with all those involving the money invested in inventory are to be included. Inventory holding costs are calculated by first quantifying as many factors as possible as narrated under elements of inventory carrying earlier in this chapter. Many will have to extrapolate from total costs and prorated based on inventory value and/or space.

For example, insurance costs are not likely to be specifically identified with the inventory; rather the total premium paid will have to be allocated based on proportion of the total assets that inventory constitutes. This is also true security and housekeeping costs. Similar exercise can bed one for costs relating to material handling of inventory cost of space utilized for stores and cost of capital tied up in inventories or opportunity cost. Since these factors have been quantified as accurately as possible, the next step is to summarize them.

This involves the combination of investment in rupees and percentages; the money invested in inventories must be divided by current inventory value to convert them to percentages. These percentages are then added resulting in total percentage.

S. No.	Description	% of work load	Monthly expenditure in Rs.	Yearly Expenditure in Rs.
I	**Salaries & Wages**			
	A) Materials Manager	25	60,000	1,80,000
	B) Pharmacy Manager	20	50,000	1,20,000
	C) Dy. Materials Manager	80	40,000	3,84,000
	D) Stores Officer	100	25,000	3,00,000
	E) Supervisor (Stores)	100	15,000	1,80,000
	F) Stores Assistants (6)	100	84,000	10,08,000
	G) Contract Labour (8)	100	32,000	3,84,000
	Sub-total I			**25,56,000**
II	**Other Expenditure (Fixed)**			
	Statutory Payments like, PF, Bonus, gratuity paid to stores personnel			6,39,000
	Taxes & Insurance			3,60,000

Contd...

II	**Other Expenditure (Fixed)**			
	Travelling, Telephones & Stationery			3,10,000
	Depreciation on Buildings Stores Racks & Handling equipment's etc.			3,57,000
	Sub-total II			**Rs. 16,66,000**

III	**Other Expenditure (Variable)**			
	a) Interest charges @ 15 percent on average inventory of Rs. 690 lakhs			82,80,000
	b) Evaporation/shrinkage/scrap & obsolescence at 2 percent on average inventory of Rs. 690 lakhs			13,80,000
	Sub-total III			**96,60,000**

Grand Total = Sub-totals (I + II + III) = Rs. 1,38,82,000.00

Monthly closing value of inventories

S. No	Month	Value
1.	April	642
2.	May	751
3.	June	707
4.	July	747
5.	August	703
6.	September	685
7.	October	755
8.	November	854
9.	December	723
10.	January	668
11.	February	566
12.	March	478
	Total =	Rs. 8279

Average In ventory = 8279/12 = Rs. 689.92 lakhs (Say Rs. 690 lakhs)

Percentage of inventory carrying cost for the year on the average inventories held during the period.

Total expenses incurred on stores actively in a year/ Average value of inventory held during the corresponding period = 1,38,82,000 / 69,00,0000 = 0.2011 or 20.11 percent. Say 20 percent per annum on the average value of inventory held.

WORKED OUT PROBLEMS

1. Snigdha super-speciality hospital incurred following expenditure on stores and purchasing activity.

		Amount in Rs.
1	Salaries and other payments made for receiving and inspection of materials	1,10,000
2	Cost of collection of materials	95,000
3	Cost on account of deterioration due to low shelf items	50,000
4	Cost of advertisement and tender documents for vendor development	75,000
5	Stationery, typing expenses incurred for procurement	1,25,000
6	Losses on account of evaporation and breakages	25,000
7	Cost of electronic data processing relevant to procurement	75,000
8	Follow up cost on account of expediting supplies including travel cost	1,60,000
9	Salaries and other statutory payments like PF, bonus, gratuity incurred on stores personnel	7,50,000
10	Cost moving items from point of storage or usage	1,05,000
11	Cost of matching the invoice to receiving document	55,000
12	Rentals or opportunity costs incurred on the area used for purchasing activity	50,000
13	Loss due to wastage, breakages, spoilage and, pilferage	1,30,000
14	Insurance cost towards fire, theft, and burglary on the value of average inventory	2 percent
15	Salaries and wages and other payments made to purchasing personnel	9,00,000
16	Electronic data processing for maintaining inventory records	1,25,000
17	Proportionate salaries paid for guarding store and stores audit staff	1,50,000
18	Advertisement costs for imports in newspapers and trade journals	75,000
19	Rentals/opportunity costs on store space	2,25,000
20	Proportionate salaries and wages incurred on tender committee for processing orders	90,000
21	Communication costs for procurement follow up viz. post, telephone telex, telegrams fax, satellite communication and VHF costs	1,20,000
22	Cost of different documents such as GRN, KRDEX etc.	1,95,000
23	Expenses incurred on purchase tenders opening formalities	65,000
24	Depreciation on office furniture and other equipment used for purchase activity	1,25,000
25	Opportunity cost on investment on inventories	20 percent
26	Depreciation on material handling equipment	50,000
27	Cost of security services for guarding inventories	1,15,000

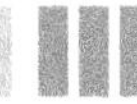

28 Depreciation charges on bins, racks, furniture and office equipment and other devices 2,50,000

29 Cost of completing a requisitions and reviewing then 75,000

The hospital on an average maintains inventory to a tune of Rs. 200 lakhs and issues 2,000 orders in a year. Find out for Snigdha Super-specialities Hospital

Cost per order and inventory carrying cost as percentage on average inventory held by the hospital

SOLUTION

Step I - Calculation of Ordering Cost

		Amount in Rs.
1	Salaries and other payments made for receiving and inspection of materials	1,10,000
2	Cost of collection of materials	95,000
3	Cost of advertisement and tender documents for source development/supplies	75,000
4	Stationery and other typing expenses incurred for procurement	1,25,000
5	Cost of electronic data processing relevant to procurement	75,000
6	Follow up cost on account of expediting supplies including travel cost	1,60,000
7	Rental or opportunity costs incurred on the area utilized for purchase activity	50,000
8	Salaries, wages and other statutory payments made to purchase personnel	9,00,000
9	Advertisement costs for imports in news papers and trade journals	75,000
10	Proportionate salaries and wages incurred on tender committee inward inspection, bill passing etc.	90,000
11	Cost of matching invoice to receiving documents	55,000
12	Cost of moving items from point of storage to usage	1,05,000
13	Cost of completing requisitions and reviewing then	75,000
14	Communication costs viz. post, telephone telex, telegrams, fax, satellite communication and VHP costs for procurement and follow up	1,20,000
15	Expenses incurred on purchase tender opening formalities	65,000
16	Depreciation on office furniture, PCs and other equipment used for purchase activity	1,25,000
	Total Expenditure	23,00,000

$$\text{Cost per order} = \frac{\text{Total expenses incurred in purchase activity}}{\text{Number of orders issued during corresponding period}}$$

$$= \frac{23,00,000}{2000} = \text{Rs. } 1,150$$

Thus, cost per order is Rs. 1,150

STEP II - Calculation of Carrying Cost

		Amount in Rs.
1	Cost due to deterioration on account of low shelf life items	50,000
2	Losses on account of evaporation and leakages	25,000
3	Salaries and other statutory payments like PF, bonus, ESI incurred on stores personnel	7,50,000
4	Loss due to wastages, breakages, spoilage and pilferage	1,20,000
5	Insurance cost towards, fire, theft burglary on the value of average inventory at the rate of 2 percent on average inventory of 200 lakhs	4,00,000
6	Cost of electronic data processing for maintaining inventory records	1,25,000
7	Proportionate salaries paid for guarding store and stores audit staff	1,50,000
8	Rentals/opportunity costs on storage space	2,25,000
9	Cost different documents such as GRN, KARDEX	2,25,000
10	Opportunity cost on investment in inventories at the rate of 20 percent on the average inventory of 200 lakhs	40,00,000
11	Depreciation on materials handling equipment	50,000
12	Depreciation charges, on bins, racks, furniture and office equipment etc.	2,50,000
Thus total expenses incurred on stores activities		63,70,000

$$\text{Inventory carrying cost} = \frac{\text{Total expenses incurred on stores activity in a year}}{\text{Value of average inventory during corresponding period}} \times 100$$

$$= \frac{63{,}70{,}000}{2{,}00{,}00{,}000} \times 100 = 31.85.\ \text{Say 32 percent}$$

Inventory carrying cost is 32 percent on the average inventory value of inventory held.

SUMMARY

Analysis of inventory problems is based on a simple common-sense observation. Inventory management is associated with opposing costs. There are always costs associated with "too much "or "too little" inventory. Optimum decision depends on how often a commodity is ordered and how much quantity is ordered. The useful objective of inventory management is optimization of total costs involved and not simply minimization of one or other opposing costs. The hidden costs are not carrying inventory at all or carrying less than required, called "Under stocking cost" or "Stock out cost" and cost of carrying more than required quantities called "Over stocking costs".

Various internal and external factors influence levels of inventory. Internal conditions start from forecasting a requirement, so that required material is available only at the right time.

External conditions include supplier's lead time, environmental conditions, government rules and regulations, credit availability, market conditions etc. All these factors, which influence on the inventory, could be summed up in the following categories: Ordering cost, inventory carrying cost, over stocking cost, under stocking cost, service level, obsolescence, scrap, waste, lead time.

Ordering cost is incurred before the inventory is received. Activities, which constitute cost of ordering (Co), ordering cost or set up cost are those involved in processing an order such as handling charges, inspection and testing charges, transportation and receiving costs, postage costs and special expediting costs. Activities pertaining to procurement of materials consume executive and non executive time, stationery and communication charges, which have to be borne by the organization, thus giving, rise to the ordering cost. Salaries, wages and other statutory payments made to purchasing personnel and follow costs constitute major expense items in the purchasing activities. Total costs incurred on purchasing activities in a year divided by number of orders issued during corresponding period would give the estimate of average ordering cost per order.

When a commodity is self supplied that ordering cost will be referred to as "set up cost" (i.e., in the case of production). This takes into account, the idle cost of labour, tooling involved from one job to other. This is mainly found in jobbing type of industries and has to be taken into account for scheduling production. This is expressed as cost per set up. Inventory carrying cost or holding cost occurs after arrival of the inventory into the organization. Inventory holding costs are related to storage and handling of the goods and are calculated by first quantifying as many of the relevant costs as possible. Major element in inventory carrying cost is interest or opportunity cost on inventory. It is usually expressed as percentage of average investment in inventory.

Inventory carrying cost is usually represented as percentage on average value of inventory held and is the ratio of total expenses incurred on stores activity in a year and value of average inventories held during the corresponding period. Inventory carrying costs are calculated as percentage of average inventory carried. Adding up inventories held at the end of each of the twelve calendar months and then dividing the result by 12 gives the figure of average inventory. In some cases, stock as on 1st of April and as on 31st March of succeeding are added and divided by 2. This type of calculation is not very accurate.

Measurement of over stocking cost is comparatively simple. This cost is basically due to investment in inventory for longer periods than necessary i.e., the demand for the item has terminated or becomes excessive. This cost is called "over stocking cost". Interpretation of this cost differs in accordance with the inventory problem, whether it is static or dynamic decision has an impact on subsequent decisions and it is necessary to take some inventory decisions, essentially made only once during its usage time and are called static decisions or one shot decisions.

Any inventory decisions of similar nature, which are taken several times for sufficiently long span of time, are termed as dynamic. The two opposing costs, viz. ordering cost and carrying cost will enable the inventory controller to optimize no. of orders and quantity inventory per order to order (i.e., EOQ).

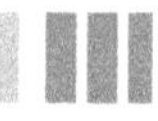

Dynamic inventory situations are of two kinds. In the first case, there is a standard demand for certain materials for certain reasons found to be procured in excess. In such a case, this item will be ultimately used provided it has enough shelf life to be used at a later date. This can be equated to "Carrying cost". In the second case, items which cannot be used after a certain period (on account of low shelf life or obsolescence), the cost will be the difference between purchase price of item + cost incurred on ordering it + cost of carrying it till it is salvaged or disposed - salvageable value.

Cost of not carrying inventory i.e., a commodity is not in stock at the time when it is required is known as out of stock or under stocking cost. Price of the commodity has no impact on the stock out cost. This is usually measured in terms of 'Opportunity cost' due to loss of production or revenue by keeping the line idle. If a stock out results in expedited orders, the extra charges incurred will be added to this cost. There are some other intangible elements also, which cannot be measured directly. Some of them are: inconvenience, lay off to labour, delay in shipment of sale orders, rift among various departments, dislocation of entire works, loss of goodwill and reduction in future revenue, loss of morale and increased laziness of workers etc. Computation of this cost is quite tricky. However, many organizations include only profit foregone due to loss of production. Over stocking and under stocking helps to determine service level that has to be maintained to minimize if not all together to eliminate these two costs.

Service level is a measure of stock control effectiveness. It is a function of demand (in terms of quantity or value) routinely met from stock.

Efficiency of inventory control is normally measured against negative scale i.e., by the number of stock outs. On the other hand, achieving zero stock outs requires very high idle investment and even then such service cannot be measured. Solution to this problem is to fix the service level as percentage depending upon criticality of items and availability of material. The two opportunity costs related to service level are over stocking cost and under stocking cost.

Service Level = Ku/(Ku + Ko)

Where Ku is cost of under stocking and Ko is cost of over stocking. The service level is generally expressed in terms of percentage.

Some tropical diseases are seasonal and availability of some products is also seasonal. The prices are usually lower at the time of harvest. Inventory manager will have to balance holding costs vs. lower prices in deciding the inventory levels for these classes of items. Apart from that, the shelf life of the item has to be taken into consideration while stocking seasonal products. In a free market under perfect conditions, price would change as dictated by the disparity between demand and supply.

Items, which are held physically intact but cannot be used due to lack of need are termed as obsolete items. Without a proper identification, causes obsolescence that cannot be controlled. A regular movement analysis FSN should give the indicator of status of inventory.

Surplus is similar to obsolete inventory. When an item in stock is more than is reasonably necessary to provide an adequate service to an operational activity. Excess over the normal is said to be surplus. This has same meaning as redundant. The term surplus material includes obsolete material that will have economic value.

Any manufacturing or operational process will generate scrap, because we do not have 100 percent efficient system which can convert all input into an output.

Scrap is usually of 3 (three) categories: ferrous, non ferrous and non metallic. All non metallic scrap is called waste such as paper, corrugated boxes, oils, bags, plastics, rubber, wood, etc. One of the most cogent arguments against rapid increase in the use of disposables is the belief that it affects ecological balance and pollutes. This is a problem for hospitals struggling with tons of waste materials daily and seeking ways to control waste and decrease pollution.

Efficient inventory control methods can reduce, but not altogether eliminate business risk. Risk in business as elsewhere is essentially a measure of uncertainty concerning the future. Inventory planning and control procedures can only help the business assess the risk and plan a strategy as far as production and purchasing plans are concerned so as to accept the risk on the most favourable terms consistent with the basic policies and objectives of business. The power of improved inventory management is limited further by the basic nature of conflict among objectives of a business i.e., better projection of occupancy rate through improved services to customers vs. lower costs through smoother operations. Lower investment needs through reduced inventories are all legitimate business aims, but they are in fundamental conflict with other objectives

Seasonality can be natural or man-made. Natural seasonality is most common in agro based industry. Man made seasonality mainly arises because of operations of an organization as reflected in books of accounts. Purchasing and sales activity will be at its peak as financial year nears its end.

Supply Seasonal: Example agricultural produce such as food grains, vegetables, cereals and pulses etc.

Demand Seasonal: Agricultural implements, fertilizers, paints construction material etc. are treated as seasonal demand and their sales are low during monsoon. Normally purchase executive is not concerned with seasonal demand and uniform supply. He is faced with a peculiar problem when supply is seasonal and demand is uniform

REVIEW QUESTIONS

1. Explain in detail the elements of inventory carrying cost and ordering cost. State how the costs are arrived at?
2. What are under stocking costs and over-stocking costs? How are they relevant to inventory control?
3. What are the elements of ordering cost and how you arrive at cost per order
4. As a materials manager, what factors you will consider to arrive at inventory carrying costs on average value of inventory held in your hospital?
5. Define term obsolescence. How obsolescence takes place in hospitals?
6. Write short notes on
   a) Dynamic inventory situations
   b) Service level
   c) Measurement of efficiency of inventory control

d) Seasonality-its impact on inventory
e) Causes for obsolescence
f) Static purchases
g) Set up cost
h) Hospital waste

7. Calculate ordering and inventory carrying costs for a hospital whose accounts reveal the following data

Purchase department expenses	Rs. 2,00,000/-
Stores personnel expenses	Rs. 2,00,000/-
Obsolescence	Rs. 60,000/-
Rental charges of warehouse	Rs. 1,40,000/-
Collection cost	Rs. 40,000/-
Receiving cost	Rs. 35,000/-
Inspection cost	Rs. 50,000/-
Stores material handling costs	Rs. 1,50,000/-
Bill payment expenses	Rs. 75,000/-
Interest charges	14.5 percent
Insurance charges	2.0 percent
Number of orders placed	5000
Average total inventory	Rs. 100 lakhs

Check your answer

Ordering cost = Rs. 80 per order

Inventory carrying cost = 22 percent on the average inventory held

8. The books of accounts of a nursing home revealed the following information on costs associated with inventories

Staff salaries of purchase department	Rs. 2,50,000/-
Expenses incurred in warehouse personnel salaries	Rs. 2,75,000/-
Cost of security for warehouse	Rs. 80,000/-
Travelling and purchase follow up expenses	Rs. 80,000/-
Taxes and insurance	1.0 % p.a.
Interest rate on inventory value	20% p.a.
Cost of bills payment	Rs. 30,000/-
Cost of materials handling in store	Rs. 1,50,000/-
Obsolescence and pilferage	Rs. 20,000/-
Cost of in-wards inspection	Rs. 48,000/-

The nursing home on an average maintains inventory of Rs. 60 lakh and placed 3400 orders in the year of review. Based on the above data, calculate cost per order and inventory carrying cost as a percentage on average on inventories held.

Check your answer:

Ordering cost = Rs. 120 per order

Inventory carrying cost = 29.75 percent on the average inventories held

PART - III

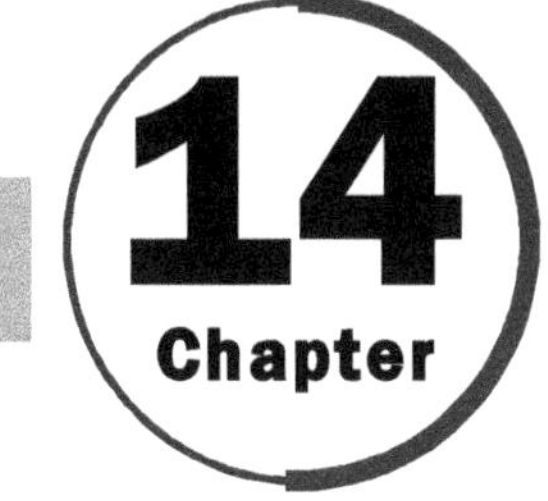

Economic Order Quantity

Contents

CHAPTER - 14

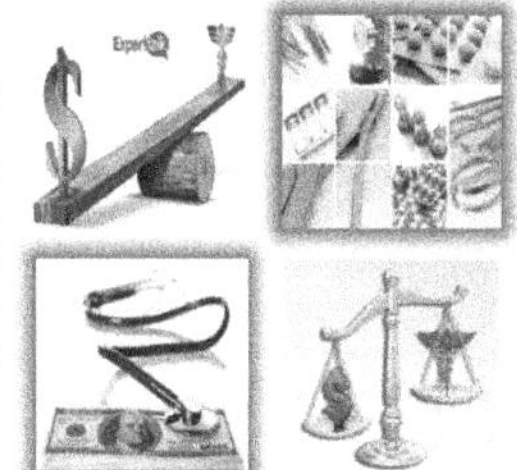

Economic Order Quantity

INTRODUCTION

Solution to any inventory problem is to find appropriate levels of holding inventories and ordering sequence and the quantities so that total cost incurred is minimized. In every inventory problem, there are three important issues that have to be tackled viz.,

1. How much inventory should be stocked?
2. When a fresh order is to be released?
3. How much quantity to be purchased at a time?

In this chapter, we are going to discuss how much quantity to be purchased at a time. We are aware, the bigger the order quantity, the bigger the average inventories investment. The policy of buying in large quantities also has its virtues, as unit prices usually are lower. In addition, the larger the unit quantity, fewer the number of orders that must be processed and fewer the shipments that need to be handled, this reduces costs. Consequently, the materials manager is torn between desires to keep inventories low by ordering in small quantities and availing quantity discounts by ordering large quantities. **EOQ helps to balance the cost of carrying inventories i.e., "Cost of possession" and cost of purchasing and processing order (also called as "Cost of acquisition or Cost of ordering").** One of the most important goals in Materials Management is to strike most economic balance between cost of possession and cost of acquisition in determining order quantity. This balancing function will answer the question: How much quantity is to be purchased at a time?

SUPPLY AND DEMAND

Supply and demand conditions impose certain limitations within which relevant costs are to be optimized, so that sum of ordering cost and inventory carrying cost is minimum. Inventories are built to act as a cushion between supply and demand. Supply can be either static or dynamic.

Inventory decisions, which are made only once during usage time of an item, are called static or one shot decisions. For example, a decision concerning oxygen plant capacity in a hospital must be made when the plant is first installed. Subsequently plant expansions may be taken up. However, the time lag is usually long enough to categorize it as an independent decision. In one shot decisions, it is not necessary to consider effect of one decision on subsequent decisions. Alternatively, supply situation can be continually variable in nature or dynamic. When repeat orders for procurement of same commodity are placed on a continuing basis, it is a case of dynamic supply conditions. Any inventory decision, which is one of a series of similar decisions spread over a sufficiently long time span, is termed as dynamic. In the continuing process, outcome of one decision has an effect on subsequent decisions and it is necessary to take this into account in the analysis.

Demand on its part can be known, partly known over a range of probable values or be totally unknown. When demand is known, the level of knowledge available to decision maker is complete. When it is partly known, the level of knowledge can be expressed in terms of probability of distribution. When demand is unknown, the level of information is least and it is difficult to express in terms of probabilities. In such cases of unknown demand, the subjective probabilities decided by decision makers could be used as starting point.

Combining the two possible supply conditions and three possible demand scenarios, following six inventory models can be perceived:

Table 14.1 Possible Supply and Demand Conditions

S.No	Supply	Demand
1	Static	Known
2	Static	Partly known
3	Static	Unknown
4	Dynamic	Known
5	Dynamic	Partly known
6	Dynamic	Unknown

Static supply demand known model is very obvious where one time supply is needed to meet a known demand allowing for the lead time, the quantity can be ordered so that it is received when needed. When supply situation is either static or dynamic but demand is unknown, stocking of those inventories can be avoided. Hence, models at 3 and 6 above are not generally put to use.

For remaining three models namely, supply static demand partly known, supply dynamic demand known and supply dynamic demand partly known, we have to take into consideration the relevant costs that affect these three models, as are shown in Table 14.2.

Table 14.2 Cost Considerations for Several Supply Demand Situations

Inventory Situation	Under-stocking cost	Over-stocking cost	Inventory carrying cost	Acquisition cost
Supply static-demand partly known	✓	✓	-	-
Supply dynamic-demand known	-	-	✓	✓
Supply dynamic – demand partly known	✓	✓	✓	✓

We shall now discuss the cost considerations for several supply demand situations.

STATIC SUPPLY SITUATIONS

A) Demand Known

In a static supply situation, when the demand is precisely known, we have 95 percent to 100 percent accurate information on quantity, description and time schedule of the materials requirement. In such conditions, buyer has to place the order for entire quantity taking into account the lead time. This will enable the supplies to reach in time, when requirements are needed.

For example purchase of magnetic resonance imaging (MRI) equipment. This is one time job and the requirements are fully known, specified before procurement. This falls under the above mentioned static certain where demand is fully known category.

B) Demand Partly Known

In this situation, the level of knowledge about demand pattern as available to decision maker is partial or incomplete and this level of knowledge can be expressed in terms of probability of distribution. Examples in this category are:

1. Service contracts for maintenance of equipment and machinery.
2. Buying of capital and insurance spare parts, which are normally purchased along with original equipment.
3. Manufacturing artificial limbs for patients in an orthopaedic hospital.

Depending upon the past behaviour of demand for such items, we can approximate a set of probabilities for different demand figures.

C) Demand Unknown

In situations like supply static and demand unknown, the level of information is so scanty, that it cannot even be expressed in terms of probabilities. In such cases, the subjective probabilities

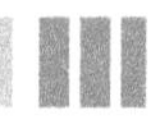

given by decision maker could be used as a starting point. Under static uncertain conditions, Purchasing decision may have to be taken but the information of various strategies to be adopted are neither logically available nor it is possible to estimate probability of occurrence of each of those strategies. In such situations executive should not be confused with total ignorance. He will certainly have some knowledge of the strategies, though his knowledge may not sufficient to obtain explicit data on which calculation of probabilities of different strategies could be based.

In such situations, a regret matrix is mainly useful to an executive who is likely to vacillate in his choice of strategies. In this matrix, we compute the regret i.e., sum of pay offs, expenses or losses for each strategy under different environmental conditions of demand. The decision rule is to select the strategy for which the aggregate regret is minimum.

DYNAMIC SUPPLY SITUATIONS

A) Demand Known

Dynamic supply conditions enable us to place as many orders as we need. Consequently, the total ordering cost incurred will be direct function of number of orders placed. The demand from consuming centres is fairly well established. We can meet this demand either by having a few orders and large inventory or holding low inventories, and correspondingly increasing the number of orders. Example: procurement of medical stores inventories

B) Demand Known Either Partially or Fully

Dynamic inventory problems are characterized by two features: There is a possibility of number of orders and there is also known probability distribution of demand. This is most often inventory problem that occurs which the materials managers are required to handle. In this type of inventory problem, all major kinds of costs are involved in decision making. They are:

1. Ordering cost is involved since alternative frequencies of ordering are possible.
2. Opposite of this possibility of varying order frequency, we have the carrying cost.
3. Since there is possibility of distribution of demand, there is possibility of not having sufficient stocks; in such a case, the materials manager has to take note of under stocking cost.
4. The other situation that items of highly seasonal demand, there may be possibility of excess stock with corresponding over stocking cost.

C) Demand Unknown

It should be noted that unknown demand conditions tend to repeat themselves, the knowledge about them increases over a period of time and they tend to become partly known and then fully known. In such cases, EOQ is applicable.

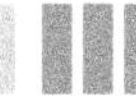

RELATIONSHIP BETWEEN NUMBER OF ORDERS AND INVENTORY HELD

When there are many supplies, we have more number of orders resulting in increase in the ordering cost. Alternatively we can have very few supplies and carry inventory, incurring inventory carrying costs. The relationship is as shown below:

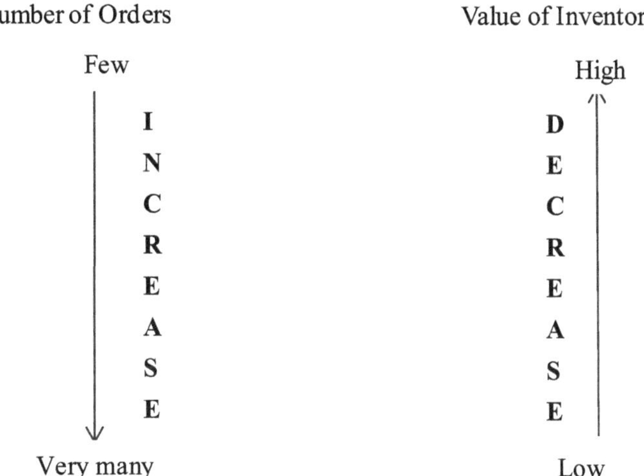

Figure 14.1 Relationship between Number of Orders and Inventory Held

Or in other words, when cost of ordering increases, cost of carrying decreases and vice versa is also true.

Relationship between cost of getting and carrying charges may be likened to an **Apothecary's scale** as shown in Figure 14.2.

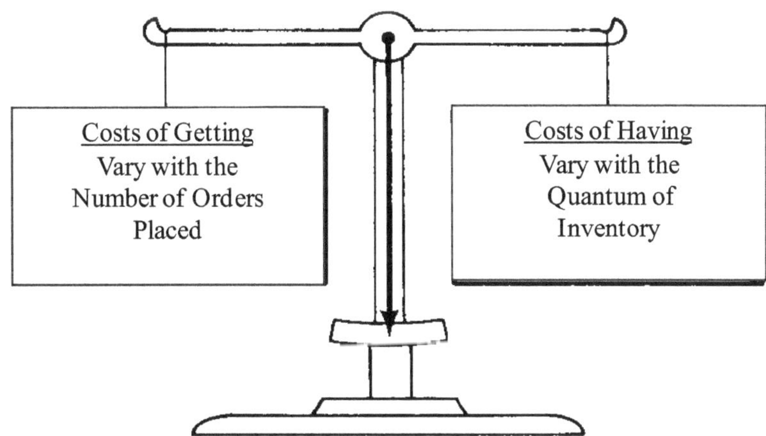

Figure 14.2 Weighing the Cost of having Inventory against the Cost of Getting

We can neither afford to have high ordering cost or high inventory carrying cost. Therefore, we have to strike a balance between the two where we have to order such a quantity so that sum of both costs is minimum i.e., the number is most advantageous.

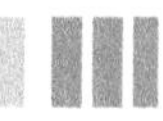

To determine best or most profitable order quantity, it is necessary to weigh cost of getting against cost of having inventory. To illustrate how these costs affect one another, consider the following example under different circumstances, an item could be ordered.

Let us consider an item with an annual consumption of 10,000 units and let price per unit be rupee one; inventory carrying cost 30 percent per annum on the average inventory and ordering cost as Rs. 60 per order.

We shall now determine optimal costs by "Trial and Error". Let us compare these various order quantities. For instance, if we order 10,000 units, then only one order will be placed in a year resulting in Rs. 60 as ordering cost since average inventory will be 5,000 units; carrying charges will be Rs. 1,500. The total costs would be Rs. 1560.

These results are tabulated below

Table 14.3 Relationship between Ordering Cost and Carrying Cost

Sl. No	Quantity Per Order	No of Orders	Ordering cost in Rs.	Average Inventory in Nos.	Inventory Carrying Cost in Rs.	Total Cost in Rs.
1	10,000	1	1 x 60 = 60	5,000	$\frac{5000 \times 30}{100 \times 1} = 1500$	1560
2	5,000	2	2 x 60 =120	2,500	$\frac{2500 \times 30}{100 \times 1} = 750$	870
3	4,000	2.5	2.5 x 60 =150	2,000	$\frac{2000 \times 30}{100 \times 1} = 600$	750
4	2,000	5	5 x 60 = 300	1,000	$\frac{1000 \times 30}{100 \times 1} = 300$	600
5	1,000	10	10 x 60 = 600	500	$\frac{500 \times 30}{100 \times 1} = 150$	750
6	500	20	20 x 60 = 1200	250	$\frac{250 \times 30}{100 \times 1} = 75$	1275

Since the objective is to minimize the inventory costs, we arrived at the optimum quantity of 2000 units per order. In this case, ordering and carrying costs are equal and total cost is optimum.

Thus, we can define ECONOMIC ORDER QUANTITY (EOQ) as that quantity, where ordering and inventory costs are equal and sum of the two is minimum (optimum).

EOQ model is however based on the assumption that consumption pattern is fully known and supplies can be had whenever required. This is very idealistic situation.

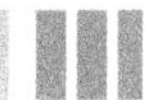

The above figures are graphically illustrated to determine optimum order quantity and shown below (Fig. 14.3).

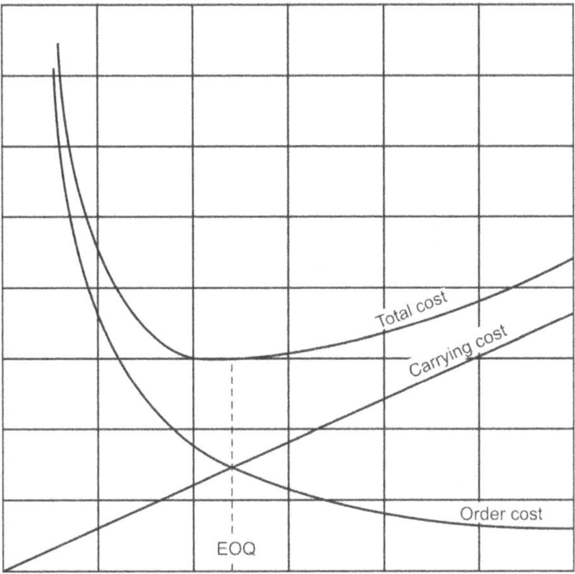

Figure 14.3 Behaviour of Ordering and Carrying Costs

DERIVATION OF ECONOMIC ORDER QUANTITY FORMULA

Step I

Calculation of Ordering Cost

As seen from the earlier Table 14.2, we observe that:

$$\text{No. of Orders} = \frac{\text{Annual Demand}}{\text{Qty. ordered per order}}$$

Total Ordering Cost = Cost per Order x No. of Orders

Step II

Calculation of Inventory Carrying Cost

Average Inventory = (Quantity per Order / 2)

Cost of Carrying Inventory = (Average Inventory × Price per Unit × Inventory Carrying Cost)

Total Cost = (Ordering Cost + Carrying Cost)

Step III

Let us now work out the Optimum Ordering Quantity:

LET

'D' Denote Annual Demand in Units

'P' Denote the Price per Unit

'Co' Denote Ordering Cost per Order

'C_C' Denote Carrying Cost in percent per annum on the average inventory

'Q' Denote Quantity to be ordered per Order

$$\text{No. of Orders} = \frac{\text{Annual Demand}}{\text{Qty. ordered per order}} = \frac{D}{Q}$$

Total Ordering Cost = Cost per Order × No. of Orders = Co × D/Q

If Q is the quantity ordered per order and is consumed uniformly till next order quantity is received, then we can consider Q/2 as average inventory held throughout the year. It may be noted that we are assuming that supplies can be had as and when we want and the consumption is uniform.

Therefore,

Carrying Cost = Average Inventory × Price per unit x Inventory Carrying Cost as percentage on average inventory

$= Q/2 \times P \times C_C$

At optimum condition, these two costs are equal.

$$C_0 \times D/Q = Q/2 \times P \times C_C$$

$$2 \times CO \times D = Q^2 \times P \times C_C$$

$$Q^2 = \frac{2D \times C_O}{P \times C_c}, \quad Q = \sqrt{\frac{2D \times C_O}{P \times C_c}}$$

Therefore,

$$EOQ = \sqrt{\frac{\text{2 Annual Demand in units X Cost per order}}{\text{Price per unit X Carrying Cost as percentage on average inventory held in a year}}}$$

DERIVATION OF EOQ FORMULA MATHEMATICALLY

Let,

'D' Denote Annual Demand

C_0 Be Cost of Ordering

C_C Be the Carrying Cost in percentage per annum

'P' Denote Price per unit

'Q' Be the Quantity per order

Total ordering cost when order placed for a quantity of Q is = $C_0 \times \dfrac{D}{Q}$

Average Inventory carried in between two supplies is Q/2

Annual Inventory cost $= Q/2 \times P \times C_C$

Total Cost $= C_0 \times D/Q + Q/2 \times P \times C_C$

In this equation, the only unknown factor is Q; hence for costs to be at minimum, we have to differentiate with respect to Q and equate it to zero to get total minimum cost.

$$[-D/Q^2] \times C_O + \tfrac{1}{2} \times P \times C_C = 0$$

$$D \times C_O = Q^2 \times P \times C_C \times \tfrac{1}{2}$$

$$2D \times C_O = Q^2 \times P \times C_C$$

$$Q^2 = \frac{2D \times C_O}{P \times C_c} \; ; \; Q = \sqrt{\frac{2D \times C_O}{P \times C_c}}$$

Substituting the figures of earlier example (Table 3.14.2), the Economic Order Quantity is

$$Q = \sqrt{\frac{2 \times 10{,}000 \times 60}{1 \times 30/100}}$$

$$= \sqrt{\frac{2 \times 10{,}000 \times 60 \times 100}{30}}$$

$$= \sqrt{2 \times 2 \times 10 \times 10 \times 100 \times 100}$$

$$= 2 \times 10 \times 100$$

$$= 2{,}000 \text{ units}$$

ASSUMPTIONS MADE IN EOQ MODEL

EOQ formula is based on certain simplifying assumptions. These may appear to limit its usefulness, particularly in the context of imports. These assumptions are as follows:

- Demand over the period (e.g., a year) is given and remains unchanged.
- Price including transport cost does not change with order size. E.g., no quantity discounts apply and remains constant throughout the year.
- Order processing costs are traceable, and remain constant.
- Lead time is zero, or accurately predictable, and does not vary (i.e., there are no delays, etc.)

LIMITATIONS OR PRACTICAL CONSIDERATIONS IN THE APPLICATION OF EOQ

1. Often inventory holding costs and ordering costs cannot be identified precisely and properly.
2. EOQ calculated often results in inconvenient number.
3. Use of EOQ usually leads to orders at random points of time resulting in suppliers receiving an irregular stream of orders.
4. EOQ applied without due regard to possibility of fall in demand can lead to a high volume of obsolete inventory.
5. EOQ may not be applicable when requirements are asymmetrical or where there is impeding price rise.
6. Available space for storage. It is often impractical to use EOQ, formula for low cost/low usage, bulk items.

This is where human judgement is an important factor. Techniques in management do not always give 100 percent results. Every decision depends upon environmental conditions i.e., those relating to technology, imports and exports, consumer tastes and myriads of other items, all of which play a vital role in taking a decision. As such, every decision is to be taken on merits of the problem, and EOQ formula should not be treated as gospel.

Since EOQ is a quantitative technique, it fixes the quantity and therefore, timing of order placement becomes variable, depending upon actual demand. Fixed order quantity of EOQ has been criticized for having two shortcomings. One is that EOQ assumes a fixed purchase price of each item and offers little consideration for quantity discounts. For this reason, total annual unit cost should be calculated using discounted prices and then compared with the standard methodology in a hospital.

The second criticism is that EOQ does not take packaging quantity into consideration. In response, the consideration of the use of common sense is offered. It is obvious that when EOQ results in an order quantity of 95 each for an item that is packed 100 per case, the EOQ has to be adjusted to meet the case quantity. For items where the calculated EOQ is significantly less than the case quantity (i.e., EOQ = 6000 units, case quantity = 10,000 units), consideration should be given to purchasing the item from another source. Similar consideration should be given to finding out if this item is really needed. Experience shows that this situation occurs primarily with low volume C items. Overall, EOQ is a sound inventory management technique that achieves the objective of inventory and buyer's lower annual cost.

REASONS FOR DEVIATING FROM EOQ TO SUIT REAL LIFE SITUATION

EOQ obtained will have to be adapted to suit to conditions of individual items:

1. Permissible upper limit of ordering quantity is bound by the shelf-life of the item and consumption rate. Example for perishables, foods and beverages.
2. Market may force us to order only in terms of packaged quantities. Here again, we have to deviate from Economic Order Quantity. Example: Say instead of ordering 900 disposable syringes, the order quantity can be for one carton containing 1000 syringes. Other examples are for items, which are known to be sporadically used in large quantities like burn care supplies and dialysis solution; in such situations EOQ should be suitably adjusted. Here, the objective of patient care must override economic factors.
3. EOQ may be deviated to suit transport requirement in order to optimize freight rates, e.g., a full wagonload or truckload. Saving in freight may compensate more than the extra inventory cost.
4. We may have to buy seasonal goods and store them in large quantities. Procurement of seasonal goods is governed by factors like, market environment, availability of transport facilities etc., and may influence purchase quantities. In such situations, appropriate weightage should be given to judgment.
5. Socio economic problems like strikes, lock outs, will force the buyer to buy extra inventory.
6. If space is limited, the buyer should not buy more quantity than can be stored in the space available. Example: refrigerated stores have limitations.
7. Convenience: Instead of ordering 14 times a year, one may order once in a month. This factor should be carefully examined to ensure that it is not to be used to cloak inertia or laziness.
8. Vendors, at times may offer substantial price discounts when bulk purchases are made or attractive freight charges may suggest larger quantities. Purchaser should carry cost benefit analysis, before decision is taken.
9. If the product is about to be discontinued and last run is made, purchase quantity is limited to actual quantity needed by manufacturing for the last run.
10. Likelihood of obsolescence, if EOQ for a specific item meets six months demand, but technology is changing quickly, it may be desirable to reduce order quantity.
11. A tight cash flow situation may make it impossible to purchase in most economical quantity. It may be necessary to reduce the size of expenditure.
12. Priority: When there is time constraint, EOQ analysis should start with A items, then B items; it may be most practical to establish a maximum re order quantity. Example: No more than 3 months supply of medical, surgical supplies will be ordered regardless of calculated EOQ.

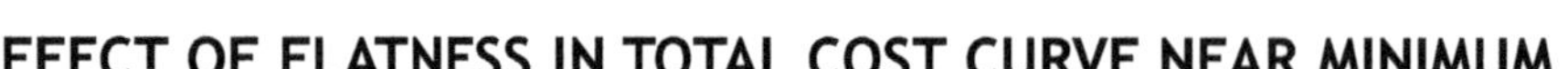

EFFECT OF FLATNESS IN TOTAL COST CURVE NEAR MINIMUM

In the graphic presentation Fig. 14.3, total cost curve is nearly flat near minimum. There would not be large variation (increase) in costs for a moderate deviation from economic order quantity. This is because the total cost depends upon square root and not directly upon cost figures. Further, it is possible to round off the ordering cost. It does not adversely affect inventory carrying cost. When order quantity deviates from EOQ, the typical values of cost increase; various values of deviation are given in the following table:

COST PENALTIES FOR DEPARTING FROM EOQ

Table 14.4 Cost Penalties for Deviating from Economic Order Quantity

Variation of Order Quantity			Typical Increase in Costs
Sl. No	**Percentage of Variation in EOQ**	**Ratio of Ordering Qty. to EOQ**	**Percentage of Addition to Minimum**
1	**2**	**3**	**4**
1	10	1.1	0.50
2	20	1.2	1.70
3	30	1.3	3.50
4	40	1.4	5.70
5	50	1.5	8.30
6	60	1.6	11.20
7	70	1.7	14.40
8	80	1.8	17.80
9	100	2.0	25.00
10	200	3.0	67.00
11	300	4.0	112.00

EXAMPLE COST PENALITIES FOR DEVIATING FROM EOQ

EOQ : 2,000 units

C_O : Rs. 60

C_C : 30 percent per annum

Effect of 10 percent increase on EOQ of 2000

$$\text{The new order quantity} = 2000 + 2000 \times \frac{10}{100} = 2000 + 200 = 2200$$

$$\text{No. of Orders} = \frac{10,000}{2,200} = 4.55$$

Ordering Cost = 60×4.55 = Rs. 273

Saving on Ordering Cost = (300 – 273) = Rs. 27

Extra Inventory Cost = = 1100

Average Inventory $= \dfrac{2200}{2} = 1100$

$= 1100 \times \dfrac{30}{100} = 330$

Total Costs = 273 + 330 = Rs. 603

Total cost if procured at EOQ i.e., 2000 units = Rs. 600

The additional cost by increasing EOQ by 10 percent = 603 – 600 = Rs. 3

Percentage of increase $= \dfrac{3}{600} \times 100 =$ 0.5 percent

It is clear that large variations in order quantity cause relatively small increase in costs. The sum of procurement costs and stock holding costs will not be as low as it could be, but it will still be only about 6 percent above the minimum, if the order quantity is about 40 percent above the optimum.

OTHER USES OF EOQ

EOQ can be adopted to calculate 'Optimal lot size', in case of scheduling the production in batch type of production. In this case, ordering cost is replaced by set up cost. Set up cost is the out of pocket cost associated with a machine set up. E.g. production of IV fluids.

Banks and financial institutions can make use of Economic Order Quantity model to calculate daily currency requirements to meet the demand. In this case, carrying cost includes interest charges and amount spent on guarding the money. Ordering cost will include amount spent on collection of money and other related expenditure.

Staggering of delivery schedules is one of the strategies adopted by inventory managers to reduce carrying costs. In this case, instead of finding EOQ, we have to calculate "Economic Receipt Quantity" (ERQ). While Cc will not change significantly, Co can be different. In case of staggering deliveries, there is one single order. Cost incurred by these activities should be divided by number of deliveries to obtain a new ordering cost. It should be noted that inspection and recurring activities may also increase and this cost will have to be taken into account.

EOQ AND QUANTITY DISCOUNTS

In EOQ formula, the sum of ordering cost and inventory carrying cost is at optimum. However in real life situation, we get discounts if we buy more quantities than EOQ. One would ask a question as to whether to go in for the discounts and buy more than EOQ or not to accept discounts.

If the optimal quantity required to be ordered (EOQ) is greater than the minimum quantity required to be ordered for availing the discount, there is no problem. However, if EOQ is lesser, there arises need to take decision to accept or reject the offer.

1. If we avail discount facility, we buy more quantity i.e., quantity per order will be more and subsequently number of orders per year will be less. If numbers of orders are less, we get saving in ordering cost and there will be reduction in total payment (i.e., because of price discount).
2. Contrary to it, when number of orders is less and quantity ordered is more, average inventory is more. Subsequently, inventory carrying cost increases. So we have the following situation before accepting or rejecting discount offer. Discount offer can be availed only if it reduces the total cost.

Total saving = Savings in Discounts + Savings in ordering cost – loss due to extra Inventory cost

DIFFICULTIES FACED BY ORGANIZATIONS IN IMPLEMENTING EOQ SYSTEM

1. EOQ formula assumes that usage of materials is both predictable and evenly distributed. If usage varies unpredictably, it becomes ineffective.
2. Faulty basic information: EOQ calculations are based on certain calculations and they are only as accurate as ordering cost or carrying cost information on which they are based. It is not easy to accurately estimate cost of acquisition and cost of possession. It is no easy job to calculate average ordering cost and in practice actual ordering cost varies from commodity to commodity.

Examples

1. An order for critical supply (those having most effect on customer service) requiring special handling would cost more than an order for an off the shelf maintenance item.
2. In case of imported items, ordering cost will always be more than locally procured items. In many cases, lack of accurate and timely data nullifies the advantages of complex systems.
3. Both carrying and ordering costs include elements of fixed and semi variable costs that should be incurred over a short term regardless of procurement action taken. E.g., salaries, wages, interest on inventory holding etc.
4. Erratic usage: In the EOQ formula, we have assumed that usage of materials is predictable and evenly distributed. When this is not the case, formula becomes useless. More complex formula can be developed for wide swings in usage, so long as these swings can be predicted. But if usage varies unpredictably, as it often happens, no formula works.
5. Price fluctuations: When price is subject to large fluctuations, watching the market and seizing opportunity at an appropriate moment can contribute to much greater cost reduction than what balancing of internal costs could yield.

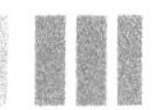

6. Where deliveries are unpredictable: When deliveries are unreliable, ensuring supplies matters more.

7. Government restrictions imposed by considerations of government EXIM policy, shipping facilities, freight charges; customs duties etc. could substantially affect order quantity.

8. Market conditions: Market conditions including economic and political factors may result in larger or smaller purchases.

These are some of the indications of practical problems, which could affect order quantities. Normally, the aim should be to order nearest quantities approximating to economic order quantity. Where large deviations are considered necessary, each case must be carefully examined to ensure that deviation is really necessary and it is more economical in the long run. However every endeavour should be made to maximize ordering according to EOQ formula. Also as soon as conditions return to normal or nearly normal, EOQ should be ordered again.

MAKING EOQ TO SUIT THE BUDGET

So far we have confined ourselves by applying the formula to individual inventory item. **Dean Ammer** had enlarged the scope of application of EOQ formula for control of overall inventories and brought out a simple solution by applying EOQ formula to control of overall inventory.

Methodology adopted by him is narrated with an illustration.

Suppose the top management takes a decision to reduce average inventories by 10 percent because of financial constraints, or due to drop in anticipated sales earnings or for increasing liquidity position without change in safety stock levels. It is cumbersome to review each and every item in stock to check whether ordering more frequently could reduce the stock. Arbitrary cuts in safety stock or order quantities are not scientific. EOQ formula permits more analytical approach.

When there is an increase in borrowing rates, inventory carrying cost in the EOQ formulae should be revised to reflect this change for use of more expensive capital.

Suppose the existing inventory is Rs. 12,00,000 including Rs. 2,00,000 safety stock and that EOQ had been computed with 16 percent carrying cost. Management wants a 10 percent (or Rs. 1,20,000) reduction in inventory investment, without any change in safety stock. This means that average inventory due to order quantity must be reduced from Rs. 10,00,000 to Rs. 8,80,000. From EOQ formulae, we know that order quantity varies inversely with square root of carrying cost (Cc). We also know that average inventory exclusive of safety stock (AI) is determined by order quantity.

Therefore,

$$\sqrt{\frac{Cc_1}{Cc_2}} = \frac{AI_2}{AI_1}$$

$$\sqrt{\frac{16}{Cc_2}} = \frac{8,80,000}{10,00,000}$$

$$\sqrt{Cc_2} \times 8,80,000 = 4 \times 10,00,000$$

$$\sqrt{Cc_2} = 4.55$$

Cc_2= 20.70 percent

The new EOQ figures can be calculated using 20.7 percent carrying cost instead of 16 percent. As the calculations above demonstrate, the EOQ for new carrying cost is 88 percent of that for the old. Hospitals that use Electronic Data Processing Systems to control inventories would simply programme in the new 20.7 percent carrying cost and the computer would automatically generate appropriate Economic Order Quantities (EOQs) for all items held in the hospital.

Worked Out Example I

Sandhya Super specialities Hospital requires an item whose annual demand (consumption) is 1, 60,000 units; price is 40 paise per unit. Ordering cost is estimated as Rs. 60 and carrying cost as 30 percent per annum on the average inventory held. Vendor offers a discount of 5 percent if 80,000 units are purchased. What should be ordering quantity? Do you accept the discount structure?

Annual Demand (D) or Annual Consumption	Rs. 1, 60,000
Cost of Ordering C_0	Rs. 60 per order
Cost of Carrying C_C	30 percent per annum
Price of the Component (P)	Re. 0.40 paise per unit

Step I

Determination of EOQ and number of orders per annum

$$EOQ = \sqrt{\frac{2DC_0}{PC_C}}$$

$$EOQ = \sqrt{\frac{2 \times \text{Annual Demand in units} \times \text{Cost per order}}{\text{Price per unit} \times \text{Carrying Cost as percentage on average inventory held in a year}}}$$

$$= \sqrt{\frac{2 \times 1,60,000 \times 60}{0.40 \times 30 / 100}}$$

$$= \sqrt{\frac{2 \times 1{,}60{,}000 \times 60 \times 100}{0.40 \times 30}}$$

Therefore, EOQ = 12649.1 units; say 12650 units

No. of orders per annum = 1, 60,000/12,650 = 12.648; say 12.65

Step II

Let us now analyze the consequence of buying 80,000 units at 5 percent discount. The situation would be as follows:

1. Number of orders is less; consequently the ordering costs are less.
2. Average inventory is more, so inventory carrying costs are more.
3. Savings on account of quantity discount offered by vendor in price.

The total saving, some amount saved form price discount plus amount saved in ordering exceeds extra cost incurred on account of carrying excess inventory than discount can be accepted.

Step III

Savings in ordering cost

$$\frac{1,60,000}{12,650} - \frac{1,60,000}{80,000} \times 60$$

$12.65 - 2 \quad = 10.65 \times 60 \quad = \quad$ Rs. 639

Step IV

Savings on account of price discount

$$1,60,000 \times 0.40 \times \frac{5}{100}$$

$1{,}600 \times 2 \;=\;$ Rs. 3200

Step V

Saving on account of ordering higher quantity than economic order quantity

$3200 \quad + \quad 639 \quad =$ Rs. 3,839

Step VI

Loss due to carrying extra inventory

$$(80{,}000 - 12{,}650) \times \tfrac{1}{2} \times 0.40 \times \frac{30}{100}$$

$$33675 \times 0.40 \times \frac{30}{100}$$

$$13470 \times 0.3 = \text{Rs. } 4041$$

Step VII

Conclusion

Since cost of holding extra inventory is higher than savings due to ordering cost and price discount. Hence reject the offer.

SHORT CUT METHOD

Under this method, the ratio of new price to old price is compared to the ratio of extra inventory over EOQ to average monthly consumption multiplied by carrying cost in percentage.

i.e., $\frac{\text{New Price}}{\text{Old price}}$ is compared to $\frac{\text{Extra inventory over EOQ}}{\text{Average monthly consumption}} \times C_C$

If the ratio of new price to old price is higher than extra inventory cost, then the discount offer can be accepted.

Step I

$$\frac{\text{New Price}}{\text{Old price}} = \frac{0.38}{0.40} = 0.95$$

Old Price 0.40

Step II

$$\text{Average monthly consumption} = \frac{1,60,000}{12} = 13333.33$$

$$\text{Extra inventory cost} = \frac{80,000 - 12,650}{13333.33} \times \frac{30}{100} = 1.515$$

Step III

Ratio of extra inventory cost is higher than price ratio. Hence reject the offer.

Worked Out Example II

Usha Maternity Hospital (UMH) purchases a disposable item at a price of Rs. 10 per item. The annual demand quantity for the item is 9000. The UMH carrying cost is 30 percent per annum and that of ordering cost is Rs. 240 per order. Find out Economic Order Quantity, and Total Costs.

The vendor offers 2 percent discount if 3,000 are purchased at a time. What is the total cost? Do you accept discount offer?

Solution

Saving on account of ordering cost and price is Rs. 2880, and extra holding cost is Rs. 2700. Hence accept the offer.

Annual demand	9,000
Cost per unit	Rs. 10
Cost of carrying	30 percent
Cost of ordering	Rs. 240 per order

$$\text{EOQ} = \sqrt{\frac{2 \times \text{Annual demand in units} \times \text{Ordering cost in Rs. per order}}{\text{Price per unit} \times \text{Cost of carrying as percentage per year}}}$$

Step I: Calculation of Economic Order Quantity

$$= \sqrt{\frac{2 \times 9000 \times 240}{10 \times 30/100}}$$

$$= \sqrt{\frac{2 \times 9000 \times 240 \times 100}{10 \times 300}}$$

$$= \sqrt{14,40,000} \quad = 1200 \text{ No.s}$$

Step II: Calculation of Total Cost

$$\text{No of orders in a year} = \frac{9000}{1200} = 7.5$$

Total ordering cost $= 7.5 \times 240 = \text{Rs. } 1800$

$$\text{Inventory cost} = 1200 \times ½ \times \frac{30}{100} \times 10$$

$$= \text{Rs. } 1800$$

Total cost $= 1800 + 1800 = \text{Rs. } 3600$

Step III: Impact of buying extra inventory to avail discount

Let us consider consequence of buying 3000 numbers at 2 percent discount. The situation would be as follows:

1. No of orders will be less and ordering costs will be less.
2. Savings in special discount i.e., in price.

Average inventory is more and inventory-carrying cost will be more. The total savings from amount saved from price discount plus amount saved in ordering exceeds extra cost incurred on account of carrying excess inventory than discount can be accepted.

Step IV: Calculation of savings on account of reduction in number orders and price discount

$$\frac{9000}{1200} - \frac{9000}{300} \times 240$$

$(7.5 - 3) \times 240 = 4.5 \times 240 = 1080$

Savings on account of price discount

$9{,}000 \times 10 \times 2/100 =$ Rs. 1,800

Total savings on account of ordering increased quantity

$=$ $1080 + 1800 =$ Rs. 2880

Step V: Calculation of extra inventory carrying cost

Loss due to extra inventory $= (3000 - 1200) \times \frac{1}{2} \times \frac{30}{100} \times 10$

$$= 1800 \times \frac{1}{2} \times 10 \times \frac{30}{100}$$

$$= 900 \times \frac{30}{100} = \text{Rs. } 2{,}700$$

Step VI: Conclusion

Since cost of carrying is less than savings on account of ordering cost and price discount. Hence accept discount.

WORKED OUT PROBLEMS

1. A large healthcare organization for its fleet of vehicles purchases spark plugs at the rate of Rs. 25 per piece. The annual consumption of spark plug is 18,000. If the ordering cost is Rs. 250 per order and carrying cost is 25 percent p.a., what would be EOQ? If the supplier of spark plugs offers a discount of 5 percent for order quantity of 3,000 per order, do you accept the discount offer?

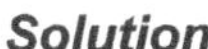

Solution

a) Calculation of EOQ

Annual demand (D) = 18,000 .

Unit price = Rs. 25

Ordering cost per order (C_O) = Rs. 250

Carrying charges (as percent) (C_C)= 25 percent

$$\text{EOQ} = \sqrt{\frac{2DC_0}{PC_c}} = \sqrt{\frac{2\times 18,000\times 250}{25\times 0.25}} = \sqrt{\frac{20\times 18,000}{0.25}}$$

$= 100 \times 12 = 1200$ units

b) Decision regarding discount offer for Q = 3000

(i) EOQ option

Total cost of materials plus Cost on materials per annum $= DP + \frac{D}{Q}C_0 + \frac{Q}{2}PC_c$

$= (18,000 \times 25) + (18,000/1200) \times 250 + (1200/2) \times 25 \times (25/100)$

$= 4,50,000 + 3750 + 3750$

Total Cost TC_{EOQ} = Rs. 4,57,500

(ii) Discount option

Discount offered for order qty. (Q_1) of 3,000 units = 5 percent on unit price New price after discount, $P_1 = 0.95 \times 25 = 23.75$

Total cost of materials plus cost on materials

$$TC_{(Discount)} = DP_1 + \frac{D}{Q_1}C_0 + \frac{Q_1}{2}P_1C_c$$

$= 18,000 \times 23.75 + (18,000/3000) \times 250 + (3000/2) \times 23.75 \times 0.25$

$= 4,27,500 + 1500 + 8906.25$

$TC_{(Discount)}$ - Rs. 4, 37,906.25

(iii) Decision rule

If $TC_{(Discount)} \leq TC_{EOQ}$ → Accept discount

If $TC_{(Discount)} \geq TC_{EOQ}$ → Reject discount offer

In this case, since $TC_{Discount}$ (i.e. Rs. 4,37,906.25) is less than TC_{EOQ} (i.e., Rs. 4,57,500), discount offer of 5 percent on unit price for ordering 3000 units per order is acceptable.

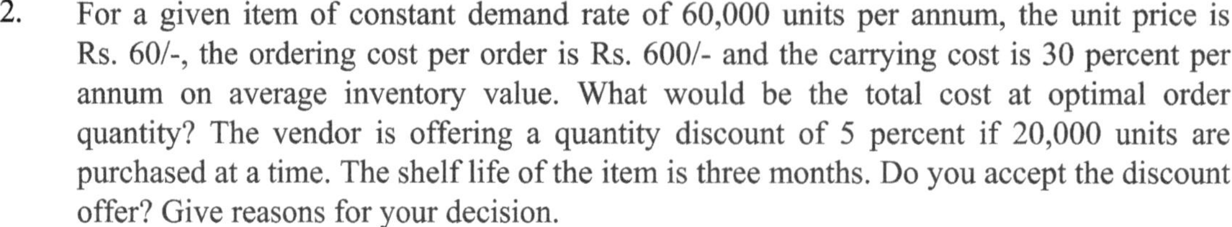

2. For a given item of constant demand rate of 60,000 units per annum, the unit price is Rs. 60/-, the ordering cost per order is Rs. 600/- and the carrying cost is 30 percent per annum on average inventory value. What would be the total cost at optimal order quantity? The vendor is offering a quantity discount of 5 percent if 20,000 units are purchased at a time. The shelf life of the item is three months. Do you accept the discount offer? Give reasons for your decision.

Solution

Annual demand	60,000 units
Cost per order	Rs. 600
Carrying cost	30 percent per annum
Price per unit	Rs. 60

Discount offered 5 percent on 20,000 units and above.

Step I

Calculation of economic order quantity (EOQ)

$$\text{EOQ} = \sqrt{\frac{2 \times \text{Annual demand (units) x Ordering cost per order}}{\text{Unit price} \times \text{Inventory carrying charges (as \%)}}} = \sqrt{\frac{2DC_0}{PC_c}}$$

$$\text{EOQ(Q)} = \sqrt{\frac{2 \times 60{,}000 \times 600}{60 \times 0.30}} = 2000 \text{ Units}$$

Step II

Total cost at optional order quantity (i.e., EOQ)

$$\text{Total cost } TC_{EOQ} = \frac{D}{Q}C_0 + \frac{Q}{2}PC_c$$

$$= \frac{60{,}000}{2000} \times 600 + \frac{2000}{2} \times 60 \times 0.30$$

$$= 18{,}000 + 18{,}000 = \text{Rs. } 36{,}000$$

Step III

Decision regarding discount offer:

Quantity to be ordered to avail discount of 5 percent on unit price $(Q_1) = 20{,}000$ units

Discount unit price $= (1 - 0.05) \times 60$

$= 0.95 \times 60 = \text{Rs. } 57$

Result of discount

i) Savings in cost of material.

ii) Savings in ordering cost per year due to reduction in number of orders per year.

iii) Loss due to increased holding cost per year, due to higher average inventory.

iv) Loss due to obsolescence if the order qty exceeds the total consumption during the shelf life of the item..

Step IV

Calculation of savings in cost of material:

Savings in cost of materials per annum $= 5/100 \times 60 \times 60{,}000$

$= \text{Rs. } 1{,}80{,}000$

Step V

$$\text{Savings on account of reduced no. of orders} = \left[\frac{60{,}000}{200} - \frac{60{,}000}{20{,}000}\right] \times 600$$

$$= (30\text{-}3) \times 600$$

$$= 27 \times 600 = \text{Rs. } 16{,}200$$

Step VI

$$\text{Loss on account of higher avg. inventory} = \frac{Q_1}{2} \text{ x } P_1C_i - \frac{Q}{2}PC_i$$

$$= \left[\frac{20{,}000 \times 57}{2} - \frac{2000 \times 60}{2}\right] \times \frac{30}{100}$$

$$= 10{,}000 \times 57 \times 0.3 - 1000 \times 60 \times 0.3$$

$$= 1{,}71{,}000 - 18{,}000 = \text{Rs. } 1{,}53{,}000$$

Step VII

Calculation of loss if ordered quantity exceeds the total consumption during shelf life:

Annual demand	=	60,000 units
Monthly demand	=	5000 units
Shelf life	=	3 months
Consumption during shelf life	=	$5000 \times 3 = 15{,}000$ units
Order quantity to avail discount	=	20,000 units
Qty that becomes obsolete	=	$20{,}000 - 15{,}000 = 5{,}000$ units
Loss due to obsolescence	=	$5000 \times$ unit price
	=	$5000 \times 57 =$ Rs. 2,85,000/-
Total savings if discount offer is accepted	=	$\begin{pmatrix}\text{savings in cost}\\ \text{of materials}\end{pmatrix} + \begin{pmatrix}\text{savings on account of}\\ \text{reduced no. of orders}\end{pmatrix}$
	=	$1{,}80{,}000 + 16{,}200$
	=	Rs. 1,96,200
Total loss if discount offer is accepted	=	$\begin{pmatrix}\text{Loss due to higher}\\ \text{average inventory}\\ \text{carrying cost}\end{pmatrix} + \begin{pmatrix}\text{loss due to}\\ \text{obsolescence}\\ \text{if any}\end{pmatrix}$
	=	$1{,}53{,}000 + 2{,}85{,}000$
	=	Rs. 4,38,000/-

Since total loss is greater than the total savings, there will be a net loss of (Rs. 4, 38,000 – 1, 96,200) i.e., Rs. 2,41,800. Hence, the discount offer is not acceptable.

SUMMARY

Causes of inventory problem is to find appropriate levels of holding inventories and ordering sequence and the quantities so that total cost incurred is minimum. In every inventory problem, there are three important issues which have to be tackled viz., how much inventory should be stocked, when a fresh order is to be released, and how much quantity to be purchased at a time? This chapter has dealt with how much quantity has to be ordered.

Demand and supply conditions impose certain limitations within which relevant costs are to be optimized i.e., to have a minimum cost so that neither ordering cost nor inventory carrying cost increases.

In the supply front, there are two possibilities, which can be termed as (a) static and (b) dynamic. Some inventory decisions essentially made only once during its usage time are calledstatic decisions or one shot decisions. From demand point they could be fully known (certain), partly known (risk) completely unknown (uncertain); similarly from supply point also it could be certain, risk and uncertain thus, one can be perceive six inventory models (2 × 3).

In static situation, the demand is certain. We have very high percentage of accurate information 95 percent to 100 percent on the quantity, description and time schedule of the materials requirement. In static certain conditions, the requirements are known full. In static risk situation, the level of

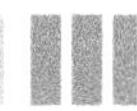

knowledge in static situation available to decision maker in risk situation is partial or incomplete and this level of knowledge can be expressed in terms of probability of distribution. In the uncertain situations, the level of information will be least and it will be difficult to express in terms of probabilities. In such uncertain cases, the subjective probabilities given by decision maker could be used a starting point.

When repeat orders are issued for procurement of same commodity on continuing basis, it is called "dynamic purchasing". In dynamic certain, we have the possibility of many supplies against certain demand. EOQ model is based on the assumption that consumption pattern is fully known and supplies can be had whenever required. This is very idealistic situation. In the "uncertain situations", the level of information will be the least. In dynamic uncertain cases, the subjective probabilities given by the decision makers could be used as starting point.

We can neither afford to have high ordering cost or high inventory carrying cost. Therefore balance has to be struck between the two where we have to order a quantity so that both the cost are optimum i.e., the quantity where total costs are minimum, which is Economic Order Quantity. Economic order quantity is given by the EOQ formula.

The EOQ obtained will have to be adopted to suit to conditions of individual items in real life situations. In the graphic representation, the total cost curve is flat near minimum. There would not be large variation (increase) in costs for a moderate deviation from economic order quantity. Even if you deviate from EOQ by 40 percent, the overall cost is increased by 5.7 percent.

Other uses of EOQ are:

EOQ can be adopted to calculate 'Optimal lot size' in case of scheduling the production in respective batch type of production. In this case, ordering cost is replaced by set up cost.

For EOQ, ordering cost and inventory carrying cost are at optimum. When we get discounts if we buy more quantities than EOQ, one would ask the question as to whether to go in for the discounts and buy more than EOQ or not to accept the discounts.

EOQ formula can be made use of as a useful tool for top management to control overall inventory levels.

REVIEW QUESTIONS

1. Supply and demand conditions impose certain limitations within which relevant costs are to be optimized. Discuss.
2. Discuss the cost considerations for several supply demand situations.
3. a. Draw a relationship between number of orders and inventory held.

   b. Derive Economic Order Quantity formula.

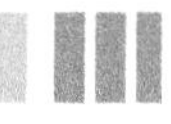

4. What are various assumptions made in EOQ model? Explain practical considerations in the application of Economic Order Quantity formula.

5. Under what circumstances you deviate from Economic Order Quantity in real life situation?

6. Discuss possible effects of low stock holding and high stock holding in a healthcare enterprise.

7. Write short notes on

   a) Other uses of EOQ

   b) Effect of flatness at the bottom of total cost curve

   c) EOQ and quantity discounts

   d) Cost penalties for deviating from Economic Order Quantity

   e) EOQ suiting the budget

   f) Assumption made in EOQ model

PROBLEMS

1. Nivya Natural product buys 80,000 shipping containers per year. Price of each container is Re. 0.40; cost of purchase is Rs. 80 per order; cost of holding one container per year = Re. 0.10; Bank rate of interest is 15 percent including a charge for taxes and insurance. Calculate

   a. Economic order quantity and time between orders based on 220 working days per year.

   b. Minimum variable cost per year.

   Check your answer

   a) EOQ = 9000 units

   b) Minimum variable cost per year = Rs. 1440/-

2. For a clinic, the annual demand for cotton rolls is 20,000 numbers. The cost of placing an order is Rs 100 and the inventory carrying cost is 20 per cent. The price per roll is Rs. 10. The supplier offers 1 per cent discount if 4,000 rolls or more are purchased and 3½ per cent discount if 10,000 rolls or more are purchased. What should be the ordering quantity and would you accept the discount?

   Check your answer

   EOQ = 1440 units

   Savings Rs. 8, 240/-

   Additional inventory costs Rs. 8560/-

   Since additional costs are greater than the savings, reject the discount offer. The order quantity should therefore be 4,000 units.

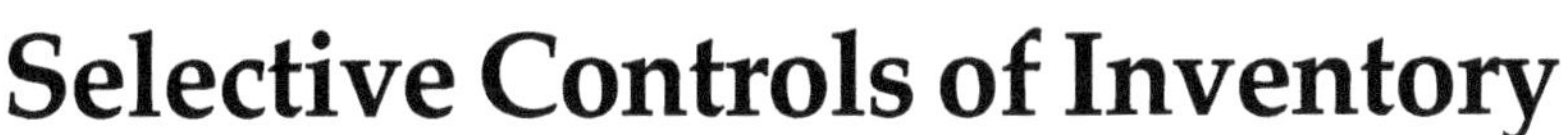

PART - III

15 Chapter

Selective Controls of Inventory

Contents

CHAPTER - 15

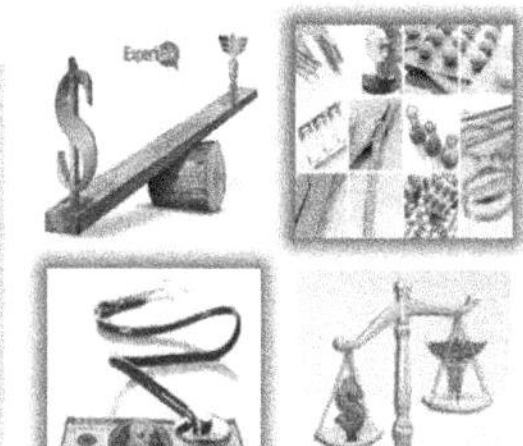

Selective Controls of Inventory

INTRODUCTION

While purchasing for an organization, material management deals with large number of items. For example, a refinery has over 50,000 items; whereas the defence services deal in millions of items. To assemble a single Boeing aircraft, it requires over 2, 35, 000 items. In a multi superspecialities hospital with bed strength of 500, number of inventory items will be somewhere around 40,000 to 50,000. Importance of each item is a major parameter while procuring it. As number of items increases, effective time spent on each item diminishes. If we add to existing manpower, too many cooks will spoil the broth. To overcome this defect, we can adopt selective control techniques to increase purchasing efficiency. Professor P Gopala Krishnan says that the motto of inventory control should be, **"Take care of pound, the penny will take care of itself."**

Common sense approach to solving any problem is to tackle important aspects more rigorously. Similarly in inventory management, classification is adopted so that a major portion of effective managerial time is spent on those materials, which are more important. Motive behind any selective control is that equally detailed analysis of all items is very expensive. Moreover such a concentration on all items will have diffused effect regardless of the priorities. Selective inventory control can indicate where a manager should concentrate his efforts. Wherever there are multiple problems clamoring for attention, there is a natural tendency to spend least time on most important problems because they are fewest in number. Management by Objectives (MBO) concentrates on identifying key result areas and performance standards and 50 percent of these are usually covered by 20 percent of his activities.

SELECTIVE INVENTORY CONTROL (SIC)

Fundamental motive behind selective control technique is to put the efforts where results are likely to be. It is well known that even though the world consists of about 7.25 (July 2015) billion people, only a handful of them determine the destiny of all the rest. Similarly, even if an organization uses millions of items, only a few items are really important. An item may be important because of its cost, criticality, availability or high consumption value. There are a number of methods available for selective control of inventory. Each method emphasizes on a particular aspect of control leading to identical conclusions i.e. Management by Objectives.

Some of them are narrated in the following paragraphs:

- **J M Juran** in November 1954, in an article titled "Universals In Management Principles and Controlling," published in American Management Review goes on to say that it is important for any control system that the **"vital few be segregated from trivial many".** This concept is applicable to inventory as in any area of management of control. ABC analysis or classification emphasizes on value of consumption. Value is defined in terms of financial worth of the quantity consumed annually and not in terms of unit price of an item. VED analysis emphasizes criticality of an item. SDE analysis is based on availability etc. In fact the very pyramidal structure of any organization is a reflection of the ABC principles.
- **P J H Baily** quotes that, **"One law for lion and the lamb is oppression."** One stock rule for Class 'A' and Class 'C' is similarly inappropriate.
- **P G Menon** suggests "Separation of significant few from comparatively unimportant many."
- **Peter Baily** is of opinion that selective control can be achieved on the principle of **"Divide and conquer".**
- **According to R L Anand,** "Traditional systems of management and control gives equal importance to all items regardless to their importance, but **if everybody is some body then nobody is anybody.**" This is a most glaring and apparent phenomenon in case of inventory.
- **C Northcote Parkinson and M K Rustomji** affirm that policing never aims at getting something done. It is meant to prevent wrong things from happening. The question that should be always asked is: How much are we likely to lose if we do not police? Is it more than the cost of policing? If the answer is yes, then do it with the least amount of effort by taking statistically valid samples rather than by checking every transaction.
- **John, H Campbell and Richard T Tersine,** say that **"Control can be a two edged sword".** Intense control is just as undesirable and costly as under control **"A Carte Blanche".** Attitude towards new sophisticated control system can be very costly. New systems that save hundreds but cost thousands of dollars are unhealthy investments.
- **Peter F Drucker** advocates that, **"One must look to the area where results are, not where work is."** A control system (systems) should be installed on the basis of its cost benefit relationship and not to achieve control as an end in itself.

BASIS AND USES OF DIFFERENT TYPES OF SELECTIVE INVENTORY CLASSIFICATIONS

Various methods are available which emphasize on particular aspect e.g., ABC classification emphasizes value of consumption; the VED classification emphasizes criticality of a material or a spare part and so on. According to nature of the inventories carried by an organization, a

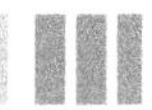

suitable method of classification should be chosen. For example, spares intensive organization like transport or mining industries would rely on the VED classification. Moreover it may be advantageous to use more than one method in conjunction. ABC and VED classifications are used for spare parts and XYZ and FSN classification for reducing obsolescence etc.

Table 15.1 lists out available classification methods, their basis and their uses.

Table 15.1 Basis and Main uses of different types of Selective Controls

S. No.	Type of Control	Basis	Main Use
1	ABC (also known as Always Better Control, Pareto's Law or Alphabetic approach)	Value of consumption of items concerned. It has nothing to do with the unit price of the item.	To control raw materials, components and work in progress in normal course of business.
2	H M L (High, Medium, Low)	Unit price of the materials (This is opposite of ABC analysis; does not take into account the consumption.)	Mainly to control purchases.
3	X Y Z	Value of items in storage.	To review the inventories, their uses etc. at scheduled intervals.
4	V E D (Vital, Essential, Desirable)	Criticality of an item.	To determine the stocking levels of spare parts, pharmacy items and critical raw materials.
5	F S N (Fast Moving, Slow Moving, Non-Moving)	Consumption pattern of items in stores.	To control obsolescence.
6	S D E (Scarce, Difficult and Easy to obtain)	Problems faced in procurement.	Lead time analysis and purchasing strategies.
7	G O L F (Government, Ordinary, Local and Foreign sources)	Source of supply of materials.	Procurement strategies.
8	S O S (Seasonal and Off-Seasonal)	Nature of supplies	To establish Procurement and holding strategies for seasonal products.
9	PQR	Shelf life of the items	To monitor the shelf life of perishable products

ABC ANALYSIS

ABC analysis is a basic analytical management tool, which enables the top management to place its effort where the results will be largest. **"It looks like cook book approach. Here is recipe**

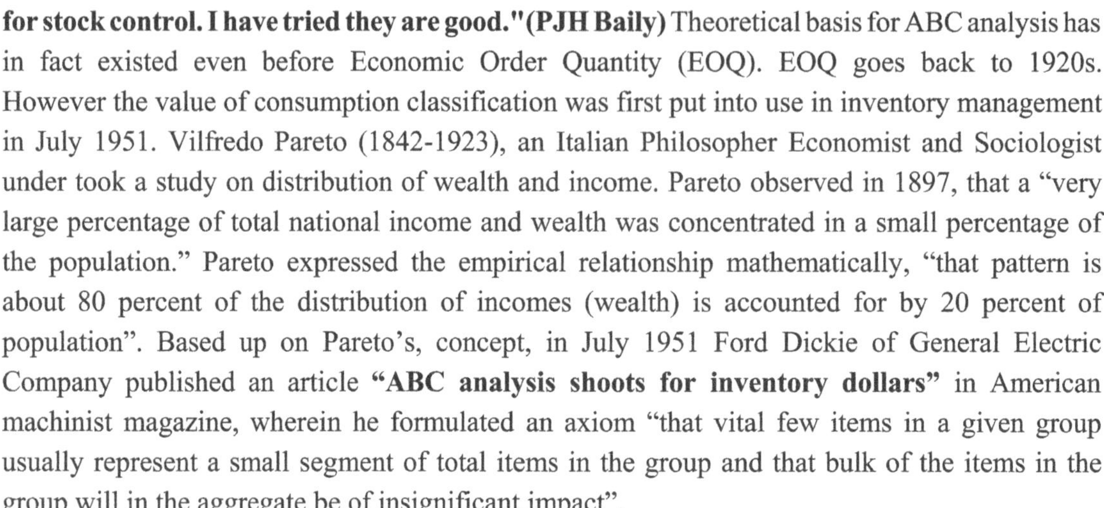

for stock control. I have tried they are good."(PJH Baily) Theoretical basis for ABC analysis has in fact existed even before Economic Order Quantity (EOQ). EOQ goes back to 1920s. However the value of consumption classification was first put into use in inventory management in July 1951. Vilfredo Pareto (1842-1923), an Italian Philosopher Economist and Sociologist under took a study on distribution of wealth and income. Pareto observed in 1897, that a "very large percentage of total national income and wealth was concentrated in a small percentage of the population." Pareto expressed the empirical relationship mathematically, "that pattern is about 80 percent of the distribution of incomes (wealth) is accounted for by 20 percent of population". Based up on Pareto's, concept, in July 1951 Ford Dickie of General Electric Company published an article **"ABC analysis shoots for inventory dollars"** in American machinist magazine, wherein he formulated an axiom "that vital few items in a given group usually represent a small segment of total items in the group and that bulk of the items in the group will in the aggregate be of insignificant impact".

ABC analysis, commonly known as **"Always Better Control" or Alphabetical approach** or Pareto's principle has universal application in many areas of human endeavour. ABC analysis as a indispensable logical tool enables top management to lay its efforts where the results will be highest. About 10 percent of the items contribute to 70 per cent of value of consumption, 20 percent of items to 20 per cent of value and the remaining 70 percent of items contribute to the remaining 10 percent value of consumption. Top 10 percent of items are called 'A' items, middle 20 percent are 'B' class items and bottom 70 percent items are called 'C' items. Obviously effective managerial time should be spent most on 'A' items since greatest monetary benefit will come by controlling 'A' items.

METHODOLOGY OF ABC CLASSIFICATION

Procedure to classify items as A, B, and C categories is as follows

- Calculate rupee value of issues. This has to be done for all items in inventory by multiplying landed cost with number of units issued in an year. Basic assumption made here is that issues and consumption are same
- Arrange all items in descending order by annual issues in rupee consumption value.
- Organize a list from these ranked items, indicating item code number, landed cost, annual issues and annual rupee value of units issued.
- Starting from top of the list, work out a successive total item by item quantity issued and the value of consumption
- Lastly work out for every item, cumulative percentages and cumulative annual issue value.

Format for ABC classification is shown in Table 15.2

Table 15.2 Format for ABC Classification

Sl. No.	Item Name or Item Code Number	Quantity Used	Unit Value	Total Value	Cumulative Value
1	2	3	4	5	6

When classifying items as A, B and C, the following issues be addressed

- In case substitute items are used or available, they should be treated as one item.
- Hospital utilises large Varity of inputs for clinical, non-clinical and housekeeping operations. While classifying inventory as A, B or C all inputs must be considered together. Separate classification such as consumables, medical stores, foods & beverages, operation theatre, materials, lab chemical and reagents etc. may not always be appropriate.
- In case of hospital inventories Period of consumption need not necessarily be one year. It can be half yearly or quarterly or even a month especially in case of drugs and pharmaceuticals.
- Traditional classification of inventory in to three groups i.e. A, B and C is not mandatory.
- Suppose a hospital is holding 20,000 items in its inventory, depending upon control practices that are in vogue, items can be re grouped into 4 or 5 groups.
- When there are large in number items in 'A' category, items can be further sub divided as A1, A2, A3 or super A and A and so on

Typical consumption patterns of most of these items conform to following pattern.

- About 10 percent of items account for about 70 percent of cumulative value of consumption are termed as 'A' items.
- Around 20 percent of items in terms of number constitute 20 percent of total consumption value. These items are known as ''B'' items.
- Residual 70 percent of items account for 10 percent of total consumption value is called as 'C' items.

ABC analysis should be periodically reviewed so that changes in product mix, prices and consumption are taken into account. The whole exercise is designed so that control exerted is proportional to consumption value of an item.

Table 15.3 gives an idea of the selective control procedure to be adopted for A B and C items.

Table 15.3 Selective Control Procedures to be Adopted for A, B and C Items

Sl.No.	Procedure	A - Items	B - Items	C - Items
1.	Type of control and authority	Very strict control. The controller should have high authority.	Moderate control; controller may be from middle management.	Low control, powers can be fully delegated to the user department to determine stock levels.
2.	Quantity of safety stock	Very low or practically nil safety stock combined with frequent ordering and/or staggered supplies.	Low safety stock; ordering can be done monthly or quarterly.	High safety stock and bulk ordering - half yearly or annual orders to take advantage of bulk discounts.
3.	Consumption control	Consumption control and flow should be regular – weekly or daily.	The period can be extended to a fortnight or a month.	The period can be extended to a quarter.
4.	Material planning & Inventory data base	Material planning should be accurate and database should be up to date.	Past consumption can be used as a basis for planning; data can be 10 to 15 days old.	Rough estimates are sufficient and data can lag behind by a month.
5.	Application of value analysis & other cost reduction techniques	A concerted attempt should be made at value analysis, waste reduction.	Moderate attempts are sufficient.	Annual review would suffice
6.	Number of sources of supply	Centralized purchase and stores and reduce lead-time.	2 or 4 reliable sources, combined purchase with moderate attempt to reduce lead-time.	1 or 2 reliable sources, annual or half yearly purchases. Decentralized and reduce clerical work.
7.	Lead time reduction	Maximum efforts should be made to reduce lead-time.	Moderate efforts	Minimum clerical efforts.
8.	Centralized or decentralized purchasing	Centralized purchasing	Combination of centralized & decentralized purchasing	Decentralized purchasing
9.	Priority	High priorities in all activities of procurement.	Normal processing. High priority only when critical.	Lowest priority.

Control policies and procedures to be such that, maximum concentration is bestowed up on A category items right from pre design stage to source development, market research purchase, value analysis, and follow up. Placing of orders for stores items should be based on the ABC principle. Generally 'A' items are ordered more frequently and in small quantities or annual orders with staggered deliveries in small quantities, while 'C' items are ordered just once or twice a year for entire year's requirement. A via media path can be adopted for 'B' items. Graphic presentation of ABC analysis with cumulative percentage of number of items on 'X' axis and cumulative percentage of consumption value on Y-axis is illustrated in Figure 15.1.

M. G. Loreng originated a graph showing cumulative percentage of income on the vertical axis (Y-axis) and cumulative percentage of population on the horizontal axis (X-axis) using ordinary graph paper not the log paper as used by **Pareto Gini.** This seems to be model for the so called Pareto curves drawn for stocks and many other things of interest to management.

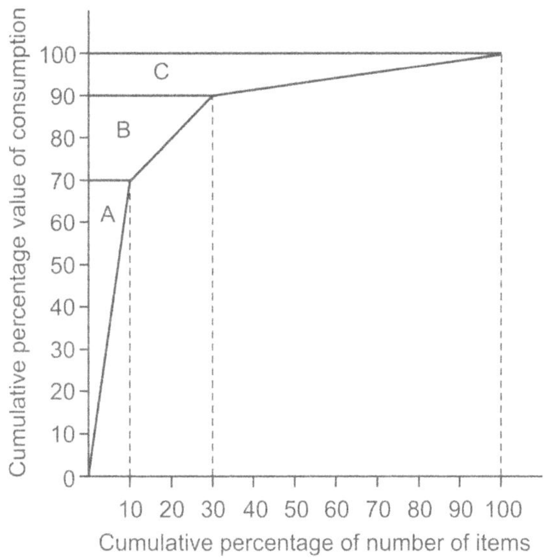

Figure 15.1 Relation between Cumulative Percentage of Items and Value of Consumption

ADVANTAGES OF ABC ANALYSIS

- When management is confronted with control of lakhs of items ABC analysis will help to focus attention merely limited number of items where results significant
- By Controlling 'A' items through, appropriate inventory analysis moribund inventories can be weeded out routinely.
- Application of ABC analysis enables the management to evolve strategies for improving inventory performance and cost reduction programmes.

- It is unfeasible to give equal attention for all A, B and C items when organization is confronted with large verities items and controls not only become very expensive but also have diffused effect on monitoring.
- Many hospitals are making use of ABC controls to reduce clerical work and resulted in efficient planning and improved inventory turnover.

For example, let us consider three items I_1, I_2, I_3 of annual consumption value of Rs. 60,000, Rs. 6,000 and Rs. 1,000 respectively, each being ordered 4 times in a year giving equal importance to all items irrespective of value of consumption.

Table 15.4 Non-rationalized Purchase Orders

Items	Annual consumption in Rs.	No. of orders	Value per order in Rs.	Average inventory in Rs.
1	2	3	4	5
I_1	60,000	4	15,000	7,500
I_2	6,000	4	1,500	750
I_3	1,000	4	250	125
TOTAL	**67,000**	**12**	---	**8,375**

By rationalizing number of purchase orders for A, B and C items, the average value of inventory can be reduced as shown in Table 15.5

Table 15.5 Rationalized Purchase Orders

Items	Annual consumption in Rs.	No. of orders	Value per order in Rs.	Average inventory in Rs.
I_1	60,000	8	7,500	3,750
I_2	6,000	3	2,000	1,000
I_3	1,000	1	1,000	500
TOTAL	**67,000**	**12**	---	**5,250**

It could be seen that total number of orders are not changed, but recognizing that 'A' items should be ordered more frequently reduces average inventory significantly.

- **Control aspect of ABC lies in separating significant few from 'trivial many'.** Concentrate on A items instead of spending time and efforts in making improvements, where benefits are marginal ('C' class items).

- Summum bonum of ABC analysis is "One must look to the area where the results are, not where work is".

LIMITATIONS OF ABC ANALYSIS

- ABC analysis will not be fully effective, in absence of standardization and codification. Same item might be held in stock with multiple names depending upon type of usage and department, which uses it.
- ABC classification ignores effectiveness or criticality aspects of an item. Importance to an item is given based on its consumption value alone and not on criticality. Hence such a classification can lead to overlooking the need for a spare part or a drug which is critically high but consumption value is low.
- Periodic review of ABC analysis is essential so that changes in prices, product mix and rate of consumption are taken into account. Periodicity depends upon fluctuations in price and consumption. Example: It is common experience that an item like diesel oil might be a class 'C' item when power supply is adequate and regular, but becomes one of the most high consumption value class "A" item during power crisis.

Short cut method to determine cut off points for ABC items

This is very quick and rough method may have to be adjusted in the light of experience or when a sample analysis or complete analysis is made later. But it would give a starting point. Calculate the average consumption value by dividing total usage value per year or month by number of items. Multiply by a factor of 2.5 to get the boundary between class A and class B. The boundary between class B and C is taken as half the average consumption value.

HML CLASSIFICATION

HML classification is akin to ABC classification. However, instead taking in to consideration "consumption value" of items, unit price forms basis for this classification. Cutoff points for H, M and L depends up on number specialities. For example, sterile cotton will be a less value item for a big hospital but a high value item for a clinic. Focus of this classification is directed to control purchase prices. Hence the procedure to be adopted is that items should be listed out in a descending order of unit value and the management may fix the cut off points. On that basis, the management may decide and delegate authority to various subordinate officers.

HML analysis helps to

- Assess storage and security requirements e.g., high price items like stents and pacemakers etc. are required to be kept under lock and key.

- Keep control over consumption at departmental head level.
- Determine frequency of stock verification as high cost and small in size are prone to pilferage.
- Evolve buying policies to control purchases.
- Delegate authority to the executives at different levels of hierarchy in the department.

XYZ CLASSIFICATION

ABC classification has value of consumption as basis, but basis for XYZ is closing value of inventory held in stores. Review of inventories, their uses etc is undertaken at pre meditated intervals. This exercise normally is done once a year at the time of annual stock taking X items are those items whose stock values are high roughly 70 percent Z items are those items whose stock values are marginal, apparently Y items fall in between. X Y Z classification helps to pin point items that are being excessively held in stock. If management is unaware, it may not be surprising that 'C' items in X category. ABC and XYZ controls in conjunction will help the managers to pin point inventory performance. Table 15.6 provides control measure that can be applied on the items according to AX, BY or CZ categories and so on.

Table 15.6 Control Matrix for ABC and XYZ Items

Class of Item	X-Items	Y-Items	Z-Items
A-Items	A critical analysis is needed for reducing the stocks.	Attempts must be made to convert these items to 'Z' category	Items are well under control.
B-Items	Consumption and stock control must be reviewed more frequently.	No further action in control may be necessary.	May be reviewed half yearly.
C-Items	Action can be initiated to dispose off excess stocks.	Controls should be tightened.	Can be reviewed annually.

XYZ analysis helps to control obsolescence. It tells how the values are distributed amongst materials in stores. Procedure to carry out XYZ classification is very simple. After annual stock taking, the closing stock values of items are arranged in descending order according to their values. Cumulative totals are entered against each item. Descending number of item is found as percentage of total value of all items in stores.

VED CLASSIFICATION

This sub topic of VED analysis is discussed here in two parts. First is it's application in spare parts management and the second its application to drugs and pharmacy inventory.

VED classification helps to identify operational/functional criticality of a spare part. This analysis is particularly essential for scientific study of spare part. If a C class item is neglected from control point of view and not available, the operations of an equipment or machine may stop if spare part is vital.

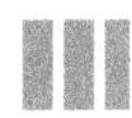

Application of VED classification was earlier limited to spare parts inventory control. Later manufacturing organization extended this classification to control critical raw materials also. VED classification approach with some modifications can also be applied to control of drugs and pharmacy inventory.

APPLICATION OF VED CLASSIFICATION TO SPARE PARTS INVENTORY

Stocking of spare parts is based on strategies different from those of regularly used material for day to day operations of hospital. Consumption of different inputs depends directly on the bed strength and occupancy rate and inpatient turnover. Demand for spare parts, on the other hand, depends upon the performance of plant and machinery. Therefore, the method of classification designed for one type of inventory will not be compatible to another type of inventory. Statistically, it has been noted that demand for spares follows Poisson distribution. Hence, VED classification is resorted to for spare parts management to overcome this shortcoming.

Acronym VED stands for **Vital, Essential and Desirable.** 'V' class spares are reasonably large quantum of stocks that might be needed to ensure smooth operations of a hospital. Absence of vital spares can cause havoc and bring the diagnosis & therapeutic equipment to a grinding halt. Some risk can be taken in case of 'E' class spares. Stocking of desirable (D) can be dispensed with, if the lead time for procurement is low. **In certain exceptional cases, criticality of a spare part changes under different circumstances.** For example, windscreen wiper in a transport organization is vital during monsoon, essential in winter and desirable in summer. It is essential that VED classification is done with the assistance of those in charge of maintenance operations.

VITAL

VITAL spares are those, which may cause stoppage of either a plant or service operations. Downtime cost or consequential losses in absence of these spares are very high. E.g. break assembly or a spark plug for an automobile.

ESSENTIAL

Essential spares are those in which stock out will result in substandard performance and cause minor disruptions for a short period. E.g., ID fans, FD fans etc. in thermal power stations or hospital laundry.

DESIRABLE

These are spares, whose non availability may not adversely affect plant performance but increases the maintenance time e.g., ED electrodes soot blower etc. in a thermal power stations cartridge for a printer or radiator for ambulance.

This classification is especially useful in capital intensive processing industries. Moreover, 'ABC' and 'VED' analysis matrix can be new to control spare parts inventories. Control plan for VED spares in combination with ABC classification can be seen from the following table.

Table 15.7 Control Plan by ABC and VED Matrix

Classes	V	E	D
A	Constant control and regular follow up	Moderate stocks	Nil stocks
B	Moderate stocks	Moderate stocks	Very low stocks
C	High stocks	Moderate stocks	Low stocks

As 'VED' classification is based on criticality of an item, combination of VED and XYZ method can give an idea of what are the items that should be disposed off to trim the inventories.

Like spare parts, plant and machinery can also be classified as Vital, Essential, Important and Normal (VEIN). Suppose a machine or equipment is at the starting point of operations, feeding at a large number of machines or service to the patient care is vital (e.g. stretcher, or cardiac monitor in cardiology department). If VED and VEIN classifications are combined, there will be 12 different classes. Vital spares for vital plant and vital spares for essential plants etc. Obviously, the criticality reduces from V to D and V to N in the classes. Hence a finer control is possible if these two classifications are applied in conjunction.

APPLICATION OF VED CONTROL MEASURES TO MEDICAL STORE INVENTORIES

ABC analysis is a concept frequently applied in inventory management. ABC analysis facilitates to identify high consumption value and highest utilization. ABC analysis pin points the items that need to focus attention so that control of these items has greater impact on inventory value and service levels as well. To administer control on drugs; it will be worthwhile to go beyond ABC concept. It would be useful to understand the objective of criticality of each product in terms of how essential it is to patient care. There are several approaches that attempt to quantify criticality of each item and include this factor in determination of stocking policies.

Criticality determination of a drug is the starting point for planning the procurement. Determination of criticality is the process where, one attempts to scientifically and systematically pinpoint and list most important steps by determining how important is their healthy functioning for well being of the whole system of patient care so that they can be given correct weightage in terms of patient care.

Following methodology can be adopted to determine the critical drug:

Criticality determination of an item is an exercise to be performed collectively through a brainstorming session by the concerned persons of i.e., both of user departments and materials management department. Team can be selected on the basis of a representative cross section of the user depending upon size and complexity of both hospital and its inventory.

Some important areas to be looked into while determining criticality are:

- Severity of utilization

- Stand by availability
- Downstream affects
- Hazards involved in the event of non availability of the drug.

Basically criticality may be gauged by posing following few simple questions:

- What would happen if a particular drug is not available?
- Whether any standby is available?
- What would be the far reaching repercussions in absence of the particular drug?
- What alternatives are available in case of emergency?
- Will it be possible to treat the patient with an alternate drug?
- What is the intensity of demand for drug?
- What is the lead time for procurement?
- Are there any difficulties faced in procurement?

If alternatives are easily available, then obviously that particular drug is not critical.

From the above factors, the drugs can be classified as Vital, Essential and Desirable.

It should be noted that criticality of the drug is not based on unit price or value of consumption.

Developing the criticality of drugs

Drugs can be classified into vital, essential and desirable by applying following criterion.

Vital-drug: There are no acceptable substitute drugs. Stock outs of such drugs are not tolerated in the patient care process. Life saving drugs falls under this category.

Essential-drug: These are essential and have readily available substitutes but not as satisfactory as original product and stock out lasting more than 48 hours could compromise patient care process.

Desirable-drug: These are desirable items, readily available substitutes as acceptable. Stock-outs lasting longer than 48 hours could compromise patient care.

The above VED classification of determination of criticality is based on ABC criticality indexing method developed by Michigan hospital, US.

After determining drug criticality, the author suggests drugs have to be regrouped by adopting following procedure

Physicians drawn from different specialities will constitute a panel. Each member of panel will furnish a list of critical drugs used in their respective specialities this data forms as basis to decide criticality for all drugs used in hospital the methodology is as follows

- Drugs, which reflect concurrently in all specialities are termed as Vital.
- Drugs, which, emerged as vital in one department and in other as essential are to be classified as vital.

- Drugs which reflect together vital and desirable should be treated as vital
- Similarly those which come out as essential and desirable are to be classified as essential drugs.
- The extent of procurement and control measures reduces from vital drugs to desirable drugs.
- Adequate stocks of vital drugs should be kept in stock to meet emergencies.
- For essential drugs some amount risk can be taken.
- Desirable drugs have alternatives and are easily available in the market at short notice.

FAST, SLOW AND NON MOVING (FSN) CLASSIFICATION

Movement of inventories forms the basis in FSN analysis. Inventories are classified as fast, slow and non moving based on their usage pattern. Starting point for this analysis is last date of receipt or the last date of issue, whichever is earlier is taken into account and period in terms of months that has elapsed since last movement is recorded. If there is rapid change in technology, the classification will have to be updated more often. FSN analysis is especially useful to prevent obsolescence, whether of spare parts or raw materials or other types of inventories. Cut off points as fast or slow or non moving, usually depend upon the type of product, the technology, process of manufacture or type of service rendered and peculiarities of the organization etc. For example if there are no issues during past two years may be positioned in non moving category; up to 10 issues in previous 2 years may be classified as slow moving and in the event the issues exceeds 10 can e placed in fast moving category.

Spare parts are normally classified as follows:

Fast moving

Items, which have moved at least once in 1-2 years, are classified as fast moving. E.g., normally boiler spares which are required for preventive maintenance fall in this category.

Slow moving

Items, which have moved at least once in a period of 2 to 4 years, are slow moving. Spares for diesel engines and generators for captive power generation normally fall in this category.

Non moving

Items, which have not moved even once in 4 to 5 years duration, are classified as non moving. XYZ and FSN analysis can be combined to control obsolete items. Disposal of obsolete items gains importance as the organization becomes older or where frequent technological changes take place. It is well known that unscrupulous traders dominate scrap market and the organizations have the choice between sunken investment in obsolete items or preventing obsolescence. **XYZ and FSN classification exercise will help in the timely prevention of obsolescence.**

The following table shows how controls are to be exercised for different classes of items:

Table 15.8 Action Plan for Control of Fast, Slow and Non-moving Items

Class of Items	F	S	N
X	Tight inventory control.	Reduce stock to low-level.	Quick disposal of items at optimum price.
Y	Normal inventory control.	Low level of stock.	Should be disposed off as early as possible.
Z	Can reduce manpower cost by maintaining higher level of stocks.	Low level of stocks.	Can afford to dispose off at lower prices.

FAST, MEDIUM AND SLOW MOVING (FMS) ANALYSIS OF DRUGS

This is very much akin to FSN analysis in narrated earlier. It is based on monthly consumption patterns of drugs. Number of units of each individual drug that had been consumed in a month is listed, and its distribution studied, in order to arrive at the cut off points, for classifying drugs as fast (F), medium (M) and slow (S) moving drugs. With rapid technological changes that are taking place in pharma industry, movement analysis assumes a greater importance to combat obsolescence and surpluses.

It is easier to increase than to decrease inventories and the tendency to do so is omnipresent. If there is a question of having a large quantity or being out of an item, a materials manager will choose the former every time since he becomes the centre of complaint when there is a shortage, but is never admonished when supplies are overstocked.

STEPS TO BE TAKEN BEFORE DISPOSAL OF NON MOVING STORES

Art of disposing scrap, surplus and other obsolete materials aims at getting the **best out of bad bargain, "waste not, want not"** is an old adage which in present business environment has to be modified as **"waste less, want less".** Since wastes are inevitable, evil.

Before an organization embarks upon disposal programme, the following points have to borne in mind:

1. Possibility of use of surplus with in the organization should be explored with or without modifications.
2. In order to get maximum price, the material should be segregated as surplus, obsolete, scrap as mix up will fetch low value.
3. As surpluses are source of revenue, proper account should be maintained.
4. Surpluses can be disposed by various methods. returns will vary depending upon the agency used.

 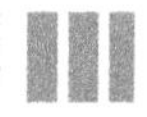

There are number of specific techniques are available for reducing excess inventories. Some of them are

1. **Use within the organization**

   Reuse of materials is in one of the methods of reclamation. A hospital can derive considerable value. Worn out linen can be cut and used as napkins. Such savings are generally substantial although some incidental extra costs may be involved. In case of surplus material which cannot be reclaimed, explore possibilities whether material can be modified for some purpose other than intended.

2. **Return to suppliers**

   Sometimes surplus materials can be sent back to original suppliers. To return excess and/or non moving materials to vendors for refund, credit, or exchange for items, which are used routinely. It is possible to use leverage with vendors to convince them to take back these items. A vendor who is anxious to increase his turnover of business is generally willing to make concessions of exchange or credit for excess inventories in conjunction with a greater commitment of sales from the hospital. Caution should however be exercised to ensure that such an arrangement is mutually advantageous (as opposed to a one sided agreement which essentially amounts to a "blackmail").

3. **Consume excess materials before reordering further quantities.**

   Revise the reorder point and enforce for future orders. It is preferable to use the excess materials if the vendor is unwilling to take back or wants to pay a very low price for the same.

4. **As is where is sales to other users.**

   As is transactions are those in which selling firms makes no express or implied warranty as to fitness of product.

   It is quite possible that another hospital may be using those items, which are in excess. In such a case, most probably these items can be sold or traded for items that are used regularly. Such sales often bring relatively high prices.

5. **Sale to scrap dealers.**

   Sell excess and/or non moving materials to a salvage dealer. This generally results in a loss. However, if the items are in significant excess and are also not likely to be used again, it is probably better to bear the loss and get rid of them.

Control Matrix General Guideline

Combination of various selective controls can be used in different matrices to achieve results. More controls are required to be exercised in the top most left corner of the matrix and being diluted as one moves away from top most left to bottom most right as seen from Figure 15.2.

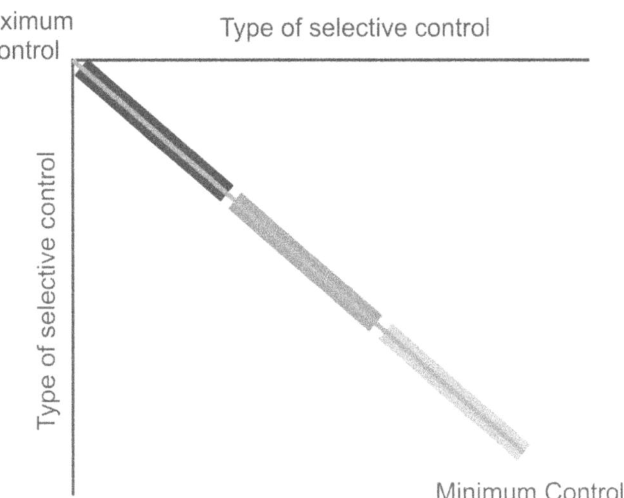

Figure 15.2 Matrix for Controls

The methods of selective controls classifications discussed earlier were based on value of consumption unit price value of inventory in storage criticality and their consumption pattern. In addition there are other methods which are directed towards controlling purchases, lead time, shelf life of items and supply management. One cannot disregard the inventory levels that depend upon source of supply, availability, seasonality etc.

S.D.E CLASSIFICATION

Scarce, difficult, and easy (SDE) classification is based on the difficulty of procurement. So far, we dealt only with classification methods based on values or criticality of items or their consumption pattern. There are other methods, which are primarily directed towards controlling purchase, lead time and related supply source problems. However, it should not be overlooked that inventory levels are also dependent upon source of supply. A scarce item with long lead time must surely have a higher safety stock than a locally available item for a given consumption level.

SDE analysis is based on problems of procurement namely:

- Non availability
- Scarcity
- Longer lead time
- Geographical location of suppliers
- Reliability of suppliers etc.

SDE classification is one such system of classification, in which materials are classified as scarce to obtain, difficult to obtain and easy to obtain.

Scarce Items are those which are

- Not freely available in the marketplace and forces need for source development
- Complicated to manufacture

- Single source supplies or very limited number of manufacturers who require supply orders to be placed several months in advance

For a scarce, 'A' category item, stocking has to follow a different pattern. It is absurd to procure it repeatedly, considering the time, effort and the expenditure involved. It would be best to obtain it once in 3, 6 or 12 months.

Purchase department employs SDE analysis for following purposes

- To decide method of buying e.g., forward buying may be followed for some items in scarce group.
- To fix responsibilities of buyers e.g., senior buyer may be given responsibility of 'S' and 'D' group items. Junior buyers may handle E category items.

G.O.L.F. CLASSIFICATION

Government, Ordinary, Local, Foreign (GOLF) classification is based on general type of suppliers. Nature of suppliers determines the quality, quantity and continuity of supply, lead time, payment terms and clerical work involved.

Government agencies as suppliers (G)

Government agencies as suppliers include government departments, canalizing agencies like S.T.C or M.M.T.C, or institute preventive medicine and public sector undertaking (PSUs). Transactions with this category of suppliers involve more clerical work and long lead time, credit facilities usually will not be allowed and payment has to be made in advance.

Ordinary suppliers (O)

'O' category of items, forms bulk of suppliers. Quality and continuity of supply from these suppliers will be good especially if sources have good standing in the market. Credit availability from these sources cannot be generalized. Usually 30 days credit may be available.

Local suppliers (L)

Cash purchases are generally made from 'L' category suppliers in commercial areas of cities.

Foreign suppliers (F)

Dealing with foreign sources involves lot of documentation. Initially government clearance, such as import licence must be obtained before foreign source of supply is tapped. After orders have been placed, a letter of credit must be established, shipping must be followed up and port clearance work to be done. Therefore the coordination involved is much more than in other cases. Imported items are accorded a special treatment as they belong to a unique category of items i.e., totally different from indigenous items.

SEASONAL, OFF SEASONAL (S.O.S) CLASSIFICATION

Nature of supplies is basis for SOS analysis. Seasonal items fall under two categories viz. seasonal and available for a limited period only. In other case, the products consumption is seasonal but it's availability is throughout the year. However the consumption is for limited period only.

Availability of agricultural products is bound by seasonality, cropping pattern and monsoons and necessitates special procurement and storing strategies. Prices of agro products will be lower at the time of harvest and gradually increases till the arrival of next crop. Thus inventory controller has to strike a balance between inventory carrying cost vis-a-vis with lower prices at time of its' availability. Application of EOQ formula may be inappropriate in dealing with seasonally items.

PQR CLASSIFICATION

This PQR classification is applied to classify items based on shelf life of the items. Shelf life is defined as the length of a material that may be stored without affecting its ability or saleability of the items. Items which have low shelf life and require perpetual attention are classified as "P" items. Items having very high shelf life and require least attention are classified as "R" items. Justifiably the items that do not fall in P and R category are called Q items. Time period in which to define P, Q & R varies from item to item. It is very much useful in healthcare institutions in patient care.

It could seen from above discussions that different methods of categorization of inventory, facilitate the manager to selectively manage methods, efficiently apply his energies to the crisis areas, thus ensuing in best possible use of efforts perceptibly. Executive has to make optimum use of all the methods and should not be guided by a **"tunnel vision"** using only one method **(Gopala Krishnan).**

WORKED OUT PROBLEMS

1. From the following data, draw an ABC analysis graph after classifying the items as A, B & C class (GDMM Exam-Dec 98).

Item	Unit Price Rs.	Annual Consumption (Units)
1.	200.00	3,000
2.	2.00	60,000
3.	500.00	20
4.	12.50	200
5.	9.00	350
6.	25.00	6,000
7.	1000.00	40
8.	70.00	300

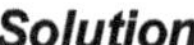

Solution

Step I:

Item	Annual consumption (units) × Unit price (Rs.)	Annual consumption value (Rs.) (ACV)
1.	3000 × 200	6, 00,000
2.	60,000 × 2	1, 20,000
3.	20 × 5000	1, 00,000
4.	12.5 × 200	2,500
5.	9 × 350	3,150
6.	25 × 6000	1, 50,000
7.	1000 × 40	40,000
8.	70 × 300	21,000

Step II: Rearrange the items in descending order of annual consumption value and calculate ACV.

Item	Annual consumption value (ACV) in descending order	Cumulative ACV
1.	6, 00,000	6, 00,000
6.	1, 50,000	7, 50,000
2.	1, 20,000	8, 70,000
3.	1, 00,000	9, 70,000
7.	40,000	10, 10,000
8.	21,000	10, 31,000
5.	3150	10, 34,150
4	2500	10, 36,650
	Total 10, 36,650	

Step III: **Since cut off points for ABC classification is not given in the problem, assume following cut off points as for the ABC analysis.**

Category	Percentage of total ACV
A	70
B	20
C	10

70 percentage of total ACV = 0.70 × 10,36,650 = Rs. 7,25,655

Since this value is near to cumulative ACV of Rs. 7,50,000, categorize items 1 and 6 under 'A' category.

A and B above together account for 90 percent of ACV

90 percentage ACV = 0.9 × 10, 36,650 = Rs. 9,32,985

Since this value is nearer to cumulative ACV of Rs. 9,70,000, categorize items 2 and 3 under 'B' category. The remaining items, 7, 8, 5 and 4 are categorized under 'C' category.

Step IV: Construction of ABC analysis graph

Exact percentage of ACV of A' category items $\frac{7,50,000}{10,36,650} \times 100 = 72.35$ percentage

Exact percentage of (A + B) items = $\frac{9,70,000}{10,36,650} \times 100 = 93.57$ percentage

Percentage of ACV of 'B item = 93.57 – 72.34 = 21.23 percentage

Percentage of ACV of 'C item = 100 - 93.57= 6.43 percentage

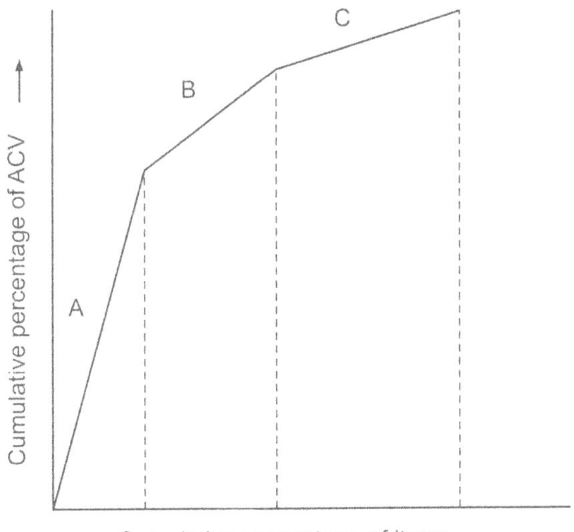

2. Find out from the following data A, B, C items when

Group	No. of items per group	Monthly consumption (units)	Unit price (Rs.)
I	40	3000	90
II	20	270	100
III	100	1700	5
IV	200	1500	4
V	60	340	50
VI	300	2500	1
VII	250	2000	2
VIII	30	170	500

- 'A' item accounts for 85 percent of consumption value
- 'B' item accounts for 10 percent of consumption value
- 'C' item accounts for 5 percent of consumption value

Solution:

Step I: Calculation of monthly consumption value (MOV)

Group	No. of items per group	Monthly consumption (units)	Unit price (Rs.)	Monthly consumption value (MCV) (Rs.)
I	40	3000	90	10,80,000
II	20	270	100	5,40,000
III	100	1700	5	8,50,000
IV	200	1500	4	12,00,000
V	60	340	50	10,20,000
VI	300	2500	1	7,50,000
VII	250	2000	2	10,00,000
VIII	30	170	500	25,50,000
			Total `	89,90,000

Step II:

Rearrange the groups in the decreasing order of MCV and calculate cumulative MCV for each group.

Group	MCV in descending order(RS.)	Cumulative MCV(Rs.)
VIII	25,50,000	25,50,000
IV	12,00,000	37,50,000
I	10,80,000	49,30,000
V	10,20,000	58,50,000
VII	10,00,000	68,50,000
III	8,50,000	77,00,000
VI	7,50,000	84,50,000
II	5,40,000	89,90,000

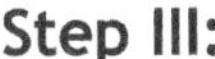

Step III:

Classifying the group as A, B & C based on MCV

85 percent of total MCV = 0.85 × 89, 90, 000 = Rs. 76,41,500

Since this value is nearer to cumulative MCV of Rs. 77,00,000, the groups VIII, IV, I, V VIII and III are categorized under group 'A'.

(A + B) comprise 95 percent of MCV

95 percent of MCV = 0.95 × 89,90,000 = Rs. 85,40,500/-

Since this value is nearer to Rs. 84, 50, 000, group VI is under category 'B' and group II is under category 'C'.

SUMMARY

Selective inventory control facilitates where the manager should concentrate his efforts. The fundamental idea behind selective control techniques is to put the efforts where results are and not where work is. All selective controls are based on the principle of management by objectives. In fact, the very pyramidal structure of any organization is a reflection of the principle of selective control.

There are 9 types of selective controls, namely ABC (Always Better Control, HML (High, Medium, Low), XYZ, VED (Vital, Essential, Desirable), FSN (Fast moving, Slow moving, Nonmoving), SDE (Scarce, Difficult and Easy to obtain), GOLF (Government, Ordinary, Local and Foreign sources) and SOS (Seasonal and Off seasonal) and PQR control based on shelf life of the materials helps to monitor on the shelf items.

Theoretical basis for ABC analysis has in fact existed even before Economic Order Quantity (EOQ). EOQ goes back to 1920's. ABC analysis is a basic analytical tool, which enables top management to place its efforts where the results will be greatest. ABC analysis should be periodically reviewed so that changes in product mix prices and rate of consumption are taken into account. Control measures to be formulated in such a way that, maximum concentration is bestowed up on 'A' items are ordered more frequently and in small quantities or annual orders with staggered deliveries in small quantities while 'C' items are ordered just once or twice a year for entire year's requirement. 'B' category items follow a middle path.

HML classification is similar to ABC classification. But in this case, instead of "consumption value" of items, unit price is the criterion. While ABC classification has value of consumption as the basis, XYZ has the value of inventory store as basis on a particular date. XYZ analysis helps to control obsolescence. It also tells how the values are distributed amongst materials in stores. VED classification is applicable to a large extent in spare parts management. This criticality aspect can also be applied to drugs in pharmacy. These items are classified as vital, essential and desirable. As 'VED' classification is based on the criticality of the item at times, it can also be used in the case of some special raw materials, which are difficult to obtain. A combination of VED and XYZ methods can give an idea of what are the items that should be disposed off so as to trim the inventories. Like VED analysis for spare parts, plant and machinery can also be classified as vital, essential, important and normal (VEIN). If VED and VEIN classifications are combined, there will be 12 different classes.

Movement analysis forms the basis for FSN classification. Items are classified as fast moving, slow moving and Non moving based on their consumption pattern. A slightly modified version, FMS analysis is applied to drugs. If there is rapid change in technology, the classification will have to be updated more often. XYZ and FSN analysis can be combined to control obsolete items. Disposal of obsolete items gains importance as the organization becomes older.

In SDE classification, the purchased items are classified as Scarce to obtain, Difficult to obtain and Easy to obtain. SDE analysis is employed by purchase department to decide the method of buying, fix responsibilities of buyers. GOLF is another system where materials are classified according to nature of suppliers as Government, Ordinary, Local and Foreign.

Raw materials can also be classified as seasonal or off seasonal items SOS systems. Agricultural products have seasonal availability pattern depending upon the monsoons and time of harvesting. Prices will be lower at the time of harvest and hence the inventory system will have to balance between holding cost and lower prices at which it will be available in dealing with the levels of these classes of items. One cannot apply EOQ here.

Natural resources that the world is left with should carefully be exploited and preserved as long as possible by resorting to recycling the waste. It is the need of the hour to control obsolescence of material effectively. As surplus material leads to obsolescence, the disposal of surplus and scrap material requires a proper approach on the part of management.

There is no rule of thumb to determine stock level or to determine type of strategy to be employed for procuring and stocking. No common procedure can be made applicable for all the items. There would be special peculiarities for each item and as such a special treatment would have to be meted out to overcome the problems or difficulties in respect of each type. Different types of classifications suggested above would give the executive a clear idea as to what are the implications and this would give him necessary clues. Prof. P. Gopala Krishna suggests that, "The executive will have to make best use of all methods and should not be guided by "tunnel vision" of using only one method."

REVIEW QUESTIONS

1. Define the term "selective inventory control"? Describe various types of classification that are used? Describe how ABC analysis is made?
2. Describe the technique of ABC analysis? What control measures you would suggest for A, B, and C items? Explain the advantages and limitation of ABC analysis.

3. Briefly describe various approaches to selective inventory controls systems, highlighting the basis and main uses of each type of control.

4. "ABC" analysis is an effective method of pegging down inventory - Discuss.

5. Traditional management and control gives equal importance to all items regardless of their importance. This is most glaring in inventory control. How various selective controls helps to overcome this problem?

6. XYZ analysis will give only value and distribution of inventory in stores on a particular day and nothing more than that. How this classification helps you to control inventories?

7. What is the need for effective drug management? What procedure you would adopt to determine criticality of drug?

8. Write short notes on

   a) Criticality of a drug

   b) FMS analysis of drugs

   c) Disposal of non-moving items

   d) As Is Where Is sales

   e) SDE classification

   f) GOLF analysis

   g) PQR classification

PROBLEMS

1. Data regarding materials consumed in a hospital with their prices is furnished below.

Item Code	Unit Cost (Rs.)	Annual Consumption (units)
3637	11.20	6850
8061	8.60	371
3195	13.18	1292
2321	91.80	62
4023	3.20	12667
4094	10.18	9625
4881	1.27	7010
3121	0.88	5100
6846	62.25	258
8355	18.10	862
1726	0.38	1940
0093	2.20	657

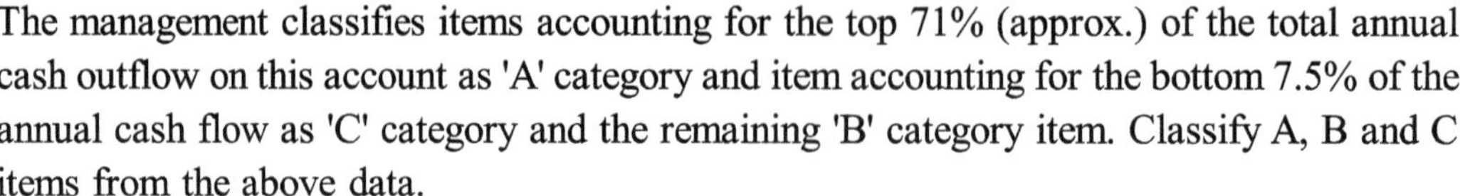

The management classifies items accounting for the top 71% (approx.) of the total annual cash outflow on this account as 'A' category and item accounting for the bottom 7.5% of the annual cash flow as 'C' category and the remaining 'B' category item. Classify A, B and C items from the above data.

Check your answer:

A category items: 4094, 4023, 3195

B category items: 6846, 8355, 4881, 3637

C category items: 2321, 3221, 8061, 0093, 1726

2. Classify the following 14 items in to ABC categories.

Item No.	Monthly Consumption (Rs.)
V-100	451
V-101	1052
V-102	205
V-103	893
V-104	843
V-105	727
V-106	412
V-107	214
V-108	188
V-109	172
V-110	170
V-111	5056
V-112	159
V-113	3424

Check your answer:

A category items: V-111, V-113, V-101, V-103

B category items: V-104, V-105, V-100, V-106

C category items: V-107, V-102, V-108, V-109, V-110, V-112

PART - III

Lead Time Management

Contents

- *Introduction*
- *Definitions*
- *Variations in Lead Time*
- *Effect of Long Lead Time on Costs and Profitability*
- *Elements of Lead Time*
- *Classification of Lead Time*
- *Internal Lead Time*
- *External Lead Time*
- *Other Factors that Contribute to Higher Lead Time*
- *Lead Times Analysis*
- *Managing Lead Times*
- *Dealing with Inconsistent Lead Times*
- *Summary*
- *Review Questions*

CHAPTER - 16

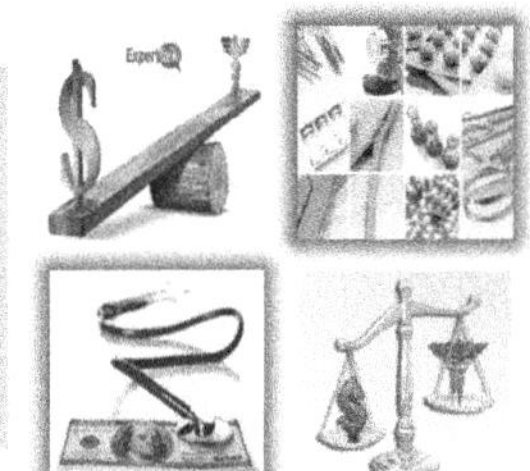

Lead Time Management

INTRODUCTION

The famous adage, **"Justice delayed is justice denied"** is a common complaint in courts of law. Similarly, supply delayed is supply denied is a common complaint of most customers, and users of healthcare institutions. They invariably complain to warehousing, purchasing and materials department, that items, which should have been delivered some time ago, are yet to arrive. In this context, users of materials must appreciate the concept of lead time from the date of receipt and acceptance of an indent to the date of receipt and acceptance of materials. There is bound to be some time gap between identification of need and the satisfaction of the need.

Lead time for supply is a balance between what the supplier wants and what the customer wants. If suppliers are powerful, they will specify a long lead time (such as a one year firm programme). If buyers have upper hand, they will expect to be supplied immediately, without any commitment. Both these extreme cases increase total operating costs. The compromise is lead time, which gives suppliers sufficient supply time, but does not force customers to commit themselves further than they can predict. Accuracy of the forecast of their requirements reduces rapidly as they look further and further ahead. This produces an order pattern, which is irregular and subject to change. Stocks are needed where the patient care lead time is shorter than the supply lead time.

If this can be altered so that supply lead time becomes less than sales lead time, stockholding can be avoided. Lead times for purchasing are governed by production and transport, lead times for manufacturing result from capacity, material availability and production planning, and lead times required by customers depend upon availability and policy.

In inventory management, lead time is one of the basic variables that determine the amount of inventories a company carries. For inventory operations, other variables which are to be considered are the following:

1. Order quantity.
2. Quantity of safety stocks.
3. Quantity of reserve stocks.

There is always some time lag between determination of need for material and the time when material is actually manufactured and delivered. This period is called 'Lead time'.

A common mistake in determining lead time is to ignore the time between when a requisition is generated and actual order placement. Normally, materials managers tend to consider only the time between order placement by purchasing and its receipt. The primary reason for this mistake is that an assumption is made that order will be placed by purchasing on the same day the requisition is received. Often this is not the case.

DEFINITIONS

Lead time can be defined as a period between decision to request for purchase of an item to the time it arrives in stores or delivery to user/customer.

Prof. P. Gopala Krishnan and Sandilya defined lead time as "The period that elapses, between recognition of need to its fulfillment."

P J H Baily defines that "Lead time is the total time it takes to get things."

Maynard defines lead time as, "The length of time that is allowed to obtain a lot quantity of an item."

George W Aljian defines lead time as, "The period of time from date of ordering to date of delivery which the buyer must reasonably allow the vendor to prepare goods for shipment."

Burton E. Lipman defines lead time as, "The time interval needed to complete a portion or all of the activities in a replenishing cycle." It includes the time to identify a replenishment requirement, process the orders and receive the item in stock, ready for use.

According to **William L. Scheyer,** Former Director of Supply, Bethesda Hospital Inc Cincinnati, U.S, lead time is total of both internal and external lead times. Internal lead time is the time required from requisition to process a purchase order typed and signed, and the order is placed with vendor. External lead time is the time required for vendor to receive the order, enter it, pick and ship goods, to the time arrives at the requesting facility.

Arnold Reisman of Case Western Reserve University, USA, states that the time interval needed to complete a portion or all the activities in replenishing cycle. It includes the time needed to identify a replenishment, requirement, process the order and receive the item in stock, ready for use.

H L Chadda defines lead time as, The time between origin of an indent for a material and the receipt of material by the indenter for use."

Norbert L loyd Enrick in his book on "Inventory Management Installation, Operation, and Control" states, "Lead time is the period that lapses, and occurs usually in months, between order placement and merchandise receipt."

A R Palit states: "Lead time is the total time taken for replenishment of the item from the time a requisition or an indent for it is submitted to the stores or purchase department to the time material is received after inspection as to quality and condition, at the stores for storage or at a using point for actual use."

Whatever may be the definitions, **one thing is certain that there is a time lag between demand and supply.**

VARIATIONS IN LEAD TIME

Lead time is generally short for those items, which a local supplier has in stock off the shelf for immediate delivery. Even in such cases, in Indian conditions, a company usually allows a week's lead time between the day on which a purchase requisition is made and stipulated delivery date in purchase order, to permit both buyer and supplier to process the order efficiently and economically. When there is an immediate need for an off the shelf market item, however, lead time usually can be shortened to less than one day.

Much longer lead times are necessary for items made to order by out of station suppliers and for more complex items. For example, dealer of diagnostic equipment accept orders with a lead time of 60 to 90 days. Medical store supplies distributors often allow their supplier i.e., pharmacy companies as much as 2 to 3 months, for complex piece of custom made equipment may go up to couple of years.

Lead times also vary for identical items. One supplier may require greater lead time for a given item than another supplier and the same supplier may have different lead times for a given item at various stages of business cycle. When business is depressed and supplier is operating well below capacity, with almost no new orders forthcoming, the lead time will be short. When the supplier is working at capacity and has large amount of orders as backlog, the lead time will be long. Variations in lead times can be quite substantial. For example, pharmacy manufacturers may require only two weeks lead time, when business is depressed but at the peak of a boom, the lead time may run into several months.

EFFECT OF LONG LEAD TIME ON COSTS AND PROFITABILITY

Most important impact of lead time on purchase function is inventory levels. When an order is placed, the first issue to be ensured is that one must have adequate stock on hand till further supplies are received. Obviously, the longer the lead time, the more stock of inventories is needed to be maintained. In business activities where people's productive time is limited, time is a scarce input. It is very relevant in this context that unduly long lead time can escalate costs.

For example:

1. Delay in finalizing purchase order may increase cost of materials or services being procured.
2. Delay in getting supplies may render men and materials idle and cause underutilization of production facilities.

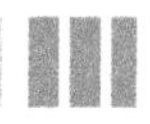

3. "A stock out is a forceful reminder that lead time has lengthened;" in contrast, a shorter lead time that causes excessive inventory investment may never be detected (Dean Ammer).

4. Long lead time automatically raises reorder levels' resulting in excess capital tied up in inventory investment. It not only reduces return on investment but leaves little or no funds available for the business to prosper and grow through investment in new products or various internal improvement projects.

5. Delays in payment of bills due to long procedural lead time may force the vendors to revise their payment terms and/or prices.

6. Long lead times during manufacturing process will build excess work in progress. The longer the manufacturing cycle, the more will be the work in process inventories.

7. It may also happen that right material is not available at the right time for the production process and this upsets the entire schedule. What is significant here is that the work-in-progress inventories are as expensive as other inventories.

ELEMENTS OF LEAD TIME

Lead time is linked to purchasing cycle, which deals with various elements involved in purchasing activity. The elements that affect lead time are:

1. Nature of purchases made.
2. Volume and varieties of purchases.
3. The degree of specialization needed to make purchase, especially for sophisticated items.

The organization of purchase department and procedures followed will vary considerably not only from organization to organization, but from item to item and industry to industry. They vary according to policies and objectives of the company; important among them are:

- Extent of powers delegated to materials manager and his subordinates. In some organizations, delegation of powers exists only on paper, but in practice, there might be neither trust nor confidence reposed on the purchase department. In actual practice, the top management might decide the matters.
- Decisions are taken only by top management in some organizations.
- The systems best suited to a hospital may not suit an engineering industry or vice-versa.
- Procedures followed by public sector organizations may not suit private sector organizations.

As in every aspect of management, there cannot be a standard method of organising a purchase department, or having a standard set of systems and procedures. Each set up has to be tailor made to meet the specific requirements of a particular hospital, healthcare centre, and institution. However, there are some basic elements in every purchase transaction, which are common and have an effect on lead time. **They are summarized as under:**

1. Need for materials is recognized by the user department or stores, or material planning department and the determination of requirement is the starting point.

2. Detailed specifications for materials are spelt out in case of job order or custom built or maintenance, repair and operation (MRO) items.

3. User department, stores or material planning department prepares a purchase requisition and towards it, to purchase department.

4. Purchase department makes out a plan for source selection and floats enquiries. At times, need for developing a new source may arise.

5. After receipt of offers, they are scrutinized and evaluated by purchase department or by a committee constituted for the purpose. Sometimes, there may be a need for negotiations with suppliers.

6. A purchase order is issued to supplier spelling out quality, quantity, price, delivery schedules, payment terms, and conditions of contract.

7. Suppliers order acceptance is obtained.

8. Purchase department does follow up with the supplier to ensure prompt delivery of right quality and quantity of materials at the appropriate time.

9. If goods are available ex-stock the supplier will ship immediately from ex-stock, otherwise the goods be manufactured and delivered.

10. Goods, quite often delivered by rail or road or any other mode of transport and goods are to be cleared by shipping and clearing department. Sometimes, vendor may deliver goods at buyer's stores.

11. If supply documents are negotiated through bank, purchase department arranges for clearance of documents by the finance department. Goods when received are first checked for physical quantities and later offered to quality control department for quality check. Occasionally goods may be inspected at vendor's plant.

12. Supplier's invoice is checked against purchase orders and after inspection the goods acceptance or otherwise is documented.

13. Goods, which are accepted, are sent to issue stores or at times to indenter directly (e.g., office furniture or material for a project) or to user department directly, when materials are in short supply.

The time taken for completing the above narrated activities constitutes "lead time" and as well referred as **purchasing cycle.**

CLASSIFICATION OF LEAD TIME

As already stated, the total time taken for identifying the need for items, placing order, and dispatch by supplier, shipping and transport, receipt and inspection can be broadly classified into internal and external lead times. Internal lead time is further classified into administrative lead time and inspection lead time. External lead time comprises of manufacturing or supplier's lead time and transportation lead time. (See Figure 16.1).

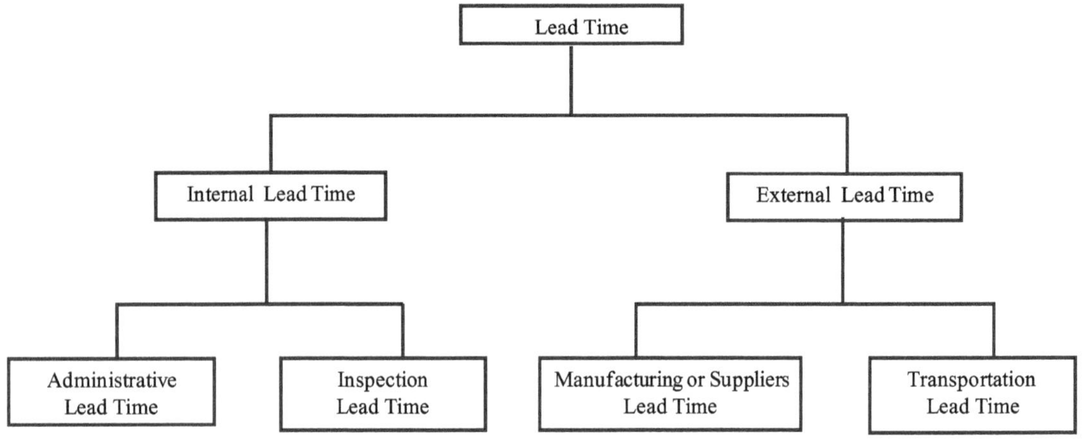

Figure 16.1 Classifications of Lead Time

Time spent on each of the four types of lead times will vary from item to item and organization to organization as stated earlier. Causes for increase in lead time can be described as delays that occur during internal and external lead times. Before we embark upon the control measures, we should classify the delays and identify causes for delays in each classification.

INTERNAL LEAD TIME

Administrative Lead Time

Administrative lead time can be stated as, "The time that elapses between recognition of need to placement of order." Material requirement has to be identified before it can be ordered. At this indent stage, material planning department has to compute the requirement of various materials over a time horizon. For regularly consumed materials, projections are based on basic of past consumption figures, modified to changes in technology and demand.

For items which are not regularly used in addition to computing the quantity of requirement, specifications will have to be drawn up, thereby increasing the need identification time. Thus, the activities are 'techno economic' in nature. The actual computing time may be half an hour. But planning department may take two to three weeks to raise an indent. This may be due to discussions, consultations, meetings, and approvals. So also is the case of new materials. Average lead time taken by a government hospital to convert an indent into an order is high compared to corporate or private hospital.

Next activity is identification of prospective sources of supply. This can be done by referring to a data bank or calling for quotations or by tendering. The time taken will be high if tendering system is adopted. It may even extend to 2 to 3 months, if open tendering system is adopted because the advertiser has to give reasonable time to publish in the newspapers, and to bidders, to submit quotations, opening of tenders, preparation of comparative statements etc.

Sometimes, the need may arise for negotiation of terms and conditions of supply. In case of new items with close tolerances, the technical departments will have to be involved in the negotiations. Once negotiations are completed, there have been instances when even the clerical formality took 3 to 6 days.

Possible reasons for delay in administration which are well within control of the organization can be attributed to following factors:

- Excessive paperwork.
- Poor O M systems.
- Cumbersome procedures.
- Poor delegation leading to delays.
- Poor communication systems.
- Wrong selection of source.
- Over worked staff and different priorities.
- Faulty tender procedures.
- Absence of proper management information system.
- Unnecessary negotiations.
- Delay in convening tender committee meetings.
- Poor buyer and seller relationships.
- Inadequate knowledge of market.
- Vague specifications resulting in vendors seeking avoidable clarifications.
- Lack of coordination with other departments.

Inspection Lead Time

Second part of internal lead time is the time taken from the date of receipt of material at receipt section to the date on which they are sent to storage bins in issue stores. This includes the time taken for inspection of materials for quality checking etc. Inspection lead time becomes bottleneck in quite a few organizations. One of the most common reasons is non availability of a standard with which, to compare the quality of materials received. Even otherwise, in inefficient organizations, goods remain at the receiving bay for a couple of weeks. This problem will be more acute in centralized purchase organizations and warehouses where the distance between indenter and purchaser is substantial. This leads to communication gaps regarding quality requirement and inspectors at warehouses will have to wait for clarifications. In the case of special custom made equipment, the indenter may have to depute quality inspection personnel, at regular intervals to check the quality of materials used as well as to keep track of programme of manufacture which naturally increases lead time. **A pertinent factor that has to be taken note of is that, if an item is rejected during inspection, lead time will increase to the extent of the time, which would be taken for obtaining replacement.**

We can summarize reasons for inspection delays as follows:

- Non availability of standards to compare the quality of material received.
- Complex design.
- Unnecessary hold ups at goods receiving bay, even in well organized and efficient hospitals. This problem is more acute in centralized purchasing organizations and warehouses.
- Items procured based on brand and or trade names.
- Piecemeal or adhoc purchases.
- Incomplete drawings or specifications.
- Sometimes, tests have to done outside at some test centres.
- On certain occasions, inspectors may have to be sent to supplier's plant.
- Poor communication between receipt section and inspection teams.
- Lack of coordination.
- Undue importance given to non critical items.
- Lack of knowledge of inspection procedures.
- Lack of adequate inspection equipment.
- Rejection of approved materials by user departments.
- Test certificates not received.
- Delayed reporting.

EXTERNAL LEAD TIME

Manufacturing Lead Time

This is the time lag between placement of order and despatch of materials by suppliers. Once a purchase order is placed, the purchaser has to wait till supplier delivers the goods. Manufacturing lead time, to a large extent, depends upon the supplier. Even if purchaser is unable to hasten the supply, he can at least prevent several delays by regular follow up. In case of custom built items ordered on small industries, supplier may not be able to procure a handful important raw materials or components. This often occurs in the case orthopedic hospitals manufacturing artificial limbs. The purchaser may be able to bail the supplier out through his contacts.

Some of the common causes for increase in manufacturing lead time can be attributed to following:

- Complex design.
- Lack of appropriate technology.
- Frequent power and machine failures.
- Inadequate plant capacity.
- Development time for tooling.
- Delay in supply of bought out items.
- Waiting for economic batch quantity.
- Frequent changes in production schedules.
- Customers specifications are not clear or vague or too general.
- Non availability of raw materials.
- Inputs for manufacturing may have to be imported.
- Lack of adequate inspection facilities.
- Financial constrains.
- Low profit margin.
- Workers absenteeism.
- Strikes, lock outs, etc.

Transportation Lead Time

Transit time is bound to be considerably more for rail transport than for road transport. Even in road transport, identifying correct transport agency also plays an important role. Transit inventories would be high if the transit lead time is high. Thus in some cases, reliance on air transport may work out to be cheaper than road and rail transport systems. In many cases, transport becomes a bottleneck. Rail wagons may not be available readily or trucks may be scarce in peak season. By experience, one can predict this type of occurrences that may happen and initiate preventive action by stocking higher quantities to prevent stock out. One has to analyse causes for excessive lead time and take positive action to bring them under control. This depends upon the mode of transport. Here **speed and economy are indirectly related.** Therefore selection of air, road, and rail transport depends on the urgency of requirement, formalities such as issuance of sales tax forms, time needed for retiring of documents from bank. The activities should be undertaken in parallel so that materials can be cleared on arrival at the destination without incurring demurrages. In case of imported consignments, transshipments will have to be made at ports and customs formalities will be added to lead time.

Some causes that contribute to long transportation lead time are:

- Selection of wrong mode of transport.
- Wrong choice of road transport carriers.
- Poor documentation.
- Inefficient clearing and forwarding work.
- Delays in settlement of transport bills.
- Lack of legal knowledge of transportation and rail/road/air transport regulations.
- Detaining of vehicles at entry tax/sales tax check posts.
- Seasonal fluctuations in demand for transportation services.
- Safety and security of goods.
- Wrong routing patterns.
- Improper packing.
- Long distance haulage resulting in trans shipments.
- Load planning problems.
- Bad conditions of roads.
- Waiting for building up economic loads.
- Traffic restrictions at city/towns entry points.

OTHER FACTORS THAT CONTRIBUTE TO HIGHER LEAD TIME

- Lead time varies for item to item even though they are from the same supplier.
- For off the shelf items, the supplier may not take much time to deliver goods. But if they are to be manufactured, then problems and uncertainties may arise.
- Quite often suppliers wait for composite load to save transport and handling costs.
- Opposite may also happen, vendor may despatch one item so that he can collect his money soon. However, the buyer does not gain as all these items are to be used in sets.

It is because of this factor that one has to plan the requirements carefully and decide where one wants the deliveries to be made, in close coordination with user department and supplier.

purchase department can determine best possible lead time. **The fact to be remembered is that "Lead time is not fixed time;"** it varies and in most cases can be adjusted to one's requirements. Hence it calls for close coordination with the suppliers. In some cases, it may happen that raw materials used by the supplier for manufacture are to be imported, or a special alloy is to be used for manufacture of an item like stent used in cardiology department. The lead time for this item will therefore depend upon lead time of raw materials required by the supplier. At times, help from buyer may solve the problems of supplier.

LEAD TIME ANALYSIS

In order to make any analysis, one must have knowledge of the essentials of lead time and also facts and figures. It is easy to get broad facts such as dates of the indents, purchase orders, delivery documents and invoices to get facts relating to lead time.

Analysis of Administrative Lead Time

Elements of administrative lead time are:

- Scrutinizing the indent.
- Floating enquiries.
- Receipt of quotations.
- Consideration of offer.
- Final decision on placement of order.

If administrative lead time is long, one has to investigate why it took so much time. In order to arrive at causes of long administrative lead time, the manager has to examine delays in each stage of purchasing cycle.

- Time lag between receipt of indent and floating of enquiries or tender notices.
- Preparations of comparative statement of quotations after bids have been received.
- Delay in convening tender committee meetings.
- Time taken by the committee in arriving at conclusions.
- Delay in issue of purchase order after purchase decision is taken.
- Delay in inspection after receipt of goods.

After finding out reasons for delay at each stage, one must initiate corrective action in regard to each element where unnecessary delays occur and lay down normal time for processing at each stage. Materials manager should also bring to the notice of various departmental personnel consequences of delays in lead time i.e., extra inventory to cover lead time consumption.

General reasons for high administrative lead time are as follows:

- Faulty tendering procedures.
- Wrong or inadequate quality specification.
- Poor delegation leading to delays in decision making.

To overcome these problems the buyer can adopt following measures:

- Laying down clear cut policies in regard to adoption of open tenders, limited tenders and purchase without tenders. Government hospitals have to go for public tender when once exceeds certain pre determined amount for purchases say five lakh, whereas the advertisement cost in newspapers may be Rs. 50,000. In other words, the hospital spends 10 percent of the purchase value on advertisement alone. This is a waste. Limited tenders should be adopted wherever possible. Up to date list of approved contractors or suppliers from whom quotations may be called is extremely helpful.
- If specifications are not clear, vendors will be quoting for different product and not for the same product. Unnecessary time has to be spent on clarifications and negotiations. Specifications must be explicit and fully stated. Specifications are to be cleared by engineering/ production and user as well as the case may be, before floating enquiries. One must ensure that vendors understand the specifications. Soft copies of drawings may be provided wherever possible.
- Study and analyze decision making and recommend adequate delegation commensurate with responsibility. Officers should be empowered to take decisions within their authority and must not send papers unnecessarily to their superiors.
- Decision making can be streamlined by laying down broad policies which can act as framework for decision making by lower level managers. Accountability should be prescribed.

Analysis of Inspection Lead Time

Normally this should take hardly one or two days. However if it takes longer time, it calls for analysis of the flow chart of activities. Once this is known, corrective action can be easier. One can appreciate vendor's complaint about delayed payment especially where payment terms are 30 days from date of dispatch. Sometimes goods are to be inspected by buyer's representative at vendor's plant or by third party before they are shipped. This often causes undue delays. High inspection lead time may be due to inadequate inspection of materials purchases, both at pre delivery (manufacturing) and post delivery stages.

Solution lies in the following measures:

- Have qualified inspection personnel.
- Ensure close coordination and proper relationships with inspection if inspection is not under the materials department.

- If inspection causes delays for no valid reasons, bring to the notice of management and point out resultant higher inventory arising out of increases in inspection lead time.
- Evaluate cases of rejection by production or user department after inspection has passed materials, and find out exact reasons for corrective action.
- Check on inspection costs and ensure that they are not high.
- Random sampling procedures for inspection have to be adopted wherever possible.
- No inspection needs to be normally done for proprietary items manufactured by reputed firms.
- Use skilled inspectors. Give them adequate training.
- Arrange test house inspection, where necessary.
- Expedite inspection reports.
- Rejection/rectification procedures to be streamlined.

Experience can save costs. Materials supplied by a vendor who is consistently okay, need be inspected only once in a way or on a random basis.

Analysis of manufacturing lead time or supplier's lead time

Supplier's lead time can be divided into following elements.

1. Productions lead time.
2. Transit lead time.
3. Pre delivery inspections lead time.

In most cases, the supplier may start production only after purchases order is received by him.

In such a situation, the following suggestions will come handy to buyer:

1. Vendor may be informed in advance before sending confirmed purchase order by phone, SMS, fax or email so that 3 or 4 days can be saved.
2. Enter into long term contracts such as system contract.
3. Where the demand is known, a letter of intent may be given to vendor to plan for procurement of his production material.

Analysis of Transportation/Transit Time

This depends upon the mode of transport. Procedures followed in many organizations are outmoded and needlessly time consuming and unproductive. It is not generally realized that these procedures increase inventory levels and delay availability of materials for production.
Comparative cost analysis and choice of right mode of transportation call for:

Comparative cost analysis and choice of right mode of transportation call for:

- Market research to identify seasonal fluctuations.
- Prompt settlement of claims.
- Proper assessment of rates of different modes of transport.
- Tariff analysis.
- Knowledge of statutory laws about transportation by road, rail, air, and port regulations.
- Routing patterns.
- Choice of reliable road transporters.
- Economics of own transport vs. public transport.
- Efficient clearing and forwarding work.
- Long term contracts with transport operators.
- Avail container service facilities.
- Planning of transport requirements in advance to avoid rush jobs.
- Safety and security of goods.
- Analysis of demurrage costs and control of such costs.
- Prompt documentation.
- Vehicle replacement policy if owned.
- Information regarding large fleet owners own garage or hired garage?
- Utilization of vehicles (two/three shifts per day) by transporters.

MANAGING LEAD TIMES

We have seen earlier that actual supply lead time contains some elements of administration in addition to lead time quoted by the supplier. In stock control equations, the supply lead time is assumed to be constant. It is significant that estimated lead time in the system reflect true lead time. If the supply lead time changes, then the lead time in the calculation should be changed to reflect this. It is a continuous task on the part of maintenance of stock systems, placement of orders and stock reaching low stock levels; changes can be normally made by groups of items from same source, or by using actual lead time to up to date standard lead time.

Setting the lead times

If a very short lead time is set for stock control, it may result in stock outs, as the level of stock will be kept too low. On other hand, if the lead time is set pessimistically, it results in overstocking. Compromise for setting the lead time is a fine judgement for inventory controller.

Minimizing the lead time

Longer lead times cause forecasting more difficult and increase the safety and reserve stock. Reducing the lead time is therefore warranted and can lead to ultimate goal of stockless supply if supplier's lead time is short enough. Inventory management should, therefore, aim to reduce overall lead time. **One of the simplest ways of reducing lead time is to specify it more precisely. 'Delivery in the month of November' as a request gives the supplier plenty of leeway. 'Delivery on 2nd Nov 11.00 a.m.' suggests an entirely different expectation and is likely to gain a much better delivery performance.** The author's numerous experiments attempting this have shown that a bulk of suppliers will improve their delivery precision greatly, simply by being asked.

Healthcare institutions also find that supplier reliability is often affected by lead time. With a lead time of one day, if a supplier of an A class item is a day late, this can be a most important issue. If lead time is 12 weeks and the supplier is a day late, this is often expected, or even considered as on time. One day's worth of stock is held to offset this. The perception of delivery performance is as a proportion of lead time. However, from an inventory perspective, one day's worth of stock is the same value, whether it is added to an extra 6 weeks' worth or to one day's worth of total inventory.

From the analysis of lead time above, total lead time should be minimized by:

- Prompt posting of information into stores computer systems without delay.
- Entering into long term contracts for major suppliers.

It is important to minimize the time lag between:

- The stock getting low in the stores and the supplier receiving the pur-chase order.
- Receiving the delivery and the event being displayed on the hospital computer system.

Once these elements of lead time are small enough, the suppliers' lead times should also be examined. Supplier's lead time as discussed earlier consists of actual physical transport time, manufacturing time in some instances and organizational time. Lead time should be a negotiated time, not something that happens at random.

For example, if a supplier quotes a 4 week delivery, it could denote:

1. All the existing stock is set aside for someone else.
2. There is a stock out because insufficient safety stock or the re ordering system failed.
3. The supply cycle time is 4 weeks to get supplies from their supplier.

Let us analyze the above three situations

In the first two cases, the 4 weeks are caused by priorities. In the first instance, order is not jumping the queue and in the second, situation supplier does not consider the order important enough

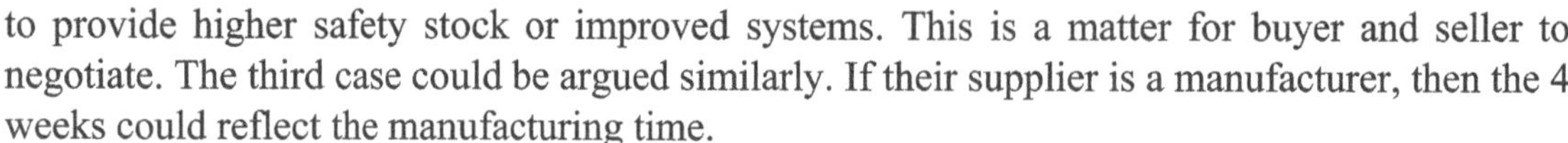

to provide higher safety stock or improved systems. This is a matter for buyer and seller to negotiate. The third case could be argued similarly. If their supplier is a manufacturer, then the 4 weeks could reflect the manufacturing time.

However, only a small part of manufacturing time is taken up with production. The production lead time taken for the work to pass through the manufacturing plant is generally much longer than the actual manufacturing time per unit assessed by work measurement. It is usually more than ten times the measured work content. Hence, there is potential for manufacturing lead time to be reduced. Again, collaboration with suppliers may enable them to reduce their own lead time.

Because of large numbers of items in inventory, reduction of lead time has to be carried out for selected types of items. These are initially 'A' class items.

DEALING WITH INCONSISTENT LEAD TIMES

With closer partnerships and higher expectations, inconsistent delivery is not the problem that it used to be. However healthcare industry customers are more sensitive to supply reliability, so strategies should be considered for that supplier where delivery is inconsistent and changing the supplier is undesirable.

When forecast of lead time is not accurate, it is difficult to set reasonable stock levels or to provide good customer service. The policy on inconsistent lead times should be determined by the impact of problem, and on whether the financial risk is high or low. For high consumption value items like 'A' class items, inconsistency has to be resolved through scheduling and working more closely with vendors to smoothen out the inconsistencies. The objective should be to smoothen out the variations rather than to improve the updating, since each time lead time is updated, stock parameters will be changed and order quantity modified.

For low value consumption items (C class), the situation is not so important unless there are many inconsistent suppliers. The strategy for avoiding the problem for routine supplies is to use pessimistic lead time in calculations. This will cause higher stocks, which may be necessary if the item is important. However, as the purchase quantity is probably large, there are only a few chances of stock out and C class items may not be worth the investment in extra stock to provide the extra availability.

SUMMARY

Lead time is defined as, **"The period that elapses between recognition of need to its fulfillment."** "Justice delayed is justice denied" is a common complaint in courts of law. Similarly, supply delayed is supply denied is a common complaint of most customers/users. In inventory management, lead time is one of the basic variables that determine the amount of inventories a company carries. Lead time varies from item to item, supplier to supplier. When the supplier is operating below installed capacity, the lead time will be short. When the supplier is working at capacity and has large amount of orders as backlog, the lead time will be long. Unduly long lead time can escalate costs.

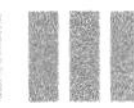

Elements that affect lead time are: Nature of purchases made, volume and varieties of purchases, the degree of specialization needed to make purchase, especially for sophisticated items.

Lead time can be classified into internal lead time and external lead time. Internal lead time is further classified into administrative lead time and inspection lead time. Similarly external lead time is further subdivided into manufacturing or supplier's lead time and transportation lead time.

Administrative lead time is the time that elapses between recognition of need to placement of order. The inspection lead time is the time taken from the date of receipt of material at receipt section to the date on which they are sent to storage bins. Supplier's lead time consists of production lead time and pre delivery inspection lead time. Transit lead time depends on the mode of transport and distance.

Management of lead time involves that any change in suppliers lead time should reflect in stock control systems i.e., the system reflect true lead time. While setting lead times, it should neither be too short nor too long to avoid under and over stocking situations. The compromise for setting the lead time is a time judgement for inventory controller. Reduction in total lead time is achieved by inputing information to stores and computer system, the purchase order without delay and partnership with major supplies.

Long and/or inconsistent lead times make it difficult to forecast demand accurately and generally lead to higher inventories. Hence all possible efforts should be made to minimize internal lead times by following efficient administrative processes in ordering and inspection. Efforts should also be made to partner with suppliers to reduce the manufacturing and transit delays by proper planning, coordination, and control.

REVIEW QUESTIONS

1. Control of lead time could lead to reduction of cost on materials. Discuss.
2. What is "lead time"? Explain its impact on the company's working capital?
3. Justice delayed is justice denied is a common complaint in course of law. Supply delayed is supply denied is a common complaint from most of customers and users. Discuss.
4. Define the term lead time. What are the elements of lead time?
5. What do you understand by the term external lead time? What is the role of materials manager to reduce external lead time?
6. What is the role of materials manager in managing the lead times especially in healthcare environment?
7. "A stock out is a forceful reminder that lead time has lengthened." Discuss.

8. Write short notes on

    a) Variations in lead time
    b) Administrative lead time
    c) Effect of lead time on stock holding
    d) Suppliers lead time
    e) Classification of lead time
    f) Dealing with inconsistent lead times
    g) Managing lead time

PART - III

Designing of Inventory Control Systems

Contents

- *Introduction*
- *Objectives of Inventory Control Systems*
- *Types of Control Systems*
- *Two Bin System*
- *Minima-Maxima Inventory Control System*
- *Imprest Stock Control*
- *Open Access Bins System*
- *Fixation of Re order Point (ROP) or Re order Level (ROL)*
- *Determination of Safety Stock*
- *Practical Inventory Systems*
- *Perpetual Inventory System (Q system)*
- *Advantages of Q Model Inventory System*
- *Limitations of Q Model Inventory Control*
- *Periodic Inventory System (P System)*
- *Advantages of Periodic Inventory System*
- *Limitations of Periodic System*
- *Comparison of Q and P Systems of Inventory Models*
- *Materials Requirement Planning (MRP)*
- *Prerequisite Inputs for MRP*
- *MRP Output Reports*
- *Benefits of MRP*
- *Hospital Requirements Planning*
- *Inventory Systems Features*
- *Summary*
- *Review Questions*

CHAPTER - 17

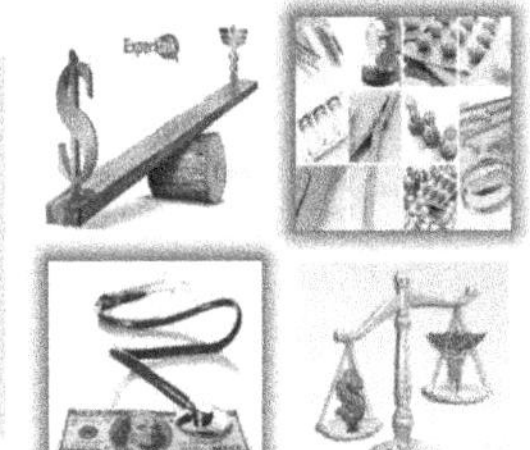

Designing of Inventory Control Systems

INTRODUCTION

A good control system provides for self control and requires attention only on exceptional basis. An analysis of the objectives of intended systems is the starting point in developing a control system. This analysis discloses the critical activities in the operations where control can be most effective. Inventory control systems, have advanced beyond the rudimentary concepts of design of control systems. They are now well established, but they still experience the usual control problems.

In this chapter, the emphasis is on control procedures for total inventory held in stock, wherever it may be stored. A hospital may have one or more control systems for managing it in various locations. It is imperative that control mechanism satisfies the service objectives of the entire healthcare institution at lowest possible cost. Selection of control system is the responsibility of top management. **The type of inventory control system selected will have an impact on almost all activities of the organization.**

OBJECTIVES OF INVENTORY CONTROL SYSTEMS

An inventory control system is a coordinated set of rules, for routinely answering following questions.

- What to order?
- When to order?
- How much to order?
- At what frequency to order?

The system should indicate how routine and non routine situations are to be treated via predetermined rules and procedures.

An effective system will accomplish the following:

1. Ensure that sufficient inventories are available.

2. Identify excess, fast and slow moving items.
3. Provide accurate, concise, and timely reports to management.
4. Expend least amount of resources in accomplishing the above mentioned three tasks.

A comprehensive inventory control system involves much more than quantitative inventory models, all aspects of the system must be considered.

There are six vital areas viz.

1. Development of demand forecasts and correction of forecast errors.
2. Selection of appropriate inventory models for the hospital
3. Measurement of inventory costs (ordering, holding over stock and stock out).
4. Methods used to record and account for inventories
5. Methods for receipt, handling, storage, and issue of inventories.
6. Information procedures used to report exceptions.

Use of sophisticated mathematical techniques by itself does not necessarily result in an effective system. Precise, highly mathematical techniques are of little use unless the information to be fed into the models is available at a realistic cost. Systems that select approximate, reasonable inventory levels with low data processing costs are often preferable. In many cases, lack of accurate and timely data nullifies the advantages of complex control systems. It should be remembered that a breakdown in any one of the above six vital areas (not just the inventory model) can undermine the efficiency of the entire system.

TYPES OF CONTROL SYSTEMS

There are several types of inventory control systems in use today. Nevertheless, it is impossible to distinguish among the systems most frequently used.

Common types of inventory systems used in healthcare institutions are:

1. Two Bin System
2. Minima-Maxima Inventory System
3. Imprest Stock Control system
4. Open-access Bin System
5. Perpetual Review System
6. Periodic Review System
7. Material Requirement Planning (MRP-I)

TWO BIN SYSTEM

In this system, two bins are kept having different capacities When the stock in the first bin is exhausted, it is time for replenishment. The second bin is like a reserve or safety stock and the demands are met from second bin. Before the stock in second is exhausted, it has to be replenished.

It is not always necessary to maintain stocks in two physical bins. The term 'Two bin system' should be restricted to visual method of stock control instead of using two actual bins; one bin can be divided at 'two levels'. One section is only used at a time and on its completion, the material is issued from second level. Steps are also taken to replenish it when the stock touches second level.

Two bin system is simple to operate because there is no need for records. Only requisite for successful operation of this system is that the order point of reserve stock be physically separated from the balance stock. This often can be done quite simply. Suppose usage of certain medicine averages four boxes a week and maximum lead time is one week. The reserve supply in two bin system might be five boxes including one box as safety stock for including unexpected changes in usage or lead time. The supply need not physically be kept in two separate bins. Simply putting a rubber band around it and then using up other boxes in inventory first can identify it. When the stock drops down to the point where it is necessary to use boxes held by rubber band it indicates that the order point has been reached. Figure 17.1 shows how and when the re order level is fixed in terms of normal lead consumption plus safety stock, the actual re-order point automatically regulates itself.

Two bin system is best suited for items of low value, fairly consistent usage and short lead time. The two bin system is actually a primitive version of conventional perpetual inventory control system.

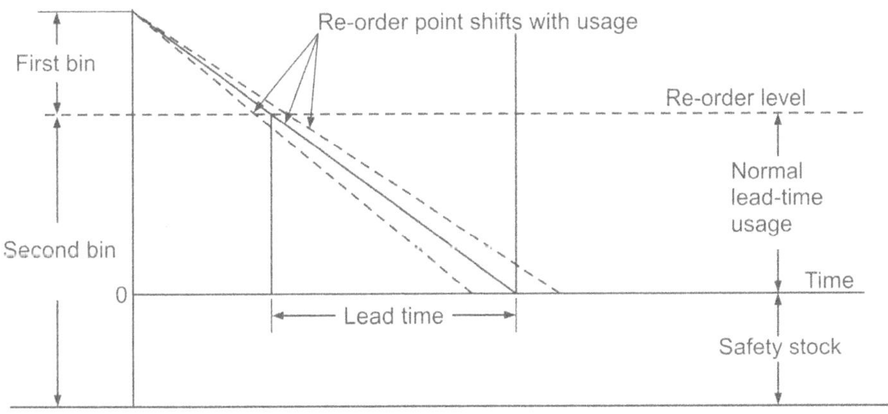

Figure 17.1 Two Bin System Showing the Automatic Regulation of Reorder Point with Rate of Usage

MINIMA-MAXIMA INVENTORY CONTROL SYSTEM

This is one of the extensively used inventory control systems. It is also known as Optional Replenishment System (s, S). The term minima-maxima is applied to any stock control method in which some maximum and minimum figures are set for stocking of each item. Theoretically, minimum inventory level could be zero. When the last unit is consumed, a new shipment arrives; maximum inventory could be economic order quantity. In practice, it is not advisable to adopt such an extreme policy. In minimum-maximum inventory system, a safety factor is established which forms basis for minimum stock level below which, inventory should not dip under normal circumstances. Maximum inventory stock is set high enough to allow for delivery time on the new shipment and provides for enough safety stock in case of delay or unexpectedly heavy usage. The extent of this safety factor depends on the importance of a particular item to process, value of investment, and availability of substitutes at short notice. A high safety factor is provided for any item, the lack of which would cause operations to come to standstill.

Under minimum-maximum system, rate of usage of an item is determined by past experience and forecasts and length of time required to obtain delivery is secured from the inventory control records and studies of alternative source of supply. An order minimum or re order point is established. This point is equal to usage multiplied the delivery time in months or weeks plus safety factor. A graphic illustration is shown in Figure 17.2.

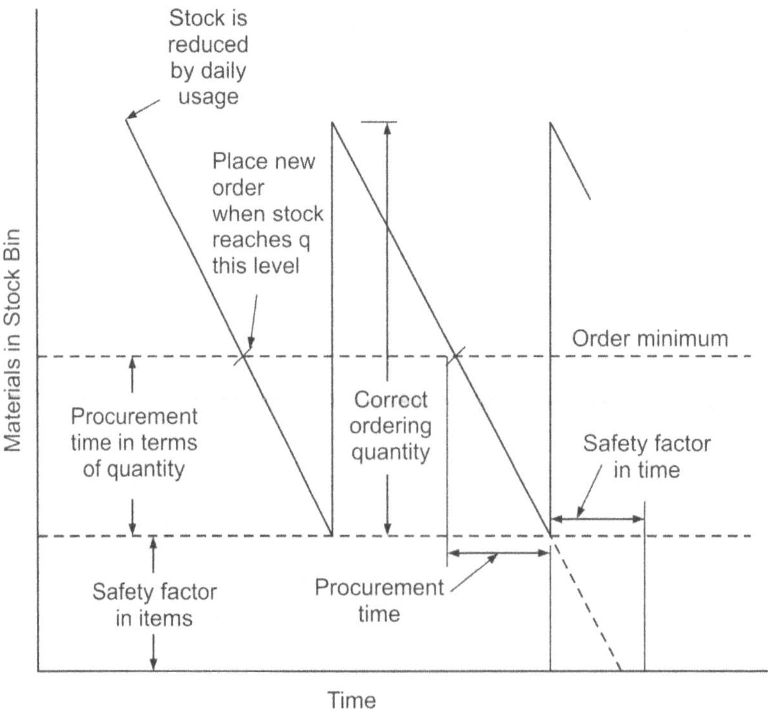

Figure 17.2 Graphic Illustration of Minima-Maxima Inventory Control

Source: Purchasing management materials in motion by wasting, Fine and Zenz.

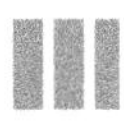

This system provides a regular procedure in that at a specified time, in terms of rate of usage, a replenishment order is released. This order quantity is planned in accordance with the procedures laid down. It may not be out of place to mention here that, **no inventory control system can be a complete substitute for executive judgement.** It is applicable only to such items as are purchased routinely. Good judgement is required in establishing the control, and the good judgement is required continuously to make adjustments for changes in the size of the safety aspect, usage rate, and price. No automatic system can guard against all possible changes.

Weakness of minimum-maximum inventory control system:

1. Junior staff generally have a tendency is to overestimate usage rate while fixing order levels, which in turn results in higher holding costs.
2. Re order points and safety stocks often are not changed for years.
3. Posting delays in records make the system futile for control. Re order of a critical item can be held up until the stores assistant gets around to posting the last withdrawal, indicating that the re order point has been reached.
4. When a new control system is developed, it may work well in the initial stages. But with the efflux of time, things change. People are reluctant to go back and rework the control system, when once it is outdated; it loses part or all of its effectiveness. This system is appropriate for use in small hospitals (less than 100 beds).

IMPREST STOCK CONTROL

This is the simplest method of stock control and involves determination of a maximum level for the bin and periodic inspection of stock levels in the bin. As we saw earlier, the bin is the receptacle, which holds the materials. The bin is then topped up as required immediately to the maximum level.

Usually the imprest stock control method is limited to 'C' class items of low consumption value and those where replenishment can be obtained immediately. System is practiced in post offices is a good example, where a fixed quantity of stamps is kept; at the end of each week (or first thing to be done on Monday morning), the quantities remaining are examined and brought back to the maximum level. In this case, there is no need for reserve quantity and maximum level need only be bare estimated weekly requirements. A stock out before the weekend could easily be rectified, because 'unlimited' supplies of stamps are continuously available from the main post office.

On the other hand, a too frequent occurrence of stock out conditions could indicate either that the maximum levels needs adjustment or that demand should be looked into in case there has been a case of pilferage. In setting the stock level, replenishment costs must be borne in mind.

OPEN ACCESS BINS SYSTEM

Let us take the requirement of sterile cotton and bandage cloth rolls in a hospital or dispensary. It will be a terrible waste of time accounting for each pack. In this case, the items are kept at the work point and staff members are free to pick them as and when needed. This system is called open access bins.

Imprest stock control can be used along with 'open-access bin'. Open access bins for materials may be used singly or in multiples situated around the units adjacent to the stocking point. The staff members help themselves to stocks without having to build records. This saves their time, which can be used for other useful activities and also eliminates cost on unnecessary paperwork. This system is very satisfactory because replenishment of the bin can be made direct from the main stores to the open access bin. In a case where there are a number of such bins, a stores vehicles may travel round the bins at fixed times, making replenishments and bringing the levels up to the desired maximum levels. Quantity replenished is taken as the quantity consumed. Stock control is not applied at the point of use and detailed control and record of each transaction is not necessary. Overall control can be maintained at the point from which replenishment is made. The stock control section normally records the volume issued on topping up the open access bins by imprest.

If therefore, the quantities drawn appear excessive or if frequent stock out occurs, these will be reflected in the overall record. Controller of stores can then make inquiries that whether any irregularity has occurred.

Sometimes it may happen that an excess consumption was merely due to a change in demand of which stores was not informed. Such a case may reveal the need to improve interdepartmental communications.

FIXATION OF RE ORDER POINT (ROP) OR RE-ORDER LEVEL (ROL)

Economic order quantity just tells us how much to order and number of orders per year. But it does not indicate when to place an order. Apparently, lead time plays a deciding role in this regard depending upon the consumption rate. Rate of consumption during lead time period can be:

1. Lesser
2. Equal or
3. Greater than Economic Order Quantity

Let us examine these three situations assuming lead time as constant.

Lead time consumption quantity is less than EOQ

The simplest solution is to place an order, when inventory is depleted to a lead time consumption level. This is diagrammatically shown hereunder in Figure 17.3

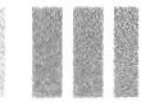

Figure 17.3 depicts a situation wherein lead time consumption is less than EOQ. In this case, whenever inventory level reaches lead time consumption quantity, we place an order equal to "EOQ", which will be received when inventory is exhausted.

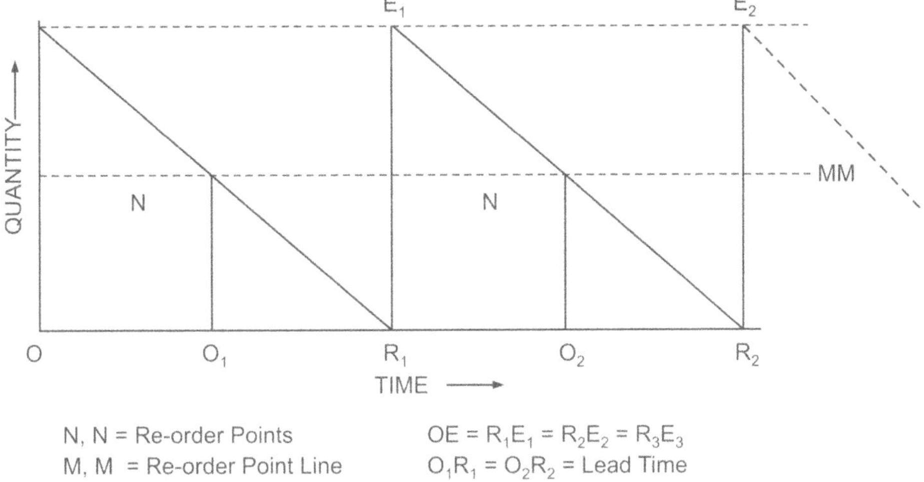

Figure 17.3 Inventory Replenishment System - When EOQ is More Than Lead Time Consumption Quantity

Lead time consumption quantity equals EOQ

In such a case, we start with EOQ and simultaneously release an order for EOQ. Fresh order is placed as soon as material against previous order is received.

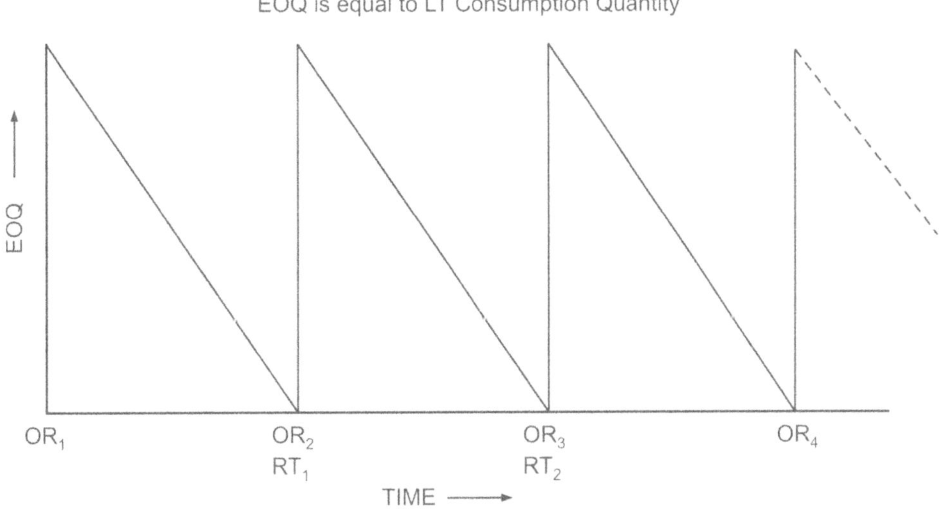

Figure 17.4 Inventory Replenishment When Lead Time Consumption Quantity is Equal to EOQ

$OR_1 = OR_2 = OR_3 = OR_4$ = LT Consumption Quanity, $RT_1 = RT_2 = RT_3$ = Receipts equal to EOQ

Lead Time Consumption Quantity More Than EOQ

In this situation, we have to establish a method to take care of long lead time with sufficient initial stock and then follow it up regularly with economic order cycles. We can see this situation in the following Figure 17.5.

Suppose the lead time for procurement of an item is 90 days and economic order quantity can feed for 30 days. If we start at time 0 with 90 days stock, we are covered for lead time consumption. In order to avoid stock out on 90th day, an order equal to EOQ (30 days' consumption quantity) should be placed on day 0 so as to receive on 90th day at RT_1. But it will meet 30 days requirement only. If we have to avoid stock out on 120th day, we should release our second order OR_2 so as to receive on 120th day. At RT_2 again place third order OR_3 to be received on 120th day at RT_3. This process is repeated once in 30 days from 90th day, our maximum stock would be Economic Order Quantity and follow ordering once in 30 days and receive supplies once in 30 days. From this we can generalize that we have to place an order when total quantity on hand plus total quantity on order is equal to lead time consumption. **This sum of stock on hand and quantity on order is called as "Virtual stock" (Prof. P. Gopala Krishnan).**

Position of 'Virtual stock' at every 30th day can be had from the following table

Table 17.1 Virtual Stock Position at every 30th day

	Stock on Hand in Days Consumption	Stock on Order in Days Consumption	Total in Days Consumption
OR_1	90	30	120
OR_2	60	60	120
OR_3	30	90	120
OR_4	30	90	120
OR_5	30	90	120
OR_6	30	90	120

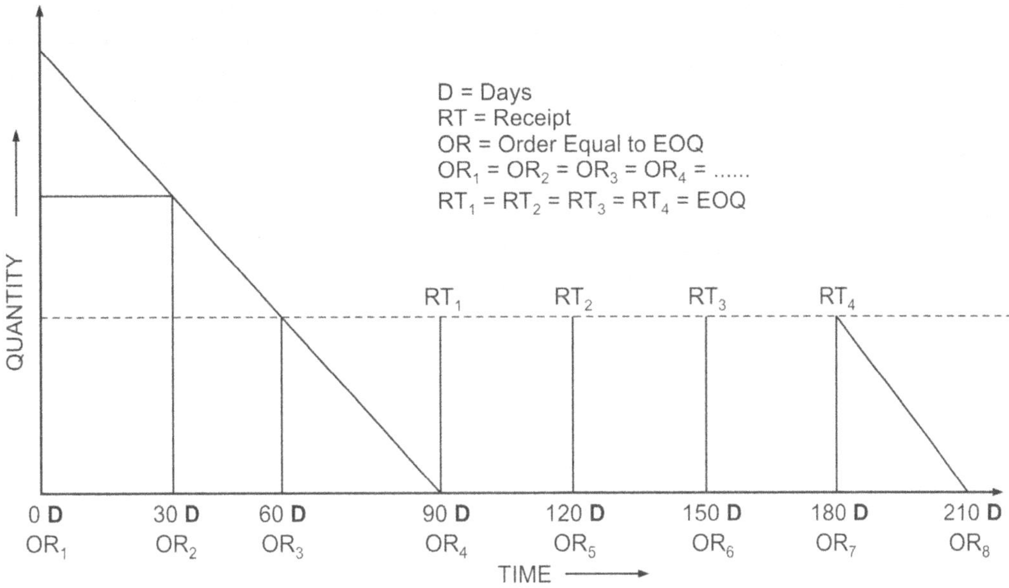

Figure 17.5 Inventory Replenishment when Lead Time Consumption Quantity is Greater than Economic Order Quantity

DETERMINATION OF SAFETY STOCK

In the economic order system, the basic assumption made among other things is supply can be had as and when required

In majority of cases, such an idealistic situation does not just exist and we have to take decisions with lesser knowledge and more uncertainty.

Problems are generally attributed to the following factors:

- Lead time is not constant and can increase without notice.
- The consumption rate may increase.

These two situations may lead to "shortages". Conversely if consumption rate or lead time reduces, we land up in a situation of "over stocking". Inventory manager has to take note of these variations and inventory system should be developed in such fashion so as to optimize between over stocking and under stocking costs and decide on the requirements of average inventory and safety stock. This forces him to deviate from simple economic order quantity model.

The term 'safety stock' is being used more in general way to take care of requirements of lead time and increase in lead time and consumption rate during lead time.

Different authors have used terms in different context leading to confusion viz.

- Minimum stock
- Safety stock
- Buffer stock
- Insurance stock
- Contingent stock
- Review level stock
- Reserve stock etc

Whatever be the terminology used by different authors, the purpose of safety stock is the lower limit below which stocks should not normally be allowed to fall under normal circumstances. **Safety stock may be compared to a 'suspension' system of an automobile.** Safety stocks absorb ups and downs in consumption and delivery period, just as leaf spring absorbs bumps due to uneven road surfaces.

In order to have clarity from confusion, **Prof. P Gopala Krishnan** used certain taxonomy for lead time consumption quantity, consumption during increase in lead time and also increases in the consumption rate as well. These requirements are met through:

- Buffer
- Reserve
- Safety stocks

This terminology later adopted by the **Indian Institute of Materials Management,** a premier professional body in the field of Materials Management in India, though this stock has been variously referred.

Buffer: provides for average consumption during average lead time.

Reserve: provides for increase in consumption rate during the lead time.

Safety: provision for possible increase in lead time.

Buffer Stock

Buffer stock provides for normal consumption during average lead time, we can obtain its value directly by multiplying average lead time by average consumption rate.

Therefore, buffer stock = Average lead time × average consumption during lead time.

For example average lead time is 9 weeks and average consumption during lead time is 100 units per week then buffer stock would be $9 \times 100 = 900$ units.

Reserve Stock

Reserve stock protects against variations in the consumption pattern. When dealing with consumption control, we observe that the pattern for majority of items will follow normal distribution curves with their respective means and standard deviations. But usually consumption patterns are in terms of daily or weekly or monthly data and the lead time will be a multiple factor of this span. Then, to find the standard deviation in consumption for lead time period, we have to multiply the standard deviation of given time span by square root of multiplying factor

Suppose the standard deviation in consumption for a month is 100 and lead time is 4 months.

Then, standard deviation for the lead time period = $100 \times \sqrt{4} = 200$ units.

The consideration of under stocking and over stocking costs enables us to specify the service level and is given by:

$$\frac{Ku}{(Ku + Ko)}$$

Where Ku is cost of under stocking and Ko is cost of over stocking. This is also given by cumulative probability. Therefore to find reserve stock, we decide on service level.

Reserve stock = $SD\sqrt{LT} \times$ Ordinate of service levels

Thus, if we decide on a 99 percent service level, the corresponding ordinate is 2.3 approximately. For a service level of 99.9 percent level, the ordinate is 3.1 approximately.

It could be seen from the above example:

- For a service level of 99 percent, the reserve stock is $100\sqrt{4} \times 2.3 = 460$ units.
- When service level is 99.9 percent, the reserve stock would be $100\sqrt{4} \times 3.1 = 620$ units.

So, buffer stock provides for normal rate of consumption during lead time, reserve stock provides for reasonable maximum usage.

Safety Stock

Lead time is not constant and varies over certain range of days. We have to provide for any possible increase by means of safety stock. Maintaining data on past behaviour of lead time can do this. Safety stock is given by average demand during maximum delay multiplied by probability of its occurrence i.e., we are taking expected value of requirement.

Thus, safety stock = Average demand during maximum delay . probability of its occurrence

For example, if lead time is 10 weeks, consumption during lead time is 100 per week. The maximum delay that occurred was 2 weeks and its probability of concurrence to be 0.25. Then safety stock will be $2 \times 100 \times 0.25 = 50$ units.

PRACTICAL INVENTORY SYSTEMS

Frequently used inventory systems are: Perpetual Inventory System (Q model) and Periodic Inventory System (P model).

Two major variables have to be borne in mind while establishing an inventory system. They are:

1. Ordering quantity
2. Frequency of the ordering process.

If one of variables is held constant, the other tends to fluctuate. Perpetual inventory system holds order size constant and lets the frequency of ordering fluctuate according to demand requirements. Where as periodic inventory system holds the frequency of ordering constant by establishing a fixed period and lets the order size fluctuate according to demand requirements.

PERPETUAL INVENTORY SYSTEM (Q SYSTEM)

This system is also known as Order Point System or Constant Review System. In this system, **whenever the stock is depleted to re order point (ROP) or re order level (ROL), an order for a fixed quantity is 'triggered' off.** The re order point is set as under. It is a sum of buffer, reserve and safety stocks. System requires constant review to see whether a particular stock reached ROP. Quantity ordered will obviously be of Economic Order Quantity. Demand fluctuations are met by varying order period. Thus if there is a faster consumption, next order will be placed earlier. Consumption during lead time, requirement during extended lead time, and increased consumption during lead time is catered. Figure 17.6 illustrates the concept of Q model inventory system.

It can be seen from the figure that **ROP is equal to sum of buffer, reserve, and safety stocks.** Whenever stock level touches ROP, an order equal to EOQ is placed. This is shown on the time axis (X-axis) by OR_1; the ordered quantity is received at RT_1; by that point of time, stock has reached 'reserved' stage. In this situation, the consumption rate and lead time have behaved as anticipated. In the next stage, RT_2 is received before stock levels reached reserves. This shows that the time period between OR_2 and RT_2, the consumption rate and/or lead time is reduced or both but on the whole such fluctuations will be insignificant. If there is any frequent dipping into reserves, then the re order levels will have to be modified in tune with the fluctuations in demand and or lead time. **For efficient functioning of this system, continuous monitoring as to whether inventory level has reached ROP or not is most indispensable.**

Thus the information system, whether through manual or computer files should be well run without difficulty and stock levels should be compared with ROP levels and orders triggered off as and when necessary. In the present discussion, we have considered a position where LT consumption is less than EOQ. If it is greater than EOQ, then the system can be operated with the help of **'virtual**

stock i.e., the order for EOQ will be placed whenever the sum of stock on hand and stock on order touches the re order level.

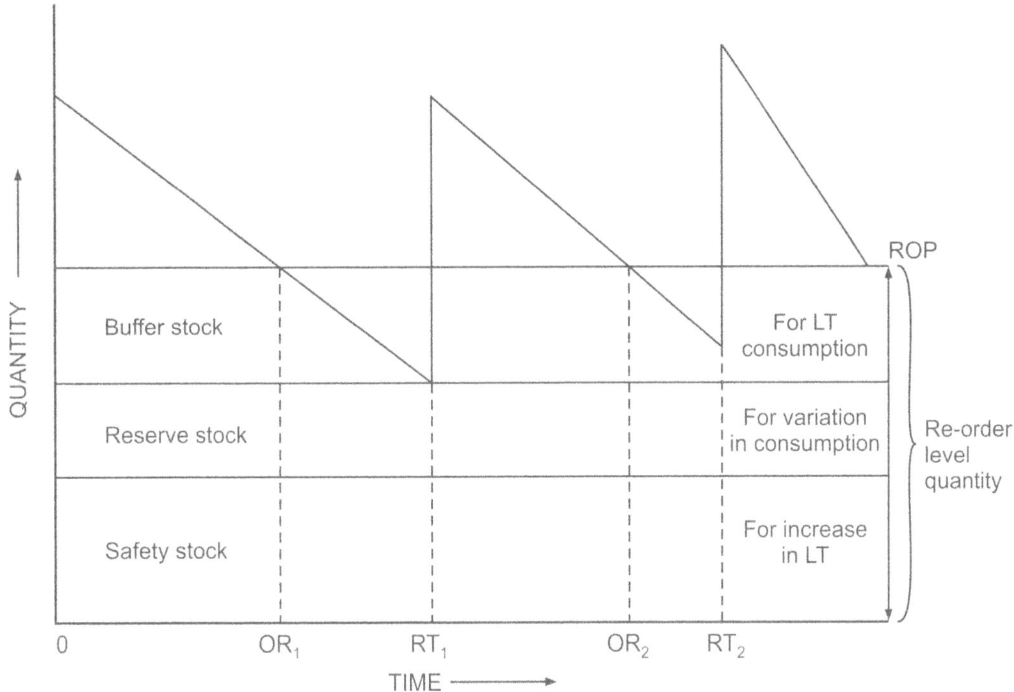

Figure 17.6 Perpetual Inventory System for a Single Item

Thus in Q system,

- **Re order Point** = Buffer + Reserve + Safety stocks
- **Maximum Inventory** = ROP + EOQ
- **Minimum Inventory** = (ROP – Buffer stock)
- **Average Inventory** = ½ × (ROP + EOQ + ROP – Buffer)

  = ROP + ½ × (EOQ – Buffer)

Prerequisites for efficient operation of Q system

Stock cards/computer files must be kept up to date and accurate for receipts and issues. Essentials of this system are:

1. Incoming materials and those returned from user departments must be deposited into appropriate bins and their stock must be posted for the physical quantities received.
2. Items should be issued in correct quantities to the requisitioners.
3. Balances on the stock cards should be periodically tallied with the physical stocks.
4. Entries must be made correctly at appropriate fields.
5. Data base must be free from clerical errors.

Operation of Q system inventory can be seen from Figure 17.7.

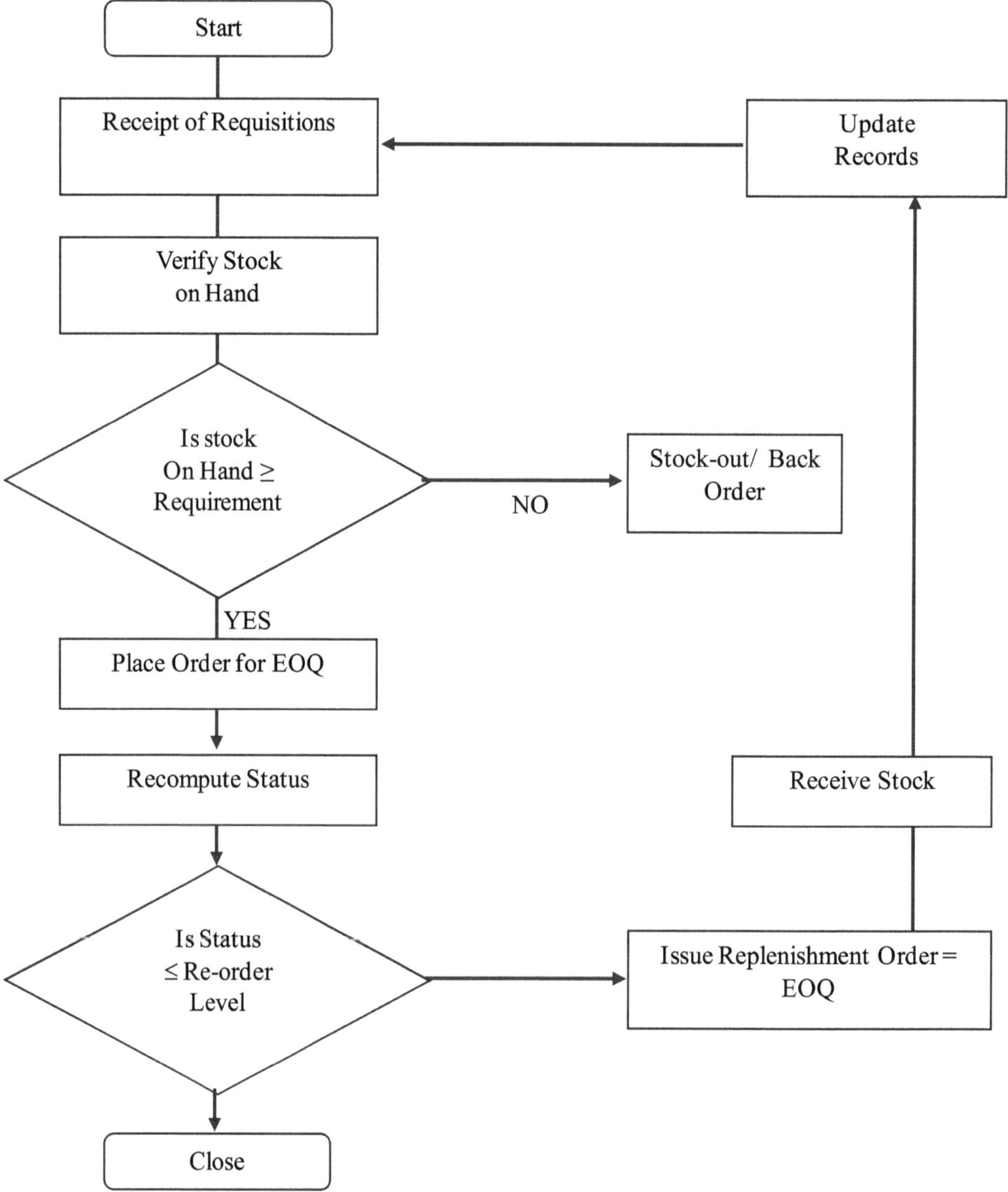

Figure 17.7 Flow Chart for Q Model Inventory System

ADVANTAGES OF Q MODEL INVENTORY SYSTEM

1. Fixed order size system with perpetual inventory records is excellent for high cost, high consumption items needing close control.
2. It calls for an efficient and meaningful order quantity; quite obviously it would be EOQ.
3. Safety reserve stocks are provided for increase in lead time and increase in consumption during lead time to avoid stock outs.
4. Relatively insensitive to forecast errors and parameter changes.
5. Less focus on slow moving items.
6. Provides for continuous control over physical stocks.

LIMITATIONS OF Q SYSTEM OF INVENTORY CONTROL

Perpetual system can have following weaknesses:

1. System requires constant monitoring results increasing operating costs.
2. It is not cost effective to adopt this system to control all categories of items. Hence its usage is mainly limited to 'A' class items.
3. The system is incapable unless order quantities, buffer, reserve, safety stocks are not periodically reviewed
4. Delays in posting of transactions can render the system useless for control.
5. Errors in posting can make the system unproductive.
6. Numerous independent orders result in frequent transportation and high freight changes due to part loads.
7. Large combined orders, which can frequently result in quantity discounts based on rupee value, must be unavoidable.
8. Since the re order points in different items occur at different times, they cannot be ordered at one time.
9. Replenishment orders are released at irregular intervals, which may be inconvenient to suppliers.
10. In case of items with long lead time, more than one order could be pending with supplier at a time and there is every possibility that he may fill up all pending orders at one time.
11. If managers do not take time to study inventory levels of individual items, order quantities tend to be established by junior staff who would like to play safe by overestimating usage rate.
12. Re order points order quantities and safety stocks may not be re-studied or changed for years.

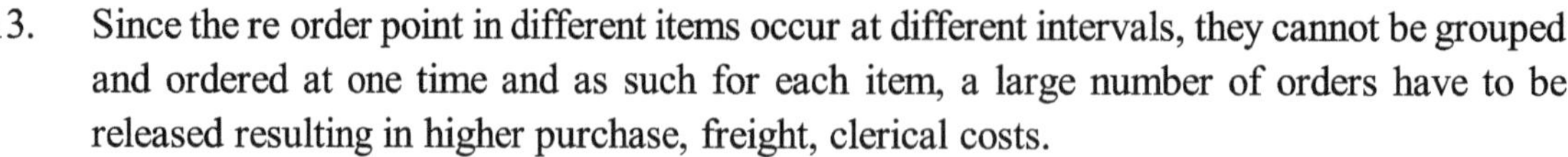

13. Since the re order point in different items occur at different intervals, they cannot be grouped and ordered at one time and as such for each item, a large number of orders have to be released resulting in higher purchase, freight, clerical costs.

PERIODIC INVENTORY SYSTEM (P SYSTEM)

This system is also known as fixed periodic review system or variable order quantity system or cyclical order system or fixed interval order system, it is more popularly known as P-system of inventory control.

In this system, the period between placements of orders is fixed, while order quantity is varied. Whereas in Q system, we have taken care of variations only due to increase in lead time, and change in lead time consumption; in P system, we have to, in addition, provide inventories for any increase in consumption between two orders and also consumption during the review period. Obviously the average inventory held in P system will be greater than that held in Q system. But the advantage lies in reduction of monitoring costs and facilitates bunching of orders. In periodic review system, number of orders in a year remains fixed because the review period is fixed. The review period is the order interval, fixed with the help of EOQ. Annual demand divided by EOQ gives number of orders in a year. Reciprocal of this number is the length of review period in units of years. Multiplying it by 12 or 52, review period is arrived at in terms of months and weeks respectively.

For example, review period in years can be fixed in the following manner:

$$\text{No. of orders} = \frac{\text{Annual Demand}}{\text{EOQ}} = \frac{D}{\text{EOQ}}$$

Where, D is annual demand.

Thus review period in years would be

$$= \frac{1}{\text{No. of Orders}}$$

$$= \frac{1}{D/\text{EOQ}} = \frac{\text{EOQ}}{D}$$

Replacing EOQ by its formula, we get review period in a year.

$$= \frac{\sqrt{\dfrac{2D \times C_O}{P \times C_C}}}{D}$$

$$= \sqrt{\frac{2D \times C_O}{P \times C_C} \times \frac{1}{D^2}}$$

$$= \sqrt{\frac{2C_O}{C_C} \times \frac{1}{P \times D}}$$

$$= \sqrt{\frac{\text{Constant}}{P \times D}} = \sqrt{\frac{\text{Constant}}{\text{Value of annual consumption}}}$$

Therefore, review period is inversely proportional to square root of annual consumption value.

Application of EOQ to set review period An Illustration

If demand (D) for an item is 2000 units per year, the price is Rs. 125 per unit, the cost of placing an order (Co) is Rs. 1000, and the yearly inventory carrying cost (Cc) is 20 percent, then

$$\text{EOQ} = \sqrt{\frac{2AD \times C_O}{P \times C_C}}$$

$$= \sqrt{\frac{2 \times 2000 \times 1000}{125 \times 0.2}} = 400$$

Optimum review interval between orders is therefore,

= EOQ/ D = 400/ 2000 = 0.2 years

= 2.4 months (i.e., every two months and one week or every 9 weeks)

Fixation of Desired Inventory Level (DIL)

It is also described as Target Stock Level (TSL) or Projected Maximum Level (PML) by some foreign authors.

Next stage in design of P model of inventory system is to establish 'Desired Inventory Level' (DIL). Every time the system is reviewed on the designated review date. Inventory on hand plus quantity on outstanding orders (i.e., the 'virtual stock') is compared with desired inventory level. Quantity ordered at each review date is given by the difference between DIL and the virtual stock.

Desired Inventory Level is given by the sum of:

1. Average consumption during average lead time plus review period.
2. Consumption during possible extension of lead time.
3. Excess consumption during average lead time and also review period.

Thus,

Buffer Inventory = Consumption Rate × [Average Lead time + Review Period (R.P.)]

Reserve Inventory = Standard Deviation × Square root of LT plus R.P. × Ordinate of Service Level (SD × $\sqrt{LT}$ + R.P × Ordinate of Service Level)

Safety Stock = Consumption during increase in lead time and probability of it's occurrence.

There is no change in safety stock as review period is fixed and not varied and hence we have to cater only to increase in lead time. But buffer stock is increased to cater to consumption both during review period and lead time. As average inventory carried is higher to meet increase in reserve stock and buffer for the review period consumption, the total cost of inventory in P system will be more than Q system.

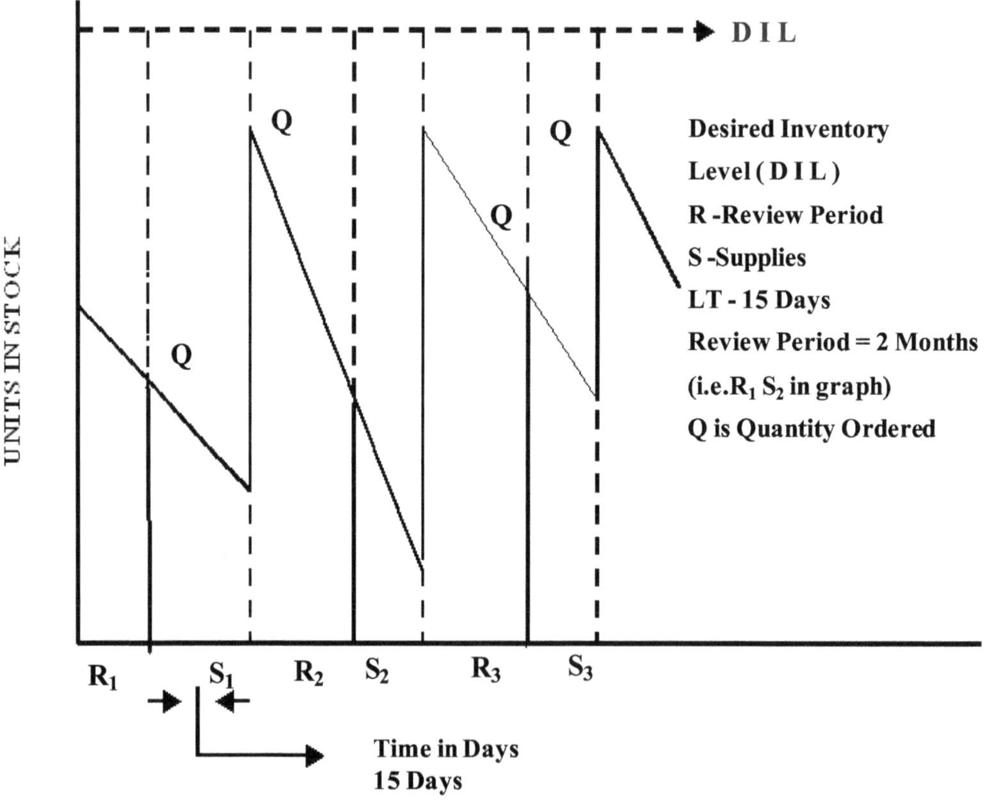

Figure 17.8 Graphic Representation of Periodic Model of Inventory Control

Perpetual inventory system monitors inventory items continuously and treats each item independently whereas periodic system treats them discretely and dependently. Frequently it is worthwhile to treat items in a dependent manner and order them in groups.

ADVANTAGES OF PERIODIC INVENTORY SYSTEM

1. Even distribution of workload over the year as review dates for each item/class of items can be actually laid down.
2. Periodic system is well suited for inventory control when the supply sources are few or when a central warehouse is used.
3. Reduction in ordering cost may be possible because items are processed under a single order.
4. Shipping costs may appreciably be decreased if an order is of suitable size such as truck load. Simultaneous ordering of several items can result convenient sizes.
5. Automatic data suppliers may offer quantity discounts exceeding a given volume of business. Grouping of several items in a single order may result in quantity discount.
6. Shipping costs may be significantly decreased if an order is of convenient size, such as container, higher capacity commercial vehicles.
7. It provides a stricter control on inventory, as at each review, order quantity varies, keeping the changing requirements in view.

LIMITATIONS OF PERIODIC SYSTEM

1. Presumption in periodic system is some sort of physical count, made at the time of review. In practice, records of transactions (indent/receipt slips) are available, but accuracy of the information system may require actual count for verification. (Lost or stolen or misplaced items are not apparent from transaction records.)
2. Some accommodation must be made for errors in transactions accounting for lost items, stock shrinkage etc.
3. Periodic system is completely defined by order period and the maximum inventory levels. In the periodic system, buffer stock represents protection against demand fluctuations both during the review period and lead time. This means that periodic system will require a larger safety stock for a given item than perpetual system.
4. It requires excessive and skilled manpower for reviews and adds to cost.
5. Reviews cannot be delegated to lower levels of staff.
6. It may lead to instability in the inventory levels due to overreaction of materials managers when fixing order quantities based on usage fluctuations and trend. As a result, order quantities may vary considerably during each review causing problems to suppliers.

The operation of P-model is shown in Flow chart 17.9.

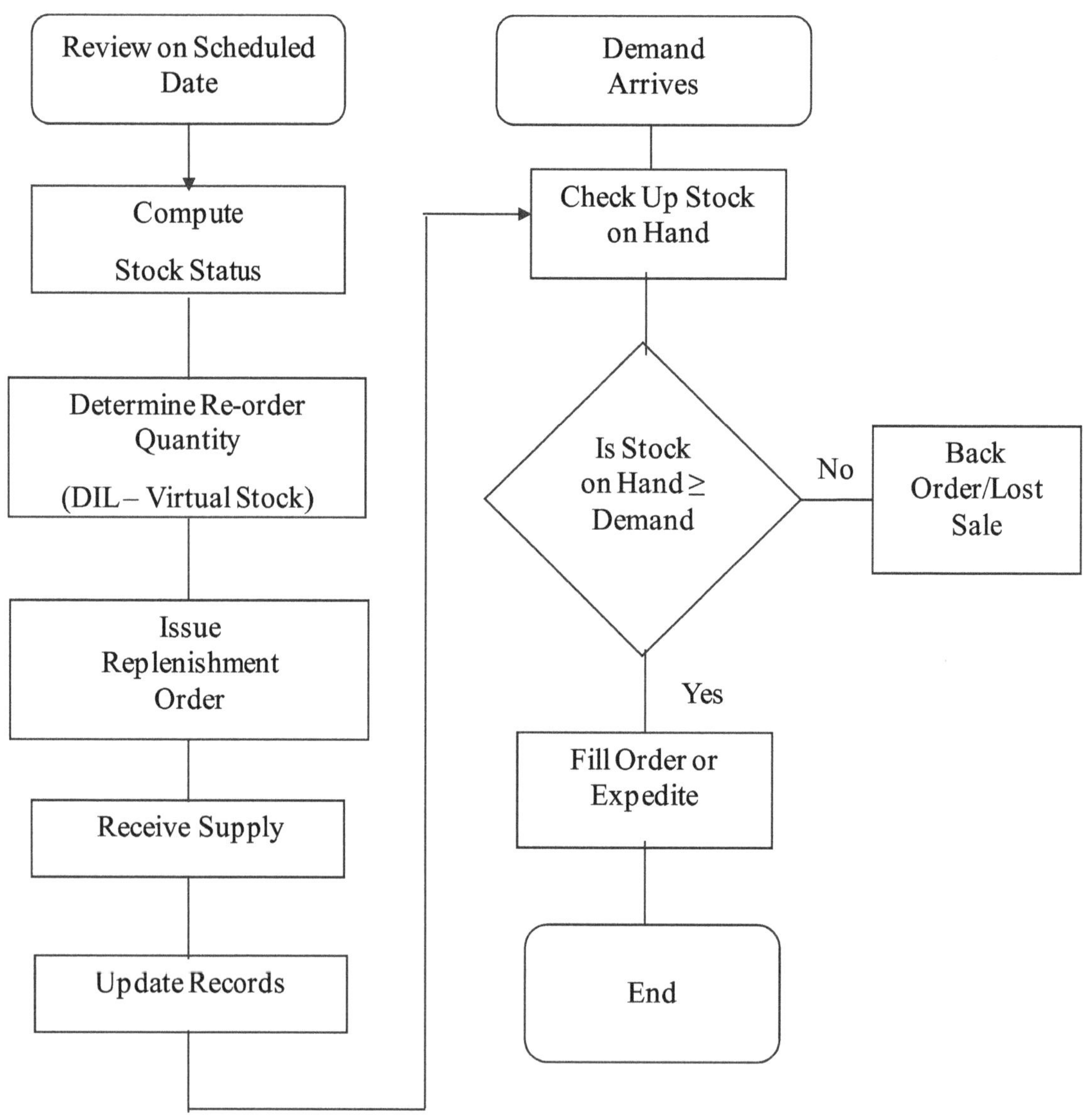

Figure 17.9 Flow Chart for P Model Inventory System

COMPARISON OF Q AND P SYSTEMS OF INVENTORY MODELS

Table 17.2 Comparison of Q and P systems of inventory models

Factor	Fixed Order Quantity System (Q)	Fixed Period System (P)
Replenishment action	Initiated when virtual stock falls to re order point.	Initiated on the designated review date at the end of prefixed interval, called review period.
Re-order quantity	Always same and is usually the economic order quantity.	Varies. It will be equal to the difference between DIL and virtual stock.
Safety stock	Kept to meet the demand during extended lead time.	Kept to meet demand during extended lead time.
Reserve stock	Meant for increased consumption during lead time.	Meant for increase in consumption during LT and RP.
Buffer stock	Meant for lead time consumption.	Meant for lead time consumption and RP.
Ordering quantity	Fixed	Varies
Ordering cycles	Varies. All items in stock are ordered according to different cycles.	Fixed. Review period is fixed for each individual item or for group of items.
Average inventory	Will be lower than in P system.	Will be higher than in Q system.

MATERIALS REQUIREMENT PLANNING MRP

Material Requirement Planning (MRP) refers to systems that keep track of requirements and plan operations of hospital in discrete time intervals. Usually the term includes explosion of net requirement on subordinate items.

Computer support is a basic requirement to operate system, even in smaller hospitals. With continuing expansion of the microcomputer and personal computer markets, many of them now operate in online, real time environment. Material managers must stay abreast of changes in computer support to remain competitive in healthcare industry of the future.

Forecasting models and other techniques, such as Material Requirements Planning (MRP), which have been well established in manufacturing industries, are modified for use in healthcare. Standardized material requirements are established for each diagnosis and procedure at each hospital. As projected admissions of patients and surgery cases are scheduled, computer network generates lists of required materials. The lists so generated are compared to stock on hand and on order quantities and the required purchase orders for replenishment of stocks are generated automatically by the system.

The use of direct computer to computer communication between healthcare facilities and major vendors is bound to increase with time. In addition, bar codes and **optical character recognition (OCR)** devices are used for streamlining the handling of the materials. This requires an increasingly effective interface between manufacturers and users of medical products.

Materials Requirement Planning (MRP) is defined as scientific method of planning for arriving at time phased requirement of materials for meeting demand at the stipulated time. Sometimes, this is also referred as dependent demand inventory system.

However, MRP uses a slightly different method in handling ordering problem. The order point system assumes that each item in inventory is independent of all other items and can be ordered independently. MRP treats items as if their priorities are dependent and it calculates future demand.

PREREQUISITE INPUTS FOR MRP

The three prerequisite inputs for making MRP work clearly are as follows:

1. Master schedules - what is planned?
2. Bill of material (BOM) - How it is done?
3. Inventory status - What has been done?

With these three inputs, MRP can determine what needs to be done in terms of what, how much, and when.

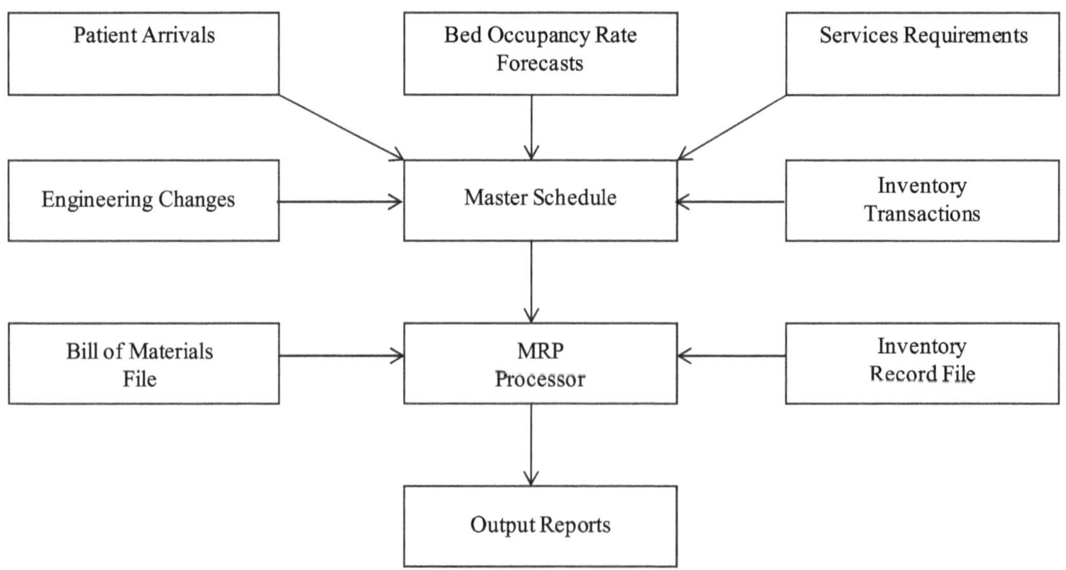

Figure 17.10 Structure of a Material Requirements Planning System

This diagram shows flow of data into the MRP processor and its conversion into useful output reports.

MRP OUTPUT REPORTS

Material requirements planning programme generates a variety of outputs that can be used in planning and management of operations. These outputs include:

1. Order release note, to place orders that have been planned by MRP system.
2. Reports showing planned orders to be released in future periods.
3. Rescheduling notices, indicating changes in due dates for open orders.
4. Cancellation notices, indicating cancellation of open orders because of changes in the master schedule.
5. Reports on inventory status.

In addition, secondary output reports can be generated by the MRP system at the user's option. These reports include:

1. Performance reports of various types, indicating costs, item usage, actual versus planned lead times, and other measures of performance.
2. Exception reports, showing deviations from schedule, orders that are overdue, scrap, and so on.
3. Inventory forecasts, indicating projected inventory levels (both aggregate inventory as well as item inventory) in future periods.

BENEFITS OF MRP

There are many advantages claimed for a well designed, well-managed material requirements planning system. Among these, the benefits reported by MRP users are the following:

- Reduction in Inventory: Industry circles have claimed a 30 to 50% reduction.
- Improved Customer Service: Some MRP proponents claim that late orders are reduced 90 percent.
- Quicker response to changes in demand and in the master schedule.
- Greater Productivity: Claims are that productivity can be increased by 5 to 30 percent through MRP.
- Labour requirements are reduced correspondingly.
- Better utilization of facilities.
- Increased revenue and reductions in expenditure.

Logic of MRP is a simple arithmetic equation $X = (A \times B) - C$ where X is action needed, A is a master production scheduled quantities, B is bill of materials quantities, C is inventories quantities available.

HOSPITAL REQUIREMENTS PLANNING

If hospitals are to survive in stiff competitive environment, healthcare institutions have to develop better cost finding and identification methods. From materials management perspective, it is also important to develop better forecasting and inventory control methodologies to help hospitals to lower the costs. Materials requirement planning (MRP) is a system long used by manufacturing firms as a way to plan for dependent demand items; good system for healthcare materials management provided that a computer is available. MRP systems logic is in fact applicable to healthcare requirements using MRP as a guide. **Hospital Requirement Planning System (HRPS)** was developed. Standardized materials requirements will be established for each diagnosis and procedure at each hospital. As projected admissions and surgery cases are scheduled, the computer will generate required bill of materials. These will be compared to on hand/on order quantities and replenishment orders will be generated automatically.

Thus the flow or consumption of materials will be tied directly to actual work flow of the institution. The necessity to build up these standard material requirements will act as a spring board to facilitate improved communication between materials managers and clinical managers. This will also speed up all parties appreciative of the unified nature of every one's input towards unswerving patient care. As a consequence, every healthcare facility will be motivated to adopt standard cost accounting practices. This will not only ensure critical care of the patient ("the product line") as well as provide an acceptable level of quality and at a profit. Efficient and effective healthcare institutions will have to adopt an inter disciplinary team approach to develop standards and managing costs. The members should include representatives from finance, clinical, medical records, and material management departments.

Use of direct computer to computer communication between healthcare facilities and major vendors will increase. In addition, use of **bar code** and **Optical Character Recognition (OCR)** devices will generally be used in reorganization of materials handling. The interface between manufacturers, distributors and users of medical products will be very effectual.

MRP in its wake brought many challenges and opportunities to hospital materials management professionals to ensure that it does not result in increased stock outs. It will be in the best interest of manufacturers, distributors and users to work together to find effective method that can satisfy every one's profit needs while meeting patient's need for quality care at reasonable cost.

Some features of the common types of inventory systems are shown in Table 17.3.

All the inventory systems have advantages and disadvantages as well as different areas of application.

INVENTORY SYSTEMS FEATURES

Table 17.3 Inventory System Features

Inventory Systems / Factor	Perpetual[a]	Two-Bin[a]	Periodic[b]	Optional Replenishment[c]	Material Requirements Planning[d]
Order Quantity	Fixed	Fixed	Variable	Variable	Variable
Reorder Point	Fixed	Fixed	Variable	Fixed	Variable
Review Period	Variable	Variable	Fixed	Fixed	Fixed/Variable
Demand Rate	Fixed/Variable	Fixed/Variable	Fixed/Variable	Fixed/Variable	Fixed
Lead Time	Fixed/Variable	Fixed/Variable	Fixed/Variable	Fixed/Variable	Fixed/Variable
Safety Stock	Medium	Medium	Large	Very large	Small/none

(Source: "Modern Materials Management" by Richard Tersine & Campbell)

Perpetual and two bin systems: Review inventory status with each transaction. If inventory I $\leq$ re order point, order EOQ quantity. If inventory I > re order point, do not order.

Periodic system: Review inventory status at intervals of T. Order quantity equal to DIL - virtual stock on each occasion.

Optional replenishment system (E, T, B): Review inventory status at intervals of T. If Maximum inventory is $\leq$ reorder point, order Maximum inventory level Virtual stock. If the inventory is > Re order point, do not order.

Materials requirement planning (MRP) system: Order items to meet production schedules.

WORKED OUT EXAMPLE 1

Sahayu Super speciality Hospital purchases crocin tablets from a manufacturer. It is one of their major consumption item costing 80 paise per tablet with an annual requirement of 3,20,000 tablets. Lead time for the item is 6 weeks. The demand for the item was normally distributed with a weekly average of 6150 units and a standard deviation of 600 units per week. The hospital wishes to maintain a service level of 95 percent. Lead time was fluctuating even though the normal lead time was taken as 6 weeks. The maximum lead time was 10 weeks and the cumulative probability of its occurrence i.e., 7, 8, 9 and 10 weeks was 0.25. Based on this information design, Q and P systems of inventory control for this item.

Sahayu hospital has estimated the normal cost of ordering as Rs. 120 and that the carrying cost as 30 percent per annum.

Step I

$$\therefore \quad EOQ = \sqrt{\frac{2 \times \text{Annual demand} \times \text{Cost of Ordering}}{\text{Price} \times \text{Inventory Carrying Cost as percentage on average inventory}}}$$

$$= \sqrt{\frac{2 \times 3,20,000 \times 120}{0.80 \times \frac{30}{100}}} = \sqrt{\frac{2 \times 3,20,000 \times 120 \times 100}{0.80 \times 30}}$$

= 17888.5 tablets say 17,900 tablets

The order quantity (EOQ) = 17,900 tablets

Step II Fixation of Re order Point or Re order Level (Q system)

It is given as sum of Buffer + Reserve + Safety stock. Buffer stock caters to the lead time consumption.

Buffer stock $= 6150 \times 6$ weeks

= 36900 tablets

Reserve stock caters to the variation in demand during lead time and is given as SD × LT × Ordinate of service level.

Standard deviation during lead time = $600 \times \sqrt{6} = 1469.69$ say 1470 tablets.

For a service level of 95 percent, the ordinate from the normal tables is 1.64.

Reserve stock = $1470 \times 1.64 = 2410.8$, say 2410 tablets

Safety stock = Average demand during maximum delay × Probability of the occurrence of the delay

$= 4 \times 6150 \times 0.25 = 6150$ tablets

Re order point = Buffer stock + Reserve stock + Safety stock

$= 36900 + 2410 + 6150 = 45460$ tablets

Step III

Under Q system, whenever stock on hand and stock on order (i.e. Virtual Stock) touches 45460 units, we have to release an order equal to EOQ, i.e., 17900 tablets

Step IV - Fixation of Review Period (P system)

Review period in weeks is given by 52 / No. of orders i.e., 52 / (AD / EOQ)

$$= \frac{52 \times EOQ}{AD} = \frac{52 \times 17{,}900}{3{,}20{,}000} = 2.90 \text{ weeks}$$

Step V

This has to be rounded off to 2 or 3 weeks based on the total costs incurred.

For 2 weeks review period, ordering cost = 52/2 × 60 = 1560.

Annual inventory carrying cost can be considered proportional to the average order quantity which is given by the demand divided by the number of orders.

Annual carrying cost = (3,20,000/26) × ½ × 0.80 × 0.30

= Rs. 1476.9 say Rs. 1477

∴ Total cost for a 2 weeks review period

1560 + 1477 = Rs. 3037

Similarly, for 3 weeks we obtain,

Ordering cost = 52/3 × 60 = Rs. 1040

and carrying cost = 3,20,000/17.3 × ½ × 0.80 × 0.30

= Rs. 2219.6, say Rs. 2,220

∴ Total cost for a 10 week review period = 1040 + 2220 = Rs. 3260

The total cost, when we adopt 2 weeks review period is lower than that of 3 weeks. Hence, we choose 2 week as review period. Now we have to calculate the desired inventory level (DIL).

DIL = Buffer stock + reserve stock + safety stock

Buffer is given by average consumption during lead time plus review period.

= 6150 × (6 + 2) = 49200 tablets

Reserve stock is $SD\sqrt{LT + RP}$ × Ordinate of service level

At 95 percent service level, the reserve stock will be

$$600 \times \sqrt{6+2} \times 1.64 = 2783.17 \text{ say } 2783 \text{ tablets}$$

Safety stock = Average demand during lead time × Probability of the occurrence.

$$= 6150 \times 4 \times 0.25 = 6150 \text{ tablets}$$

$$\text{DIL} = 49200 + 2783 + 6150 = 58133 \text{ tablets}$$

Thus, under P system, we review the stock status once in two weeks and top inventory up to 58133 tablets.

WORKED OUT EXAMPLE 2

Sandhya Super Speciality Hospital annual requirement of a medicine is 16000 tablets. Average lead time for this item is six weeks. Demand for the item is normally distributed with a weekly average of 310 and a weekly standard deviation of 50 tablets. Hospital stipulates a service level of 95 percent. The maximum lead time is ten weeks with cumulative probability of 7, 8, 9, 10 weeks; lead time is estimated as 0.25. Estimated cost of ordering is Rs. 600 and that of carrying charges as 30 percent per annum. Design P and Q systems of inventory control.

Step I Find out EOQ

$$\text{EOQ} = \sqrt{\frac{2 \times D \times C_o}{P \times C_c}} = \sqrt{\frac{2 \times 16{,}000 \times 600 \times 100}{1 \times 30}} = 8000 \text{ tablets.}$$

Hence, the Economic Order Quantity is = 8000 tablets.

Step II Q system

Fixation re order point for Q system of inventory model

Reorder points is = Buffer + Reserve + Safety

Buffer stock = average demand during average lead time

$$= 310 \times 6 = 1860 \text{ tablets.}$$

Reserve Stock = SD $\sqrt{LT}$ × Ordinate of service level

Standard deviation during lead time 50 ($\sqrt{6}$) = 122.5 tablets.

The ordinate from normal table for a service level of 95 percent is 1.64.

Thus, Reserve stock is (122.5) (1.64) = 201 tablets.

Safety stock is given by average demand during maxim in delay multiplied by the probability of occurrence of delay = 4 × 310 × 0.25 = 310 tablets.

Thus, ROP is 1860 + 201 + 310 = 2371 tablets.

Step III Operation of Q System

Whenever stock on hand and stock on order touches 2371 tablets, an order equal to EOQ at 8000 tablets have to be released (virtual stock).

Step IV P SYSTEM

Determination of Review Period

In P system, we have to determine the review/period which is

52 / Annual Demand / EOQ

$$= \frac{52}{16000 / 8000}$$

$$= \frac{52 \times 8000}{16000} = 26 \text{ weeks}$$

If this period is estimated in decimals, then we have to round off by considering the total of annual inventory costs and ordering charges.

Step V

Fixation of Desired Inventory Level (DIL)

DIL = Buffer + Reserve + Safety

Buffer in P system is given by average consumption during (lead time and review period)

$= 310 \times (6 + 26) = 310 \times 32 = 9920$ tablets.

This stock shoots up heavily since the review period is large denoting a low consumption value item.

Reserve stock caters to fluctuations in consumption during lead time and review. Standard deviation is (50 and ordinate of service level is 1.64).

$50 \times \sqrt{(6 + 26)} = 282.8$ units $\times\ 1.64 = 463.8$ say 464 tablets.

Safety stock is average demand in extension of lead time multiplied by probability of its occurrence, i.e. $310 \times 0.25 \times (10 - 6) = 310$ tablets as before.

DIL = 9920 + 464 + 310 = 10694 tablets.

Step VI

Every time stock is reviewed once in 26 weeks and top it to 10,500 tablets in the periodic review system. Obviously the stock level is higher as we are going to monitor the item only once in 26 weeks.

SUMMARY

Management's responsibility is to manage organization's assets, both human and nonhuman, in the light of defined goals. Inventory tends to have an impact upon all functional areas. It should not be surprising that the inventories are bothersome and contentious in view of their diverse influence.

Design of inventory management systems can be approached from diverse angles. Often emphasis is put on specific control models rather than the relevant systems. The decision to institute Materials Management system can be just as significant as the choice of the particular models for the system. Too frequently an organization is adapted to a mathematical model rather than vice versa. System designers must tread a straight and narrow path between the pitfalls of oversimplification and the muddle of over complication.

Problems of inventory and Materials Management are omnipresent and multifaceted. No simple formula takes into account all of the variables encountered in real situations. The value of good approximations in permitting a practical and understandable solution to a problem is often far greater than any loss caused by lack of accuracy or precision. Aggregate inventory analysis is not a precise science.

All inventory systems have advantages and disadvantages as well as different areas of application. The two bin system has application where constant review is not necessary because of low activity and/or low unit cost. Two bin system defers action until a reasonable size order can be placed, but it can result in relatively high freight costs. It is not always necessary to maintain stocks in two physical bins. The term 'two bin system' should be restricted to visual method of stock control instead of using two actual bins; one bin can be divided at 'two levels'.

In open access bin system, items are kept at the work point and staff members are free topick them as and when needed. Open access bins for materials may be used singly or in multiples situated around the units adjacent to the stocking point. The staff members help themselves to stocks without having to build records. This saves their time, which can be used for other useful activities and also eliminates coston unnecessary paperwork.

Impreat stock control is the simplest method of stock control and involves determination of amaximum level for the bin and periodic inspection of stock levels. The bin is topped up as required mmediately to the maximum level. Usually imprest stock control method is restricted to 'C' class items of low consumption value and those where replenishment can be obtained immediately.

Under minimum maximum system, the rate of usage of an item is determined by past experience and forecasts, and the length of time required to obtain delivery is secured from the inventory control records and from studies of alternative sources of supply. The system works fairly well if the inventory control executives generate orders, when the stock level touches average inventory level. However if the hospital inventory control executive uses maximum monthly demand instead of average monthly demand, amounts to provision of extra buffer stock.

In fixed order system (Q model), whenever the stock touches the re order point (ROP), an order for a fixed quantity i.e., EOQ is 'triggered' off. The re-order point is sum of buffer, reserve, and safety stocks. The system requires constant review to see whether the particular stock reached ROP. The perpetual system is well suited to high cost items as well as a class items where constant review is desirable.

In periodic review system, the period between the placements of orders is fixed, while order quantity is varied. This system finds applications where 1. there are many small issues of items from inventory, so that posting records for each issue is impractical, as in retail stores, supermarkets; 2. purchase orders are placed for many different items from one source or a central warehouse; 3. transportation and ordering costs can be reduced significantly by combining orders. The cost of maintaining the periodic system may be higher because of larger safety stock and the review cost.

Whereas the periodic system involves higher holding costs, the perpetual system tends to cause higher processing costs due to its close control over every transaction (inflow and outflow). The perpetual system with fixed order sizes will be more appropriate if: 1. The number of transactions is low compared to annual demand, 2. Transaction paperwork costs are low compared to ordering costs, 3. The unit cost of the item is high, 4. The stock-out cost is high, 5. Demand fluctuations are great and difficult to predict, 6. Holding costs are high.

If the above conditions are reversed, the periodic system will be preferred. Periodic system has been used extensively in the past. It is probably the most widely used system because of its application at the retail level. With the advent of computers and other less costly business machines, perpetual posting of inventory is becoming more prevalent. At the retail level, a device is replacing the cash register that electronically updates inventory levels from the point of the cash or credit transaction. Application of computers permits the manager to determine inventory levels and investment almost instantaneously. They also make available a substantial amount of information that was previously unavailable or too costly to obtain, with which they control inventory levels and make decisions. Development and implementation of an inventory control system to meet the needs of a specific organization is a customizing operation. Inventory management is not an island unto itself; the system must serve the goals of the organization as well as service objectives of other departments.

Material requirements planning system requires the smallest safety stock. When demand exhibits an upward trend, the perpetual is more desirable than the periodic system. With an upward trend, the perpetual system orders more frequently and the orders get larger and larger, and more safety stock is required.

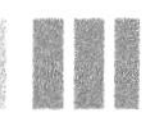

MRP is a scientific method of planning for arriving at time phased requirement of materials for meeting demand at the stipulated time. Sometimes this is also referred as dependent demand inventory system.

MRP calculates the requirement of materials and schedules of supply demand pattern. The usual questions asked in inventory management are what to buy, how much quantity to buy, when to buy, at what frequency to buy. EOQ gives answer to how much quantity to buy. And MRP is required to answer the other questions such as: when to buy and what frequency to buy. The prerequisite for MRP are master production schedules, bill of materials, inventory status records. MRP inputs covers master production schedules, production structure file or bill of materials file, and inventory records file. Structure of a material requirement planning (MRP) system comprises of revenue forecasts, patient arrivals, master schedule, engineering changes, inventory transactions, and inventory record files. If hospitals are to survive in the competitive environment, MRP is a good system for healthcare Materials Management. MRP as a guide in Hospital Material Requirement Planning (HRMP) system can be developed. The need to develop these standard material requirements will act as spring board for improved communication between materials managers and clinical managers and will also accelerate all parties understanding of interrelated nature of everyone's contributors to direct patient care.

REVIEW QUESTIONS

1. What is inventory control system? (a) What an effective inventory control system should accomplish? (b) What typical areas should be considered in developing a comprehensive inventory control system?
2. Define MRP. Installing MRP system tends to bring an integration of materials management, clinical management and vendors. Discuss.
3. What are the factors that influence the size of the safety factor to be used in setting in minimum and maximum inventory levels?
4. Define lead time. Assuming lead time as constant, how will you fix re order levels when,
   a. EOQ more than lead time consumption quantity
   b. EOQ equal to lead time consumption quantity
   c. EOQ less than lead time consumption quantity
5. Design 'P' and 'Q' systems of inventory control by means of a sketch. Describe the importance and limitations of two systems.
6. What is perpetual review system? How will you fix the re order level? And explain how the system operates with a diagram.
7. Describe how will you fix desired inventory level and explain how a periodic review system operates with the help of a diagram.

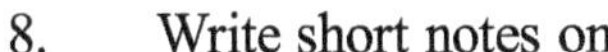

8. Write short notes on
    a) Derived demand
    b) Reorder point
    c) Minima maxima inventory system
    d) Desired inventory level
    e) Two-bin system
    f) Imprest stock control system
    g) Open access bin system
    h) Pre requisite inputs for MRP
    i) Buffer stock
    j) Reserve stock
    k) Benefits of MRP

PROBLEMS

1. Determine safety stock, reserve stock, and buffer stock for the data given below:

Normal usage	=	100 per week
Lead time	=	4 to 6 weeks
Minimum usage	=	50 per week
Maximum usage	=	150 per week
Re-order quantity	=	600 units

Also calculate the re-order level, minimum and maximum levels of inventory and also average inventory level.

Check your answer

Re order level = Safety stock + Reserve stock + Buffer stock

$$= 100 + 250 + 500 = 850$$

Minimum inventory level = S.S. + R.S. = 100 + 250 = 350 units

$$\text{Max inventory level} = \begin{pmatrix}\text{Minimum}\\ \text{level}\end{pmatrix} \times \begin{pmatrix}\text{Order}\\ \text{quantity}\end{pmatrix} = 350 + 600 = 950 \text{ units}$$

Average inventory level = (Min. level + Max. level) / 2 = (350 + 950) / 2 = 650 units

2. Veena Industries, manufacturers of computer peripherals, require certain item costing Rs. 3.75 each. The annual demand is 24,000 units. Average lead time is 6 weeks and the demand per week is 460 with a standard deviation of 50 units per week. The company stipulates the policy of maintaining a service level of 95% (K = 1.64). Though normal lead time is 6 weeks, it is fluctuating and maximum lead time that occurred is 10 weeks. The cumulative probability of its occurrence, i.e., 7, 8, 9, 10 weeks is 0.25. The ordering cost is Rs. 180 per order and the inventory carrying cost is 30% p.a. Based on the above information, design fixed order quantity inventory system and explains how it operates.

Check your answer

EOQ = 2771.28

Re-order level= 460 + 201 + 2760 = 3421 units

Operation of 'Q' model of inventory control

Whenever stock on hand falls below to re-order level of 3421 units, fresh order is placed for EOQ i.e., 2667 units.

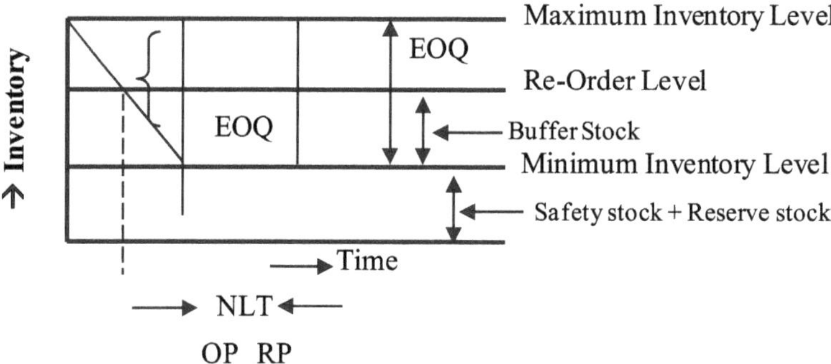

NLT – Normal Lead time : OP - Order point RP – Receiving Point

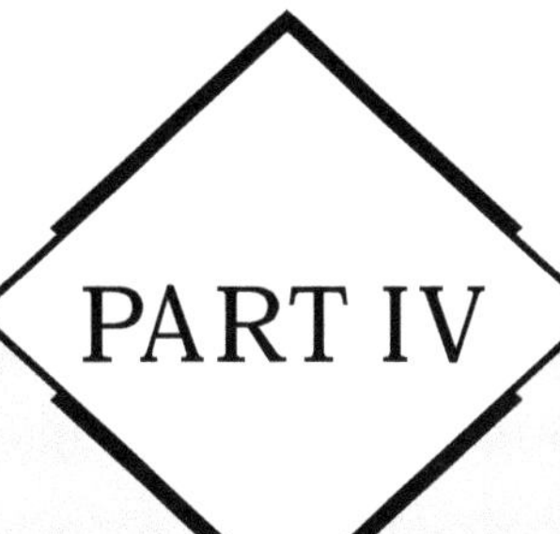
PART IV

PART - IV

Stores Organization

Contents

- *Introduction*
- *Stores Organization*
- *Centralized and Decentralized Stores*
- *Different Types of Stores in Hospitals*
- *Stores Organization in Hospitals*
- *Functions of Hospital Store*
- *Planning of Hospital Stores*
- *Indenting of Stores in Government Hospitals*
- *Functions and Duties of a Stores Incharge*
- *Control of Stores*
- *Location of Stores*
- *Summary*
- *Review Questions*

CHAPTER - 18

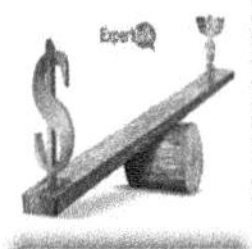
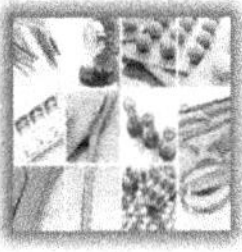
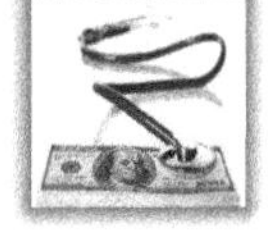
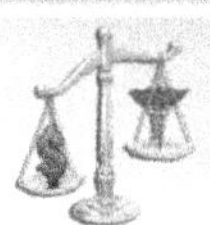

Stores Organization

INTRODUCTION

Work in a hospital is done by a large number of employees, each of whom has a specified task to peform. All the people concerned share the total quantum of work, all working towards a common objective or goal of patient care. In such a situation, each person must know precisely what he has to do. He must also know how to do it and when exactly it needs to be completed. One must also coordinate his work with that done by one or more of his colleagues in the organization. Such coordination may be with someone in the same department or in another department to whom he reports (i.e., who supervises his work or who is his boss); and also those persons who reports to him (i.e., who are his subordinates and for whose work he has overall responsibility). These requirements are met when we "organize" work. If precise definitions of work do not get laid down, no one will know who has to do what. Store is generally most neglected area in a hospital. This neglect includes lack of policies and systematic procedures. Without such policies and procedures stores operations reverts to a childhood game of 'hide and seek'. Upon receipt of requisition for goods "hidden" somewhere in store room, the store helpers have to "seek" many locations to find the items required.

Organization involves breaking down all the work necessary to achieve the objective into individual jobs or tasks, i.e., that which is capable of being done by one person; and providing a formal system of coordinating the efforts of various individuals involved. **Peter Drucker say's,** "Organization is not an end in itself, but a means to the end of business performance. Organization is an indispensable means to good management and a wrong structure can seriously impair business or even destroy it. **This structure must be designed so as to make possible the attainment of the objectives of a business in a most effective, efficient and economical manner."**

STORES ORGANIZATION

Traditionally, stores department had been attached to head of departments and even considered a part of concerned departments. Today, it has been recognized that departmental heads have interests which conflict with the basic objectives of inventory control. As such, the modern concept is to delink stores from user departments. Best practice is to place the stores under the materials manager and make it a part of materials department. Materials manager should have the same status as other senior departmental heads who report to the Chief Executive.

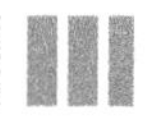

Stores organization may be defined as a systematic coordination and combination of efforts in a manner which would result in optimum efficiency with a minimum of expenditure. Some of its main tasks are formulation of a sound financial policy, efficient planning of work, effective supervision and control of personnel, receipt and distribution of various products. The way the stores department is organized will depend upon size and requirements of the organization. It may be a small store consisting of a manager, a supervisor, a couple of assistants and three or four helpers. On the other end of the scale, one may find a very big department headed by a senior executive with, may be, half a dozen or a number of stores for different types of products, or may be a large number of depots across the country. A typical organization chart of a store in a multi speciality hospital is given in Figure 18.1. The figure gives typical organization chart of stores department in a large multi speciality healthcare institution. Broad functions are given in the chart.

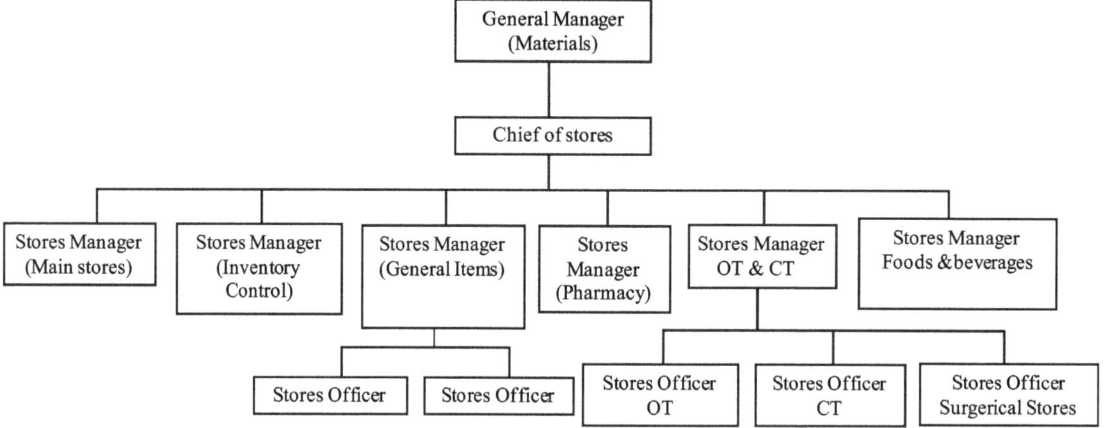

Figure 18.1 Typical Organization Chart of the Stores Department in a big Multi speciality Healthcare Institution

CENTRALIZED AND DECENTRALIZED STORES

Number of factors influence decision of centralized or decentralized stores. Some of them are administrative convenience, nature of materials, quantity of materials consumed, materials handling equipment etc. The structure of a stores department is a major factor in a hospital. A very big store having a large number of specialities may have a main store which can serve as a base, with decentralized stores for each division or unit of production, preferably located as near the unit as possible. Main store supplies to all other sub stores in the hospital. In the main stores, items are arranged department wise with a number of codes for each item groups. The range of items stored ranges between the most expensive items like pacemakers, arterial stents to low cost fast moving items such as soaps, tissue paper etc. Another possibility is that the main store can be completely eliminated and supplies delivered directly to the sub store.

A large multi speciality hospital like Apollo hospital a jubilee hills Hyderabad providing a variety of services may have a centralized warehouse at its hub location besides a large number of stock points or depots in various branches located in the city. A small hospital (say 100 bedded) on the other hand can have just one simple store from which the entire distribution can take place.

Centralization or decentralization then is a matter of convenience. However, one basic organizational feature must be observed. Entire stores set up should be under the unified control of one department with one chief of stores or controller of stores, as he is sometimes called in some organizations, in order to efficiently achieve objectives of the store.

Decentralized storage of nursing units can be broken down as shown below.

- **Linen stores:** for storage of linen supplies.
- **Clean miscellaneous stores:** for stocking miscellaneous clean items.
- **Clean holding place:** to hold portable carts or wall hung module filled with clean supplies.
- **Clean utility:** for preparation of supplies before using them on patients.
- **Soiled utility:** place to keep soiled supplies.
- **Soiled holding:** place to hold portable carts or wall hung modules with soiled supplies.
- **Medicine rooms:** storage/preparation of medicines.
- **Dietary stores:** storage of dietary carts and meal nourishment preparation.

Advantages of a Centralized Store

1. A much wider range of goods is provided for all users than is possible in a smaller store.
2. Inventory can be minimum, this is especially so, in the case of tools, jigs fixtures, equipment and spares.
3. Better control is possible.
4. Economy in storage space is possible. Goods in bulk will occupy less space.
5. Bigger storehouses enable use of better and more modern handling methods (mechanical or automatic).
6. Reduction in duplication of expensive equipment.
7. Delivery at a single point reduces cost of delivery.
8. Receipt and inspection of goods can be more efficiently organized.
9. Opportunities of standardization are enhanced.
10. Stock turnover is increased and the probability of deterioration during storage is correspondingly reduced.

11. A single accountable person in charge of total system that cuts across all the department boundaries, Policies governing function clearly stated and responsibilities are carefully delineated to hospital materials management personnel resulting in an unified management.

12. Nursing personnel is solely made responsible for patient care and supply functions are done by trained non medical personnel thereby improving personnel efficiency.

13. Unnecessary duplication of records that takes place in decentralized stores can be avoided resulting in cost effectiveness as fewer personnel will be needed for managing the stores.

    For example, one may have ten different Kardex cards for one material stocked in ten places. Similarly, accounting work is multiplied.

14. The steps and measures in each function are spelled out therefore, a particular function is performed the similar way regardless of its location, there by achieve functional and procedural uniformity.

15. Ensures the quality of supplies and equipment product standardization reduces total number of items in inventory.

Disadvantages of a centralized Store:

1. Extra handling is involved and staff will be required for transport of material from main stores to the various user departments or nursing stations or units

2. If system is not well organized, there can sometimes be severe shortages at work places causing unnecessary interruptions to functioning of the hospital.

3. Inefficiency can also result in user departments/ nursing stations keeping some buffer inside the unit which can lead to cluttering of space and to pilferage because of the absence of security.

4. More internal documentation may become necessary.

5. If a fire accident occurs, there is a bigger risk, losing of entire stocks lost and bring entire operations of hospital to halt.

6. It calls for total organizational change. “It requires higher degree of management effort and expertise than a decentralied store.

7. Total organizational change is needed in retaining personnel and reorientation and a redefinition of all tasks and responsibilities; a completely new state of mind toward materials management.

Advantages of Decentralized Store:

1. Speedy issue of material, eliminating long waiting that takes place in centralized system.

2. After sanitization and decontamination of supplies and equipment, it is immediately used in that department without further transportation. Maintaining principles of asepsis

3. Since patient care is personalized service, it is beneficial to let the physician have the supplies and equipment that he needs; where he needs it and when he needs it as in the case of assembly type production.

 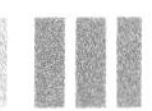

4. Extra transportation from stores to various user departments or nursing stations is minimal.
5. More internal documentation may not be necessary.
6. User departments or nursing stations, keeping unofficial inventories can be minimized.
7. Cutting space and shrinkage of material can be avoided.

Disadvantages of Decentralized Store:

1. Since different procedures are practiced in different departments, it is difficult to establish a standard of performance and measure quality of patient care uniformly.
2. Departmental objectives might come in conflict with institutional objectives when taken as a whole.
3. The islands unto themselves phenomenon intensifies, interdepartmental competition for scarce resources and causes the failure of recognised communication channels and creation of informal communication channels.
4. With each department pursuing its own functions individually, the fixed cost of performing a job or running a machine is duplicated many times. Economies of scales is foregone.
5. Usage is hard to measure; obsolescence is plentiful; pilferage and /or shrinkage are generally higher and are uncontrollable.
6. Economy in storage space is foregone in absence of bulk storage.
7. Delivery at multiple points increases costs of delivery.
8. Opportunities for standardization are bleak.

The degree to which departmental and sub stores are necessary depends upon size and rate of growth of a hospital and upon physical spread. The degree of decentralization depends also to a greater extent than is usually admitted on the personalities involved in the service given by the central stores.

DIFFERENT TYPES OF STORES IN HOSPITALS

It will be quite apparent; there can be myriads of types of materials which are stored depending upon the type and complexity of the industry which the stores serve.

There can be small items like nuts and bolts or heavy items like steel plates, there can be gases in cylinders (like LPG or medical gases), powders, liquids some of them dangerous like acids and alkalis or inflammables, like petrol and so on. The variety is almost infinite.

Very broadly stores are divided into two types on the basis of following considerations:

1. Functional i.e., depending on the use to which the materials are put to.
2. Physical i.e., in terms of size and distance like central stores, sub-stores and so on.

Functional Stores

Functional stores are further classified into different types depending upon the nature of goods stored. Some of the functional stores in hospitals are shown in Table 18.1.

Table 18.1 Types of Functional Stores in Hospitals

Pharmacy stores	Cath lab stores
Foods and beverages stores	Refrigerated store
General stores	Flammable materials stores
Linen stores	Dehumidified stores
Surgical stores	Transit
Packing stores	Transit stores
Receipt stores	Lab stores
Quarantine stores	Housekeeping stores
Finished goods stores	Consumable stores
Stationary stores	Equipment stores
Spare parts and maintenance stores	Medicines room: Storage/ preparation of medicines

Physical Considerations

There can be various types of stores based on the quantity of stocks held or distance from the point of usage like,

1. Central stores
2. Sub stores
3. Departmental stores
4. Group stores
5. Transit stores
6. Site stores

1. **Central stores:** Central stores will include all the items that have been procured and stored but not dispensed to the user departments but have been stored for distribution and use at a later date. The word "central" only denotes that it serves various units each of which may have separate sub stores or departmental stores. Central stores also exist in multi location hospitals operating under hub and spokes concept.

   One of the problems in having a central store is the handling costs involved in transferring materials to sub stores or nursing centres. Usually therefore, central store is located at the point of greater usage.

   One of the main control factors in the establishment of a central store is to ensure that unnecessary inventories are not built up by the sub stores or for that matter by the central stores.

   For purposes of inventory levels, the total stocks in the sub stores and the central stores should be considered as one.

2. **Sub stores:** Sub stores are located at the place of usage. It can be even within the nursing stations.

3. **Departmental stores:** This serves a department of a hospital. For example in a hospital, surgery requirements are served by separate store or an in patient pharmacy. The reason behind this is that each requires separate type of materials. The store becomes a specialized store. Actually there is a little difference between 2 and 3.

4. **Group stores:** In some hospitals, it can happen that several hospitals belonging to the same group are all in one compound. For example in Hyderabad, the Apollo General Hospital and the Apollo Cancer Hospital belonging to the same management are located in the same campus. One store can serve all these units. This is called a group stores.

5. **Transit stores:** As its name implies, these are stores where stores are stored for a temporary period.

6. **Site stores:** This is a store usually at a project site containing building or construction materials like machinery, cement, steel, tools, etc.

STORES ORGANIZATION IN HOSPITALS

Stores management is vital in hospitals since uninterrupted supply of many items for patient care is to be ensured at all times. There is hardly anything which will not be required in a hospital sometimes or the other.

Hence, it becomes obligatory on the part of hospital materials manager to see that:

1. All the stores are procured in adequate quantities but not in quantities so as to lock up too much capital.
2. Stored properly so that they do not get damaged during storage.
3. Used properly to ensure turnover by utilizing on FIFO stocks basis and storing fresh stocks.
4. Above all, accounting meticulously for all items.

FUNCTIONS OF HOSPITAL STORES

Primary functions of hospital stores are as follows.

1. Storcs planning
2. Receive materials as ordered
3. Inform indenting departments regarding the arrival of stores
4. Inspection of materials
5. Record keeping

6. Storage and preservation
7. Issue of materials against authorized indents
8. Bill processing of materials received
9. Physical safe custody of materials
10. Process purchase requisition for items
11. Condemnation of shelf expired items and disposal
12. Dispatch
13. Clearing and forwarding
14. Stock taking and audit

PLANNING OF HOSPITAL STORES

Hospital stores may be planned according to nature of material to be stored.

1. **Medical and drug stores:** It consist of emergency drugs, general drugs, special drugs, medical gases, chemicals capital items, consumables and so on.
2. **Surgical stores:** These store bandages, gauzes, sutures, instruments, equipments, rubber goods, glass items, cotton and general surgical items.
3. **General stores:** The items of general stores are cleansing materials like soaps and detergents, enamel wares, ward/general furniture, small electric items and so on.
4. **Linen stores:** Linen stores include textiles, synthetic fabric, woolen items, furnishings and their house keeping items.
5. **Stationery stores:** All the stationery items including medical forms and papers for medical documentation etc.
6. **Dietary stores or food and beverages:** Vegetables, fruits, tinned items, dry rations, dietary items, grocery or kitchen items etc.
7. **Engineering and maintenance:** It consists of spare parts of civil, electrical, mechanical and electronic items.

INDENTING OF STORES IN GOVERNMENT HOSPITALS

Following are different categories of indents made by different departments and sent to purchasing authority in the hospital.

1. Annual indents
2. Supplementary indents
3. Emergent indents

Annual Indents

It is a forecast of requirements for the ensuing financial year. It should be prepared carefully each year after taking into account the existing stock position, last one year's average consumption (mean of last three years) and quantities required for the next year.

It should give complete specifications of each item, likely source of procurement and approximate cost which should not exceed the financial allocations of the department for that year.

Annual indent should be submitted by 1st January each year for ensuing financial year. Indents for consumable and non consumable stores should be submitted separately.

Supplementary Indents

Normally, there should be no supplementary indents. However, if needed, it should be submitted separately, provided it is certified that items included therein could not be foreseen at the time of submission of the annual indents and are urgently required during the year.

Supplementary indents may be submitted by 1st August of every year provided the limit of financial allocation for the year has not exceeded.

Emergent Indents

This may be avoided as far as possible, and should only be resorted to when the demand is of immediate, inescapable nature and funds of the departmental allocation are available.

All demands should be signed by the officer or doctor in charge of the department concerned before forwarding to the purchase department.

An emergent indent may be submitted at any time of the year with approval of the competent authority.

Each indent should be prepared in triplicate, one kept in the department, and two sent to the purchase department.

Indenting Groups

In a healthcare institution, items in each indent may be grouped as detailed below:

1. Surgical instruments and equipment
2. Medical stores/chemicals/stains and dyes
3. Linen goods
4. Stationery stores items
5. General store items
6. Diet items

7. Engineering items Electrical goods, electronic instruments
8. Rubber goods
9. Furniture Wooden, Steel
10. Glass wares Laboratory equipment
11. Optical instruments and equipment
12. Photographic materials
13. Housekeeping items
14. Miscellaneous items e.g., spare parts for maintenance of plant and equipment

FUNCTONS AND DUTIES OF A STORES INCHARGE

Stores incharge has an important contribution to make. Productivity of the hospital to a large extent is influenced by the efficiency of the stores function. In a large hospital, broad spectrum materials have to be received and issued. Stores keeper has to ensure that incoming materials are kept as close to the user departments as possible to reduce materials handling, issuing delays and idling of operations for want of materials. He also has the responsibility to keep track of consumptions. As regards functions and duties, there is a difference between the functions of staff and their duties and activities. Duties can be looked upon as the narrow tactics of the operation, while the function can be compared with the larger strategy over a broad field.

For example, in a large multi speciality hospital store, duties of staff may be clearly divided. Order pickers will be responsible for collecting and assembling orders, checkers for counting and checking, and stores assistants for clean and good housekeeping of the hospital. The storekeeper has to maintain general supervision of various activities However, all have common functions associated with stores, such as the careful preservation of materials, observing any faults and rectifying or reporting them, etc.

Functions and duties

- To plan an efficient storage of items so as to put the available space to maximum use.
- To receive materials and keep them in store/stock room in proper manner.
- To issue materials to proper persons against properly authorized requisitions.
- Being a custodian of store, he must keep quantity account of each item showing receipts, issues and balances.
- To carry out surprise checks and ensure that bin card balances tally with physical balances.
- To ensure that all items of materials are in good usable condition.

- To provide stores officer on daily basis, list of critical items whose stock is likely to be exhausted. (Store officer in turn will inform purchase department for appropriate action.)
- To help management in inventory control by preparing lists of non moving and slow moving items.
- To take all possible precautions to prevent pilferage, theft and malpractices.
- To maintain store in a tidy manner by keeping items in their respective bins.

Other allied functions

- Projection of budgetary requirements.
- Planning and execution of stock checking activities.
- Communicate the purchase department about requirements.
- Maintain efficient and effective material handling system.
- Help in standardization and variety reduction.
- Minimize obsolescence, surplus, scrap through proper codification, preservation and handling.
- Coordination with other departments for various stores function activities including demand forecasting.

CONTROL OF STORES

Function of stores control is perhaps the least glamorous of all aspects of Materials Management and is yet so necessary. It involves receiving of materials, storing them properly and issuing them to different user areas against the duly authorized stores requisition.

Two basic systems may be used in physically controlling stores materials. They are **closed and open systems.**

Closed System

In this system, all materials are physically stored in a closed and controlled area to exercise physical control of store items by keeping them under lock and key. None other than the concerned store personnel are permitted to the store area.

Materials are received and issued from this area only after producing authorized documents. This type of system is being followed in hospitals and is designed to afford maximum physical security to stores.

Open System

This system is used in manufacturing industries where there is high, repetitive, mass production and type of operation requires continuous demand for the same materials. No store room exists and stores are received and kept as close to the point of user area as is physically possible.

In hospitals, closed system is usually followed since storage of materials is inevitable as the needs of daily utilization are variable and emergency needs are not always foreseeable. The hospital stores should be centralized for better control of materials.

LOCATION OF STORES

Hospital stores have normally been found located in areas which are either unusable by other departments or are not suitable for other functions of hospital.

Basement is one such area being used as stores. They are poorly designed for use as storage facilities with low ceilings, exposed pipes, difficult access and faulty flow design.

Storage facilities however have been given higher status and priority in a number of healthcare institutions

Location of stores should be such that it fulfils the following:

- An item should be easily accessed and when required it should be possible to issue oldest stock first (FIFO principle).
- Receipt and issues of materials within least possible time.
- Cost of transportation is economical.
- Materials are saved from pilferage, theft and fire.
- Ensures strict control over the movement of stock.
- Unnecessary fatigue and monotony of staff is avoided.
- Easily accessible to all the user areas of hospital.

For achieving the above aim, it is necessary that store building should be near to the area where the materials are required. While selecting a suitable site for a store, due consideration should be given to temperature, humidity and lighting arrangements. There should also be scope for future expansion of the store.

Role of Store Keeper is similar to Cashier

The letter M in material connotes money in kind. A cashier performs identical function as that of store keeper. The cashier has to receive cash and make disbursement, whereas store keeper receives and issues materials to user department. A comparision between store keeper and cashier is given in Table 18.2.

Table 18.2 Comparision between Store Keeper and Cashier

Store Keeper	Cashier
Receives various inputs required for operations of the hospital	Receives money from financial institutions IP, OP and casuality departments.
Issues materials to various user departments based on the requisition slips authorized by competent authority.	Makes payments to customers i.e., refund of excess payment collected or suppliers of materials and service providers.
Keeps track of materials movement in and out of hospital.	Keeps vigil on money flow in and out of hospital's different departments and bank.
Takes preventive measures to control pilferage of stock items.	Prevents any theft of money or fraud.
Store keeper maintains complete records of stores items received by the hospital and issued.	Keeps up to date and accurate record of all monetary transactions.
Check the material on their receipt and ensures that they are received are in good condition.	Cashier receives and counts the money on receipt and makes sure the currency is genuine.
On receipt and acceptance of materials, arranges them at the appropriate place allotted to the item.	Keeps money in appropriate place and in safe custody
Deals with variety of materials that are used for day to day operation of hospital.	Deals with cash only.

In addition to the above similarities, there are certain dissimilarities viz., cashier works in a small room environment, whereas, the store keeper operates, over a larger area. Discrepancies in stocks take long time to detect as compared to cash discrepancies.

SUMMARY

Structure of stores department is a major factor in a hospital. The main store supplies to all other sub stores in the hospital. In the main stores, items are arranged department wise with a number of codes for each item, groups. Entire stores set up should be under a unified control of one department with one chief of stores or controller of stores, as he is sometimes called in some organizations.

In order to achieve the objective of efficiency, stores are classified into different types depending upon to nature of goods stored. Some of the functional stores are central stores, substores, departmental stores, group stores, transit stores, and site stores etc.

Central stores will include all items that have been procured and stored but not dispensed to the user departments but have been stored for distribution and use at a later date. Central stores also exist in multi location hospitals operating under hub and spoke concept.

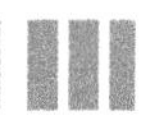

For purposes of inventory levels, the total stocks in the sub stores and the central stores should be considered as one. Sub stores are located at the place of usage. Departmental store serves a department of a hospital. It becomes a specialized store. Sometimes, it is felt that one store can serve all these units. This is called a group store. Transit stores are stores where goods are stored for a temporary period. Site store is a store usually at a project site containing building or construction materials like cement, steel, tools, etc.

Primary functions of hospital stores are planning, informing indenting departments regarding the arrival of stores, inspection of materials, and issuance of materials against authorized indents. Hospital stores may be planned according to the nature of stores. Surgical stores store bandages, gauzes, sutures, instruments, equipments, rubber goods, glass items, cotton and general surgical items. The items of general stores are cleansing materials like soaps and detergents, tupper wares, ward/general furniture, small electric items and so on. Linen stores include textiles, synthetic fabric, woolen articles and furnishings and their house keeping items. Dietary stores or food and beverages stores handle vegetables, fruits, tinned items, dry rations, dietary items, grocery, kitchen items etc.

Indenting of stores in government hospitals can be as annual indents, supplementary indents, emergent indents etc. Indents for consumable and non-consumable stores should be submitted separately. Indenting groups include medical stores/ chemicals/ stains and dyes, stationery, diet items, photographic materials, housekeeping items and general items etc.

Control of stores involves receiving of materials, storing them properly and issuing them to different user areas against the duly authorized stores requisition. Two basic systems may be used in physically controlling stores materials. None other than the concerned store personnel are permitted to the store area. Hospital stores should be centralized for better control of materials. Duties and responsibilities of each person in the stores should be clearly defined. Since the materials are money invested in the inventories, which is nothing but cash in kind, the store keeper's role is similar to a cashier since both perform some identical functions.

In addition to above similarities, there are certain dissimilarities viz., cashier works in a small room environment, whereas, store keeper operates, over a larger area. Discrepancies in stocks take long time to detect as compared to cash discrepancies.

REVIEW QUESTIONS

1. While providing service is the principle objective of stores, what are the obligations of stores vis à vis other departments so that the services provided are efficient and in the overall interest of enterprise?
2. State factors that influence the decision of centralized or decentralized stores in a 500 bedded hospital. Discuss pros and cons.
3. Describe stores function in a hospital.
4. Explain the indenting procedure in government hospitals.

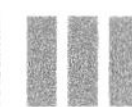

5. Discuss the similarities and dissimilarities between store keeper and cashier.
6. The productivity of hospitals largely influenced by the efficiency of the stores function. Discuss.
7. The three important functions in the stores are receipts, storage and prevention and issues. These activities have certain important responsibilities which have to be fulfilled by stores personnel. Describe them.
8. Stores function, is an important task in Materials Management. Its major activity revolves around three major functions i.e. receipt, issues, and storage.
9. Write short notes on
   a) Planning hospital stores
   b) Closed system stores
   c) Open system stores
   d) Indenting groups
   e) Central stores
   f) Functional stores

PART - IV

Stores Building and Stores Layout

Contents

CHAPTER - 19

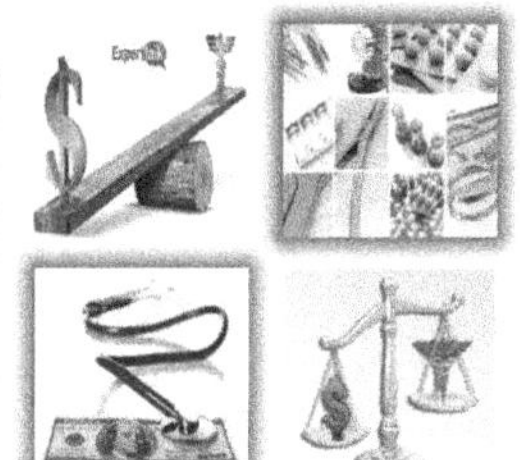

Stores Building and Stores Layout

INTRODUCTION

Businesses are interested in maintaining or improving market share and must continuously strive to reduce operating costs and investment. Failure to do so entails the risk of losing ground to fierce competitors. The most important costs and investments of a warehouse are few in number. Amongst costs of greatest importance are transport to and from the warehouse; building, equipment, human resources and inventory investment, and the operating expenses. Of these, controlling building and equipment design is a vital key to success because designs impact other operating costs. The distribution centre warehouse storeroom with the lowest cost per unit of space occupied has the best potential for reducing others costs and investments. For example, in buildings that are larger than necessary, people and automations spend more time in motion. The result is higher pay roll and equipment expenses and capital investment. In a smaller building, better space utilization makes it possible to store and process the same volume. Expenses on utilities are also proportionate to the degree of store space utilization. Ideal warehouse is no warehouse at all! However, it is difficult to achieve complete elimination of distribution warehousing of slow moving, inexpensive and small parts and products. This does not deter healthcare institutions from pursuing continuous reduction of warehousing through programmes designed to upgrade their supplier's ability to fill customer orders directly from their production processes. In the long transition period during which distribution inventories are continuously being reduced and warehouses are still a reality, it will befit organizations to reorganize their facilities to yield superior results.

STORES SITE LOCATION

Complexity of modern healthcare industry has lead to complex stores. New names have been invented for special types of stores needed in a particular situation. As far as possible; stores should be located in a central place. Stores location is the process of selecting an appropriate site for stores building in the hospital premises. It also includes decisions on how materials are to be arranged in the stores.

Good stores location principles include

- Economy in cost of transportation, approachability, efficient service to user departments.
- Minimization of fire hazards, security of stocks.
- Minimization of risk of spoilage/ deterioration.
- Flexibility for future expansion etc.
- Good layout of stores is imperative to ensure efficient timely receipts and issues of materials.
- Materials within the store should be placed considering frequency of issue, susceptibility to damage, fire hazards, cost of items etc.

A store serves its clients, be it the user department or the patients in the latter case, it becomes part of hospital distribution network. There can be one centralized warehouse or there can be a large number of sub stores located in the hospital near the consumption centres. The location of sub stores may be decided upon by the application of quantitative methods like operations research. One may choose between a centralized store and decentralized system serving specific consuming units of the hospital.

First task in locating a store, therefore, is to make a detailed plan by clearly defining objectives and evaluating several options available.

Planning includes not only location of a store but also its layout, storage methods and materials handling system.

Each store should be customized to the unique environment of the hospital.

Best possible site might not always be available for various reasons, in which case a less suitable compromise solution might be accepted.

In some other cases, one might have to locate a store quite far away from hospital's user departments for want of space. This would of course involve additional transportation costs but options might be limited.

Principles of good stores location are summarized below:

- Optimization of transportation costs.
- Efficient service.
- Minimizing the fire hazards. Proper security arrangements.
- Minimization of risk of spoilage and deterioration.
- Provision for future expansion.
- Proximity to public transport system.

Above factors have to be such that, an overall integration of all principles narrated above.

LOCATION OF HOSPITAL STORES

Stores must be located at an appropriate place in the hospital and then, it should be decided before hand how materials are arranged inside the stores (i.e., the precise spot where an item has to be placed) so as to provide efficient and prompt service to the user departments. Hospital stores are normally found to be located in areas which are either unusable by other departments or are not suitable for other functions of hospital. Basement is one such area. These areas are poorly designed for use as storage facilities. They have low ceilings, exposed pipelines, difficult access and faulty flow design. Storage facilities however have been given higher status and priority in a few healthcare institutions.

Location of stores should be such that it fulfills the following criteria:

- Items should be easily accessible when required.
- It should be possible to issue oldest stock first (FIFO principle).
- Receipt and issues of materials should be possible within the least possible time.
- Cost of materials handling should be low, as for as possible.
- Materials must be safe from pilferage, theft and fire.
- Stricter control to be ensured over movement of stock.
- Unnecessary fatigue and monotony of staff should be avoided.
- Easy access should be provided to all the user areas of hospital.

For achieving the above objectives, it is necessary that store building should be near to the area where the materials are required. **While selecting a suitable site for a store, due consideration should be given to temperature, humidity and lighting arrangements. There should also be scope for future expansion of the store.**

SITE SELECTION

Site selection is governed by various extraneous factors such as:

- Regulations of local bodies, or the government.
- Availability of services like electricity, water, skilled labour, transport, etc.
- Adequacy of roads connecting the site.
- Space available for building and maneuvering of vehicles which come to the stores. Some trailers carrying containers are up to 13 meters long.
- Cost or rental or lease of land.
- Adequacy of space for future expansion.

- Site conditions, i.e., whether, high foundation costs or demolishing of an existing structure are involved.

Location of store is of primary importance. If an unsuitable site is decided upon and a building is constructed on it, there can be never ending troubles. Many hospitals face difficulties by building a store in the space available and choosing an architect who has no clue about the specific requirements of the store. Such situations must be avoided. Quite often, storage accommodation is hired for various reasons like shortage of capital to construct one's own building, lack of space in the hospital premises, high cost of land in congested urban areas, seasonal fluctuations, etc.

Hospital must be very careful in hiring such buildings because there can be several shortcomings like inadequacy of security, inadequate floor strength, leaking roofs and seeping walls, environment problems like insects, pests, rodents, water logging etc., and lack of space for vehicles to load and unload goods. Maintenance and housekeeping need extreme care.

STORES BUILDING

There are many kinds of buildings, which are used for storage; the more important of them are described below:

A single storey building with a huge open interior divided into compartments through fixed or movable partitions.

A multi storied building saves land costs especially in the cities.

PRINCIPLES OF BUILDING DESIGN

In designing a storehouse, certain principles which must be borne in mind, are set out below:

A storehouse holds stock, which is depleted by issues and increased by receipts. Inward and outward flows are therefore of primary importance. Quick vehicle turn around is essential to efficient store keeping.

Stock yard plays an important role in keeping transport moving since it allows vehicles to manoeuvre and to queue in an orderly fashion.

Working areas, including goods inward and goods outwards, maintenance areas and packing should be grouped as closely together as is reasonably possible while retaining separate flows. This would mean the reduction of costs on providing common areas, e.g., washrooms, etc.

Location of office should be close to the working areas, to aid in communication.

Offices can be on the first floor. Ground floor is suitable for storage.

Height of the building from floor to rafters must be adequate to permit maximum floor loading. It should be somewhat greater than the maximum stocking height for commodities being stored and the capacity of handling devices being used. The costs of building for height are low compared to cost of floor and roof. Main gangways should run the length of long buildings and across short ones. Lighting is parallel to subsidiary gangways. Subsidiary gangways run off the main gangways but not necessarily at right angles. Adequate lighting must be provided to light stack faces. Doors should be wide and high enough to be well clear of loaded vehicles or equipment passing through them. Floor thickness and strength must be specified and checked during building construction. Fire precautions need to be carefully considered before the building is erected. Fire exits must be provided.

Security arrangements to control access to both buildings and yards are required and involve provision of a perimeter wall or fencing.

Main gangways are best placed to run the length of long building to give good access throughout the building. In short building, gangways should be across to economize on storage space Figure 19.1 Main gangways must be wide enough for two of the largest vehicles or material handling equipments likely to be used to pass each other without risk of collision.

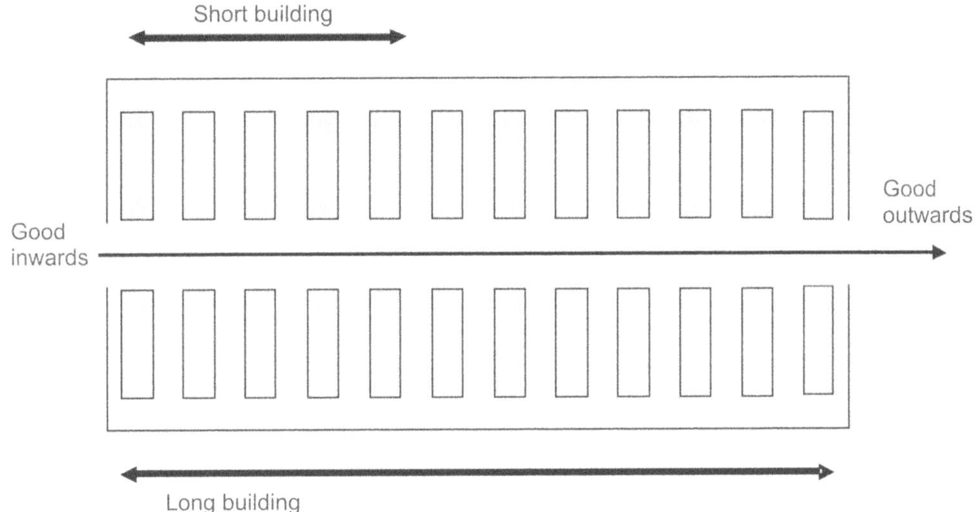

Figure 19.1 Straight through Flow

STORAGE FACILITIES

Primary factors in storage are:

Every item must be found when it is required.

It must be possible to issue the oldest stock first (first in, first out). Items should be in good condition when issued.

It should be possible to use storage equipment easily and quickly without risk to men or materials.

These requirements demand tidiness, methods and discipline. It is assumed that everyone who works in stores obeys the rules. Rules for whole storehouse should follow the same basic principles, but each type of storage has some of its own special needs. There are a wide variety of storage media, some of which are associated with particular methods of handling.

STORES PLANNING

First task in stores planning is to gather facts (as distinct from opinions).

Some questions need to be addressed are:

- Whom does the store serve?
- Where are they located?
- What are the items stocked?
- What are their maximum and minimum quantities,
- Their nature (small, big, bulky, liquid, hazardous, heavy) and
- Whether they can be kept in crates, bins, pallets, or in open yard etc and the total space they are likely to occupy?
- How are they received or dispatched?
- How much quantity per day or week?
- How many road trucks, of what sizes are involved per day?
- How many railway wagons?
- What type of materials handling equipment required?
- Number of staff, officers, supervisors, workers (or various categories)

Receiving and dispatch section requirements.

- How much space is available? (Area in square metres or volume in cubic metres).
- What type of material handling equipment is envisaged? (Forklifts, overhead cranes, or manual systems.)

Success of the stores building design will depend primarily on the facts that have been gathered and analyzed. The problem has to be studied in depth and no fact is small enough to be ignored.

Two basic considerations of a stores layout project are

1. Materials to be stored (or jobs to be handled).
2. Space available (three dimensional).

A complete study of space along with drawings to scale assists in the computation of pallet width and depth and shelf heights for pallet racks. Locations of columns in the building and their widths should also be taken in to consideration. After a space chart is prepared, a plan of the building complex which will include store buildings, loading and unloading bays, roads, open areas, railway sidings, etc. should be plotted.

Within the store building itself, the following should be planned out:

- The actual storage,
- Office and administration areas.
- Segregation of receipt, storage, issue and dispatch sections.

Overall plan of the store complex enables one to know the exact volume of storage space available and also the possibilities for expansion.

Outside and inside elevation drawings of the building should include ceiling and stacking height details, as well as floor load capacities.

PLANNING THE LAYOUT

Criteria for stores layout are based on the following factors:

1. Popularity
2. Similarity
3. Size
4. Characteristics of materials to be stored
5. Security

Popularity signifies frequency of demand and could be described using ABC inventory classification based on the value of consumption. Normally about 80 to 85 percent in terms of value of items requires 20 percent of the items stored. Items must be placed in the stores in such a way that they are easily accessible; and faster moving items must be kept nearest to issue section, and then comes, medium moving items; and thirdly, slow moving items, which must be kept at the rear end of the store. Most important advantage in this system is handling and picking.

Similarity of inventory items should be addressed after their popularity has been determined. **Similarity is a function of application or use by the same person.** Similar items should be stored

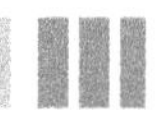

together. In addition, storing by similarity satisfies the need for taking a quick inventory and performing quick issue procedures.

Storage by size is opposite to storage by similarity or by popularity. This is important and also means, besides the unit size, volume of the total quantities stored at any time. Adequate space must be provided for the volume of items. A variety of positions to accommodate different sizes and different volumes of items must be identified. Size obviously must be considered in order to provide for proper quantities of items in proper spaces and to promote faster issues and reduce handling. However, the size of material does not alter stocking principles of popularity and similarity. A modern method of storage is to use standardized pallets for materials to be handled or stored.

Characteristics of materials: For e.g., liquids, hazardous items, small electronic parts, perishable items, gases, items in bulk, furnace oil, fuel oils etc. differ from one another. Their characteristics are such that they cannot be stored by popularity or similarity. Their storage should be by consideration for their safety. Flammables, toxic substances should be stored near overhead safety showers. Drug items that require tighter security or entail high risk should be stored in an area that can be locked and where access can be limited. One of the points to be considered is the special characteristics of some goods, especially in respect of compatibility between the various items stored. This is especially so with regard to, say, foodstuffs and chemicals.

Security: This is another important matter which has to be taken into account while designing a store. For security reasons, stores should be away from the main gate and from the factory wall of the premises. Main stores should be placed in such a way that suppliers' representatives, drivers, and others do not have very easy access.

Above criteria are summarized in the following Table 19.1

Table 19.1 Criteria for Location of Materials in Stores

Categories of material to be stored	Suggested Location in the Stores
High usage items	As close to the issue counters as possible.
Heavy items which are difficult to handle	Near the point of use, or near broad gangways or the gate or in the open.
Oils, greases, paints and messy items	In a separate storeroom.
Inflammable and dangerous items	In isolated, fireproof place with sprinkler system.
Low shelf life or perishable items	Air conditioned stores.
Costly items like stents, pacemakers etc.	In a locked cupboard and away from entrance to stores.
Bulky items impervious to weather	In open yard.

LAYOUT DESIGN

Starting point for stores layout design is a stock list containing the names of all the items that are required to be stored and the list should preferably include the characteristics mentioned earlier, which includes the volume of space that is likely to be occupied. A well designed layout will satisfy the objectives of efficient stocking and order fulfiling procedures. Each layout must be tailor made to suit existing requirements.

Two methods are normally adopted for designing store layout; namely **judgement method and scientific method**

In judgement method, floor plan is prepared for each floor of the store building where operations are to take place. Exact type of storage equipment, pallet sizes and material handling equipment are then decided upon. Entire building may be racked and palletized. The next step in designing is judgment on the basis of logic. Assuming that there are about 20 different groups of materials to be stocked say drugs, disposables, consumables, chemicals, linen, surgical items, stationery, spares etc., space should be assigned on various floors to accommodate these material groups. Judgement will be based on the ease of handling, the size of the materials, floor load requirements, speed and frequency of issue and several others of the various considerations usually applicable to stores operations.

Planner would then decide upon:

- Number and type of racks needed in that area.
- Number and sizes of pallets required for the materials.

Scientific Method: In the scientific method, the design is based on a detailed scientific study of exact requirements based on work study techniques. This will have to be done with the help of an industrial engineering expert.

The study will determine the space in terms of area and volume that would be required.

Proper method of storage of the materials, especially on the floor, will be determined on the basis of evaluation of various alternatives. Stores planning worksheet is made out, showing the exact layout and illustrating the types of storage equipment envisaged.

Two factors in determining layout are "economy and efficiency".

A store whose space is not fully utilized is a waste of capital.

One that holds too much is wasteful in terms of time and labour.

If the store is packed too closely on the ground, access becomes impossible. The same applies if it is stacked too high above the ground level.

The objective should be to maintain a work flow through the store so that it can operate continuously without hindrance caused by blocked gangways or inaccessibility to materials. In view of this it is necessary to examine the work flows themselves.

There are four main criteria:

1. Receipt and inspection of materials from suppliers and their storage.
2. Picking of materials, their issue and dispatch.
3. Stock taking.
4. Stock maintenance, stock turnover, periodic inspection, maintenance and re binning.

To these may be added, the rearrangement of storage which involves shifting of materials so that stocks are conveniently grouped and placed for efficient operation. Each task has its own work flow either beginning or ending with the location at which stocks are held. It is necessary to ensure that neither of these operations interferes with the other. Since all work flow is concerned with the location, attention must be given to the type of storage being used. This is related to the bulk and weight of materials being stored and a number of different types of storage will have to be used as necessary. Small items might be stored in bins, larger ones in racks with boxed stocks acting as reserves, block stacked boxes on pallets and heavy or awkward material in special storage. Items in any of these storage groups may move quickly, at a medium pace, or slowly. Fast moving items must be placed preferentially in relation to the other types of stock for easy access. Keeping the above factors in view, there are several possibilities that may be considered to obtain a satisfactory flow through the storehouse.

DIFFERENT FORMS FOR LAYOUT DESIGN

Design of the stores layout should follow some basic principles like straight through flow or as per consumption pattern or based on work elements grouping them together and making allowances for special treatment of materials according to their speed and movement.

Straight through flow

A straight through flow is the simplest. The goods enter through one door, are stacked in straight row, picked, moved in one direction along the length of the storehouse, and moved out through an exit. This system does not take into account the need to place working areas together, the different kinds of storage, the speed of movement and the need for areas set aside for various other functions. Clearly, therefore, this system is not good enough see Fig. 19.2. Straight flow layout is also applicable for hospital stores.

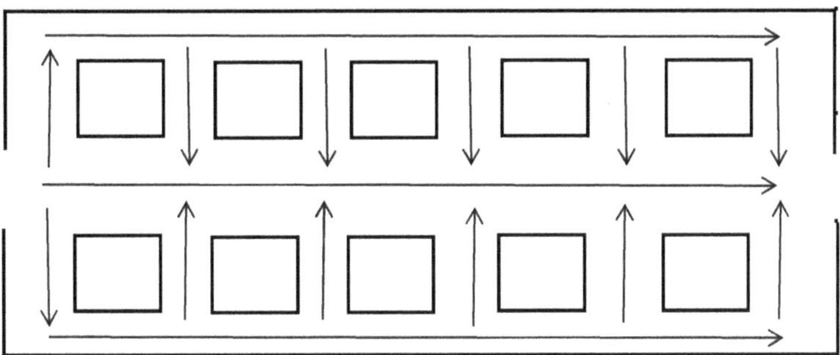

Figure 19.2 Straight through Flow Layout

In the second case of straight line flow for different types of storage, the layout is in terms of method of storage. Only receipts and issues are considered see Fig. 19.3. No attempt is made to group work areas, nor is there any means of dealing more economically with faster moving stores.

It is evident, conclusion is that, straight line flow cannot fully satisfy all requirements.

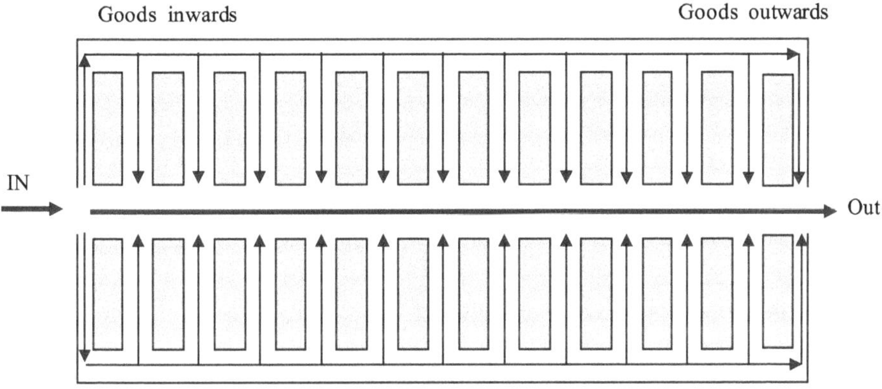

Figure 19.3 Straight - through Flow

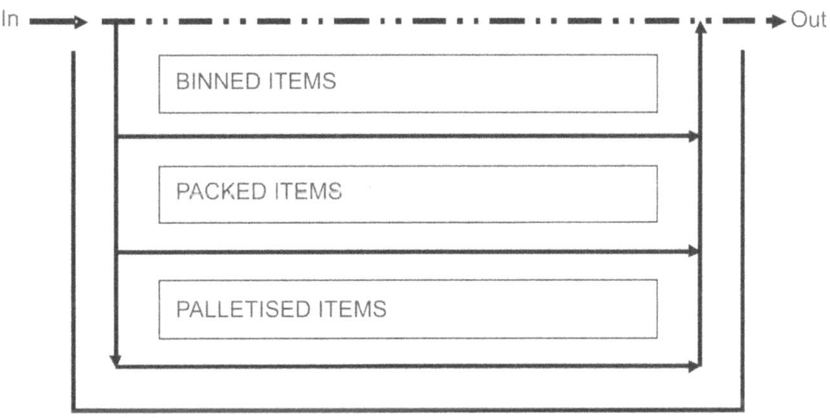

Figure 19.4 Straight Line Flow - Different Types of Storage

Element Based Flow

In this layout, items are stored either on their consumption speed, fast moving, medium moving and slow moving or other characteristics e.g., long life, perishable, expendable, nonexpendable, items requiring special low temperatures. Three possible layouts are shown in the figures below. These layouts allow for all work elements, grouping them together and making allowance for special treatment of materials according to their speed of movement. The flow is preserved regardless of whatever activities are being carried out. Flexibility is maintained because each division shown on the plan is movable. One area can be made larger at the expense of another by moving a partition or a section of stores. The only omission is the type of storage and clearly, this will depend upon the characteristics of the items being stored. Binned items are small, easily handled and a large proportion of them are likely to be fast or moderately fast moving. Reserve stocks to fill the bins will be held for a majority of the items and these will be held in racks or in the palletized area of the storehouse. Racks hold reserve items or those items which are too big or heavy for bins. Fast moving items are light enough for easy manual handling to and from the racks. The principle of minimum movement dictates that manual handling be reduced to the act of selection only, all other movements are dealt with, in bulk, by mechanical means.

Pallets are specifically designed to permit the handling of blocks of stocks as entities by fork lift trucks. Areas in which they are located must, therefore, be designed to facilitate the use of this equipment. Here, there will be a relatively smaller number of fast moving items, bulk of the items being reserve stocks or items occasionally used. Heavy lifts, etc. can block the flow unless special arrangements are made for them. They should either be held in a separate building or have their own access facilities. These items generally tend to be slow moving.

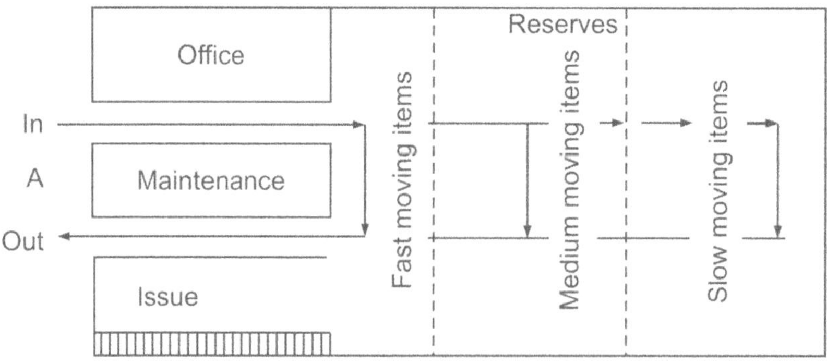

Figure 19.5 Layout based on Work Elements Type-1

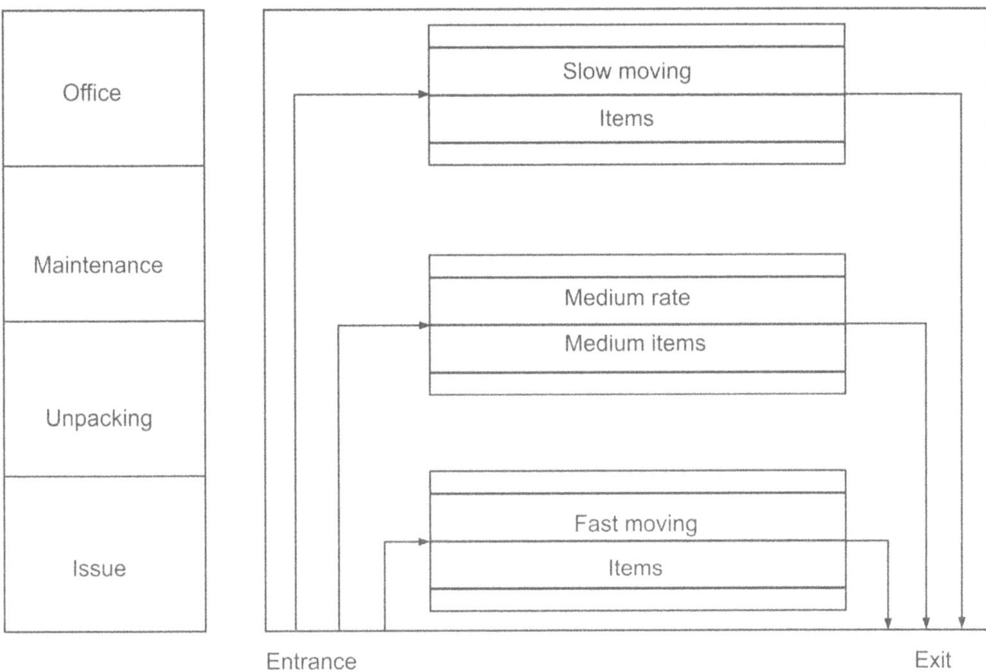

Figure 19.6 Layout based on Work Elements Type-2

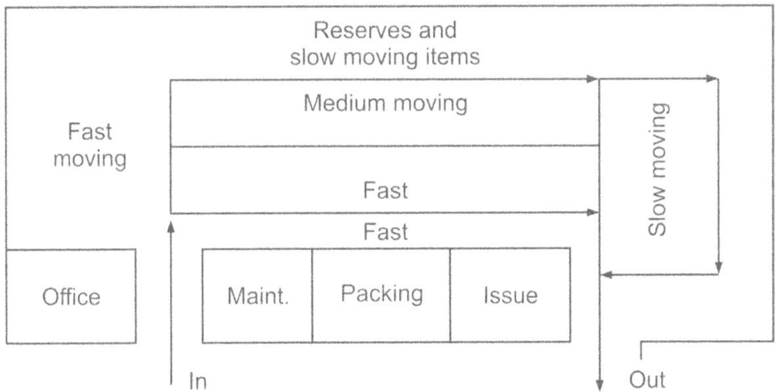

Figure 19.7 Layout based on Work Elements Type-3

SMALL STORE HOUSES

Small storehouses have limitations of space. Efficiency is achieved by deciding on the range of goods, the quantity of stock for each and the speed at which the stock can be replaced, both regularly and in an emergency.

Some of the basic necessities of a small storehouse are:

Facilities: Facility area for incoming and outgoing goods is needed. Space requirements for this are dependent upon the actual conditions, e.g., volume handled per day, type of goods kept, etc.

The turnover in such a store should be sufficiently fast.

Stock control: Supply lead time and the average usage in it are likely to be the basis of stock holding. If arrangements are made for delivery at specified hours or on specified days, it will enable the staff to organize their time efficiently. If an indicator system is attached to stock control cards to show which of the stocks have reached reorder level, the items concerned can easily be found at the end of each day.

Following rules may be observed for small storehouses:

- Formal and regular stock review is necessary to ensure that only fast moving items are generally carried.
- **Reordering should normally be on a cyclic basis.**
- An easily operated storage system with a uniform type of racking should be planned.
- A disciplined approach for issues and receipts, keeping a separate area for each, in necessary.
- Inventory control and stock accounting should be efficient.
- Stock cards should always be up to date and postings must be immediate.

INVENTORTY LOCATION SYSTEMS

An essential requirement in any storehouse is that materials be found in minimum possible time when they are needed. Location systems are the means by which it is done. Since the materials must be located manually, the person concerned must get to the right place with the minimum loss of time. To achieve this, the system must be simple, unambiguous and consistent. Colour codes cannot be easily identified when lighting is bad. Coding systems are better. For example:

1st number : designates storehouse, the storage bay or the group.

2nd number : the block of storage

3rd number : the particular item of the group

4th number : the level or shelf

5th number : the bin number

Either alphabets or alphanumeric codes can be used in the coding system. Thus:

B = Bin; R = Rack; S = Stacking area.

N/E/W/S = the four directions.

F = Front; B = Back; L = Left; R = Right.

Small case letters e.g., "a", "b", "c", "d" and "e", represent levels, etc.

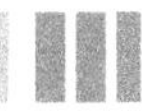

Having decided on the codes, mark the areas with large signs. These should be in a standard position. The stock cards must clearly indicate location.

Since the efficiency of a storehouse's operations depends mostly on its location system, responsibility for this should preferably be given to only one individual.

LAYOUT DESIGN

As stated earlier, the two important factors in layout i.e., **economy and efficiency** as applicable to industrial stores or warehouses also hold good in the case of hospital stores layout design.

While designing layout of the stores, following points must be kept in mind.

- Shelves must match to the type of products that are being stored.
- Rows of shelves should be parallel to the longest dimension of the room.
- Flow pattern should be optimized through the use of straight path.
- Dead ends should be avoided, otherwise personnel would have to come back in order to move from row to row and it will be time consuming.
- Flooring should be clean and dust free. Concrete floors should be cured.
- Lighting should be adequate.
- Heating and air conditioning may have significant effect on perishable and sterile items.
- Available space should be utilized properly.
- Width of aisles should be approximately twice the width of widest materials handling equipment that will be generally used in the room.

There is only one way to happiness and that is to cease worrying about things which are beyond the power of our will.

Space requirement for Hospital Stores based on bed strength

Requirement planning is one of the vital steps in hospital stores. It consists of listing every area in a proposed construction. The space requirement for hospital stores needs proper attention as far as planning is concerned.

Mc Gibony recommends an area of 20 sq. ft. (2 sq. m) per bed for hospital stores.

Housley suggested that a hospital needs about 1000-1500 Sq. ft. of central storage space as a good practice.

John. H. Holmgren and Walter. J Wentz recommended an average of 10 sq ft (1 sq. m) per bed in central stores area and 5 sq. ft. (0.5 sq. m) per bed in skilled nursing homes.

Timmappayya recommended an area of 300-600 sq. ft. (30 - 60 sq. m) for a hospital of less than 200 beds and correspondingly more space for larger hospitals.

Miglani suggested that 4-5 sq. ft. (0.5 sq. m) area per bed should be good enough to meet the requirement for storage of drugs in a large hospital having bed strength of 700 and above.

Review committee on Scales of Accommodation for Armed Forces Hospital, recommends that for assessment of plinth area, a conversion factor of 120 percent is to be added to total floor area requirement. This is to cater for circulation area including stairs, lifts, ramps and wall thickness. The area per bed varies with number of specialities, volume and number of items, lead time required to obtain the items. Keeping the above factors in mind, the store area per bed can be decided.

PHARMACY STORES LOCATION AND LAYOUT

Pharmacy stores is the pivot of three pharmacies in the hospital namely out patient, inpatient and operation theatre pharmacies. This emphasizes the need for planning and designing the pharmacy in a manner that results in efficient clinical and administrative services. Frequently, the pharmacy is not organized and managed as its importance warrants.

Factors which should be considered for designing of pharmacy stores, functions, location, facilities and space requirements are covered in detail in Chapter 2.

SUMMARY

Traditional pharmacy services are undergoing a rapid change all over the world, especially in the dispensing and distribution systems and many innovative approaches and methods have been introduced in the recent past. Though not all the hospitals can implement these changes, it is hoped that some of the larger and progressive hospitals in our country would introduce and test these newer systems and be pace setters for other hospitals to follow.

To improve market share, organizations must continuously strive to reduce operation costs and investment. The most important costs and investments are transport to and fro from warehouse; the building, equipment, people and inventory investment and operating expenses.

Of the above, controlling building and equipment design stands out as vital key to the success of operating costs.

Store serves its clients, be it the production department or the hospital's customers. In the latter case, it becomes part of the hospital's distribution network. The first task in locating a store, therefore, is to make a detailed plan by clearly defining objectives and evaluating several operations possible.

Planning covers not only the location of a store but its layout, storage methods and materials handling system. Site selection is governed by various extraneous factors such as government or municipal regulations, cost of land, adequacy of space and infrastructural facilities like air, road, water and power.

 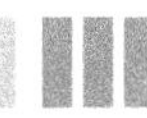

Storage accommodation is hired for various reasons; like shortage of capital to construct one's own building, lack of space in the premises, high cost of land in congested parts of urban areas, seasonal fluctuations, etc.

The success of stores building design depends primarily on the facts that have been gathered and analyzed such as quantity and nature of items to be stocked, number of handling equipments, space and items to be stocked and the maximum & minimum stocks to be maintained, etc. The two basic considerations of a stores layout are materials to be stored (or jobs to be handled), space available (three dimensional). Drawings should be made to scale.

Efficient and effective layout must be based on factors such as similarity, popularity, size, security and characteristics of materials to be stored. The two methods normally adopted for designing the layout of a store are judgement method and scientific method. In the judgement method, the first thing to do is to prepare a floor plan for each floor of the store building, where operations are to take place. In the scientific method, the design is based on a detailed scientific study of exact requirements based on work study techniques. Two factors in determining layout are economy and efficiency.

Main criteria for examining work flow are receipt and inspection of materials from suppliers and their storage; picking of materials, their issue and dispatch; stock taking, stock maintenance, stock turnover, periodic inspection, maintenance and re binning

In designing a storehouse, there are certain principles, which must be borne in mind; such as items to be stocked, work areas including goods inward and goods outward and maintenance areas and the height of the building from floor to rafters.

Small storehouses have limitations of space. Efficiency is achieved by deciding on the range of goods, the quantity of stock for each and the speed at which the stock can be replaced, both regularly and in an emergency. Basic necessities of a small storehouse are facilities and stock control.

An essential requirement in any storehouse is that materials be found when they are wanted without waste of time and issues should be made on FIFO basis. Location systems are the means by which it is done.

Hospital stores have normally been found located in areas which are either unusable by other departments or are not suitable for other functions of hospital. Basement is one such area being used as stores. They are poorly designed for use as storage facilities with low ceilings, exposed pipes, difficult access and faulty flow design.

Hospital stores location should facilitate easy access for issue of oldest stock first; transportation should be economical and ergonomics should be achieved.

While selecting a suitable site for a store, due consideration should be given to temperature, humidity and lighting arrangements. There should also be scope for future expansion of the store.

Layout should be designed taking into account factors like arrangement of shelves, use of straight path, avoiding dead ends, providing width of aisles one and half times the widest material handling equipment in the hospital. Shelves must match the type of products that are being stored. Hospitals also follow layout designs similar to industrial stores like straight-through flow, element based flow layouts.

Space planning is vital in hospital stores. It consists of listing of every area in a proposed construction. The space requirement for hospital stores need proper attention as far as planning is concerned. Various authors recommend an area of 0.5 to 2 sq. m. per bed for hospital stores and 10-15 sq. m. of central storage space. Keeping different factors in mind, the store area per bed can be decided.

Pharmacy is one of the most extensively used therapeutic facilities of the hospital and one of the few areas where large amounts of money are spent on purchases on a recurring basis. A good pharmacy is a blend of several things such as qualified personnel, supported by sound budget and support and cooperation of medical, nursing and administrative staff. A modern and progressive pharmacy calls for new methods of operations, new production approaches and new distribution techniques to achieve reduced costs and increased efficiency.

Most important functions performed by pharmacy stores are purchase, stores, compounding, packaging, labelling and dispensing pharmaceutical items and it also serves as a source of drug information to pharmacists, physicians and other healthcare personnel and patients.

In determining the most suitable location for the pharmacy, flow of out patients traffic through the hospital, flow of drugs and other raw materials into the pharmacy, flow of drugs and services from the pharmacy to the inpatient areas and other departments, needs for future expansion, should be considered. Since there is no such thing as a typical hospital, there cannot be a typical pharmacy. Therefore, each hospital has to pattern its own pharmacy, to suit its requirements. Broadly speaking, the pharmacy has four main functional areas. They are: dispensing area, production or preparation area, administrative area and the storage area.

Central stores area is required on an average 1 sq. m. per bed in hospitals and 0.5 sq. m. per bed in nursing homes.

Many a time, it is discovered that a new hospital does not have adequate storage space, once it is built. Most healthcare facilities have problems of space. There are rules, methods and equipments and materials handling systems both manual and automated available to assist in the effort of moving supplies into and out of hand within general stores area.

Many individual hospitals are groups of organizationally related hospitals renting or buying off site, in order to ensure minimum stock supplies. This is due to increase in use of disposables, an increase in beds and longer lead times, and increase in number of items without a corresponding increase in general stores area.

REVIEW QUESTIONS

1. Discuss in detail the criteria for stores layout.
2. A well designed layout will satisfy the objectives of effective stock keeping and efficient order fulfilling. Discuss in detail.
3. What are the basic principles for a good stores layout? Explain with illustrative examples.
4. List out various elements that are to be considered when deciding upon the size and location of central stores.
5. Stores location is a process of selecting appropriate site for stores building in hospital premises. What parameters do you take into consideration with respect to stores location?
6. Write short notes on
    a. Stores building
    b. Small storehouses
    c. Space requirement for hospital stores
    d. Pharmacy stores
    e. Site location
    f. Similarity of inventory in stores layout

PART - IV

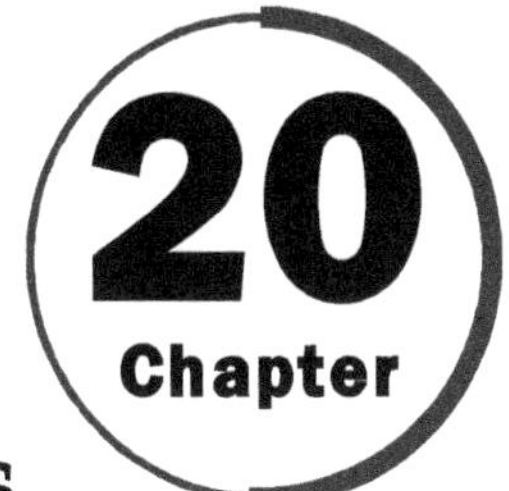

Physical Verification of Inventories

Contents

- *Introduction*
- *Purpose of Physical Inventory Taking*
- *How to Conduct Stock Verification*
- *Emergency Stock Receipt and Requisitions*
- *Cross Check and Verification*
- *Methods of Stock Taking*
- *Comparison among Three most Popular Methods of Stock Taking*
- *Investigation into Discrepancies, Reconciliation, Stock Adjustment and Write Offs*
- *Summary*
- *Review Questions*

CHAPTER - 20

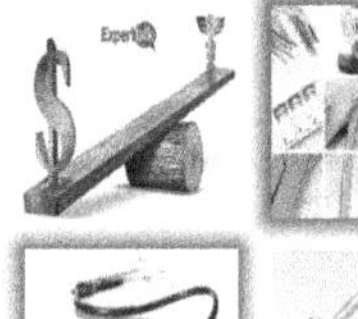
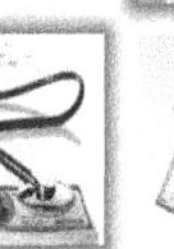
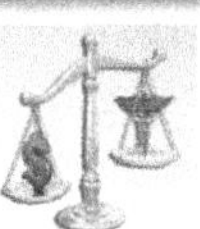

Physical Verification of Inventories

INTRODUCTION

Stock taking or stock verification can be defined as a process of physical counting, weighing, measuring the stock of materials that is held and making a record of these figures. Thus the stock verification is the basis for authentication of correctness of performance statements.

Physical verification of inventory is a measure of how much quantity of each item is actually available on hand and in stock records. Physical verification of inventory allows actual cost adjustments to be made on all supplies purchased. It is also a means of evaluating the efficiencies of inventory control and material handling for an organization. Other factors related to inventory verification are appropriate security for materials that are susceptible to shrinkage (i.e., pilferage, evaporation losses, etc.), stock rotation, lot control, and environmental conditions affecting the shelf life. It is also a statutory necessity since inventory figures appear in asset column of organization's balance sheet. Auditors must certify that book figures reflect the true and fair value of stocks actually held by the organization. This is required for revealing any weaknesses in the overall storage system, so as to make improvement and to enable better inventory control.

Stores controller has the physical custody of materials and is responsible for its safe upkeep. He must constantly review stocks, update accounts and reconcile physical stocks with book stocks. The magnitude of this problem can increase because errors can happen in each transaction and this can accumulate into major discrepancies. Other factors that have to be considered are containment of pilferage, obsolescence, damage due to different causes or improper storage and other losses. Stores controller must verify stocks regularly so that anything that is amiss comes to his notice for necessary corrective action. This verification should be accompanied by proper valuation and auditing exercise so that monetary values of items stored and their utilization can be known.

Stores represent money and should be carefully protected, checked and valued at the close of accounting period. Value of stocks is usually very much greater than that of cash held at any time. It is necessary to verify it from time to time in order to ensure that materials purchased and stored are intact in the store house and their quality and quantity have not deteriorated during storage. Hence physical verification is necessary.

PURPOSE OF PHYSICAL INVENTORY TAKING

Stock verification serves the following:

- To verify accuracy of stock records postings.
- To support the value of stocks, shown in the balance sheet by physical verification.
- To disclose the possibility of fraud, theft or pilferage etc.
- To reveal any weakness in the system for the custody and control of stock.

Discrepancies do occur between physical stocks in the store and those indicated in the stock cards in every enterprise, even, in the one with the best systems. Discrepancies in stocks arise due to various reasons.

Some of the reasons are:

1. Incoming goods placed in the bin, but goods inward note (GIN) or material requisition note (MRN) not posted in the stock card.
2. Posting errors in receipts and issues.
    a. Errors in posting i.e., entry of receipts made in issue column or vice versa.
    b. Addition or subtraction errors while, posting in manual systems.
    c. Variations due to human errors in receipts and issues. E.g., bulk handling.
3. Pilferage especially attractive items or costly materials like electronic components etc.
4. Materials issued but stock cards not posted.
5. Incorrect quantities issued i.e., issue of more quantity or less quantity than what was indented or noted in the bin card or stock card.
6. Errors in quantity posted. E.g. 521 metres posted as 52 yards or 204 posted as 402.
7. Evaporation losses etc.

Errors lead to problems. In order to avoid stock discrepancies, physical checking of stocks or stock taking is very necessary. Apart from this objective, checking of entries is vital from the point of view of accountability because **stocks represent money and as such, like cash, they have to be safeguarded,** constantly checked and accounted for. In addition to these basic reasons there are various other purposes which physical, controls and procedures. Size and number of surpluses and deficiencies that are revealed by stock taking is a good indicator of efficiency and effectiveness in store keeping methods.

HOW TO CONDUCT STOCK VERIFICATION

Where, physical stock verification is to be carried out and to conduct the actual count accurately, the process must be planned so as to cause minimum interruption to the ongoing activities of patient care.

Procedure

Personnel must be trained to undertake stock verification operations. The need and importance for stock verification must be explained to all the hospital staff in advance. Clear and effective procedures must be established to meet exigencies of emergency supply requisitions while the inventory verification is on. Documents that are to be used for conduct of stock verification must be designed, printed, and kept in folders. Services of hospital's internal audit and Information Technology departments be utilised to design formats. This activity should commence at least two months in advance of scheduled date for verification of inventory. Instructions in writing for conducting stock verification should also, be prepared, along with written schedule showing dates for stock verification in each location should be produced and distributed to all functionaries of the hospital. Selection and training of personnel to conduct the verification of inventory is vital. It is recommended that in addition to the coordinator of stock verification programme there be an assistant coordinator with specific responsibility for emergency issues and receipts of supplies during the exercise. There should also be an audit assistant, probably assigned by the internal audit department that is responsible for the security of counting materials. All materials should be distributed by and returned to the audit assistant. Teams of two office assistants should do the actual counting. Supply supervisors, assigned by the inventory coordinator, should be responsible for maintaining orderly arrangement of items at each location and assisting the counting teams to ensure that every item is counted and no item is counted more than once. Auditors, assigned by the chief of internal auditing, must oversee the entire inventory verification procedure, verifying physical counts and releasing each inventory location for return to normal activity.

Preparations for Stock Taking

The hospital's inventory master file (probably computer maintained) should be complete before the stock verification exercise is commenced. It should include all items that are to be verified. Each item in the file should be identified by a stock number, and the stock numbers should be clearly posted on the stock at each location in the hospital. One day before stock taking, each location should be cleaned up, with materials arranged and stored in clean containers.

Signs should be pasted at prominent locations to identify the inventory locations for the count teams. The inventory coordinator should inspect each area with supply supervisors the day before the inventory. All stock deliveries received up to the day before stock taking must be entered into automated inventory recording system and transferred to the store room prior to the completion of the workday. Likewise, issuing of requisitioned stock should be stopped one day before stock taking and all requisitions on hand should be completed and batched for entry into the automated system by the end of the day. All stock requisitions on hand should be completed and batched for entry into the automated system by the end of the day. Departmental and central receiving sections, as well as receiving dock, should be shut down on the day of stock taking as their personnel will be involved in stock verification activities.

Detailed planning procedure for organizing stock verification

1. Review previous year's notes and conduct a critical review on the stocks to be verified; assign responsibilities.
2. Schedule a date for stock verification and organize, coordination meeting at least 60 days in advance with internal auditors and computer services:
   a. Allocate duties to particular individuals in the department for all areas and clean up the same a day before inventory.
   b. Go round the area to be inventoried along with stock verifiers to ensure readiness. And it should be accomplished the day before the stock verification commences.
3. Prepare a schedule of deadlines to be met and communicate these deadlines viz., closing or cut off date of stock taking to all user departments within the hospital.
4. Explain how emergency indents are to be processed during this period. This schedule shall include cut offs for receiving as well as for inventory posting.
5. Prepare a written booklet of instructions to be followed for taking the physical inventory. Assign to each stock verification team leader specific areas. Each team leader is apprised of the instructions 30 days in advance.
6. Organize training for all the stock verifiers' team at least one week before physical verification work commences.
7. Identify all stock items with a stock number in the automated or manual inventory system.
8. Use bright colours to mark stock code number.
9. Clearly indicate on all those items that are not for verification "DO NOT INVENTORY."
10. Neatly stack the items to facilitate accurate and speedy counting.
11. Keep materials in clean containers prior to the start of the inventory.
12. A two week advance planning is made to identify all items to be verified
13. Ensure location signs posted to avoid confusion to verifications teams.
14. Classify the inventory in separate line stock items, stock keeping units (SKU) per shelf space, bin, or row. Segregate areas within the inventory by demarking the floor to identify the boundaries between adjacent areas.
15. Ensure that all items to be verified are on the inventory master file so that count cards can be printed. (Deadline for entering new items on to the master file is two weeks prior stock taking) This is the responsibility of the store room, inventory control, and central supply supervisor.
16. Use a pre printed stock verification tag (count card) with the stock number written on the tag to be used by the stock verifier teams. Use a special tag such as a bright coloured one, which is readily noticeable, to identify "unidentified items."

17. Indent inventory verification cards two weeks before stock verification commences and the card are:

- Central stores cards
- Blank cards or have signs printed that read "Blank card no of items removed after inventory count."
- Alpha listing central stores - eight copies.
- Numerical listing central stores - eight copies.

How to Organize Stock Taking?

Physical inventory should be performed by the designated count teams; each consisting of two persons, one would do actual physical counting, and other to record.

Each team should receive from the audit assistant a bunch of count cards to be used in a specific location. See Figure 20.1.

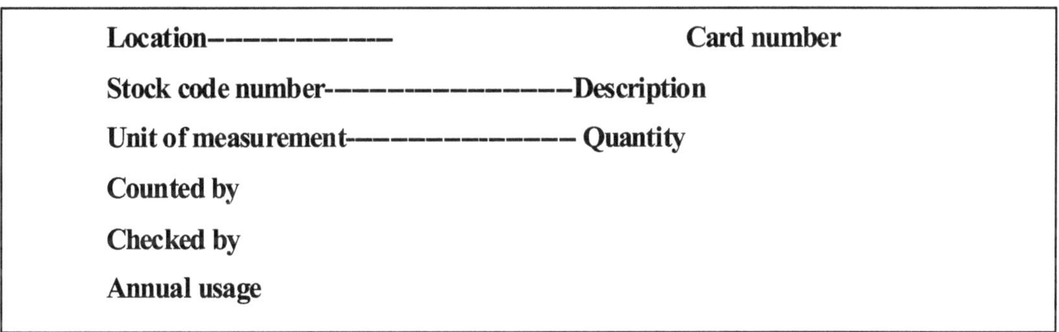

Location------------ **Card number**

Stock code number-----------------Description

Unit of measurement--------------- Quantity

Counted by

Checked by

Annual usage

Figure 20.1 Format of Physical Stock Count Card

After the number of cards is verified on the packet control form, which is left with the audit assistant, the count team proceeds to the indicated stock location and begins the actual counting. If an item is present for which there is no count card, the supply supervisor for that area will identify the item and complete a blank count card. The supervisor will fill in the stock number, item description, and unit of issue from an alphabetical list of all stock to be inventoried. The count team will record location, quantity, and its team number. The top copy of each count card will be torn off and attached directly to the stock to assist in subsequent verification of the count. The bottom copy will be turned in to the audit assistant after all count cards are completed. The audit assistant will check the packet control form to be sure that the number of cards returned equals the number distributed.

After cards are returned to the audit assistant, they are turned in to the data processing department, where review by the auditors is possible. The auditors randomly survey and recount items to measure the percentage of accuracy and effectiveness of Materials Management. The absolute difference between book value and physical value is the true measure of discrepancy.

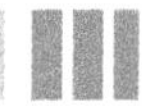

EMERGENCY STOCK RECEIPT AND REQUISITIONS

Stock items are to be physically received and issued to requesting departments, if absolutely necessary. The processing of the receipt and issue of these items into the automated inventory system is to be conducted at the completion of the physical inventory. All packing lists entered into the automated inventory after the completion of the physical verification should be stamped after stock verification.

When an emergency requisition is received during the physical verification, every attempt should be made to provide an opportunity for the requestor to borrow from another department.

If this is not possible, then the following guidelines should be followed:

- If the stock item has not been counted, the requested item and quantity should be removed from the storage area and a blank count card completed for the item and quantity removed.
- Quantity should be removed from the storage area and a copy of the requisition attached to the shelf location.

CROSS CHECK AND VERIFICATION

Audit assistant releases all completed count cards to computer services department. Cards are sorted according to the type of inventory to ensure that stock number and other codes are valid, to eliminate duplicates, and to incorporate corrections including those made by the inventory auditors. The discrepancy report should contain a list of those items on the inventory master list for which the accounting records' quantity on hand differs from the count taken during the physical inventory. See Figure 20.2.

A cross check may be done on inventory items that have been classified as high value items so that the value of these items can be measured against the ledger balance. Rechecks should be done on those items for which there is a high value discrepancy between the physical count and the book inventory. Stock adjustments in various records should be carried out after obtaining sanctions from the appropriate authority. The card balance should then be corrected as soon as possible so that the hospital's accounting records reflect the true value of the inventory on hand.

Sl. no	Stock code number	Description of the Item	Physical stock quantity	Quantity as per records	Adjustment	Average cost	Total cost
1							
2							
3							

Figure 20.2 Physical Inventory Discrepancy Report Format

It is extremely important that each small step in the preparation and execution of a physical inventory be carefully planned. This approach described has been effective in producing an orderly, accurate physical inventory.

METHODS OF STOCK TAKING

Various methods of stock verification can be adopted. The actual technique used depends upon the size and value of stock held and their complexity. Some of the methods commonly used are described below:

1. Annual stock taking
2. Periodic stock verification
3. Perpetual inventory method
4. Daily stock checking
5. Checking by stores in charge

Annual stock taking

Annual stock taking is a process of making a complete count of stores once in a year by a team consisting of accounts, store, and engineering and other staff. This is done at the end of each financial year by closing down the stores for a certain number of days. As per statutory requirements, each item must be physically checked and counted, and the auditors must be satisfied that physical checking has been carried out meticulously.

Advantages

a. This is the simplest and most convenient method of stock verification.

b. The stock verification is done on or near the date of balance sheet. Hence, the value of closing stock provided to the accounts department for incorporating in the balance sheet is more reliable.

c. Annual stock taking does not require permanent staff as in the case of perpetual method of stock taking. Personnel from other departments can be drafted for stock verification.

Disadvantages

a. It necessitates closing down the stores for a few days.

b. In the case of finished goods, the business might have to be interrupted for a few days.

c. Errors come to light only at the end of the financial year. This has repercussions on proper inventory control.

d. Since the entire process is carried out in a few days, thorough checking is not possible.

e. It creates a peak load work and hence overtime working becomes unavoidable.

f. Finalization of accounts at times gets delayed.

Periodic stock verification

This method is a halfway between annual checking and perceptual checking. Checking is done by accounts and stores at regular intervals say, once in three months or half yearly. However, issues and receipts are not interrupted and production shops are not closed. This method ensures that stocks are properly recorded and year end rush of work is also avoided.

Periodic stock verification is practiced by organizations registered under cooperative societies Act. One can expect the periodic stock verification to have advantages, disadvantages, akin to both annual stock taking and perpetual inventory.

Perpetual inventory method

If the stores happens to be very big and very large number of materials are stocked, year end stock verification would be a very difficult task unless a large number of stock verifiers are employed. A technique to overcome this problem is perceptual inventory system of stock taking. This needs usually a team of 2 or 3 stock verifiers, who take up a few items each day and check the stocks. Discrepancies are recorded and immediately investigated. The stock check should be planned in such a way that all items are checked at least once in a year and the important items checked two, three or four times a year. Costly or attractive items or those classified as 'A' items ould need more frequent checking, while 'C' class items or very heavy equipment may be checked only once or twice in a year.

There are several advantages in this system; important among them are:

a. Usually, the direct cost of perpetual inventory checking is lower than that of the annual inventory checking method.

b. Work is done by specialized staff, whereas in annual stock taking method, inexperienced people have to be inducted to do checking quite often, and they do so in a very routine manner or cut corners because the work is unusually boring.

c. In perpetual inventory method, the work is done at an 'expert' level. Greater diligence is also possible since verifiers are not racing against time and have to check only a limited number of items every day. The checking is also more accurate.

d. Losses due to stoppages of operations during the year end stock taking period are virtually eliminated.

e. Discrepancies can be detected and solved more often. People usually remember what happened during last few weeks rather than what happened one year ago. This helps in speeding up reconciliation of discrepancies. Correct stock figures avoid last minute production hold-ups.

f. It acts as an effective deterrent to malpractices, as pilferage is detected quickly. There is also a greater inducement to keep records up to date, than in case of annual stock verification.

g. Deteriorated and obsolete stocks are also easily detected.

h. Checking records and comparing with standard inventory norms ensures adequate stock provision and facilitates the preparation of annual accounts expeditiously.

Some small hospitals, nursing homes adopt a system of checking the balances every time receipt or issue is made. This is very not easy in stores where a large number of items are stocked. Immediate reconciliation of discrepancies is vital to this system. Stock adjustments in various records should be carried out after obtaining sanctions from the appropriate authority.

Daily stock checking

In this method, store keepers are required to check 10 to 15 items a day at random. This enables stores to locate discrepancies, as the storekeepers are conversant with possible areas/items where such discrepancies are likely to occur. This also eliminates any tendency on the part of the store keeper to overlook possibilities of malpractices.

Checking by stores in charge

This method is similar to the one described above except that checking is done by stores in charge. Discrepancies are immediately scrutinized and necessary corrective actions taken.

COMPARISON AMONG THREE MOST POPULAR METHODS OF STOCK TAKING

Comparison of three types if stock verification methods is shown in Table 20.1

Table 20.1 Comparison of the Three Methods of Stock Verification

Influencing factors	STOCK TAKING METHODS		
	Annual stock taking	**Periodic stock taking**	**Perpetual stock taking**
Impact on the operations of the hospital stores	At the time of annual stocktaking, routine activities such as movement of materials into the stores and out of stores are disrupted.	Issues and receipts are not interrupted and hospital operations are not closed.	Dislocation of work is minimized as the stocktaking is undertaken when the stores activity is not at peak.
Accuracy of stock verification	In annual stock taking, entire stores have to be verified in a short period, which causes a lot of stress on the stock verifiers and prone to errors.	Errors are few because the stocktaking is undertaken at different times.	It is error free as limited numbers of items are verified every day.

Table 20.1 *contd....*

Influencing factors	STOCK TAKING METHODS		
	Annual stock taking	**Periodic stock taking**	**Perpetual stock taking**
Time lag in noticing discrepancies in stocks	Errors come to light only at the end of the financial year. This has repercussions on proper inventory control.	Errors come to light periodically, can be corrected and it minimizes need for reconciliation.	Discrepancies come to light early and it eliminates disruptions.
Rectification of discrepancies.	Physical control of the stocks may not be very effective as it is an annual exercise.	Discrepancies can be detected and solved at regular intervals of time.	Discrepancies can be detected and solved more often.
Work load on junior staff	Work load is minimum as stock taking is done once in a year.	Work load is neither too low nor too high as in the case of annual or perpetual stock taking.	Work load is maximum as stock taking is done throughout the year.
Cost involved	Low	Medium	High
Application	Best suited for seasonal industries as stock verification can be done during off season.	Fairly adaptable for batch production industries.	Continuous process industries can best make use of perpetual system without disrupting the operations.

INVESTIGATION INTO DISCREPANCIES, RECONCILIATION, STOCK ADJUSTMENT AND WRITE OFFS

If the quantity in stock as found by physical examination does not tally with the balance on stock records, there is a discrepancy. If stock found exceeds the recorded figure, there is a surplus. Conversely, if the physical stock is less than the book figure, there is a deficiency. These discrepancies have to be reconciled before finalization closing stocks

Minor Discrepancies

There are limitations to accuracy of stock taking, particularly where large quantities are to be counted, weighed or measured. For example, in measuring 100 steel bars of random lengths, no two persons are likely to get the same result to the nearest meter. If therefore discrepancies of small proportions are be found in such circumstances, it is advisable to leave the book balance unaltered unless the value involved is significant.

Store Keepers' Agreement

Stock verifiers should not declare a discrepancy on any item without first giving the store keeper concerned the opportunity of investigation.

There are several reasons for this viz:

1. Often there are duplicate locations of which checkers are not aware, but of which store keeper knows.
2. The store keeper usually has a better practical knowledge of the stocks than anyone else and may be able to correct errors on the part of stock verifiers, particularly errors of identification.
3. It gives the store keeper an opportunity to explain or correct the difference if possible, and ensure an awareness of discrepancies, which may reflect on performance of duty.
4. When storekeeper is unable to explain a discrepancy, stock sheet should be signed to indicate an agreement that discrepancy is genuine.

Major Discrepancies

After stock is taken and store keeper has agreed that a discrepancy exists, the procedure to follow depends upon nature and value of discrepancy.

The following steps are to be taken in investigation of discrepancies:

1. Examine the stock record since the date of check to make sure that there are no arithmetical or data entry errors, obvious omissions and or duplication in posting.
2. Scrutinize the record to see that there has been no mistake over the units of issue.
3. Examine the items kept in neighbouring bins to find out if a balancing discrepancy exists on another item.
4. Check basic documents (i.e., receipt, issue, transfer, and return to stores note) for any exceptionally large or apparently unusual transactions.
5. Check all basic documents on which action has been taken since the last stock taking.
6. Have physical stock taking verified by an independent person.
7. Investigate the results of earlier stock taking to find out whether there was a discrepancy on that occasion too. In some odd cases, it may be found that a deficiency at earlier stock taking is followed by a surplus on the next stock taking and it may be the first check which was inaccurate.
8. Question the storekeeper concerned to find out if he has any explanation or suspicion as to how the discrepancy might have occurred.
9. Make inquiries with consumer department in case there have been any issues from or returns to stores without documentation, outside normal working hours.

10. In serious cases, where theft or fraud is suspected, call the police.
11. Wherever necessary, review and tighten up physical security measures and documentary procedures.

After investigation, both the stock records and accounts will require adjustments, in regard to the discrepancies after the necessary administrative approvals are obtained. For any reconciled lapses, write off should be done and stock records adjusted accordingly.

SUMMARY

Stock taking or stock verification is the process of physical counting, weighing, measuring the stock of materials that is held and making a record of these figures. It is a basis for authentication of correctness of performance statements.

Physical verification of inventory is a measure of how much quantity of each item is actually available on hand and in stock records and allows actual cost adjustments to be made on all supplies purchased.

Other factors related to inventory verification are appropriate security for materials that are susceptible to shrinkage (i.e., pilferage, evaporation losses etc.), stock rotation, lot control and environmental conditions affecting the shelf life. It is also a statutory necessity since inventory figures appear in asset column of organization's balance sheet.

The stores controller has the physical custody of the materials and is responsible for its safe upkeep. He must constantly review stocks, update accounts and reconcile the physical stocks with book stocks.

Stores represent money and should be carefully protected, checked and valued at the close of accounting period. Value of stocks is usually very much greater than that of cash held at any time.

In every enterprise, even, in the one with the best systems, discrepancies occur between physical stocks in the store and those indicated in the stock cards.

The size and number of surpluses and deficiencies that are revealed by stock taking is a good indicator of efficiency and effectiveness in store keeping methods, controls and procedures.

Various methods of stock verification can be adopted. The actual technique used will depend upon the size and value of stock held and their complexity. Some of the methods commonly used are:

1. Annual stock taking, 2. Periodic stock verification, 3. Perpetual inventory method, 4. Daily stock checking, 5. Checking by stores in charge.

Discrepancy on any item should be declared only after giving the store keeper concerned the opportunity of investigation. After store keeper has agreed that a discrepancy exists, steps are to be taken in regard to investigation. After investigation, both the stock records and accounts require adjustments in regard to the discrepancies with prior administrative approvals.

REVIEW QUESTIONS

1. What is the purpose of physical stock taking? How it is conducted?
2. Describe in detail preparation for stock taking.
3. What are the various techniques of stock taking? Describe advantages and disadvantages of each type of stock taking.
4. What are usual causes of discrepancies in stocks? How are they set right?
5. Differentiate between periodic counting and cycle counting methods of physical stock taking.
6. Write short notes on
   a) Handling of emergency, stock receipts and requisitions
   b) Discrepancies' in stock taking
   c) Store keepers agreement
   d) Daily stock checking
   e) Checking by stores in charge

PART - IV

21

Chapter

Inventory Valuation

Contents

CHAPTER - 21

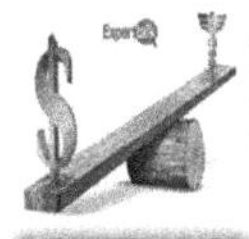
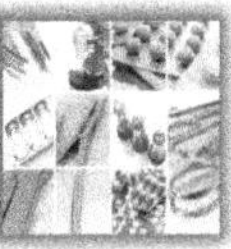
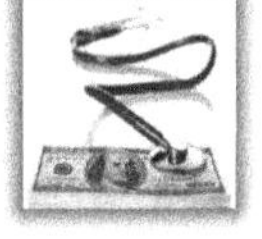
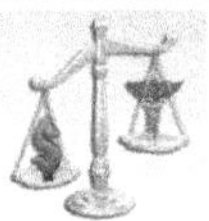

Inventory Valuation

INTRODUCTION

Maintaining inventory is associated with many financial implications. In the earlier chapters, the discussions mainly centered on lowering inventory costs, safety stocks and inventories held on hand. This chapter addresses the need for valuation of inventories to enable the hospitals to know and confirm its knowledge of financial strengths and weaknesses. Stores valuation converts physical inventories into monetary figures. Stock verification validates the existence of stocks. These two basic tools form the basis of measuring efficiency of the hospital. Since materials form the major input in the operations of the hospitals, their valuation becomes very crucial in judging performance of the hospital. Since materials cost constitutes a major component of the product or service cost, the valuation of materials consumed in day to day operations of hospital and stocks held at the end of the financial year must be valued properly.

Valuation process can be classified under the following heads:

1. Valuation of incoming materials
2. Valuation of materials consumed
3. Valuation of materials returned from various operating departments to stores.

NEED FOR VALUATION OF INVENTORY

Valuations of inventories are required for different purposes and valuation varies according to purpose for which the valuation is applied for, they are as follows:

1. **Valuation for insurance**

   Here, stock is valued on the basis of having to replace it, but in addition may consider the value lost to the hospital as a result of it not being available.

2. **Costing to establish the actual cost to the organization of manufacturing a product or providing service:**

   Purpose here is to arrive at the value of stock i.e., what the hospital paid for it, but also includes a cost for labour, storage and other overheads involved in holding it.

3. **Value of inventory as a book entry**

   Hospital may have to choose as to whether to value stock at its replacement value or at what it costs.

4. **Value of inventory on sale after liquidation proceedings**

   Organization will be selling at a discount, but in addition, there may be some items which have been custom made for organization alone, have only a scrap value.

5. **Preparing estimate for tenders**

   Hospital may be looking ahead, it wants latest available price which, maybe factorized to give a forecast to some point in the future.

   Example: entering in to contracts with medical insurance companies.

6. **Value of items purchased as an investment:**

   The reason for purchase is to maximize profit which is set out by:

   Profit = Selling Price less (Purchase Price + Cost of storage, transport, etc.+ interest over the period on the purchase price + tax on the transaction).

   Value varies according to the circumstances and time. For each of these valuations, different data is required. Generally speaking, cost of doing these separate valuations is not worth the effort and hospitals select one or two methods on which all costing and valuations will be based.

VALUATION OF INCOMING MATERIALS

Valuation of incoming materials is relatively easy as compared to valuation of materials consumed. Invoice or supply bill received from the supplier forms the basic document and also the starting point in the valuation of the receipt of materials.

Following points are considered for the purpose:

1. To start with, materials are valued as per purchase order price. Different vendors raise invoices differently; namely, net price, basic price with discounts, suppliers' ex-works, FO.R. (Place of dispatch), F.O.R. (Place of destination), Buyers' works, at site etc. While arriving at the landed cost, the buyer must take into consideration the appropriate expenses incurred required to be added to the basic price to arrive at the actual cost incurred (i.e., landed cost). For the purpose of costing, discount is deducted from the basic price and all other expenses billed by the vendor (i.e., excise or customs duty, sales tax, octroi, transport, insurance charges etc.) are added.

2. In the event, where vendor's invoice consists of more than one item of supplies, the expenses jointly incurred (viz. freight, insurance, octroi, carriage inward etc.) for all items are distributed on the basis of weighted average to arrive at correct values.

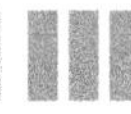

3. Valuation of imported materials is done differently by taking into account the cost of material i.e., basic price (which is stated in foreign currency and needs to be converted into Indian currency), customs duty, clearing charges, freight, and local transport charges, octroi etc.

4. Use of computers reduces clerical work considerably. Cost of material can be calculated by developing software incorporating break up of various cost elements such as basic price, discounts, packing and forwarding, excise duty, sales lax, freight, insurance, octroi, etc.

5. For normal credit period. Cash discounts are generally ignored as it represents opportunity cost of the money.

Illustration -1 Valuation of indigenously procured equipment

Particulars relating to, purchase of electro medical apparatus model 9018-90-99 for interferential therapies with stimulator vectrostim standard with standard accessories is as follows:

1	Quoted pric	Rs. 24,500
2	Discount	10 percent
3	Central excise duty	5 percent
4	Surcharge oil excise	0.50 Percent
5	Packing and forwarding charges	3 percent
6	VAT	5 Percent
7	Freig	Rs. 500
8	Transit insurance	0.25 Percent
10	Educational cess	0.1 percent
11	S.H.E cess	0.05 percent
12	Octroi	2 percent
13	Delivery charges from transporters godown to the buyer's place	Rs. 150
14	Unloading charges at site	Rs. 50

Calculate: 1. Total cost of material purchased

2. Unit cost of material to be considered for valuation of receipts.

Calculation of landed cost:

a) Statement showing cost of materials

	Figures in Rs.
Basic cost	24,500.00
Less discount offered 10 percent	2,450.00
	22,050.00

Packing and forwarding cost		
@ 3 percent		661.50
		22,711.50
Central Excise Duty		
At 5 percent of 22,711.5 = Rs. 1136.00		
Surcharge on excise duty at		
[0.5 percent on Rs. 1136	6.00	
	1142.00	
Educational Cess 0.1 percent		
on excise duty	22.71	
S.H.E Cess 0.05 percent	11.35	
	1176.06	(+) 1,176.00
		23,887.50
VAT @ 5 percent on 23,887.50 =	1194.37	(+) 1,194.00
		25,081.50
Other costs		
Freight	500.00	
Transit insurance @ 0.25		
Percent on Rs. 25, 081.50	62.70	
Octroi at 2 percent		
Rs. 25, 081.50	501.63	
Delivery charges from transporters		
godown to the buyer's place	150.00	
Unloading charges @ site	50.00	
	1264.33	(+) 1264.50
		Rs. 26,346.00

Illustration II : Valuation of imported equipment

Supplier: M/s	KAWB & DT. 5504503072/8-8-13	Exchange rate:65.35
	SAWB & DT.	IGM No.
	INVOICE No. SO-521015/ 18-7-13	PK/KGS:

IMPORTER: M/s

Item Description	Thompson Retractor for Liver Transplant with Standard Accessories
Quantity	1
Unit Rate	$31760.00
CIF Invoice	$31760.00
FC Miscellaneous	0.00
Invoice CIF	$31760.00

	Rupees
Indian Rupee on CIF	2075516.00
Freight	0.00
Insurance	0.00
CIF in Indian Rupee	2075516.00
Landing charges 1Percent	20755.00
Total	**2096271.16**
Assessable Value	**2096271**
Customs Tariff Head (CTH)/Central Excise Tariff Head (CETH)	90189025
Duty Rate	5+6+0+3+4* if the machine is being imported for own use it attracts SAD (Special Addl. Duty)too.
Basic Custom Duty	104813.56
Additional?	132065.08
Cess on Addl. Duty?	Nil
Cumm.Edn.Cess ?	7106.36
Total	**243985.00**
SAD @ 4% ON TOTAL (VALUE+Duties)	93610
DUTY AMOUNT	**337595**
TOTAL LANDED COST(Assessable Value + Customs Duty)	**20962 71.16+ 337595 = 2433866**

Illustration III: Valuation of imported drug

Supplier: M/s	KAWB & DT. 5504503072/8-8-13	Exchange rate: 61.55
	SAWB & DT.	IGM No.
	INVOICE No. SO-521015/18-7-13	PK/KGS:

IMPORTER: M/s

Item Description	Ptoclaim 7.5MG, Blister pack of 56 Tablets (German Origin ;7 No's)
Quantity	420.0
Unit Rate	1.7296
CIF Invoice	$726.45
FC Miscellaneous	0.00
Invoice CIF	$726.45

		Rupees
Indian Rupee on CIF		44713.00
Freight		0.00
Insurance		0.00
CIF in Indian Rupee		44713.00
Landing charges 1 percent		447.13
Total		45160.13
Assessable Value		45160
CTH (Customs Tariff Head)/CETH (Central Excise Tariff Head)	30049039	
Duty Rate	10+6+0+3+4	
Basic Custom Duty		4516.01
Additional ?		2980.57
Cess on Addl. Duty ?		Nil
Cumm. Edn. Cess ?		224.90
Addl. Duty		2115.26
Total		9836.74
DUTY AMOUNT		9837.00
TOTAL LANDED COST(Assessable value + Customs Duty)	**45160+9837 =**	**54997.00**

UNIQUE FEATURES OF HOSPITALS INVENTORY VALUATION

In a manufacturing and retail organization, the inventories are held at different stages like raw materials, work in process, sub assemblies, finished goods etc., whereas retail companies have one type of merchandize available for sale; in the organization reflect in their books of accounts till such time the goods are sold. In either case, inventories are treated as assets. However, the approach to inventory accounting by hospitals is unique and inconsistent. That means both official and unofficial inventories exist throughout the healthcare institutions. Healthcare institutions generally consider those inventories that are maintained in central stores, central supply, pharmacy and dietary etc. Inventory issued and utilized by any of the departments mentioned is immediately charged off to the department that requisitioned it. Unofficial inventory generally constitutes stocks held by nursing units, laboratory, maintenance etc. that are kept in stock for use. However, it is not under the control of official inventory departments. Thus, unofficial inventory includes all those items, which are requisitioned from official inventory (i.e., from main stores) and items which are issued for use by various departments i.e., everything expensed upon issue or receipt. Such expensing of items by hospital can be attributed to the reason that hospitals view inventory not as an asset but as a liability.

Concept of expensing as much and as soon as possible in practice encourages investment of large capital in unofficial inventory than necessary. These unofficial inventories further lock up working capital for the hospital and represent a primary source of cost containment through reduction of unofficial inventories.

Thus, if a hospital switches over to accounting of inventory until it actually is consumed, it results in:

- Value of official inventory increases dramatically.
- Hospital inventory permits an accurate accounting.
- Adoption of this procedure is a stepping stone for reducing inventory and gaining better leverage on hospital supply cost.

A survey conducted by Edward Sanderson revealed that in many US hospitals, purchasing practitioners have indicated that improper inventory accounting is a source of misunderstanding and confusion.

Much of this misunderstanding is from trying to apply pure accounting theory to actual practice without understanding the theory itself. In hospitals, stock valuation will have to address various methods of accounting and their impact on inventory systems, patient charges, supplies and proper record keeping.

METHODS OF VALUATION MATERIALS ISSUES

Valuation of issues is far more complex than valuation of receipts, especially if the material is to be issued out of different lots purchased at different prices, problem arises in deciding as to which receipt prices should be used to value the material issue.

There are different methods of valuations of materials and they are:

1. FIFO (First in First Out)
2. LIFO (Last in First Out)
3. HIFO (Highest in First Out)

4. NIFO (Next in First Out)
5. Base stock method
6. Simple average price method
7. Periodic simple average price method
8. Moving simple average price method
9. Weighted average price method
10. Periodic weighted average price method
11. Moving weighted average price method
12. Market price method or Replacement price method
13. Standard price method
14. Inflated price method
15. Reuse price method

Various methods of inventory valuation narrated above can be grouped into four broad categories. Viz specific price, actual cost, average price, notional price and is shown Table 21.1

Table 21.1 Classification of Methods of Stock Valuation

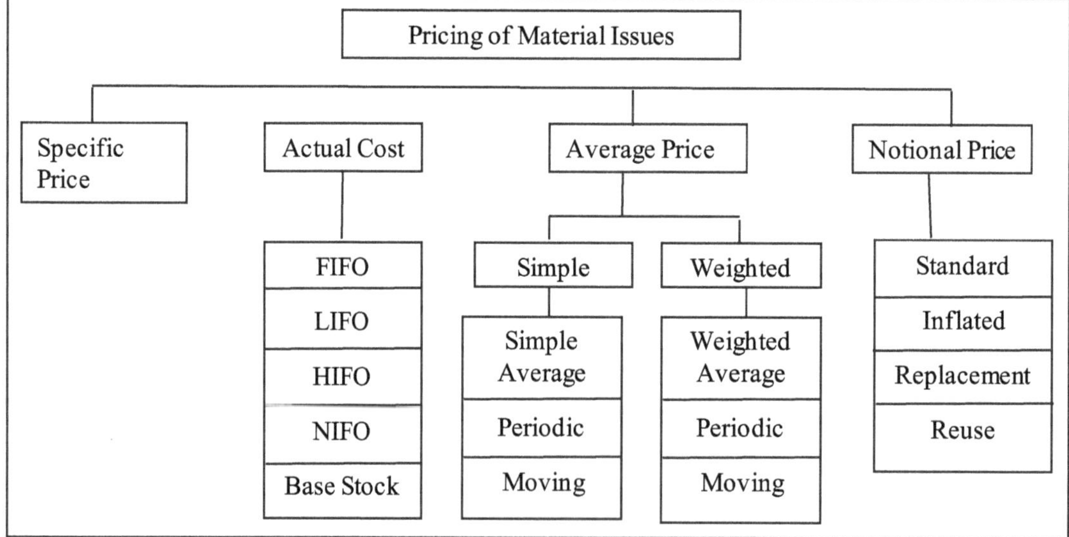

1. FIRST IN FIRST OUT (FIFO) METHOD

First In First Out method operates on the assumption that the materials are issued to user departments in the same sequence in which they are received into the store. In other words, the earliest consignment is first issued to user department and therefore, the issues are valued by taking into account the price of the oldest consignment and once it is exhausted, the price of the next oldest consignment is charged. The sequence of issue is only on paper under FIFO and not in reality i.e., physical issue of materials is not done. Only materials at the earliest rate are charged first.

It will be noticed that valuation of the issue is same as the value of receipts as they came into stores. Issues are in the same chronological order of the receipts and the same original values are given.

Operation of FIFO Method (Table 21.2)

Data below gives the details of purchases and issues of materials of store of company between months of April to September of first half the year.

Table 21. 2 Illustration of FIFO Method of Valuation of Inventories

Date	Receipt Units	Unit Value (Rs.)	Issue Units	Units Value (Rs.)
1st April	200	100		
2nd June	200	110		
6th June			50	100
9th June			150	100
11th June			80	110
1st August	200	120	20	110
5th August			100	110
30th September	100	120	100	120
			80	120

Advantages

1. In the case of slow moving materials, bulk items and the materials of high unit cost, this method is more appropriate.
2. This method has the advantage of adhering strictly to cost and recovery actual costs from operations of hospital in the order in which it is incurred.
3. This method is simple to operate and can be gainfully used where number of transactions are limited.
4. All values reflect cost of purchase and therefore no adjustments are made for the cost of replacement or for rises and falls in value.

Disadvantages

1. Number of calculations complicates the accounts and increases human errors in accounting system.
2. More than one price is often required to use, to evaluate one requisition.
3. Effect of current market price is not reflected in the cost of production.
4. If prices are fluctuating, every batch production will have different material cost and hence comparison becomes pointless.
5. When prices are falling, materials charged for patient care is high and cost of stock replacement is low and conversely when prices are raising the charge to patient care will be low while replacement costs of materials will be high.
6. Under inflationary conditions, this method inflates profits and therefore higher amounts are to be paid towards advance tax payment.
7. In actual practice, occasions may arise when physically FIFO is not followed. For example, materials may sometimes directly be transferred from goods receiving bay to user section. Even though stock received earlier may be available in the stores, this step is taken so that double handling is avoided.
8. It is an accurate way of measuring cost historically but has disadvantages if it is used for preparation of quotations.
9. When excess material is returned from user departments or nursing stations to stores, the adjustment will create complications in case of issues with more than one price.

2. LAST IN FIRST OUT (LIFO) METHOD

The LIFO valuation method also uses actual prices but in this method uses the value and charges for issues at the price of most recently received consignment until it is used up. That is, **LIFO method assumes that the last receipt will be issued first from the store, even though the physical issue of the material is not made out of the said lot.**

This method also ensures that materials are issued at actual cost except it is reverse of FIFO method. This method is also suitable where price fluctuations are not very many. Inventory valuation in LIFO method is shown in Table 21.3.

Table 21.3 Inventory Valuation Last in First Out Method

Date	Receipt Units	Units Value in Rs.	Issues Units	Units Value in Rs.
01-06-01	100	100		
02-07-01	100	110	25	110
06-07-01			75	110
09-07-01			40	100
17-07-01			10	100
01-09-01	100	120		
05-09-01			90	120

Advantages

1. This method is simple and easy to understand.
2. Product or service cost reflects current prices.
3. In this method, production is charged at latest prices and product cost reflects market conditions so long as receipts have been recent. Hence, price changing decisions can be taken more realistically.
4. LIFO method postpones the recognition of income, consequently rescheduling of tax payment.
5. Useful when prices are on escalating trend.
6. It prevents the necessity of ascertaining replacement price of materials.
7. Since this method uses latest price, tends to be better for preparation of quotations, especially relevant in inflatory market.

Disadvantages

1. Calculations become complicated if stocks are received frequently and at varying costs.
2. May give wrong results during periods of falling prices.
3. Stock will be at cost but will not represent correct price level; hence during falling prices, loss will have to be written off.
4. It may be noted that occasions may arise where LIFO may not be physically feasible. For example, in case of perishable or items with low shelf life, it is always preferable to consume first the lots which were received first even though LIFO may be adopted in accounting.
5. When stock is being run out, it calls for adjustments in stock values if they have risen abnormally or dropped markedly.
6. Akin to FIFO method, useful comparison of material cost of one job to another is not feasible, where price fluctuations are too recurrent.
7. As in case of FIFO method, sometimes more than one price has to be adopted for pricing a single issue of materials.
8. During the periods of falling prices, the issues are priced lower. It requires some adjustments on the principles of valuation of stock at cost or market price, whichever is lower.
9. In the event, latest receipt price is not finalized; work of pricing of issues has to be kept in abeyance.

3. HIGHEST IN FIRST OUT (HIFO) METHOD

HIFO method is in variation of above two methods. In this method, the issues are valued at highest price paid. For example, if there are three different prices for materials in stocks

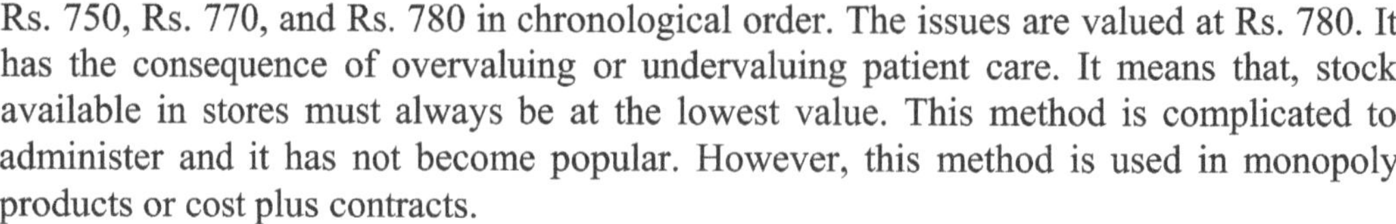

Rs. 750, Rs. 770, and Rs. 780 in chronological order. The issues are valued at Rs. 780. It has the consequence of overvaluing or undervaluing patient care. It means that, stock available in stores must always be at the lowest value. This method is complicated to administer and it has not become popular. However, this method is used in monopoly products or cost plus contracts.

4. NEXT IN FIRST OUT (NIFO) METHOD

This NIFO method also is in variation to FIFO and LIFO methods. In the NIFO method, the replacement value is taken into account. For example, if the cost of purchase is Rs. 700 but market price today is Rs. 750, then Rs. 750 is the value of issues. The hitch in this method is the price, if ruling at the time of supply differs from purchase order price. This method is similar to replacement method.

5. BASE STOCK METHOD

This method also assumes that materials are issued at cost. It is assumed that a fixed minimum stock of material is always carried at original cost and the minimum stock is never touched except in emergency. This method is akin to FIFO method except minimum stock. The minimum stock held depends upon factors such as the material, lead time, and price. The closing stock at any time consists of minimum of two components i.e., a base stock component at a fixed value and additional material held in FIFO basis. There is one point, which needs to be clarified here, physical stock of quantities kept as base stock need not be the ones purchased earlier. These are to be issued depending on the shelf life of the item. This is only notional and this concept is used for accounting purpose. As this method is used with FIFO or LIFO, all the advantages and disadvantages of FIFO or LIFO will apply depending on the method followed.

6. SIMPLE AVERAGE PRICE METHOD

In this method, issues are valued on simple average price. Average price is calculated each time whenever a new consignment is received at a new price. This is done by taking mean of prices paid per unit of stock on consignment still remaining and the price of new consignment.

For example: If the existing price of stock valued at Rs. 1000 and new stock arrived valued at Rs. 1100, it means average price is Rs. 1050. This price will be used until next change in price occurs.

Average price is calculated before the issues takes place. To avoid errors in calculations, reverse order is followed on the assumption that the issues are on first in first out basis.

Advantages

1. The method is simple to understand and easy to operate.
2. Cost distortions are not much because of adopting an average price.

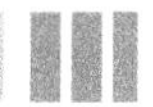

3. Simple average price is useful when purchases are made in fixed lots (say EOQ) and price does not vary vastly.

Disadvantages

1. This method does not consider the quantities of lots in stock. Absurd results are obtained if the quantity purchased in different lots varies. Since actual costs are not used, profit or loss results.
2. For accounting purpose, it may not highlight a true value and will require reconciliation account.
3. Average method involves considerable calculations and is therefore ideally suited for computerized accounting system and not conducive for manually operated accounts.
4. Where prices fluctuate swiftly over a fairly slender range, the average price is useful. On the other hand, if there are extraordinary rise or fall in prices, a false average may result which does not reflect the trend.
5. Since the prices are not weighted by the quantities purchased, the average prices arrived at does not give proper depiction of facts unless fluctuations are not much or quantities purchased in each order are same.
6. As this is only an approximate average, adjustments are necessary periodically.

Illustration of simple average price method is shown in Table 21.4.

Table 21.4 Simple Average Method for Price Issues

Date	Situation	Receipts			Issues			Balance	
		Qty. (Nos.)	Unit Rate (Rs.)	Value (Rs.)	Qty. (Nos.)	Unit Rate (Rs.)	Value (Rs.)	Qty. (Nos.)	Value (Rs.)
Apr 1st	Opening balance	---	--	--	--	--	--	300 @ Rs. 9.80 each	2940
Apr 5th	GRN	500	10	5000	--	--	--	800	7940
Apr 15th	SR	--	--	--	300	9.9 (10 + 9.8)/2	2970	500	4950
Apr 20th	GRN	400	10.10	4040	--	--	--	900	8990
Apr 25th	SR	--	--	--	200	10.05 (10+10.10)/2	2010	700	7035
Apr 30th	MRN	200	10.05	2010				900	9045

(GRN: Goods Receipt Note, SR: Stores Requisition, MRN: Material Return Note)

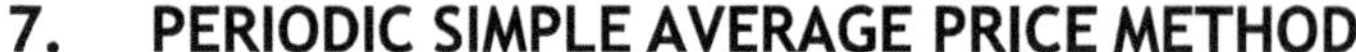

7. PERIODIC SIMPLE AVERAGE PRICE METHOD

This method follows the principle of the simple average price. A period is set over which the average is calculated periodically, say, once in a month, quarter or six months. The average so obtained is then used for pricing the materials issues of that period uniformly.

Operation of this method is illustrated below.

March 1st purchased 500 nos. @ Rs.10.00 each

March 10th Purchased 400 nos. @ Rs. 10.25 each

March 25th Purchased 300 nos. @ Rs. 10.50 each

Therefore, average price to be charged shall be:

(10.00+10.25+10.50)/3 = Rs. 10.25

Advantages

1. Periodic average price is extremely simple to operate. It is even simpler than the simple average price, since the only calculation of issue price occurs at the end of the period concerned.
2. Variations in price are considerably reduced.

Disadvantages

1. Pricing of material issues is delayed since the periodical simple average can be calculated after the period is over.
2. Because of periodic activity, there is considerable amount of work at one time since issue prices of all materials in store require to be calculated.
3. Since actual prices are not in use, profit or loss arises.

An important point to be observed in this method is that though purchases and closing stock are included into the calculations, but opening stock does not enter the calculations, since it was purchased in the last period's calculations.

8. MOVING SIMPLE AVERAGE PRICE METHOD

To arrive at moving simple average price, the issues are valued at a price which, is calculated by dividing the total of the periodic simple average prices of a given number of periods by the number of periods. It takes into account the average price of the current period and also the average prices for a given number of earlier periods. Usually odd number of months, say 3, 5, or 7 is used. This method evens out price fluctuations over a number of periods and cost distortions from one job to another job are reduced. In case of rising prices, the stock is overvalued. Profit or loss may arise due to approximations.

9. WEIGHTED AVERAGE PRICE METHOD

This method is an improved version over simple average price method since it gives weightage to the quantities of different lots in stock.

Weighted price is obtained by dividing the cost of materials in stock by total quantity of materials in the stock. In the weighted average method, whenever a fresh batch of material is received, a new weighted average price is required to be arrived at. In view of the fact that weighted price takes into account both the price and the quantity of material in stock, the absurd results are avoided.

An illustration of weighted average price of three different batches of material is in stock, when a material required is to be issued. The average price arrived at for pricing issues under this method are as follows.

1000 units of Rs. 20

2000 units of Rs. 21

3000 units of Rs. 22

$$\text{Weighted average price} = \frac{1000 \times 20 + 2000 \times 21 + 3000 \times 22}{1000 + 2000 + 3000}$$

$$= \frac{20000 + 42000 + 66000}{6000}$$

$$= \text{Rs. } 21.33$$

Alternatively, the price on receipt of fresh supply is obtained by dividing the "value of existing stocks by the quantity in stock". Issue prices, in this method, are calculated at the time of receipt of materials, and not at the time of issue of materials.

Advantages

1. It is easy to understand and simple to operate.
2. Issue prices need not be calculated every time, when issues are made.
3. In the valuation, both the cost charged to production and value of closing stock reflects reasonable market conditions.
4. Another advantage of this method accuracy, mainly where the price paid for materials fluctuate significantly. However, this method involves more calculations. To take advantage the benefit of accuracy, the calculations required to be made up to fourth decimal.
5. Though price of material does not represent actual cost price of material but it represents average cost of materials in stores, because of weightage factors, price fluctuations are evenly distributed in the valuation

Disadvantages

1. Main disadvantage of this method is that a fresh rate requires to be worked out as soon as a new consignment is received and therefore involves more calculations when prices and quantities are fluctuating significantly.

2. Profit and loss arises in the end as the actual prices are not used for pricing issues.

An illustration on the weighted method of pricing out issues is shown in Table 21.5

Table 21.5 Illustration of Weighted Average Price Method

Date	Receipt Units Nos.	Units Value in Rs.	Issues Units Nos.	Units Value in Rs.	Weighted Average Value Rs.
01-06	100	100			100
02-07	100	110			105
	i.e (Rs. 100 × 100 + 100 × 110) ÷ 200				
06-07			25	105	
09-07			115	105	
17-07			10	105	
01-09	100	120			115
	i.e (50 × 105) + (100 × 120) ÷ 150				
05-09			90	115	

Differences between simple average price method and weighted average price method can be had from Table 21.6.

Table 21.6 Differences between Simple Average Price Method and Weighted Average Price Method

Simple average price method	Weighted average price method
1. Considers only prices of different batches at the time of issue. On the other hand, it does not consider the quantity of material available in stock.	1. Both prices and quantities of batches in stock are taken into account at the time of issue of materials.
2. Whenever materials are issued, new average is worked out. Not at the time of receipt of materials.	2. Fresh average is worked out as soon as a new lot is received but not at the time of issue.

10. PERIODIC WEIGHTED AVERAGE PRICE METHOD

In periodic weighted average price method, the price is fixed taking into account at the end of the period, by dividing the total amount of purchase by the total quantity. Unlike the weighted average price method, it is easy to arrive at the prices, as number of calculations is less since it avoids the need to calculate weighted average for every supply received.

Advantages

1. Clerical work load and calculations involved in the weighted average method reduced considerably.
2. This method is more accurate than periodic simple average price method as both quantities and costs are taken care of.

Disadvantages

1. Periodical weighted average price is arrived at, after the expiry of the period. Hence, the pricing of materials issues is delayed.
2. Since actual prices are not applied, there is bound to be scope for profit or loss.

11. MOVING WEIGHTED AVERAGE PRICE METHOD

In this method, to obtain moving average, the total of the weighted average price of the current period and weighted average prices of given number of preceding periods is to be divided by the number of periods (i.e., current + preceding periods). This price is to be applied to all the issues in the current period. It is comparatively similar to moving simple average method except for that this is a moving weighted average price and hence all the advantages and disadvantages are akin to moving simple average method are applicable here also.

12. MARKET PRICE METHOD

Market price is also known as replacement costing. Issues under this method are valued at price prevailing in the market at the time of issue. This pricing method pre supposes the determination of replacement cost of materials at the time of each issue and involves considerable clerical work. It is very difficult to get market price daily for all the issues made on that date of issue and involves lot of clerical work. This method is not universally adopted since it introduces elements of uncertainty and estimates and is manly used at the time of disposal of surplus, obsolete and non moving items.

13. STANDARD PRICE METHOD

Where standard costing system of pricing is in vogue this method is best suited. Receipts as well as issues are costed at the pre determined price called standard price.

In this method, a 'forecasted' price for a period is used to evaluate issue. This forecasted price takes into account, the market conditions, transportation costs, usage rate, storage facilities, handling facilities, quantity and quantity discounts, price rise etc. It is pertinent to note that actual price will be distinctly different from the forecasted price. The standard price so fixed is kept stable for a specific period (say six months or one year). Issue of material, during this period is priced at the standard prices irrespective of the actual prices.

At the end of the period, new standard prices are set for next period. Actual price is compared with the standard price and the difference is charged to an account which is known as "price variance account".

Standard price is arrived at by considering the following factors:

1. The quantity of materials on hand.
2. The quantity of materials to be purchased and its impact on quantity discounts.
3. Prices normally paid or payable.
4. Normal purchasing cost involved.
5. Likelihood of a rise or fall in prices due to fluctuations in the market.
6. Changes in demand for the item due to changes in operations of the hospital.
7. Anticipated container charges, freight and warehousing expenses to the price of materials.
8. Price committed on the purchase orders is valid for the contracted period.

A standard price will be set for each material and is applied for all the issues in the pre- set-period, normally a year. It is compared with the actual price paid. Profit or loss may arise under this method also but it is not due to average prices.

It is on account of variances from a pre determined price set for each material. If the actual price paid exceeds standard, it is adverse variance and if the actual price is less than standard, it is favourable variance. All receipts under this method are posted at actual prices and issues at standard prices for each material. Under this method, stocks on hand is underestimated during period of rising prices and it is overestimated during period of falling prices.

Advantages

1. It is simple to operate since all the issues are priced at the same standard rate.
2. It is a barometer to measure the efficiency of purchase department.
3. It is obvious that actual price will definitely be different from forecasted price. The difference between the two helps to evaluate the performance of purchasing.
4. Further, this method is simple to operate, if pricing decisions are to take care of variance between market price and forecast price. Hence, this method is quite popular.
5. Constructive assessment of one job or process with another job or process is viable
6. Clerical costs are reduced the since the standard price will be applied to all the issues to be made in the pre determined period.

Disadvantages

1. In this case, the error is intrinsic to the system and profit or losses on issues depend on actual prices being lesser or more than the forecast.
2. Issues may not be at recent economic values and hence profit or loss may arise which has to be adjusted in the books of accounts.
3. To fix a standard price is very difficult during the period of inflation or when it fluctuates widely.
4. Value of closing stock may show incongruous figures.
5. The trend of actual prices may not be reflected.
6. Incorrect standard prices, if applied may result in depiction of production or operations cost.

14. INFLATED PRICE METHOD

The materials price charged in this method is slightly higher (i.e., higher by a small percentage) than the actual purchase price. The extra percentage is intended to counterbalance (i.e., recover) cost of wastage of material, expenses towards inspection, storing, carrying, handling of materials, and losses arising out of evaporation and breaking up bulk etc. are treated as production and operations overheads. Since all these expenses are added to determine the cost of issue, inflated price will cover the full cost of materials. This is not a separate method of pricing. Any of the prices actual, average or notional may be inflated for the purpose of valuation of issues.

15. RE USE PRICE METHOD

It is the price which is used to value a material in its reuse. This price is adopted for the issue of materials to other departments for an alternative use. Profit or loss may arise because issues are not valued at actual cost and it has to be adjusted in accounts.

Reported profits are affected by the way inventories are priced. The method of inventory valuation can have considerable effect on the analysis of all decisions about liquidity and profitability of an organization.

SUMMARY

Inventory valuation is the pricing of the receipts issues and returns of materials in store with an object to arrive at the proper cost of materials consumed for production and to determine the value of stock held at the end of the period.

Valuation of receipts of materials is relatively an easy task and is done at a rate which takes into account all the expenses, till an item lands in the company's store. For valuation of issues of materials one has to decide, based on company's policy, the receipt prices which should be considered to value material as material may be issued out of the various lots purchased at different rates (landed costs).

Methods of valuation of materials range from conservative practices such as market price or cost of procurement whichever is lower on one hand to modern development to replacement cost on the other.

1. FIFO (First in First Out)
2. LIFO (Last in First Out)
3. HIFO (Highest in First Out)
4. NIFO (Next in First Out)
5. Base stock method
6. Simple average
7. Periodic simple average
8. Moving average
9. Weighted average
10. Periodic weighted average
11. Moving weighted average
12. Market pricing method
13. Standard costing method
14. Inflated price method
15. Reuse price method.

FIFO (First in First Out) method ensures that materials are issued at actual cost, hence no profit or loss incurred by the valuation. LIFO (Last in First Out) method also ensures that materials are issued at actual cost, but it is reverse of FIFO method. HIFO (Highest in First Out) method is in variation of above two methods. In this method, the highest cost is taken for issues. NIFO (Next in First Out) method also is in variation to FIFO and LIFO methods. In the NIFO method, the replacement value is taken into account. Base stock method also assumes that materials are issued at cost. Simple average method issues are valued on simple average price. Average price is calculated each time a new consignment is received at a new price. Periodic simple average method is similar to that of simple average method, the difference is that instead of finding an average price for each issue, an average price is calculated for a period (may be monthly or quarterly or half yearly or annually) and all issues in that period are valued accordingly. Moving simple average method, the issues are valued at a price which is calculated by dividing total of periodic simple average prices of a given number of periods by number of periods. Weighted average method is almost similar to simple average method. However purchase prices are weighted by respective quantities .Periodic weighted average method is just as periodic simple average, is an extension of simple average valuation; so also the periodic weighted average method is derived from weighted average method. Moving weighted average is more or less identical to moving simple average method except that this is a moving weighted average price method.Market price method, also known as replacement price method. This method is not generally adopted due to elements of uncertainty and estimates. At the time of disposal of surplus, obsolete and non moving items, this method is used. In standard cost method a 'forecasted' price for a period is used to evaluate issue. It is a predetermined price on the basis of specifications of all the factors affecting price of materials in a future period. The factors generally considered are quantity, quantity discounts, prices normally paid payable, purchasing costs involved, changes in production operation requirements etc.

 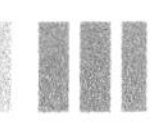

Inflated prices include over and above the invoice price. Other expenses like cost of receiving, inspection, storing and carrying etc. are treated as production operations overheads. In this method, all the above expenses are added to the invoice price. Reuse price is a price which is used to value material in its reuse. This price is adopted for issues of materials to other departments for an alternative use.

REVIEW QUESTIONS

1. Explain briefly different methods of inventory valuation. Which method would you suggest when the prices are frequently fluctuating?
2. What is stores accounting? Distinguish between FIFO, LIFO and weighted average methods used in stock valuation.
3. What is the need for valuation of inventory? How will you arrive at the landed cost of incoming material?
4. Which method of stock valuation is most suitable for perishable commodities in the hospital? Why? Reason out suitability of the method.
5. What is the need for inventory valuation? Describe the unique features of hospital inventory valuation?
6. Write short notes on
   a) Differences between simple average and weight average methods of pricing of issues.
   b) Average method of valuation.
   c) Standard price method of stock valuation.
   d) Actual cost method of inventory valuation.
   e) Base stock method of valuation.
   f) Replacement price method.

PROBLEMS

1. A hospital stores book of accounts has revealed the following medical stores transactions for September 2015. Write up the priced stores ledger on FIFO method.

Date		Quantity (Units)	Price per unit (Rs.)
Sep 1	Opening balance	25	162.50
Sep 4	Issues	8	
Sep 6	Receipts from B & Co.	50	5.75
Sep 7	Issues	12	
Sep 10	Returns to B & Co.	10	
Sep 12	Issues	15	
Sep 13	Issues	20	
Sep 15	Receipts from M & Co.	25	6.10
Sep 17	Issues	10	
Sep 19	Received replacement from B & Co.	10	
Sep 20	Returned from department material of M & Co.	5	
Sep 22	Transfer from Job 182 to Job 187 in the dept	5	
Sep 26	Issues	10	
Sep 29	Transfer from Dept. A to Dept. B	5	
Sep 30	Shortage in stock taking	2	

Check your answer

13 units at 6.10 = Rs. 79.30

15 units at 5.75 = Rs. 86.25

--------- ---------------

28 units Rs. 165.55

2. From the data given below, find out closing stock and closing values applying FIFO, and LIFO methods of inventory valuation.

Date	Receipts			Issues		
	Qty. (Units)	Cost price unit(Rs.)	Value (Rs.)	Qty. (Units)	Cost price unit(Rs.)	Value (Rs.)
Jan 1	500	8.00				
Jan 5	200	8.50				
Jan 10	--	--	--	400		
Jan 12	150	8.20				
Jan 14	--	--	--	200		
Jan 15	--	--	--	100		
Jan 19	--	--	--	100		
Jan 20	300	9.00				
Jan 25	400	8.00				
Jan 26	--	--	--	200		
Jan 30	--	--	--	250		

Check your answer:

FIFO method:

Closing stock = 300 units,

Value of closing stock = 300 units @ Rs. 8 = Rs. 2400.00

LIFO method:

Closing stock = 250 units x @ Rs. 9 Value = Rs. 2250.00

Closing stock = 50 units × @ Rs. 8 Value = Rs. 400.00

Rs. 2650.00

Total closing stock = 300 units. Total closing stock value = Rs. 2650.00

Supply and Distribution Management

Contents

CHAPTER - 22

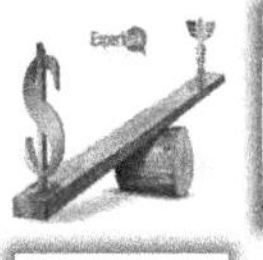
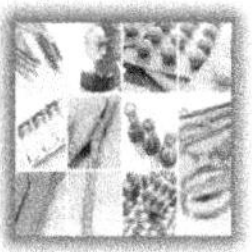
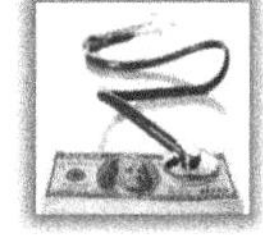
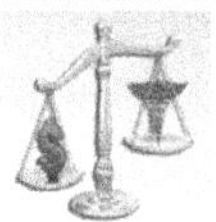

Supply and Distribution Management

INTRODUCTION

Hospital distribution system is a complex network of storage (source) and user (destination) points. In a healthcare facility, the distribution system is an integral part of a Materials Management programme and significantly affects its performance. The goal of an effective distribution system is to provide right item to the right requisition at the right time for a least total cost. **Every rupee spent to purchase an item needs another rupee in storing and moving it.** There is no one best system for all situations. Exchange cart system is perhaps the most well known method of supply distribution in hospitals. It has impressive benefits. However, there are other alternatives which could be cost effective and provide more efficient distribution. Hospitals need to take a broad systems approach. A detailed study and analysis of the entire distribution network and requirements generally reveals opportunities for streamlining it and reducing total costs. Movement of items such as food, beverages, medicines, office supplies, linen (both soiled and clean), trash, mail, equipment, and paper makes the material flow in a hospital voluminous and complicated.

OPTIMIZATION OF STORAGE SPACE

Materials managers in hospitals have historically been complaining lack of adequate storage space to maintain the inventory level, required to meet the demands of the hospital. In a majority of cases, their complaints fell on deaf ears. Administrators do have sympathy for materials manager's plight, but are generally unable to provide additional space owing to physical constraints of existing facilities. Even when expansion is under consideration, additional storage space for central stores is given low priority in deference to the needs for expanded patient care services. Seldom is the question of additional storage space considered in hospital expansion plans. Hospital materials managers must therefore become creative and improve utilization of the space currently available. They need to deal with the problem of storage on the basis of working within the confines of existing space. Movement and control of supplies throughout the hospital are major concerns for users as well as materials managers. **The subject of supply distribution is closely associated with space considerations.**

Distribution system is a key component of a Materials Management programme. It affects many other operations and functions. Supply distribution is intimately related to inventory management. This is a direct link up. An effective system can directly support the hospital's inventory management and also directly affect the amount of inventory maintained in a general store room as well as in user departments. **Edward D. Sanderson,** in his book on "Hospital Purchasing and Inventory Management", reports that numerous studies have estimated that there may be a one to three ratio for what is stored in the store room to what is in the user areas; that is, for every $1 of inventory in the store room, there may be $3 in the user areas. Frequency at which the supply distribution system replenishes stocks in user departments has a direct effect on inventory levels. **The more frequently inventories are replenished, smaller the inventories needed at user points in the hospital departments at any time.**

SUPPLY AND INTERNAL DISTRIBUTION

Problems associated with a well planned storage facility extend beyond the store room. It is not limited to the discussion of inventory management to those items that are maintained within the store room. **A logical extension of inventory management is supply and internal distribution.** The increased responsibility of the Materials Management concept has broadened the scope of inventory management to extend to the nursing units and all other departments. Those other departments were traditionally off limits to the materials managers, but the advent of Materials Management is removing the obstacles to such extended inventory management. This extension brings with it the need for MM to review and update the methods of supply and internal distribution.

With an internal distribution system in place, patient care personnel no longer need to prepare requisitions or put away supplies once orders have been filled and delivered. This can make more time available for patient care. This can be done at no extra cost to the hospital. It is merely a reallocation and better use of personnel time. Supply persons should manage the distribution system and care persons can concentrate on patients' care. The location system for items in the store room can positively affect order picking productivity. If items are stored in logical sequence (such as by product code numbers) or by broad product classifications, store room requisitions can be generated in that sequence, thus reducing the time required to locate and pick orders, whether they be for an exchange cart, par level, or standard requisition system. Store room layout and location of items inside, of course affect the order picking methods employed in supply and internal distribution. Inadequate parking space in the warehouse store room virtually eliminates using an exchange cart system. Such systems need space to park all those carts. Service levels provided to user areas can be further enhanced by implementing a proper distribution system. The system should be proactive and replenish inventories in the user areas automatically on a cycle basis. Such a system will require less user personnel time. Management of patient supply charges can also be vastly enhanced by coordination with the internal distribution system. As replenishment frequency increases, timeliness of the reconciliation for charges and the opportunity for control and management of losses are correspondingly improved. This brings about reduced losses and directly increases hospital revenue.

PLANNING OF FACILITIES

Plans for maximizing storage space must begin by identifying the physical requirements for every item to be stored. This process requires that every item be categorized by size, shape, and weight for the maximum amount of inventory. The information thus collected is used to identify the type of storage required, i.e., shelf, or pallet etc. Items are then sorted by storage requirements to determine an accurate picture of the total requirements for each type of storage unit. For example, all items requiring shelf storage are grouped together. Individual item analysis must also include total cubic requirements. Once this information is complete, the next phases of the planning process can be taken up.

Design and layout process must start by defining the physical dimensions of the storage area including ceiling height, room dimensions, location of support columns, and lighting arrangement. In many cases, the facilities maintenance department may be in a position to provide the scale drawings of the area. If drawings are not available, it would be necessary to measure the area and create scale drawings. Once the room drawings are made available, templates should be made in the same scale to represent existing shelving units and pallets. Shelving templates should identify the number of shelves per unit etc. At this point, it may be helpful to also review the types of storage units. Shelves are available in various widths, lengths, and heights. They should be selected on the basis of the type of item to be stored. Depths of 30, 45, and 60 cm are the most popular and appropriate sizes for use in a store room. Weight bearing capabilities, types of pallets to be used should also be considered. Metal pallets are ideal, whereas wooden or plastic pallets are cheaper but prone to fire hazards. Logical layouts should be considered after the templates are completed and these can be based on the use of static shelving or an active aisle system.

Uniform shelving arrangements provide maximum accessibility and orderly flow of materials. Static aisle arrangement accommodates an orderly flow of material from the receiving area to storage and also from storage to the user. **The main traffic aisle must be wide enough to accommodate various types of material handling equipment.** The stocking and picking aisles that radiate from the main traffic aisle are narrower. These aisles may vary in width to accommodate the various sizes and volumes of the material stored in the location. Active aisle concept utilizes movable carts on tracks in the aisles. This concept maximizes the footage that is normally lost to required aisles in the static concept. Manufacturers of active aisle systems claim improved utilization of floor space by more than 50 percent. Such claims may be true but materials managers considering this type of storage should compare the actual difference between the amounts of shelf space available with the active aisle system versus that available with current or proposed static shelving. Any improvements will depend upon current available square footage, room design, and the amount of available static shelving. Active aisle is a sound concept when employed for loose issue items, but is impractical for heavy bulk storage. Active aisle also more expensive, and should be reviewed with the idea of determining where the payback will come from. Finally, a properly designed store room not only maximizes use of available floor space, but also the use of available cubic space.

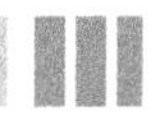

Maximizing cubic space must not be neglected during the design stage. Individual item storage must take into consideration upward as well as horizontal storage. A rule of thumb is useful. In order to maximize storage space, think upward, not spread it out.

Physical limitations of a store room extend beyond size to type of floors, walls, ceilings, lighting, etc. These characteristics are as important as available square metre area. Floors in a store room should be cemented concrete. White marble or vinyl tile floors look good, but are impractical to maintain. Walls should also preferably be concrete or concrete block painted in bright, cheerful colours. Nothing is more depressing in a store room than unpainted, grey or brown walls. Ceiling height should be at least 3 to 4 metres clear height (floor to bottom of light fixtures or fire alarm sensors); anything less will limit the available cubic space. Ceiling height is also a limiting factor on the height of shelving units. Open ceilings create excessive dirt, especially if there are concrete floors above. In such cases, provisions for continued housekeeping will be necessary. Lighting is another physical limitation. Lighting patterns should be adequate to prevent dark areas in storage areas as well as aisles. Store room personnel cannot pick items which they cannot see. Practitioners should also be aware that fire safety codes in most countries require that upward storage must be maintained at a minimum of 45 cm below lighting fixtures, ceilings, or sprinkler heads.

Storage facility should have a stock location system in order to prevent lost motion and delays in locating inventory items. A definite address for every stock item is necessary for maintaining orderliness, efficient storage, and quick order filling. A simple, efficient location system of labeling shelving and pallets is accomplished by using alphanumeric characters. A complete system also includes a file or catalogue maintained either in stock number sequence or alphabetically with location codes. This record must also be current and changes should be posted as soon as they occur.

Typically, items are stored on the basis of popularity.

Storage based upon popularity refers to frequency of demand, and usually coincides with the ABC concept. Popular A items are stored closest to the major traffic aisle or work area; Medium B movers are next, followed by slow moving C items, which are last or furthest from the traffic aisle or work area. This methodology ensures that a majority of stocking and issuing activity will be completed near the work area and limits the average travel time for the work to be accomplished. Storage by popularity should be the first consideration.

Storage based upon similarity refers to items that are frequently ordered or used by one department and are stored close to each other to avoid unnecessary travel between items. For example, items used and ordered frequently by surgery would be stocked in the same area. Storage by similarity comes second to storage by popularity.

Storage based upon size is the third possibility. In this system size of the item in question will influence how an item will be stored. Adequate space must be provided to balance the inventory requirements with the need for maximum space utilization. Both can be met by minimizing the height of shelves above the maximum height of the stock located on the shelf below.

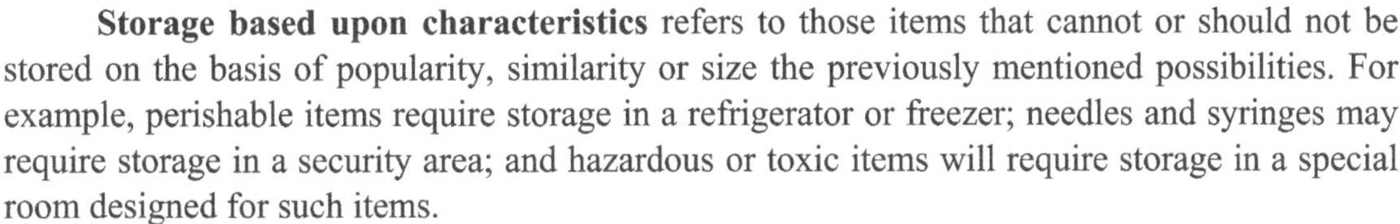

Storage based upon characteristics refers to those items that cannot or should not be stored on the basis of popularity, similarity or size the previously mentioned possibilities. For example, perishable items require storage in a refrigerator or freezer; needles and syringes may require storage in a security area; and hazardous or toxic items will require storage in a special room designed for such items.

BASIC DISTRIBUTION OPTIONS

Some of the important distribution options are discussed here under

Material Requisition System

Material requisition procedure is the oldest and most traditional method used by hospitals. The use of direct requisitions creates a second inventory for store room items, one in stores and the other in the user department. This system is basically controlled by the user. Each departmental head functions as a materials manager and keeps track of his own inventories. Whenever inventory levels in the department get low, he prepares a requisition and presents it to the central storage point. The requisition is filled, supplies are delivered to the user area, and users put the items in their appropriate place. Regardless of how the unofficial inventory is accounted for, it is usually controlled in relation to the department's comfort factor. The consistency of performance by the store room will be deciding or influencing item that determines if the comfort factor is high or low. A low comfort factor will cause the using department to maintain higher levels of supplies, in case the store room runs out. But a high comfort factor does not necessarily produce the reverse effect. Users will continue to maintain traditional levels in the event a stock out occurs in the store room. The effect of the user comfort factor usually results in excessive inventory being maintained within the user's department. Excessive inventory really means hoarding. If excessive inventory is being maintained by the user, the reason is the store room's failure to support the requirements of the user. The blame for excessive inventory is two way. If MM wants the users to reduce inventory, it must first prove to them that their requirements can be supported by the store room. With this procedure, each department determines its own needs. The order is transmitted to the store room, where it is filled and delivered to the department. **Depending upon the nature of the item, the requisition is charged either to the department or to the patient.**

The fetch and carry procedure is a slight variation of the direct requisition procedure. Only the delivery method differs. With this procedure, the user prepares a direct requisition; and carries it to the store room, picks up the material, and returns with it to the department. This procedure is normally followed by the requesting department when the material is immediately required and the need is such that they cannot wait for delivery of the order by store room personnel. This procedure can also be adopted as a normal routine for obtaining supplies. User department personnel may be required to spend more time travelling to and from the store room than in accomplishing the work they were originally hired to do.

Advantages

- Little capital investment is required.
- This system is traditional and more easily accepted.
- Some employees feel a sense of importance or power by being able to control their inventories, even though they may not have had any formal training or experience in this area.

Disadvantages

- User department labour, usually more highly skilled, higher educated, and better paid, is used to a greater degree for materials control function instead of patient care.
- More user department space may be used for storage instead of for patient care. This is brought on by general lack of control or management of the inventory because the departments may have inadequate expertise in managing inventories.
- Hoarding is also a characteristic of this system. If a department ever experiences a shortage situation, it may vow never to let it happen again and may maintain inordinately high quantities of inventory in the user area.
- This ordering and maintaining of needlessly high inventory can create artificial stock-outs in the hospital store room.
- A department may order an unusually large quantity of an item, totally depleting what is available in the store room. Even the most well conceived reorder points and safety stock levels cannot anticipate unusual or irrational ordering patterns.
- Other departments ordering this item then find it unavailable from the store room even though it actually is available in the hospital, but in a user area and unavailable to other requesters.
- This forces the store room to replenish its stock on an emergency basis and has the net effect of increasing the total inventory investment in the hospital (the store room plus the hoarding department) without improving real availability.
- Requisition system can be improved by maintaining a catalogue of what is required in each of the user areas and establishing a schedule of order intervals for all departments.
- Frequency of these intervals may encourage the users to maintain lower inventories, and the catalogue at least identifies what is generally maintained in those areas in case another department needs to borrow from them to tide over their immediate needs.

STOCKLESS INVENTORY

As a supply distribution method, stockless inventory represents an alternative to maintaining supplies in and distributing supplies from the store room. Stockless inventory is generally suited to those items that are used primarily by only one or two departments. Specifically, departments such

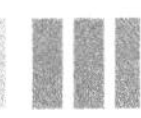

as laboratory, radiology, surgery, and other specialized departments are ideally suited for a programme of stockless inventory. It is accomplished by identifying specialized departmental supplies, establishing appropriate departmental inventory quotas, and processing orders directly to the user department without accumulating any inventory in the store room. The primary objective of stockless inventory management is to establish and maintain limited specified quantities of unofficial inventory.

Establishment of a stockless inventory programme begins by identifying those store room items being maintained by the above mentioned specialized departments. These items may then be combined with other non store room items for analysis of usage and lead times. After the identification phase is completed, initial quotas for each item are to be established in consultation with users, taking into consideration usage, lead times, turnover rates, and ups and downs in the supply cycle.

Initial quotas should be flexible for subsequent changes. Quota establishment can be based upon either the use of periodic ordering or on user departmental supply budgets. The criteria for using the budget process require dividing the user's annual supply budget by the desired number of turns per year to establish a maximum total rupee value for all items falling under the stockless inventory programme. The final step is to establish a routine order cycle and special requisition to facilitate centralized ordering through the purchasing department. Ideally, the routine order cycle should allow for two or three orders per month. The orders should be processed on a requisition similar to a PAR level requisition, which identifies each specific line item, the established maximum quota, and the quantity required to bring stock up to that quota.

Advantages

- More efficient utilization of the store room by freeing valuable space.
- Less inventory holding costs because there is less stock on hand.
- Elimination of one level of supply duplication, primarily in the store room, enables the hospital to save money through reduction in average inventory.
- Greater participation of the department head for increased effective supply utilization and cost containment.
- Reduction in inventory shrinkage and pilferage can be accomplished.
- More control over unofficial inventories.

Disadvantages

- Stockless inventory should not be viewed as a sure way to obtain an immediate reduction in official inventory, and to reduce the store room work load.
- Official as well unofficial inventory still requires the use of limited financial resources.
- Stockless inventory also requires the monitoring of user department inventories to ensure that the objectives are being met.

PAR LEVEL SYSTEM

In par level system, each user department stores supplies in an assigned location in its own area. Physical stock levels in that user area are pre-determined, based on a usage rate and the frequency of replenishment process. PAR level programme should accomplish two objectives. First is to bring user department inventories under the control of one central inventory management and the second objective is to take the user department out of the supply business i.e., to eliminate user department personnel for the functions of requisitioning, inventory management, etc. Traditional PAR programmes utilize existing shelving or cabinets within the department. Supplies are checked periodically by store room personnel and refilled to bring each item up to the established standard. At periodic intervals (e.g., everyday at designated time, once in three days, or weekly), supply personnel conduct a physical inventory of what is available, then order and obtain supplies to return the on hand levels to the pre determined or par level. Frequency of replenishment is a variable that can be adjusted to meet the specific requirements of the user. For example, a PAR programme on a nursing unit may require daily replenishment, whereas a PAR programme in radiology may require weekly replenishment. The important point is to determine with the user a reasonable schedule that will accommodate the needs of both departments.

During conversion process all storage areas should be checked for back up supplies. This includes all drawers and cabinets throughout the department. User departments are creative in storing back up supplies. For example, at one hospital, the second and third shifts had their own stock of flashlight batteries and ballpoint pens.

Establishing a PAR level programme for any department will be subject to the physical constraints of available shelves and cabinets.

Following guidelines should be followed as closely as possible when establishing the location of supplies for this programme:

1. Generically similar items should be stored together, that is, all tapes, I.V. supplies, etc.
2. High usage A and B items should be placed between waist and eye level to permit easy access and location.
3. Items like bedpans, admission kits, etc. which are large and heavy should be nearer the floor.
4. Low usage, C category and unimportant items should be placed towards the top of the cabinet or at the back of the unit.

Establishment of a PAR level programme presents an opportunity to bring unofficial inventory into the official classification. Initially, official inventory dollars begin to go up until excessive stocks are used up. When a department is converted to a PAR programme, the department should receive credit for all existing inventory. Determining when the items were withdrawn from the store room will be an almost impossible task. Therefore, credit should be based on the latest cost of inventory. Later issue of material will also be charged out at latest cost, so it will even out eventually. Credit should only be given for items that can be reissued. Any item that appears to be unusable should be thrown out.

Advantages

- Par level programme is easily implemented and requires little capital investment in terms of remodelling costs or purchase of material handling equipment.
- It also improves inventory management by establishing a standard level in all user areas and, based on the frequency of replenishment, can reduce total stock levels.
- Lower inventory levels in the user areas will need less space, possibly freeing up more area for patient care.
- Furthermore, as this system is managed and implemented by supply personnel, it places the management responsibility for inventory control and supply distribution functions where they best belong i.e., with the supply personnel.
- It eliminates need for patient care personnel to spend their time on supply and internal distribution function.
- This provides the hospital with the potential of improving patient care by providing more time for that function with no increase in cost.

This system is operated on preset intervals providing continuity and timeliness in the supply charge requisition process. Hence, the management of supply charges is also enhanced. This reduces total hospital costs and increases net revenue.

Disadvantages

- This system is more labour intensive than others. It requires several trips to and from user areas to conduct the physical inventory, return to storage point to obtain supplies, and then go back to the user area to deliver those supplies and put them away.
- Time spent on so many trips unproductive and unsupervised, and can therefore result in wasted time. There also is considerable traffic with such a system.
- Another serious disadvantage is that the inventory status in a user department usually is dynamic. It changes continuously. In the par level system, there is a time gap between the time inventory level is reviewed and the supplies are obtained and returned to the user area.
- During the intervening time, there may be a significant change in the status of the inventory. As a result, when the supplies are returned to the user area, they no longer may be adequate to bring the levels up to the pre determined par.
- When the inventory status changes between the time of the review and the time of the replenishment, return trips become necessary, making it even more labour intensive and even less cost effective.

- Proposed implementation of a PAR level programme usually invokes extreme reactions from the user departments.
- Those departments who really dislike controlling their department inventory welcome the programme.
- Some departments may object to the implementation. Their objections usually arise from a feeling of invasion of established domain and that such a programme is a threat to the operation in the form of increased potential for stock outs.

Approaching these departments and gaining their trust require both patience and tact. Here, the soft sell approach is often successful. The department's confidence is gained by agreeing to liberal maximum stock levels and working extra hard to make sure there are no stock-outs. Once a good track record is established, maximum levels are gradually reduced to more realistic levels. This process usually takes six months to achieve. This approach has been criticized because inventory reduction is not achieved immediately.

A major drawback to this distribution system is the actual replenishment of stock. This can be achieved in two ways. The first is to have stores personnel inventory in each department, return to the store room, draw the necessary stock, and return to the unit. The second procedure is to replenish common supplies from a master cart. First procedure may result in some items not being brought up to the established or agreed quantity level because the user continues to draw from the inventory during the time stores personnel is drawing stock from the store room. The second alternative of master cart is more effective, except that it is not always possible to carry adequate stock on the cart to meet the needs of all the nursing units. Both options should be evaluated and the best solution chosen for each particular hospital. There is a need to work closely with the department head in establishing stock locations. Usage determination is not based on store room usage, but on the fact that departmental personnel must identify stock locations quickly. Flexibility in location of stock is a paramount consideration for the success of this programme. Another problem that arises with either of these methods is that store room personnel must be away from their department for extended periods of time. They usually like this situation because it gives them an opportunity to visit other areas of the hospital, but it is unproductive, if left uncontrolled.

EXCHANGE CART SYSTEM

Exchange carts were traditionally used to distribute medical/surgical supplies and linen to nursing units. In some instances, surgery, emergency room, and physical therapy can also be converted to an exchange cart programme. Limitations of an exchange cart programme are those placed on it by the physical layout of the hospital. Location of stock on the exchange cart should follow the guidelines established for PAR level programme. User participation in establishing stock locations is an important part of the programme.

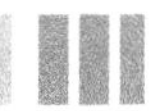

Exchange cart system is the most popular of all internal distribution systems implemented in hospitals in recent times. In this system also, there are pre determined levels and pre determined intervals for replenishing inventory to those levels as in the par system. However, in the exchange cart system, a cart is used for storage and internal distribution. A duplicate of each cart in the user area is parked in the storage area. At the pre determined time, the full cart can be taken to the user and exchanged for the depleted one. The depleted cart is then restocked and readied for delivery on the next occasion. The cycle repeats itself at agreed periodic intervals.

With most cart designs, either the user can draw from both sides of the cart, or only from a single side. The two sided system limits the physical quantity of stock that can be maintained for each line item. However, it permits improved visibility of lower usage C items. The one sided draw system allows for a larger quantity of items, but presents a disadvantage in that lower usage C items tend to be maintained towards the bottom or back of the cart. There, they are more difficult to find. In addition, stores personnel tend to overlook items normally kept on the back of the shelf, and so such items may not be replenished as necessary. For this reason, a sound quality control system is necessary to ensure that all items required on the cart are there.

Advantages

- Exchange cart programmes appear to be the most efficient method of supply distribution. Stores personnel spend most of their time in the store room because the actual exchange time is minimal.
- Productivity improves because they have more time to complete other tasks. Quality control is improved because carts can be checked prior to storage for the next exchange. A quality control programme assures user departments that established standards are being met on the full cart.
- Exchange cart system provides better manpower utilization, less time is spent travelling, and order picking time can be more productive provided it is done in an area that can be supervised under similar conditions as those prevalent on a factory production line.
- Order picking time can be minimized if carts are set up in accordance with the item location in the store room and item locations on each cart provided the two are similar. However this may not always be possible. Supply personnel oversee the carts in the stocking area.
- Management responsibility for and control over this function can be optimized. Standardizing the items on the carts and proximal locations to
- Similar items give advantages beyond order picking. User personnel who are required to move around to different user areas can locate items more easily under this system. Of course, this can also be true for par level systems.
- This system supports control of inventories through the frequencies of exchange. However, it may require almost twice as much inventory as that of a par level system because there are duplicate carts.

- Proper selection of intervals between cart exchanges will help in managing and controlling supply charges.
- Service levels to user areas improve because of the instantaneous restocking to the full pre-determined levels.
- There is no time lag between taking inventory and delivery of supplies. The full cart is delivered, and depleted one removed.

Disadvantages

- In exchange cart system, there may be a substantial capital investment required to purchase carts as well as to remodel storage areas in the general store room and the user areas to park them. Although the number will vary, the minimum requirement is two carts per user department.
- Parking space required for these carts can be significant.
- Care should be taken when specifying and selecting the cart equipment. Cart manufacturers offer many styles and materials available from. Hospital must select the material that will provide durability for long life and the design that will best meet the demands of the storage and user areas. Given the differences in costs of different raw materials used in manufacturing carts (e.g., fibre glass, stainless steel, mild steel chrome plated, or zinc galvanized), care should be taken to carefully evaluate their expected life, the aesthetics they provide, and their relative costs.
- Whether the cart will be cleaned manually or in an automatic cart washer also might be a factor to be considered.
- Interchangeability of parts and the ease with which carts are assembled and changed are key maintenance considerations.
- A hospital may require many carts to implement the system. Hence the time spent assembling and adjusting them as needs change may be considerable. Such a hospital is better off buying carts that can be assembled by hand with no special tools and can be changed easily and quickly.
- The type of caster wheel also is important and must be based on intended use. They come in different sizes, surface finishes and configurations, each with a unique application and associated cost. Again, careful evaluation is needed for the best selection.

OTHER RELATED FACTORS

Delivering merchandise on a scheduled basis eliminates infructious and avoidable trips and traffic. The best delivery route is that one which avoids retracing of steps and minimizes the total distance travelled. Hospitals also should consider delivering non stock items along with routine store room items. This obviously depends on the frequencies with which departments order and receive goods from the store room vis à vis the frequency with which they receive non stock items.

Centralization of related distribution functions can lead to improved efficiencies. The streamlining of receiving function, the distribution of non stock merchandise, and the centralization of storage facilities can complement the supply distribution system and allow it to produce optimum benefits. Scheduling these activities further improves efficiency by making the work load smooth, which leads to better handling of peak demands and genuine emergencies. Assigning each department a given order replenishment day or time helps distribution personnel to plan their work load and respond better to emergencies. Use of pre printed requisition forms for each department encourages staff members to complete the forms correctly and on time.

It is also feasible and cost effective to combine all physical distribution (supplies, linen, food, etc) into a central function. This way, personnel productivity can be improved, schedules adhered to, elevator congestion can be minimized and service levels maintained. Centralization of related functions allows standardization in the methods used. This is expected to improve the accuracy of clerical functions performed and the service provided.

MAINTENANCE OF RECORDS

Maintaining of statistics for routine supply distribution is essential. Statistics that show random requirements are equally important. Whenever a department places an emergency order, or a non emergency order that is outside the routine system, extra time and handling are required and total costs increase. Reviewing the frequencies of these requests, their sources, and the items sought can reduce or eliminate these needs. Frequently requested items can be placed in the department's normal inventory, or levels for those items can be increased. Abusers can be counseled as to how to work within the system and receive services as are intended to be provided without creating extra difficulties and increasing operating costs.

Timely maintenance of correct, true and accurate records is a key element in any successful distribution system. Records of the activities that show usage, demand, and trends are very useful. The data can be utilized to review par levels and adjust them accordingly. In stock service levels in hospitals should be determined in order to obtain data that can be used to evaluate the success of their routine supply distribution system. Maintaining statistics on what is ordered and delivered allows system performance to be measured and evaluated objectively.

EVALUATION OF EXISTING AND PROPOSED DISTRIBUTION SYSTEMS

Evaluating physical and cost factors in a hospital's existing system as it relates to the options available is simple but it does take some planning and effort to complete it in a plausible manner that provides usable information. Supply department should start by conducting a physical inventory of the user departments. This inventory should be valued at the current replacement price of each item to find the total inventory value available as a starting point. Next, demands for a given review period should be determined for each of the user departments, based on set intervals (e.g., daily, twice a week or weekly). Demands should include both random and emergency requirements. The demand inventory levels should be valued and compared to the existing physical inventory determined in the earlier step. This gives a picture of what to expect by establishing demand inventory levels and a given frequency of supply replenishment. Comparing the two inventory levels and their associated values reveals the net increase or decrease that a change in the distribution system will bring about. The hospital's inventory carrying cost factor should be applied to the difference in order to identify the potential savings in such expense that may result from a change in the distribution system.

Next step is to document the flow design in detail, including steps required in the existing distribution system. A flow chart helps. Then a hospital can compare it to the processes involved in the other available systems. Figure 22.1 **(Scheyer)** shows how a flow diagram can visually simplify the identification and evaluation of each process.

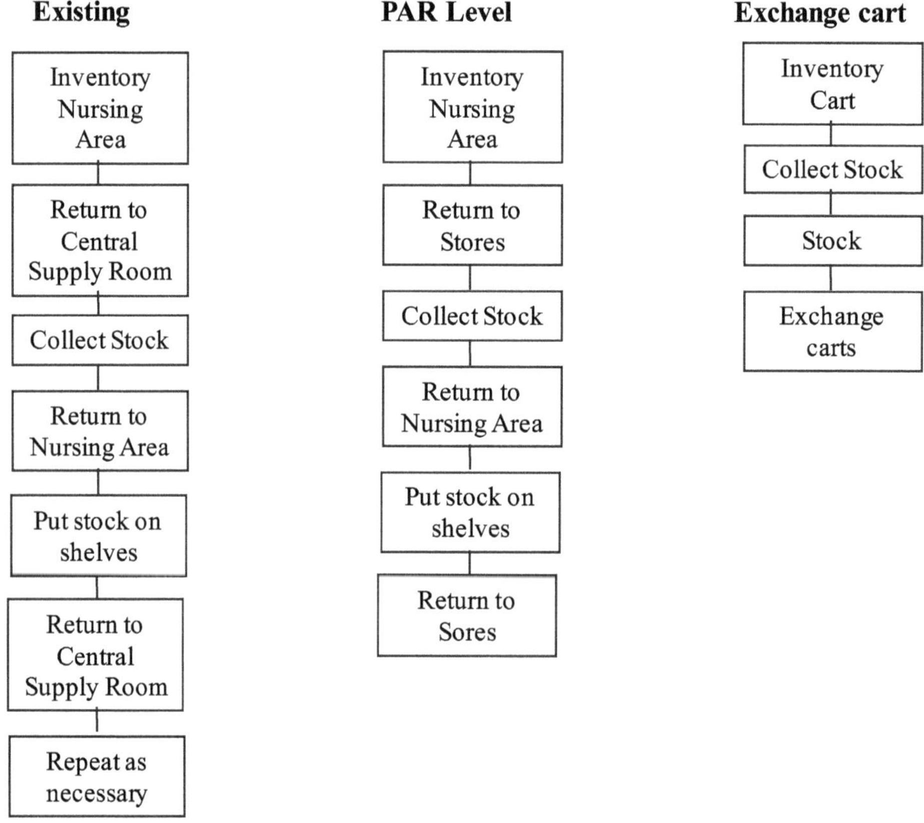

Figure 22.1 Supply Distribution to Nursing Floor Comparative Flow Diagrams

Source: William Sheyer-Handbook of Healthcare Material Management

After the flow diagrammes are studied, a detailed step by step procedure should be documented for each proposed system. Applying standard times required for each step or function in the various systems provides a means by which each can be evaluated for manpower costs. Standard times can be obtained from industrial engineering manuals or the hospital may conduct its own time and motion studies to establish standard times for each function. After those functions have been identified and the standard times applied, current labour rates should be used to cost out each step within each system for arriving at a total labour cost.

It is important to document all other costs of the existing and proposed systems for comparison. Costs of paper work, supplies, capital expenses, data collection, and physical rearranging of storage areas should be documented, annualized and compared. A research study conducted in USA shows that a substantial saving were achieved in inventory carrying costs, labour costs, and other expenses by adopting par system and exchange cart systems for central supply room and stores.

OPERATIONAL ISSUES

Operational issues should be considered. These factors are other than the financial considerations that help hospitals decide which system is best for them.

These include:

- The ability to supervise employees who provide the service and perform the distribution function.
- The assignment of management responsibility and authority for supply distribution function including inventory management.
- The traffic congestion expected in the routes that must be followed.
- Adequacy of the space for storage, working, and parking of materials handling equipment e.g., fork lift trucks, carts etc.

Some of these factors could cause a hospital to select one alternative over another, especially when the direct costs are extremely close to one another.

Costs over the Life Cycle

Total life cycle costs of the options should be evaluated. A research study conducted in US hospitals showed that at the outset, the par level system is economically superior. Assuming that labour costs increase at 10 percent per year, by the seventh year, the cost of an exchange cart system becomes less than that of a par level system. The total cost over 10 years, though, is still less for par level. (Source: Hospital Materials Management Quarterly vol. II No. 2). Return on investment (ROI) must take into consideration the continuing costs associated with a given decision. Looking beyond the first year makes a substantial difference in the selection of the final option.

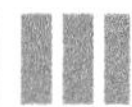

Implementation

Proper planning significantly enhances the probability of a successful conversion or change as well as achievement of goals identified in the feasibility analysis. A requisition system is not recommended as a routine means of providing supply service to medium to large consumer departments. Implementation planning is therefore required for exchange cart or par level restocking systems. Since both the systems are similar, this implementation plan also can be utilized for either.

Team Approach

Entities such as administration, finance, nursing, and medical staff should be involved in planning at various stages. Implementation planning should include various members of the hospital's management team in order to facilitate the gathering of inputs and communication process at various levels in the organization. Certainly the person to whom, materials management reports and who has the line administrative responsibilities should be involved or at least informed throughout the entire process. All departments immediately affected by any change in distribution system should be involved in the implementation planning. This would include not only the department heads and managers but certain staff members as well. Staff members in a department frequently know more about what actually is happening and what the real needs are than the department manager. Involvement also gives staff members a sense of participation and can help develop support for the system. Some changes in systems can still run into problems during the debugging phases and staff support will be essential to help resolve them. These resources can be brought together in a task force or committee type of configuration so as to provide for a formal process. This facilitates the documentation of progress and results, effective communication of the planning, progress made, and ultimate results. This group should also be charged with the responsibility for ensuring that the identified goals are in fact achieved by the conversion to whatever system is selected. Sometime after implementation, the situation must be reassessed to identify the savings and/or service improvements. Changes or modifications should be made if expected goals have not been achieved.

Steps in developing a Model for distribution

1. Determine on hand inventory levels in each affected department.
2. Identify daily supply demand/usage for each user department. High, low, and average daily demand figures for that sample should be noted.
3. Averages create a smoothing effect so the peak demands should be planned for. Finally, inputs should be sought from the users by having them evaluate the data gathered.
4. Frequently they can identify where a peak is unrepresentative of routine activity and this helps to establish more appropriate levels of inventory.
5. Draft a list of all products used by each department. This includes such information as: 1. item code 2. source of supply 3. description 4. unit of measurement for issue 5. landed

cost 6. optimum inventory level 7. charge vs. non charge status etc. This list can be prepared before taking physical counts and can serve as a master catalogue.

6. Determine frequency of supply replacement. This depends upon the type of system selected as well as targeted on hand inventory levels and turnover rates.
7. Identify functional requirements and specifications required for all exchange carts if that system is used.
8. Determine appropriate location for supplies at the user area including a con figuration for those supplies so that reordering and restocking as well as on demand item location can be facilitated. User department inputs must be included in this vital process.
9. Standardized layouts should be established as much in order to enhance productivity in ordering, restocking, and retrieval for use processes.
10. Determine the timing for inventory review, ordering, and restocking based upon the variables such as times of peak supply demand, corridor and elevator congestion, and staff availability.
11. Identify and determine the preferred methodology of individual order, batch or zone processing.
12. Establish appropriate paper work and record keeping systems including designing forms, setting up automated data systems communications, and so on.
13. Adjust layouts, configurations, and inventory levels at supply source in order to accommodate the new system.
14. Conduct in service training programmes for all personnel involved and affected by the system.
15. Establish a mechanism for tracking non-routine/random demand for supplies that occur outside the basic system to determine the continuing effectiveness of the system and assess the appropriateness of the product mix and inventory levels.
16. Establish policies and procedures for effecting appropriate changes. It is essential to ensure that inventory levels will be adjusted routinely to match changing demand.
17. Implementation can be commenced on a pilot project basis, batch or zone basis, or hospital wide. These can be equally successful, depending on the degree of complexity and sophistication of the system selected and the extent of the impact of the change.
18. Schedule meetings for reviewing progress and making any modifications that may be required.

Without adequate implementation planning, the system is destined to fail. Credibility established early in a programme is essential.

CART SYSTEM FOR OPERATION THEATRE STORES

Surgical case carts should be considered an integral part of distribution system. The most important consideration in evaluating the distribution system in the hospital is the possibility of including surgical case carts.

Bulk Replacement

The most basic supply option for surgery is a bulk replacement system. In this system, the OT manager acts as a materials manager and orders stock from several sources: general stores, central supply and outside vendors on a scheduled or non scheduled basis. The surgery department also may do its own sterile processing of instruments, basins, surgical trays, and linens. It basically is a self-sufficient operation. The inherent advantages of such a system are that it requires little interdepartmental coordination and, therefore, little conflict to deal with. With this system in place, OT is able to control its own destiny; it has virtually full authority. The major disadvantage in the system is that very expensive and highly trained staff is required.

Par Level System

A par level system can also be used to meet the demands/needs of OT as for other areas of the hospital. This system has the same advantages as those in the hospital wide distribution system. In addition, it requires less instrument inventory. Also less coordination is required so there is less interdepartmental conflict. The major disadvantage among other things is that the job done by part-time managers whereas it requires full time attention of experienced and educated personnel.

Case Cart System

Jamie C. Kowalski in his article on Hospital Distribution System defined the case cart system as one that provides all items (instruments, linens, and supplies) for a surgical procedure on a mobile cart. The cart is prepared in a storage area and delivered to the operating room scheduled for that procedure before the procedure is to begin. Items on the cart are used during the procedure. The top of the cart may be used as a back or gown table. At the end of the procedure, items to be disposed of and/or reprocessed are collected, placed on the cart, and returned to reprocessing area. **Major advantage is reduction in average inventory required for surgery and better utilization of equipment and manpower. A disadvantage of the case cart is that it requires a significant expenditure for purchase of carts. Parking space also is required.** Increased interdepartmental friction between the surgery and supply departments also can result. It is generally caused by the human errors that inevitably occur. The departments may resort to mutual bickering. While this possibility is real, a firm commitment to the programme and proper mechanisms for communication and problem solving help keep those problems under control.

Key factors for selecting a case cart

It is necessary to have a schedule showing the time and room for each procedure in order to establish and implement a successful case cart system. An ordering method that is easy to follow and provides a permanent record of what was ordered, delivered, and used is also necessary. A preference card is needed to allow the surgeon to identify items that are required because of personal choice or unusual conditions of a procedure. Standardization of sets, highly productive reprocessing, and adequate instrument inventory are vital. Equally essential is a trained staff that can effectively and efficiently assemble instrument sets and surgical case carts.

The level of accuracy with which this is done is vital. It is impossible to anticipate all items required for a surgical procedure. There should be a method for obtaining emergency items that are required and place where they are located should be known. This may be in the OT or storage area. It should be well organized, and use of these items should be well documented. Repeated requests for these back up items may signify a need to add them to the standard case cart requisition. Back up items should include supplies, instruments, and linens. Timing requirements relate to obtaining a completed and approved surgery schedule including ordering, filling, and delivering of carts and returning used items to reprocessing area and entering them into the reprocessing cycle. Requisitions, random or emergency calls, or unusual requirements beyond what is ordered through regular system must be recorded and documented.

A key factor in selecting a case cart system is the cleaning method. Hospitals with centralized processing areas frequently install automatic cart washing machines. Carts are to be washed frequently. They should be washed after each use. Cart parts should be able to withstand high temperatures and constant washing without unusual maintenance or frequent breakdown. Stainless steel generally meets these criteria. For back up carts which may not get washed very frequently, chrome or zinc plated may be acceptable, long lasting, and economical. Castors also must be selected carefully.

After the evaluation process is completed and existing system is compared to other systems, a method should be established for evaluating the results once they have been implemented (refer Figure 22.1). This should include an analysis of all of the factors that the distribution system affects and is affected by. The question of which procedure is best for any hospital is difficult to answer. The choice depends on nature of physical plant and the economic impact of operational and financial resources required, establishing and maintaining a sound distribution programme. Consideration should be given to utilizing either a PAR level or an exchange cart, or a combination of the two. The best combination for any hospital is decided on the basis of existing and expected advantages and disadvantages within the facility. Inventory management and supply distribution should be centralized under one central manager.

Equipment requirements should be based upon the following factors:

- Type of material to be handled (type, shape, and weight etc.).
- Volume of goods to be handled and number of times movement is expected to occur.
- Distance over which the materials are to be moved.
- Physical limitations: ceiling height, maximum permissible load on floor, inclination of ramps, weight restrictions on elevators, etc.
- Available equipment that is currently in use and equipment that is available but not being used presently.
- Safety precautions to be observed in order to prevent accidents or injury to employees using the equipment.

Equipment selection thus requires a detailed analysis for meeting the functional requirements associated with proper materials handling. Every effort should be made to combine or eliminate operations in order to reduce the cost and time of materials handling. Equipment should be selected such that it will aid in eliminating delays due to congestion. Maintenance of the required quantity of an equipment type will also aid in reducing congestion and wastage of productive time caused by a lack of available equipment.

Types of equipment used in a store room include, but are not limited to:

1. Platform trucks, used primarily for movement of large quantities of boxes, packages, etc. Platform trucks are available with steel or wooden decks. Sizes range from 60 cm wide by 105 cm long to 75 cm wide by 150cm long; weight capacity from 500 to 1500 kg.
2. Two wheel hand trucks used primarily for movement of case stock and loading and unloading delivery vehicles. Weight capacity ranges from 200 to 500 kg.
3. Drum truck, used primarily for loading, unloading, and transportation of barrels and drums. Available in two or four wheel models. Weight capacity is up to 500 kg.
4. Oxygen tank trucks. Movement of cylinders is the primary purpose of this special design equipment. Capacity will vary from one to two cylinders.
5. Appliance hand truck. Design is similar to general purpose two wheel truck except that this vehicle can be used for refrigerators, tile cabinets, and large pieces of furniture safely. Weight capacity is 100 to 500 kg.
6. Platform trolley, designed to move equipment, furniture, refrigerators, etc. can be made from seasoned wood or steel with varying caster sizes. Weight capacity is 500 to 2000 kg.
7. Hand pallet truck, designed specifically to move wooden or metal pallets. These are manufactured with varying widths from 50 to 70 cm, and lengths from 80 to 120 cm. Weight capacities range from 1000 to 3000 kg per load.

SUMMARY

Hospital distribution system is a complex network of storage (source) and user (destination) points. The goal of an effective distribution system is to provide the right item to the right place at the right time for the least total cost. Hospitals need to take a broad systems approach. Hospital materials managers must become creative and improve utilization of the space currently available. The movement and control of supplies throughout the hospital are major concerns for users as well as materials managers.

Distribution system is a key component of a Materials Management programme. Supply distribution is intimately related to inventory management. An effective system can directly support the hospital's inventory management and also directly affect the amount of inventory maintained in a general store room as well as in user departments. The frequency at which the supply distribution system replenishes stocks in user departments has a direct effect on inventory levels. The more frequently inventories are replenished, the smaller the inventories needed at user points in the hospital departments at any time.A logical extension of inventory management is supply and internal distribution.

Supply staff should manage the distribution system and care persons can concentrate on patients' care. The location system for items in the store room can positively affect order picking productivity. Exchange cart systems need space to park all carts. The service levels provided to user areas can be enhanced by implementing a proper distribution system. The system should be proactive and replenish inventories in the user areas automatically on a cycle basis. Such a system will require less user personnel time. Management of patient supply charges can also be vastly enhanced by coordination with the internal distribution system.

Plans for maximizing storage space must begin by identifying the physical requirements for every item to be stored. Items are then sorted by storage requirements to determine an accurate picture of the total requirements for each type of storage unit. Individual item analysis must also include total cubic requirements. Individual item storage must take into consideration upward as well as horizontal storage. Store room personnel cannot pick items which they cannot see. The storage facility should have a stock location system in order to prevent lost motion and delays in locating inventory items. Typically, items are stored on the basis of popularity. Storage by similarity comes second to storage by popularity.

Materials requisition procedure is the oldest and most traditional method used by hospitals. The use of direct requisitions creates a second inventory for store room items, one in stores and the other in user department. This system is basically controlled by user area. If excessive inventory is being maintained by user, reason is the store room's failure to support the requirements of the user. In this system, more user department space may be used for storage instead of patient care.

As a supply distribution method, stockless inventory represents an alternative to maintaining supplies in and distributing supplies from the store room. It is accomplished by identifying specialized departmental supplies, establishing appropriate departmental inventory quotas, and processing orders directly to the user department without accumulating any inventory in the store room.

In par level system, each user department stores supplies in an assigned location in its own area. The first objective is to bring user department inventories under the control of one central inventory management and the second objective is to take the user department out of the supply business i.e., to eliminate user department personnel for the functions of requisitioning, inventory management, etc. In par level system, there is a time gap between the time inventory level is reviewed and the supplies are obtained and returned to user area.

Exchange cart system is the most popular of all internal distribution systems implemented in hospitals in recent times. In this system also, there are pre determined levels and pre determined intervals for replenishing inventory to those levels as in the par system. However, in exchange cart system, a cart is used for storage and internal distribution. A quality control programme assures user departments that established standards are being met on the full cart. Order picking time can be minimized if carts are set up in accordance with the item location in store room and item locations on each cart provided the two are similar. Standardizing items on the carts and proximal locations to similar items gives advantages beyond order picking.

The supply department should start by conducting a physical inventory of the user departments. The demand inventory levels should be valued and compared to the existing physical inventory determined in the earlier step. Then a hospital can compare it to the processes involved in the other available systems.

Surgical case carts should be considered an integral part of distribution system. The most important consideration in evaluating the distribution system in the hospital is the possibility of including surgical case carts. The most basic supply option for surgery is a bulk replacement system. Case cart system is the one that provides all items (instruments, linens, and supplies) for a surgical procedure on a mobile cart. Items on the cart are used during the procedure. Equipment requirements should be based upon among other considerations on the type of material to be handled and the volume of goods to be handled and the number of times movement is expected to occur.

REVIEW QUESTIONS

1. Planning for maximizing storage space must begin with identifying physical requirement of each item to be stored. Elaborate this statement in light of hospital distribution system.
2. Discuss briefly the basic distribution options that are available to materials manager in a hospital.
3. Explain par level system of distribution. Discusses it's merits and demerits
4. Describe the importance of surgerical cart system in the overall hospital distribution system.
5. How will you evaluate the existing distribution system vis à vis proposed system in hospital distribution?
6. What are the operational issues involved in hospital distribution management Explain in detail
7. Write short notes on
   a) Optimization of storage space
   b) Supply and internal distribution
   c) Stockless inventory
   d) Par level system
   e) Case Cart System
   f) Exchange cart system
   g) Equipment requirement for stores distribution system

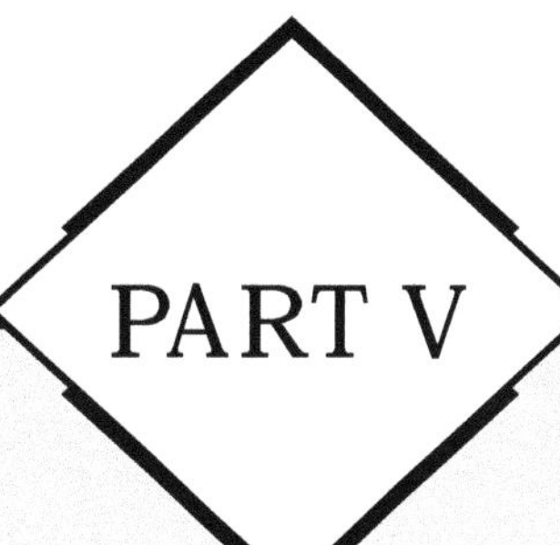

Chapter-23: Value Analysis/Value Engineering (VAVE)

Chapter-24: Supply Chain Management Relevance to Healthcare Industry

Chapter-25: Information Technology (IT) Applications in Healthcare

PART - V

Value Analysis / Value Engineering (VAVE)

Contents

CHAPTER - 23

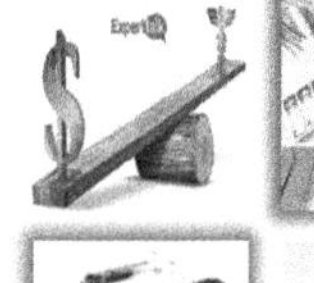

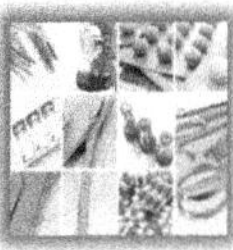

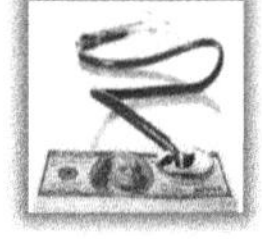

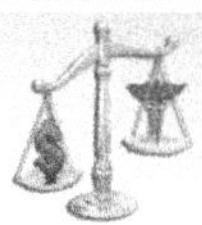

Value Analysis / Value Engineering (VAVE)

Function is the "Key" to value Engineering and the "Functional Analysis" is the "Keel" on which value analysis is built up.

- M. S. Vittal

INTRODUCTION

Liberalization, privatization and Globalization of Indian economy have brought in its wake many challenges and opportunities, but also serious problems and difficulties for Indian healthcare industry. This in turn has imposed heavy responsibilities on the healthcare managers who play a crucial role in achieving cost reduction, improved competitiveness, quality improvements, technology up gradations, and import substitution and above all, an efficient working and higher productivity of the organization.

In healthcare business, primary goal is to deliver quality care and the secondary goal is to get paid appropriately for all services rendered. Considering the complexity of healthcare billing and overall revenue cycle process, combined with increasing cost to deliver services, a hospital cannot afford to have any inefficiency in their revenue impacting activities. Any weaknesses in staffing, procedures, IT systems, and infrastructure can have a significant adverse effect on the financial status of the hospital. Many evaluations have been performed with the goal of improving hospital revenue with varying degrees of success. Fortunately a few techniques and management tools are available, to help health care managers to shoulder the responsibility. "VALUE ENGINEERING" happens to be one of the most appropriate and effective one at the present juncture.

WHAT IS VALUE ANALYSIS? (VA)

Value Analysis helps to maximize conservation of material resources and Import substitution helps, savings in valuable foreign exchange.

Examples

Conservation of utilization of material and natural resources: Use of tamarind seed starch for starching hospital linen in place of starch made from maize or tapioca and other edible food products. Tamarind seed is waste product and its use for manufacturing starch products can bring about conservation of food grains as well as reduction in cost sizing of textiles substantially.

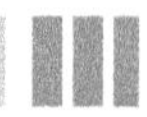

Import substitution: India was importing stents for angioplasty procedure. Stent is a small metal spring like device used for blocked heart arteries. It is pushed to the site of the block under online video camera and opened at the block so that the blood flow resumes. Stent keeps the artery open and sometimes works throughout the person's life. The price of the stent was about Rs. 65, 000. But the new stent costs Rs. 15,000. Procedure of removal blockage using the stent is known as angioplasty. **Dr. Somaraju, chairman,** Care Hospital indigenously developed a stent in collaboration with defense metallurgical laboratory under the stewardship of Dr. Abdul Kalam APJ former President of India. (The Hindu' dated, October 30th 1998). In the present case, VA not only resulted in substitution of indigenous materials for imported goods without sacrificing quality or performance, savings in cost of Rs 50000 as well as valuable foreign exchange to an extent of Rs. 65,000.

Value analysis should not be confused with price analysis or cost analysis. Value of the item is measured in terms of its function or purpose and at times, appearance of the item and its prestige. Value analysis is more basic and thorough study and once it is done it need not be repeated for same function, for some time to come unless factors emphasizing the function change significantly.

The Food and beverage department buyer is out for shopping vegetables. There are four varieties of tomatoes to choose from, costing Rs. 10, 15, 20 and 25 per Kg respectively. Qualities of all are good and they are edible. Price is obviously not same. The answer is simple; the prudent buyer will buy that quality which serves the food and beverage department's need (end use.)

Example

If hospital is hosting a dinner for its VIP guests, one of the menu items is salad for which tomatoes are required. Then Rs. 25 will be obvious choice. If it is required to make tomato soup, or Rasam, then buyer will purchase Rs. 10 quality.

In other words his choice will depend upon function which the tomato is to perform. Each of the four varieties has a value and this value depends upon functions it has to perform.

Value Analysis in Healthcare

Value analysis brings together users who have clinical product knowledge, financial analysts, and those with purchasing expertise in order to make best valued product and service acquisition decisions.

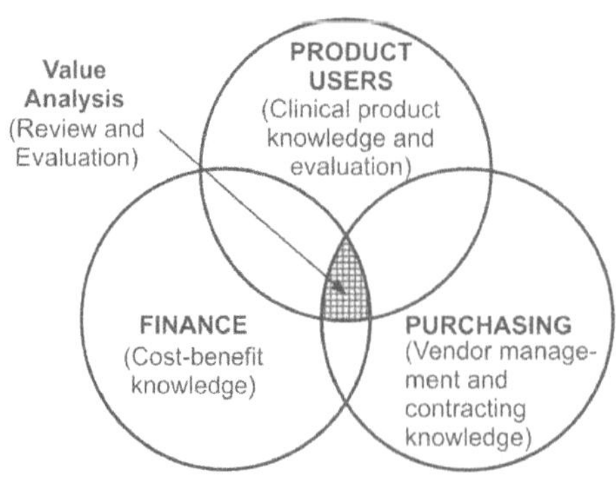

VALUE ENGINEERING VERSUS VALUE ANALYSIS (VAVE)

Value improvement programmes in health care industry are called variously as product analysis, Value improvement, Product evaluation, value control, cost analysis, vendor quality rating, value analysis, and value management.

Value Engineering comprises of a group of techniques aimed at systematic classification of "unnecessary costs" in a product or service, and efficiently eliminating them without detriment to quality and efficiency.

Initially this group of techniques was mostly used in engineering field which gave its name "value engineering". It can be applied in many other areas such as Marketing, Purchasing, Office work, services etc. and more as a general term Value analysis is used.

DEFINITIONS OF VALUE ANALYSIS

Value analysis is "engineering unnecessary cost factors out of purchased items". It assumes that there may be unnecessary cost factors built in a product that can be eliminated without lowering quality.

–John H. Holmgren and Walter J. Wentz

(Materials Management and Purchasing for Health care Facility).

Value analysis is "Study of relationship of design, function, and cost of any product, material, or service, with the objective of reducing its cost through modification of design, or material specification, manufacture by more efficient process, change of source of supply (external or internal) or possible elimination or incorporation into related item.

– Dena S. Ammer

(Purchasing and Materials Management for Health care Institutions)

Value analysis is creative substitution that could often be made that would result in reduction of unit as well as total cost without any reduction in function of materials or services in question.

–Arnold Reisman

(Materials Management for Health Services)

"Value analysis is an investigative process that systematically studies every element of material, component or service in terms of its functional and its associated cost to develop the most effective quality specifications at most cost effective price."

–Edward D. Sanderson

(Hospital Purchasing and Inventory Management)

"The essence of value analysis is the questioning and challenging of the need for the function of each product or piece of equipment; next consideration should be given to alternative ways or methods of performing the product's function."

- Charles E. Housley

(Hospital Materiel Management)

Terry Cox Director, Supply Chain Services, Texas children hospital, Houston views that. "Value analysis is not simply standardization, as a hospital might standardize on an item that is unnecessarily expensive, produces no enhanced benefit over the current item, and yet is the choice of the clinicians. One would hope, however, that the result of a good value analysis program would include standardization on the supply that has proven to be the best balance between cost and benefit."

Other comprehensive definitions related to manufacturing industry are quoted here under, which are identical to those given by some of the authors on Materials Management in Health Care Industry.

"Value Analysis is the systematic applications of recognized techniques, which identify the function of a product or service, establish monetary value for the function, and provide the necessary function and reliability at the lowest overall cost".

– Society of American Value Engineering (SAVE)

"Value Analysis / Value Engineering" is a philosophy implemented by the use of specific set of techniques, a body of knowledge and a group of learned skills. It is an organized creative approach which has for its purpose the efficient identification of unnecessary costs i.e., costs which do not provide quality, use, appearance or customer feature".

–Lawrence D. Miles

"Value Analysis / Value Engineering" is functionally oriented scientific method for improving product value by relating the elements of product worth to their corresponding elements of product cost, in order to accomplish the required function at the lowest cost in resources".

–W.D. Falcon

"Value Engineering" is the systematic, objective, analytical approach to achieve that optimum relationship of function, quality and cost, which combines in a product or service the attributes of essential function, adequate dependability, and lowest life cycle cost.

–Donald E. Parket

Thus from the above definitions it could be concluded Value Analysis is an organized procedure for efficient identification and elimination of infructuous costs without affecting quality of productor service.

ORIGIN OF VALUE ANALYSIS

Earlier incarnation of VA concepts occurred outside healthcare industry in 1946. Smoker referred to the classic perspectives of such management engineering experts as **Larry Miles** and William Edwards Deming. Miles merely coined the idea that anything not adding value to a product or service adds costs. According to Smoker. Miles applied his theory to the successful development

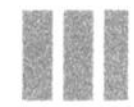

and production of "Liberty Ships," which were designed to move material and personnel to the European and the Pacific regions during World War II.

Meanwhile, Deming picked up the charge and advocated his treatise that **"quality is free,"** Smoker indicated, in that **"tight tolerances promote quality and quality control assures near zero defects."**

During World War-II, one of the most serious problems faced by companies engaged in war effort was shortage of materials. They experimented on substitute materials, often in a very unorthodox way. In many cases the experiments clicked. Surprisingly there were large numbers of instances where substitutes were much cheaper and performed more efficiently than original material.

After the World War-II in 1947 **Hary Erlicher,** Vice President, Purchasing **General Electric Company** (USA) felt that the problem of finding substitutes could be done in a more scientific way rather than by ad hoc crises approach.

He entrusted this job to a team of engineers headed by **Lawrence D. Miles,** Purchase Engineer. In fact it was he who coined the term Value Analysis and its synonym Value Engineering and off late it is also known as value management.

The team under the stewardship of **Lawrence D. Miles** pioneered and perfected it. By this the General Electric Company saved about $ 200 million over a period of 17 years. If necessity is mother of all inventions Lawrence D. Miles can rightly be called as **"the father of Value Engineering"**

In U.S. the technique is widely used and is given a great deal of importance. In fact U.S. Defence Department insists that value analysis must be applied in all contracts exceeding $ 1, 00,000. **Robert Mac** Namara, the then secretary for Defence placed on record as having said that year ending July 1965, the U.S Defence Department saved $ 4.6 million by applying Value analysis without any adverse effect on strength and combat readiness of its armed forces.

Many companies in U.S have adopted a new approach towards product development called **Design for Manufacturability and Assembly (DFMA).** Using this approach, many companies work to fashion a product that both satisfy the consumers and are easy to manufacture. This often results not only in lower costs, but also in higher quality and more reliable products.

BASIC FEATURES OF VALUE ENGINEERING

Whatever be the definition, there are certain basic features of value engineering:

I. A systematic step by step application of recognized techniques

II. A multi disciplinary team effort

III. Functional approach

IV. Application of creativity techniques

V. Evaluation and further investigation of ideas generated

I. A systematic step by step application of recognized techniques

Robert T. Yokl, president and Chief Value Strategist, Strategic Value Analysis in Healthcare, Skippack, PA, and one of the ardent advocates of value analysis cautioned "It's been our experience that supply chain managers traditionally select their VA team members by title or by their power and influence in their organization to participate in value analysis projects." We have found this type of selection method to be a roll of the dice that you are going to get the best people for your VA teams. Healthcare organizations need to be more scientific in their VA team selection, if they want them to be peak performers.

Application of Value analysis involves the following phases.

1. **Information phase:**

Define and price the function. Obtain and interpret the facts. The questions to be answered are

- What is it?
- What does it do? and
- What does it cost?

2. **Speculation Phase:**

Determine alternative solutions by asking questions such as

- How else the job can be done? and
- At what cost?

3. **Analysis Phase:**

- Determination and comparison of feasibility
- Determination and comparison of suitability
- Determination and comparison of costs

The questions that facilitate analysis phase are

- Is this bctter than that?
- How much better and why?

4. **Decision and action phase:**

- Audit effectiveness of the selection
- Use operating experience to effect further improvement
- Get departmental and managerial approvals
- Prepare new specification

5. **Evaluation Phase:**

Evaluation phase in value analysis activities are

- Review key alternatives with all departments and vendors concerned
- Select best alternative

II. A multi disciplinary team effort

Team effort greatly magnifies creativity of individual members and makes it easy to carry out project work early by sharing the 'chores'.

Team members can be drawn from clinical and business departments. Decision of a group will be more likely to be correct than that of an individual. The implementation of team's recommendations would be easier and quicker.

III. Functional approach

Functional approach focuses on what something does rather than on how it is done.

For example functioning of the battery is to provide energy.

In value engineering, instead of asking **"what is it?"** regarding an item under study, we ask **"what is it supposed to do?"** Identification and thorough analysis of the functions helps us to provide the required functions at lowest cost, or in a better way. In this process a host of unnecessary or excessive cost functions, which invariably exist in our designs, can be isolated, reduced, or eliminated.

By applying value analysis approach hospitals can facilitate agreement between two important groups of personnel who are at odds with one another e.g. clinical departments like medicine and nursing and business departments like materials department.

Another example of functional approach is **Virginia Commonwealth Health Systems (VCUHS),** adopted the product selection methodology resulting in three fold benefits i.e., a better product (improved outcomes, enhanced patient dignity, and superior customer service for patients and families), better compliance by staff (through education and involvement in the process of product choice), and better pricing for the health system (fiscal responsibility).

IV. Application of creativity techniques

This involves usage of techniques, like "Brainstorming" in order to generate large number of ideas for providing required function.

Suggestions for nurturing creativity in an organization are:

1. Avoid over managing; encourage initiative
2. Put up with small errors, punishment may stifle creativity
3. Encourage innovativeness

4. Recognize and reward creativity
5. Provide the right environment for creative efforts
6. Set personal example from the top
7. Let ideas grow; allow enough time for incubation
8. Remove mental blocks, and weed out persistent negative influences.
9. Watch out for "killer phrases"
10. Encourage positive approach
11. Depute personnel to training and development programmes on creativity and related subjects.

Important guidelines for Brain storming as an effective tool for value analysis are:

1. Selection of group members. Ideal number of members is four and it should not go beyond ten. Committee members should include representatives from clinical and non clinical departments.

   Value Analysis Facilitators (VAFs) are Registered Nurses who operate as liaisons between the clinical and business divisions. Having management experience, advanced education, and a clinical background, these VAFs speak both languages and facilitate projects that ultimately satisfy the priorities of both philosophies: Providing products that contribute to the best possible outcomes for patients (clinical) at the most responsible prices (business).

2. All members of the group should have same status. Chairman will have minimum role. Otherwise band wagon concept will prevail.
3. Domination of one person on other team members should be avoided from brainstorming group. If this not possible, the chairman has to take adequate steps restrain.

Time and agenda should be prepared well in advance of actual meeting. The agenda should be simple and well defined.

All proceedings of the meeting should be recorded including minutes of all ideas both potentially useful and useless.

Evaluation and implementation is not part of brainstorming process and would normally take place in a conventional cost reduction or value analysis meeting.

V. Evaluation and further investigation of ideas generated

This involves selection of one or two optimum solutions and recommends them for implementation. It would be very difficult to compare, judge and rank large number of attributes simultaneously. For this purpose simple technique called a paired comparison method is available. In this method each attribute is compared with all others, but with one at a time, not only to determine which is more important but also how much more important, and weights are awarded according to degree of difference.

Case 1 Example: At **Virginia Common Wealth University Health System (VCUHS),** the nursing staff experienced problems with the **Fecal Management System (FMS)** in use. An FMS is "a temporary containment device for patients with acute fecal incontinence. It was designed to safely and effectively divert liquid or semi liquid fecal matter, help protect patients' wounds from fecal contamination, and reduce the risk of both skin breakdown and spread of infection, such as infection with Clostridium difficile (C. difficile). Stool, being comprised of 30 percent bacteria, can be a major contributing factor in negative outcomes related to infections. With **Hospital Acquired Infections (HAIs)** counted on the **Centers for Medicare and Medicaid's (CMS's)** "never events" list, facilities are no longer reimbursed for the treatment associated with them. Clearly, prevention of such non reimbursed negative outcomes is a priority in any healthcare setting.

At VCUHS, the device being used was leaking and often had an unpleasant odour. These problems led to compliance issues with patients and/or their families, contributed to skin breakdown and frequent linen changes.

The Value Analysis Department and Facilitators were asked to assist.

Pricing Analysis: As with any Value Analysis project undertaken, a cost analysis was undertaken. In the 12-month period preceding the project, VCUHS spent $400,000 on Fecal Management Systems. The pricing and usage data were compared with other like sized institutions via a comparative index offered by VCUHS' membership in **University Health System Consortium (UHSC), an alliance of Academic Medical Centers (AMCs).** This index provides benchmarking data in relation to pricing and annual usage. For this product area, there were 36 AMCs purchasing the same product.

In analyzing price, 97 percent of the 36 facilities were receiving a better price while only 14 percent purchased a higher volume. Barring any convincing arguments, volume purchased (14th percentile) should have been close to price paid (97th percentile). The conclusion of the Value Analysis Department was that VCUHS's pricing was not representative of the volume and the VAF's determined that pricing required correction.

A Request for Proposal (RFP) was sent out to the three market leaders for FMS's. Each company was asked to provide their most competitive pricing in anticipation of a commitment to a majority of VCUHS' market share. A multi-year agreement was not out of the question.

Each company returned pricing that demonstrated a positive benefit to VCUHS' supply cost expense; therefore, all three companies were "allowed to play" in the clinical aspect of product selection. This financial weed out process seeks to eliminate a clinician's investment in products that have little chance of being purchased (due to exorbitant cost).

An initial average savings opportunity of $60,000 annually was realized, with Company A, giving a slightly greater savings than Companies B and C.

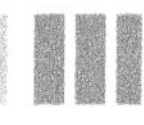

This process was accomplished prior to the clinicians seeing any demonstrations. In this way, whichever clinical option was chosen would offer significant financial savings. By the culmination of the clinical portion of the project, due to continued negotiations by the VAF's, the savings increased to a mean of $70,000. Financial analysis and negotiation were needed for competitive pricing.

In order to seek input from clinicians, a Value Analysis Ad Hoc Committee was formed, consisting of clinical experts from various units, who volunteered to participate in the decision-making process. Finding participants for this committee was not difficult. The nurses were quick to point out that HAIs have always been "never events" for clinicians. Chaired by a VAF, this committee included representatives from the Wound Care Team and several of the Intensive Care Units (ICU's). Front line staff involvement is crucial to appropriate decision making and buy in of product users. As a designated magnet facility (by the **American Nurses Credentialing Center (ANCC),** VCUHS is committed to involving direct caregivers in the decision-making process for all facets of their vocation possible. Product selection is no exception.

The committee sat through demonstrations by three FMS vendors, scoring them on a 1 to 5 scale in areas such as patient safety, improved patient outcomes, technical support, and capacity to supply, among others. Each area was weighted appropriately by the committee (i.e.: patient safety was 25percent, while R&D was 5 percent). The scoring, after demos, culminated in the following:

Company A: 4.08

Company B: 4.02

Company C 3.41.

Using this data driven decision making process, clinical trials were set up for companies A and B in two intensive care units (Surgical Trauma and Medical Respiratory). Company C was excluded. Each company provided clinicians with free product and education prior to use. Many staff nurses were involved in the trials and completed an evaluation tool while using each product. After clinical trials, comparison of the evaluations (another data driven decision making process) showed a slight clinician preference for Company A. Both products showed improvement in the odor issue and leakage was minimized. The Ad Hoc Committee gathered once more to go over the data and make a decision. The committee was then disbanded. This resolved and provided a product of acceptable clinical quality.

In this example, both clinical and business perspectives resulted in same choice: Company A. While optimal, this is certainly not always the case; had the conclusions been mixed, either product choice would have been acceptable. With the clinical evaluations so close in score, the clinicians would have supported Company B, if the clinical advantages were superior. Similarly, the financial departments would have supported Company B, if Company B had offered far greater savings. By eliminating any financially unacceptable options and allowing the final decisions to be made by the end users, this encourages the clinician's commitment to the Value Analysis process and support of future endeavours.

The decision to change products from current vendor was promoted at meetings, councils, committees, and other venues. Using an SBAR format, memos were sent to impacted departments. Special emphasis was placed on the fact that direct care staff was involved in the decision-making process. Although staff is interested in the monetary savings generated by a product change, they are far more interested in the clinical benefits to their patients.

Project Resolution and Follow Up: The Value Analysis Department followed up on the clinical Project Rationale by monitoring clinician input and reviewing incident reports related to products. The financial Project Rationale was tabulated quarterly. The Value Analysis Department tracked purchasing data to compare the estimated **"Return-On-investment" (ROI)** with the actual (annualized) savings.

(Source: www.readperiodicals.com)

VALUE ANALYSIS IN HEALTHCARE INDUSTRY IN THE INDIAN CONTEXT

Post liberalization era, a few leading healthcare institutions have implemented value engineering programmes as an ongoing activity and reaped noteworthy gains. Very few healthcare institutions are willing to make public the benefits achieved through value engineering because of fear of competition. By and large Indian hospitals are still to recognize and appreciate the relevance of value management.

Value management is particularly important to Indian healthcare Industry for the following reasons

1. Hospitals, which were established over 20 years ago with imported equipment and technology, have remained stagnant. With the advent of liberalization of Indian economy these hospitals are unable to sustain competition with major corporate hospitals especially in the absence of R and D facilities and clinical research.
2. Healthcare Industry in government sector under protective policies of the Government remained insulated from the onslaught of latest technology and real competition. In fact Technology is not just about going ahead. It is about staying ahead.
3. In changed economic scenario and fierce competition in corporate healthcare Industry in India will have to find ways and means to reduce costs and improve efficiency of their operations without which their survival will be at stake.

IMPORTANCE OF VALUE ANALYSIS AS A COST REDUCTION TECHNIQUE

Human Resources (HR) problems in healthcare institutions are undoubtedly important. But they have been given so much attention that another major and growing problem i.e. materials problem has all along been neglected. **Dean Ammer observed that hospital's salary and fringe benefits cost is accompanied by an approximately 15 percent in non-personal costs.** Hospitals are not only paying higher prices for purchases but also using more of them. **Cost reduction is pressing need of healthcare industry which is generally plagued by:**

Increased use of Purchased materials is partly due to technological changes as compared to earlier times when hospitals offered nursing care along with room and board. Progress in healthcare techniques has created new paramedical skills. Its effect has been greater, culminating into development of new materials, drugs, equipment and plethora of other items incidental to the health care.

Dean Ammer is of the opinion that aggregate healthcare man-hours per patient will not increase as much as material usage. In short, the suppliers to the healthcare institutions are almost certain to enjoy a higher growth rate than that of the healthcare institutions themselves.

Stiff competition among corporate hospitals, package schemes imposed by insurance companies for treatment of various ailments and other market constraints do not permit the unlimited passing on these escalations to the patients. Already reduced profitability further eroded by low productivity due to outdated equipment, processes and techniques, large inventories, crippling interest rates and other burdens also necessitate cost reduction programme.

For this reason cost reduction has been the primary objectives of application of value engineering, where it has been found to be exceptionally appropriate and useful. Although Value analysis is essentially a problem solving technique, because of its success, it is better recognized as a tool for cost reduction.

CAUSES OF UNNECESSARY COSTS

Since Value analysis attacks unnecessary costs, it would be pertinent to find out how unnecessary costs arise so that we may overcome or minimize these causes.

1. Lack of information

Most people who design a product or service are quite often not sure of real needs of users and usually over design the product by providing features that users do not use. (i.e., concept of err on safer side). Further technology is fast changing; new material and new processes are coming up almost every day. They create obsolescence in respect of old material or processes, costs which were considered acceptable yesterday become unnecessary today. **"In the face of competition the royal road to ruin is to adopt methods of yesterday to the business of today".**

2. Lack of ideas

A survey done some time back in U.S.A showed, that most people use less than 5 percent of their creative abilities. Most of us believe that we hardly have any time to think. and want previously tried out material, design, process and procedures. We jump at the first idea that works, and usually do not try to find out whether any better methods are possible. **Mind is like a parachute it works only when it is open.**

3. Wrong beliefs, habits and attitudes

Most of us use our judgment more than it is valid and jump to conclusions. Many of these happen to be wrong and do not stand for a moment's scrutiny if tested on the anvils of facts. But we believe them as if they were taken out of Holy Scriptures

4. Changed circumstances

Everyone likes progress but hardly anyone wants to change, especially if that change affects his work or him. Circumstances might have changed, yet one longs to be conservative and continue the same features year after year.

Value analysis aims at systematic identification and elimination of infructuous costs i.e., costs which do not improve the quality or efficiency of a product, or service or value or prolong its life or give a better appearance or provide additional utility features. **In other words value analysis results in, increased use of alternatives or less expensive materials.**

5. Cheaper designs

Less costly methods of treatment so as to provide same performance, improving quality and efficiency resulting in decrease of overall costs and consequently contributing to greater value. Application of newer techniques will results in additional bed availability. Traditionally a patient with a fracture of leg would occupy the bed for many days or weeks. Now with more advanced techniques of surgery and treatment, patient is sent home much earlier. Therefore bed turnover of surgical department goes up.

6. Creativity Killer Phrases

To generate new ideas one must overcome several mental blocks that come of innovation and creativity. **Some of typical mind stoppers are listed below**

- **We tried earlier and it did not work:** when and under what circumstances. It may now work under present or changed circumstances.
- **It will set a nasty precedent:** Mankind owes its progress to those men and women who broke this barrier
- **It will not work here:** It may work in other places or countries; it may work in Corporate hospitals and not in Government hospitals and vice versa etc. It is only escapism.
- **Costs too much:** customers may pay for it if the price is commensurate with quality and their expectations
- **Customers may not like it:** Why not if you give a better service at a cheaper price
- **It is impracticable:** If it has not been tried, how does one know It is impracticable?
- **Hospital user:** departments will have none of this.
- **We tried the best and the greatest:** we do not have to learn anything from others.
- **Why change When it works:** How long will it work?

- **There is no other source of supply:** Probably we did not know any other
- **That is not our problem:** clinical department says it is problem of nursing department, nursing puts the blame on materials department, Materials department blames indenter or design and so on, the buck keeps going round and round.
- **Management won't support it:** Who is in the management, it is you and I
- **Hospital policy:** Policy is framed by us; why not change the policy if it warrants?
- **Our hospital is too large and complicated:** If the hospital is too large and complicated is an excellent ground to initiate value analysis programme. It will turn the fragmented bedlam in to a system The size of the hospital is not a matter of constraint for application good management practices.
- **Our hospital is too small for this:** Majority of Indian hospitals are in small hospital category they need as much assistance in area of cost reduction techniques as they do for large ones. In fact a very small savings can make the difference in operating at profit or loss. In fact small can greatly benefit from value analysis programme.
- **Our hospital is different:** Regardless of size, mission, ownership, location, management expertise and objectives, through effective management, Value analysis can be implemented.
- **Why worry the corporate customer or patient pays:** Wait till some other hospital comes with a better and cheaper product or service)
- **It will not work in our hospital:** I know (This is the dim-witted argument from Mr. Know All)
- **It is not invented here:** we know everything and anything; what we do not know is not worth knowing.
- **It is a good idea but not workable:** That is lethargy, too sluggish to stir.
- **It is wonderful idea we must do. But we are right now busy:** with medical camp or expansion programme. It is not for eternity may be for a month quarter or half year or year, when there will be time for life saving changes
- **It is a military order:** no discussions will be permitted. In fact value engineering was born out of military priority requirements.
- **Collaborators design should not be changed:** But how old is the design? Perhaps collaborator might have changed long ago.
- **Let us set up a Committee to study it:** Best way to avoid decisions procrastination in practice.
- **I have bigger problem:** Value analysis is the least of my worries.

Such wrong beliefs can kill cost reduction ideas before they are christened.

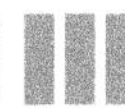

Unnecessary costs will continue to be incurred. Positive thinking, as a state of mind opens the door for each of us to develop creative ideas. Brainstorming is an excellent technique for creative ideas. Here it is worth remembering Elmer G. Letterman's quotation.**"We are today here yesterday's thoughts have brought us, and shall be tomorrow where today carrying us".**

Above list is illustrative many more creativity killers can be cited what is not needed the reasons, why something will not work but find out ways and means overcome psychological barriers.

TYPES OF VALUE

Before proceeding further on the subject of value analysis, it is necessary to have clear idea of what we mean by the word "VALUE." This word has many connotations like

- Economic value
- Moral value,
- Religious value
- Aesthetic value
- Social value
- Political value
- Judicial value and so on.

But healthcare industry is more concerned with Economic value. Cost is total sum of money spent for materials, labor, overheads etc. To produce any item, price is the amount for which service provider or supplier is willing to sell that product, and usually includes cost plus a margin of profit.

CONSTITUENTS OF ECONOMIC VALUE

Properties and qualities which relate to "Economic Value" of any item can be grouped under the following categories:

Use Value: Use value is based on the elements and qualities of any given material or service in relation to purpose of material or service. It is a monetary measure of qualities of items that contribute to its performance. For example Brake of an automobile.

Cost Value: It is sum total of cost of materials, labour and other costs required to produce an item. Cost analysis is based upon the cost of product and is normally expressed monetarily. Sometimes an item can be considered as investment because it will generate savings. Insulation that will save on energy cost is a good example.

Esteem Value: Qualities, which add prestige and make the ownership of item desirable. Esteem value is based upon the attractiveness involved through ownership of the item or use of a particular service and is subjective. An Indian Woman wanting gold embroidered sari or an American or European lady wanting platinum ring are some examples.

Exchange Value: Properties which make the object possible of being traded for other items or to be sold or exchanged or ability to withstand depreciation. Exchange value is based upon elements or quality that makes an item exchangeable for something.

For example the exchange value of a used car when it is turned in for new car. Gold or diamonds are sought after because of their exchange value.

It is obvious all these values play an important part in our personal lives. As far as health care Industry and National economy are concerned use value objective is most important. Others are subordinated to it varying degrees.

A word of caution is necessary here regarding term "perceived value", sometimes used in marketing jargons, which refers to what customer "thinks he is buying" as against "what he is actually getting".

Typical examples are the fancy containers of popular cosmetic preparations which have a big hollow at the bottom. Other examples are fancy automobile registration numbers etc.

Reuse Value applies when an item can be used for another purpose, when its original purpose is no longer served. Soft drink sold in PET bottles. Another typical example is a glass container for selling fruit jam that can be reused as drinking glass once its contents have been used up.

Loss Value is if an item has more value, when lost than it had before.

Use of value engineering techniques should be guided by following equation

Exchange value = Use value + Esteem value

To sum up, the word "value" in the context of value engineering refers to what the customer or end user thinks the product is worth to meet his minimum specific requirements.

He is not concerned with, which materials and processes have been used? What is actual cost of manufacture or how much profit margins is added?

His interest is in fulfilling his minimum functional needs at the desired place and time, at lowest cost.

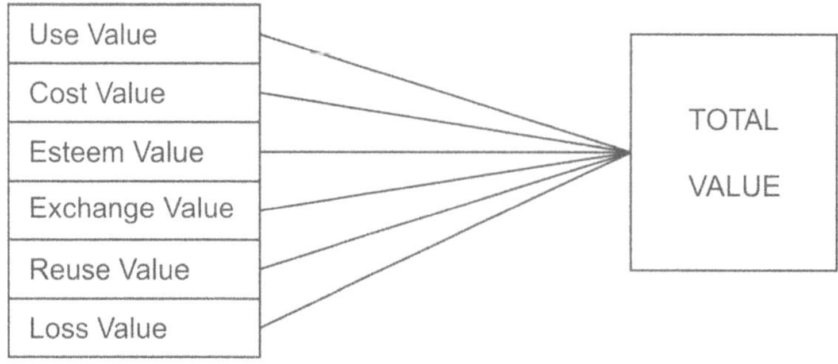

Figure 23.1 Total Economic Value

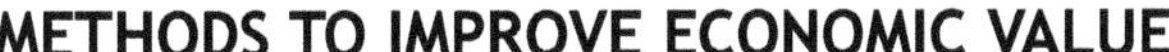

METHODS TO IMPROVE ECONOMIC VALUE

Let us consider at this stage what is meant by 'VALUE' ? Value in itself is somewhat difficult to define. It means different things for different people. Also it often confused with cost and price of a product or service.

One may define value of an item as its worth to you, compared to the price you may pay for it.

$$\text{Value} = \frac{\text{Worth to you}}{\text{Price you pay}}$$

Worth of an item purely depends upon functional utility or the end use, and more subjectively on its artistic or prestige value.

Value can therefore be improved in three ways by

1. **Improving the utility and usefulness of the item etc., i.e., improving worth, without increasing the cost**

   Example:

   Use of plastic bottles instead of conventional glass bottles, a patient admitted for diarrhea or vomiting requires administering of 10 to 12 bottles of glucose during his stay. The difference between glass bottles and plastic bottles is around Rs. 5 per bottle. Thereby on each patient, the hospital can save Rs. 50 to Rs. 60 in addition to intangible benefits such as avoiding breakages and disposal.

2. **Reducing the costs and retaining same worth.**

   Examples:

   Antibiotic policy doctors can be advised to develop an antibiotic policy wherein medicines are prescribed by generic names. Hospital can adopt a policy of acquiring antibiotics from a particular pharmaceutical establishment. This brings down costs while retaining its worth.

   Use of indigenous Stent developed by Dr Kalaam and Dr Raju as mentioned earlier.

   Other examples are replacement of copper wire with aluminum wire for household electrical wiring, tamarind starch replacing maize starch for laundry requirements.

3. **Improving the worth and also reducing the price**

   Example:

   Incorporating IV Stand with the bed itself instead of having it as a separate unit with appropriate value engineering design the need for separate IV Stand can be avoided. The tangible benefit per bed will be around Rs. 500 apart from intangible benefit like saving of space. This example will be of great use to small hospitals and nursing homes.

TECHNIQUES OF VALUE ANALYSIS OR CHECK LIST APPROACH

Lawrence D. Miles has after considerable work in this field evolved a number of techniques.

Skilful application of which will help to

- Identify unnecessary costs,
- Remove obstacles and
- Provide a course of action for developing worthwhile value alternatives

Lawrence D. Miles, father of value Analysis with the help of his colleague in General Electric company by name Roy Fountain had framed a list of 10 (Ten) questions to aid value analysis.

Most important approaches he developed are

- Function approach
- Application of creativity techniques
- Evaluation and further investigation of ideas generated

A.R. Palit, known as father of Indian Materials Management Movement had amended and amplified questions to aid value analysis. He brought out 17 questions to suit to Indian business environment. They are as follows:

1. Does the use of item contribute to end value?

This question seeks to determine whether a useful and necessary purpose exists for the item or services. Answer should clearly state the function(s) the user requires. Dean Ammer suggested that every hospital materials manager should be able to identify at least one purchase that serves no useful purpose or if it does not add value it can be eliminated altogether.

2. Is this the only item suitable for the end use? If not what alternatives are available and are any of them are better or cheaper?

According to Smoker, former director, Materials Resource Services at Well spans Health, York, PA healthcare organizations need to look at bigger picture. he cited using silver impregnated products vs. practicing effective aseptic techniques in installing scrub machines to reinforce employees returning scrubs. "Do we try to goof proof every thing which will add cost to the system instead of coaching healthcare professionals to use their heads as well as their hands.

3. Is this item a standard one, as regard to specifications, size and shape, colour, etc.?

Sanderson cites need for value analysis and emphasizes standardization. One of the problems the materials manager may encounter in establishing standardization is the 'indifference to standardization' syndrome. This syndrome is characterized by the preference for certain brands without regard quality or cost. Indifference to standardization is like a cancer; left unchecked it will consume the whole and result in pandemonium for purchasing. Every hospital should have standardization programme, that promote simplification reduction in number of types, sizes, etc, in inventory; elimination of the extra procedures necessary to purchase special items

4. **If several types are to be purchased, is it necessary to buy all the different shapes, types, colours, etc., or can number of sizes, shapes, etc. be reduced?**

Smoker said that traditional definitions and impressions of value analysis particularly in healthcare is no longer appropriate to succeed; Smoker ads on that "value analysis is used to focus primarily on product standardization and reducing overall costs" he told Healthcare Purchasing News, **"drive more volume to fewer vendors and the world will spin appropriately on its axis.** But a new twist involves clinical quality, value analysis which includes life cycle cost and clinical benefits to drive desirable patient outcomes."

5. **Is the cost of item commensurate in usefulness with terms of contribution to end product or service?**

Based upon the desired function the question is to determine whether a lower cost item will accomplish the same function. A good materials manager should be able to indentify dozens of such cases where lower cost items will do the same job.

If not can it be modified or greater economy or use-fullness or finding satisfactory cheaper substitute. All this is tied in to need for carefully reviewing quality.

6. **Can consumption of the item be cut down by value analysis Including considerations of end use?**

Using of hot air instead of paper towels. In high use areas such as public toilets and rest rooms, there is a large amount fritter away of paper towels. The materials manager in coordination with the executive of housekeeping department perform studies on these areas to determine the cost of paper towels on annual basis, then compare those figures with the cost of installing hot air hand driers. Objective here is the quantity purchased most economical? Most economical in view of cost and long term benefit.

7. **Is the item of right design? Are specifications and Tolerances too stringent? Does the item need all its features?**

Dean Ammer while stressing the need for value analysis he emphasizes importance of study of the relationship of design, function and cost of any product, materials or services with the object of reducing its cost through modification of design, or materials specifications, manufacture by more efficient process, change in source of supply (internal or external) or possible elimination incorporation into a related item. Greatest benefits accrue when a material is used in large, quantities either by virtue of a high of in one product or lesser rate of use in several products.

8. Is the method of manufacturing of the item is too expensive? Can usuable item be manufactured by cheaper method?

Can it be manufactured at a lower cost by the supplier if quantities are procured at a time are increased or If long term contracts are entered into for larger quantities enable supplier to use better tools or methods of production?

Though, this test applies to a large extent to manufacturers. Hospitals however can apply to such areas like manufacturing artificial limbs, laundry, sterilization, food preparation and production of medical gases, IV fluids etc.,

9. Obtain available costs and analyse them. Various types of costs used in cost accounting and management decisions are :

Material cost, Labour cost, Overhead costs, fixed costs, Variable costs Prime cost Decision cost Shop cost Manufacturing cost. Standard cost Incremental cost and so on.

Each of these costs may be of importance in different situations. For the purpose of value analysis most meaningful costs are considered. Meaningful costs will have some relationship to its performance.

10. Seek information from best or most authentic source :

For value analysis gather information on any aspect of cost, such as Material, Labour, Methods, Process of Manufacturing, Finishing, Packaging etc

Very often, information is obtained from knowledgeable persons, is based on old information, insufficient knowledge, pre conceived ideas, existing procedures of long standing and so on. Such information may likely to mislead the analyst.

Wherever possible the information obtained must be verified that there are no mistakes. Conscious efforts must be made to locate the best source of information.

11. Discuss with specialists and take advantage of their ideas

Specialists may be from one's own organization or from outside. Select specialists carefully.

For soliciting ideas, item can be broken down into various phases depending up on its nature.viz

- Design of the item its arrangement and appearance.
- Mechanics of item what does it comprise of E.g. electrical circuits and servo mechanism etc.
- Metals or non metals from which parts are made
- Process involved in manufacture

It is therefore necessary to seek advice from proper specialists, who are experts in their own field or technology, so that you can get from them authentic and latest know how. Administrator, along with chief of medical staff, will recommend those physicians on the staff whose specialties and personalities are best suited to contribute to medical judgement to value improvement.

12. Think Creatively

Human mind is capable of developing "new ideas" in varying degrees. The more you think of existing situation and analyze its phases, the greater will be the number of new ideas that may come to your mind as alternatives.

Till recently, creativity was thought to be 'prerogative of a gifted few', who are born genius. This myth has been exploded after extensive studies by psychologists and behavioural scientists. It is now established that normal individual with average intelligence can be trained and developed to improve his talent effectively.

Individual creativity can be developed by 'brain storming' session of few individuals to stimulate creative thinking and more alternatives may be brought to light.

To quote **Thomas Alwa Edison,** the Great Inventor - **"creativity is ten percent inspiration and ninety percent perspiration".**

13. Use Standard Parts

Standard parts are interchangeable and cheaper than specially made, (non standard) parts. This is because, that standard parts are generally made by mass production methods leading to uniformity, interchangeability and reduced costs.

14. Refine ideas

One specific way of rapidly developing any idea or group of ideas is to list their advantages and disadvantages. In this way the disadvantages, the new and smaller problems are isolated, weighed against the advantages, and then overcome by additional creative thought. In this manner the good points of many ideas are combined while disadvantages are eliminated.

15. Consult your supplier for new ideas

In the past sales representatives have been noted for their hard sell and their marketing techniques. However with the conception of materials management developing, the responsibility of salesman is changing, he should turn out to be a representative to a hospital from his company. In this role, the representative can be very valuable to the hospital. Here is an example how. Surgical sales people helped American hospitals to improve laparoscope surgeries

In any ten day period, United States surgical sales people visit every one of 5,000 U.S. hospitals where surgeries are performed. They gown up and walk right into operating rooms to coach surgeons in the use of complex instruments which their companies make. They listen to what doctors like and don't like, need and don't need. Its close connection to customers made U.S. Surgical quick to pick up on early experiments in laparoscopic surgery by inserting a tiny video camera into the body along with slim, long handled instruments. Supplier company's close connections to customers have resulted in many innovative new products. Consumers often create new products on their own, companies can benefit by finding those products and putting them on the market **(Kotler and Armstrong).**

Value analysis can focus solely on internal supply with some success, but true potential lies in applying it to external supply as well. Many firms are using this approach and are called early supplier involvement; suppliers are involved at design phase of a product or service. Suppliers provide suggestions for design changes and materials choices that will result in more efficient operations and higher quality.

In automotive industry a higher level of early supplier involvement is known as pre sourcing, where by suppliers selected early in vehicles concept development stage and are given significant, if not total responsibility for designing of certain components or systems. Pre-sourced supplies are also take responsibility for the cost, quality, and on time delivery of items they produce.

Ideas and suggestions arising out of the experience of suppliers can be of great help to buying company. As supplier may be dealing with many others who are in similar lines of business as that of buying company. Many suppliers would be willing to develop new techniques to suit your needs, to mutual advantage of both. **"Good buyer and seller relationship is essential for value analysis".**

16. Remove Road Blocks

Road blocks arise principally out of ignorance and inherent resistance to change. We should try to break these road blocks by questioning everything.

Nothing is a 'holy cow'. These must be tackled with patience, clearly explaining position of viewpoint of proposed method to individual concerned.

There are no short cuts, to overcome road blocks. Nursing staff is probably more involved in product selection and review than any other functional group in the hospital. Directors and supervisors aswell as the online staff nurse will probably be needed atmost product reviews to evaluate items from a nursing patient view point. Unless this is done it is bound to create impediments to the process of value ananysis.

For this purpose there must be willingness among its top managers individually and collectively, to review existing policies, practices, methods and techniques with a view to challenge them, where necessary.

17. Get maximum co operation from colleagues in other departments with whom you have to deal

As a value analyst one may not be fully conversant with all details of working of various departments. He has to very often rely on people working in each department in the organization. He has to keep concerned departmental people informed about the item that has been chosen for study and why he selected that particular item how much it costs to the hospital and why there is a need to reduce the cost if possible.

Value improvement programmes in hospitals would not be accomplished without some reference to importance of obtaining support for such programmes from administration, medical staff and nursing. Administrative support should be sought from chief administrative officer by the materials manager. Materials manager should also seek the help of administrator in medical staff involvement in value improvement.

Materials manager as coordinator of value analysis programme must be polite and friendly with everyone so that when time comes he has to secure their help and full cooperation from administration medical staff and nursing **"Co-operation be gets co-operation"**

ESSENCE OF VALUE ANALYSIS / MISS CONCEPT

A.R. Palit, a pioneer in the field of materials management in India has summarized the essence of value analysis in two words so easy to remember **E-K-CHANGE MISS.**

This is popularly known as **MISS** Technique.

E- STANDS FOR ELIMINATE : Can we eliminate the item altogether? In other words can we do without it?

K- STANDS FOR KEEP: when we cannot eliminate an item, we have to keep it, at the same time we must try to reduce the cost so as to obtain better value for money.

Good examples are 10 and 100 rupee notes printed on imported currency paper.

Change is necessary, when an item or method or process cannot be eliminated but has to be kept. One way of reducing the cost may be cutting down consumption but there are other ways represented by the word MISS

M-STANDS FOR MODIFY

This may mean

- A slight modification in the design,
- Specifications
- Size
- Shape
- Colour
- Elimination of an unwanted accessory
- Unnecessary feature
- Relaxation of tolerance, which is not required to perform a function

I-STANDS FOR INCORPORATE

Value can be improved by combining two or more operations or parts the cost of an item can be reduced.

S -STANDS FOR SUB DIVIDE

Sometimes a complicated item can be obtained at a cheaper price or manufacture in small parts and assembled. Then economy can also be affected at times in regard to transportation and packaging costs by ordering an item in smaller sizes.

This is exactly opposite to incorporation.

A firm in western India reduced the cost if an item required in limited quantity by having fabricated parts rather by having it in die cast in one piece as was done by foreign collaboration.

S - STANDS FOR SUBSTITUTE

Complete substitution can be affected to bring down cost or improve value we have to concentrate what else will do the function to be performed.

One of the areas where value analysis has a significant role to play is use of brand names. Proprietary Preparations are generally high priced vis à vis with generic preparations. The price difference may at times be 5 to 6 times. Value analysis of such products will ensure cost effectiveness without affecting the functionality. Value analysis is an important methodology to ensure continuous quality improvement in medical stores.

Other Examples:

For house hold electrical wiring aluminum is replacing copper.

Maize Starch is replaced by tamarind seed starch for sizing textiles.

By contributing substantially towards cost reduction, inventory reduction, import substitution, standardization, reduction in processing costs and times, cost reduction on packaging, consumables and other indirect materials etc.Value engineering has emerged as the most effective and appropriate technique available to materials managers.

SUMMARY

In these days of increasing costs and dwindling profits "VALUE ANALYSIS" has emerged as most effective and appropriate tool for achieving quick results in cost reduction, and solves plethora business problems like profitability and poor competitiveness dependence on imports and scarce materials, quality problems, production and procurement problems, low productivity etc.

However one thing is certain there is no limit to wonders that value analysis can achieve if only one cares to understand the great impact that cost reduction can have on survival and growth of one's company.

Value Engineering is of special relevance in the context of liberalization of Indian Economy, which brings in its wake not only challenges and opportunities, but also serious problems and difficulties. In spite of out dated designs and technology having an abundance of unnecessary features and costs, archaic methods and systems and in efficiency in operations, many industries survived so long under protection of tariffs and controls. Such industries now stand exposed to the onslaught of latest technology and management practices have provided the management tool to face these challenges.

Value Analysis can help to maximize: Conservation of utilization of material resources, Substitution of indigenous materials for imported goods without sacrificing quality, and performance and reduce costs substantially.

Value analysis should not be confused with price analysis or cost analysis the value of the item is measured in terms of its function or purpose primarily is that of quality, at times appearance of the item and its prestige.

Value Engineering comprises of a group of techniques aimed at systematic classification of "Unnecessary Costs" in a product or service, and efficiently eliminating them without detrimental to its quality and efficiency.

During the Second World War, companies engaged in war effort faced serious problem of shortage of materials. This leads to experimenting on substitute materials quite often in a very unorthodox way. In many cases the experiment clicked.

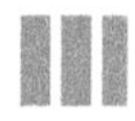

Surprisingly there were large numbers of instances where substitutes were much cheaper and functioned more efficiently than original material.

Although Value engineering is essentially a problem solving technique, because of its success, it is better recognized as a tool for cost reduction.

The word "Value" has many connotations like Economic value, Moral value, Religious value, Aesthetic value, Social value, Political value, judicial value and so on of which we are more concern with economic value

"Economic Value" of any item can be grouped under 4 (four) Categories as mentioned below: Use value, Cost value, Esteem value, Exchange value

One may define value of an item as it's worth' to you, compared to the price you may pay for it. Value = Worth to you / Price you Pay.

Value could be improved in three ways by Improving the utility and usefulness or reducing the costs, but retaining same worth, or improving the worth and also reducing the price

Lawrence D. Miles popularly known as father of value engineering framed a list of 10 (Ten) questions to aid value analysis, later Mr. A.R. Palit amended and amplified the ten questions to seventeen for use in India conditions

A.R. Palit has summarized the essence of value analysis in two words so easy to remember E-K-CHANGE MISS. Where 'E' stands for Elimination, 'K' stands for Key, 'M' stands for modify, 'I' stands for Incorporate, 'S' stands for Subdivide, and 'S' stands for Substitute.

To successfully implement value engineering programme ,the materials manager be supposed to seek the help of the administrator in medical staff involvement in value improvement project. The administrator, along with the chief of medical staff, will recommended those physicians on the staff whose specialities and personalities are best suited to contributing medical judgement to the value improvement committee's determination. Medical staff's support would be enhanced if the environment of key members of the staff were publicized through committee reports, hospital newsletters, or like information channels.

REVIEW QUESTIONS

1. Value Analysis helps to maximize conservation of material resources and Import substitution helps, savings in valuable foreign exchange. Discuss
2. Function is the "Key" to value engineering and the "Functional Analysis" is the "Keel" on which value analysis is built up. Discuss.
3. What do you understand by the terms value analysis and value engineering. Describe the basic features of value engineering.
4. Value analysis attacks unnecessary costs, how unnecessary costs arise and how you overcome or minimize these costs.
5. What do you understand by the term Brain storming explain how it is organized?
6. If necessity is mother of all inventions Lawrence D. Miles can be rightly called "the father of Value Engineering". Discuss
7. Value analysis aims at a systematic identification and elimination of unnecessary costs. Explain with suitable examples.
8. Write short notes on
   a. Value Analysis and value engineering (VAVE)
   b. Functional analysis
   c. Basic features of value engineering
   d. Causes of un necessary costs
   e. Constituents of economic value
   f. Road Blocks
   g. Creativity Killer Phrases

PART - V

24
Chapter

Supply Chain Management Relevance to Healthcare Industry

Contents

CHAPTER - 24

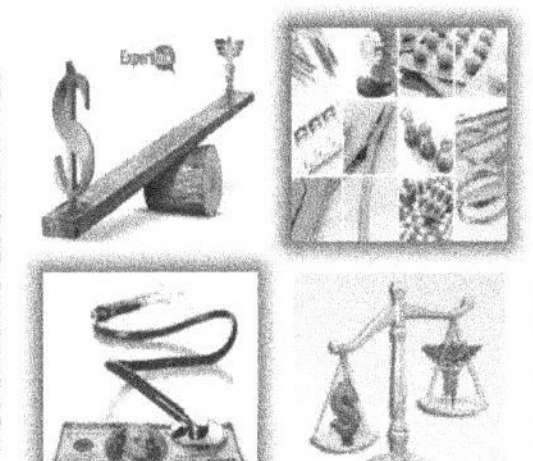

Supply Chain Management Relevance to Healthcare Industry

INTRODUCTION

The concept of Supply Chain Management (SCM) is better understood in a manufacturing environment. This chapter is dealt in two parts. First part is devoted to manufacturing scenario and second to the healthcare industry in order to have a better understanding of SCM relevant to hospital industry.

Supply Chain Management is a term that has grown significantly in use and popularity in Industry since late 1980s, although considerable confusion exists about what it actually means. Sometimes term is used as a substitute or synonym for logistics. However, the definition of supply chain management is much broader than logistics. Challenges which organizations are facing to day are vastly different from those a few years ago. **The forces of globalization of economies have subjected the national businesses to international competition.** Traditional business cycles are being affected by stiff competition. Time pressures and speed of change are constantly accelerating. **To day, every thing in business must be faster, newer and quicker.** Due to increased exposure through television media, internet and international travel, customer has lot more information now regarding alternative or competitive products available in international markets. Customers' expectations have increased substantially. Customer now expects the products cheaper yet better in quality and reliability. Most companies find their margins getting squeezed as they lowered the margins yet had to invest more resources to ensure speed and reliability. Under intensive competitive pressures integrated supply chain scenario is a tug of war, pulled on one side by customers' ever multiplying demands and on the other by company's strong urge to grow and run the organization on a profitable basis. Managers have come to realize that they have to keep the rope from snapping and yet achieve both the objectives growth and profitability. Alignment of firms that bring products or services to market has been called supply chain, demand chain or the value chain. A similar scenario prevails in healthcare industry in the first decade and of the current millennium.

Extracts of Key Note Address delivered by **Shri M. Gopala Krishna, IAS (Retd.),** former **Chairman of Andhra Pradesh State Financial Corporation (APSFC),** Hyderabad on the occasion of

National Convention of Indian Institute of Materials Management held at Hyderabad in November 99 has been the source for some of the concepts presented in this chapter. The author happend to be the chairman of the convention.

WHAT IS A SUPPLY CHAIN MANAGEMENT?

Supply chain management is integration of all business processes from tier II suppliers to end users that provide product services and information that add value for customers. A supply chain consists of all stages involved, in fulfilling a customer request. Supply chain not only includes the manufacturer and suppliers, but also transporters, warehouses, retailers, and customers themselves. These functions include, but are not limited to, new product development, marketing, operations, distribution, finance, and customer service alone. Supply chain management is the management of all key business processes across the various links in the supply chain. With in each organization, **supply chain includes all function such as**

- Customer relationship management
- Customer service management
- Demand management
- Manufacturing flow management
- Order fulfillment
- New product development and commercialization.

Supply chain is dynamic and involves constant flow of products, services, funds and information among different stages. Each stage of supply chain performs different processes in accordance with its core competence and interacts with other stages of supply chain. Supply chain activities begin with a customer order and end when a satisfied customer has paid for his or her purchase. **The term supply chain conjures up images of products, or supply, moving from suppliers to manufacturers to distributors to customers along a chain.** In supply chain, materials and products flow downstream, funds flow upstream and information flows both ways. The link may be only one player or more than one players involved at each stage. In reality, a manufacturer or healthcare institution may receive materials from several suppliers and then supply to several distributors. Therefore it is more appropriate to use the term supply network to describe the structure of most supply chains.

A typical supply chain may involve a variety of stages as described below:

- Customers,
- Retailers,
- Wholesalers / Distributors,
- Manufacturers,
- Component / Raw material suppliers.

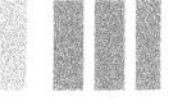

Appropriate design of supply chain will depend on both customer's needs and roles and functions of stages involved in fulfilling those needs. In cases such as a mail order company, manufacturers do not respond to customer orders directly but maintain an inventory of products from which it fill customer orders. In case of a small retail store, supply chain may also contain a distributor and wholesaler between the retail store and the manufacturer. See Figure 24.1.

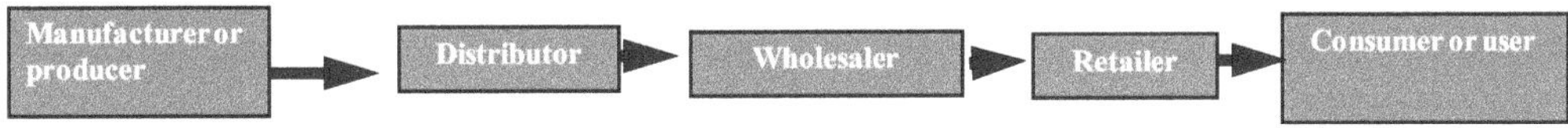

Figure 24.1 Small Retail Store Supply Chain

SUPPLY CHAIN MANAGEMENT (SCM) DEFINITION

Supply Chain Management is a process oriented, integrated approach to procuring, and delivering products and services to customers. SCM has a broad scope that includes sub-suppliers, suppliers, and internal operations, trade customers, retail customers and end users. SCM covers the management of material, information and funds flow. The process here refers to producing value for the ultimate consumer who is the end user.

It will thus be noticed from the above definition that supply chain is in fact the people and processes that deliver product/service to the consumer/the end user. Individual companies no longer compete with other as stand alone companies but one supply chain competes against other. Supply chain has come to stay because when organizations work independent of their suppliers and customers, costs and inefficiencies tend to build at the interfaces. From these considerations, the definition of supply chain management emerges as: **"An integrated management of all the linkages and value adding activities from the supplier's supplier to the customer's customer (Ultimate Customer) in such a way that enhanced customer value is achieved at lower costs".**

EVOLUTION OF SCM IN INDIAN INDUSTRY

Evolution of supply chain management in the context of Indian industry is briefly described below.

In the early years, between 1960 and 1975, emphasis in supply management was on inventory push to points of warehousing and purchase. Distribution management was the priority. The period 1975 - 1990 saw the integration of MM operations within the manufacturing companies, and the rise of power of 'consumer pull'. Emphasis shifted to lowering operating costs. The decade of 1990s recognized that the main purpose of business is the creation of 'customer' and holding him. **Customer satisfaction moved towards customer delight and customer surprise.** Enterprise wide Resource Planning moved towards Extended Enterprise Resource planning. This led to emergence of the 'virtual' companies. As we marched towards Y2K, the economic process set in motion in 1990's resulted in more intense competition world wide. Survival in business depended on strategies to survive and grow. Companies that were not well prepared to meet the newly emerged realities simply got wiped out from market place. Now companies draw sustenance from **three P's- Plans, People, Processes.** The three P's are interdependent and interact with each other to produce a business output in the shape of customer satisfaction, market share and productivity. Plan people and process also constitute three pillars supporting supply chain system. Withdrawal of support of any one of the pillars leads to collapse of the system. SCM strategy is to be evolved by taking stock of all three P's. SCM seeks to integrate all these three elements. With Information Technology (IT) and advanced computer software it has been possible to synchronize between plan and the processes. However challenges still continue to exist from people factor as the emotional factors and individual predilections are intractable in nature. Wide area networking, global sourcing and connectivity are the order of the day.

CONCEPT OF SCM

Supply chain encompasses over and above logistics, flow of materials and products to customers and also includes external organizations that are part of the process. The task of supply chain management is to integrate the entire set of operations and processes involved in product flow process into a single supra organization across organizational and some cases across national boundaries. The concept of supply chain embraces several points; important among these are providing goods and services, logistic operations, procurement, production and distribution operations and balancing costs and assets. SCM provides direction and control in a system between operations to direct scheduling and planning. **Supply chain as a management system operates at two levels i.e., corporate stage and operation stage.** As operations are defined by corporate decisions, corporate decisions can only be made on the basis of operating capabilities.

COMPONENTS OF SUPPLY CHAIN MANAGEMENT

Supply chain has two components.

1. 'Internal' chain links all company departments to execute a customer's order.
2. 'External' chain comprises of a group of companies, which work together in specified channels to deliver the product.

The common goal is to increase sales by making products to order while reducing inventory costs. This is akin to **'just in time'** instead of stocking for **'just in case'** (J.I.C). As stated earlier supply chain management is an integration of Business Processes from end users through original suppliers that provides products, services and information that add value to customers. Figure 24.2 illustrates how purchasing or its expanded role of procurement supports supply chain management.

Purchasing is primarily for inbound or upstream, channel activities, where logistics spans both inbound and outbound relationships.

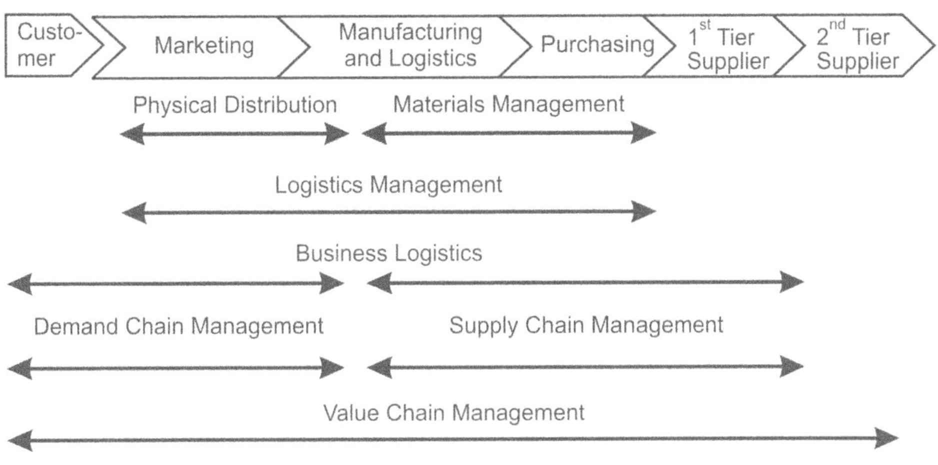

Figure 24.2 The Components of Supply Chain both Internal and External

IMPORTANCE OF SCM

SCM is extremely important in all industries in the manufacturing and service sectors under all economic conditions and continues to be important even in declining markets and during periods of economic slow down, when market growth can not conceal inefficient practices. SCM is also critical when an organization is concentrating on enlarging its business portfolio through new product and market development and when the organization is making decisions related to Supply Chain Configuration. SCM as a systems approach is highly interactive and complex, and requires simultaneous consideration of many trade offs. SCM is important at times when shareholders want pro-active action to beat the growing competition, seek high value addition, high returns, as well as creation of long term share value. SCM helps Company chief executives to optimize sales growth, reduce costs, and improve overall working capital management, performance, productivity and profitability. Companies that know how to continuously improve management of their supply chains will be the new success stories in global market places. Information Technology provides them competitive advantage in that direction by reducing costs of processing and storing information and harnessing external drivers of change through better information sharing, connectivity and seamless instant communications.

OBJECTIVES OF SCM

Main objective of managing a company's Supply chain is to ensure having at hand correct level and mix of inventory required at every point in the supply chain to meet a strategically targeted customer service level, and to meet that service level at the lowest possible cost with least amount of work load. However, **today's customers expect to have exact products that they want, when they want, at the place where they want, at a price that they want and in the**

 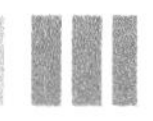

volumes that they need. An expensive and luxurious option to react quickly to varying customer demands is to keep more than adequate quantities in finished goods inventories. However in such a case, whenever demand falls, the unsold finished products become wasted money.

A well managed supply chain is expected to support strategic objectives of a business by adopting following performance objectives.

- Reduced costs
- Shorter lead times
- Quality in relation to end uses and/ or customers expectations
- Flexibility
- Improved and enhanced customer services
- Better product availability and reliability

The configuration of supply chain varies from organization to organization. The activities of supply chain include three basic elements, systems, technology, relationships. Primary objective of every supply chain is to maximize the overall value generated. The value which a supply chain generates is difference between what the final product is worth to the customer and the effort that entire supply chain expends in filling the customer's requests. Companies therefore use supply chain planning to anticipate conditions and act pro actively, not just react, to dynamically changing situations and be cost effective at all times.

SCM ROLE OF VARIOUS FUNCTIONS

To execute a company's competitive strategy, all the functions associated with internal and external supply chains must play their roles and each function must develop its own sub-strategy. The sub strategy must facilitate the best possible performance of each function. For example, a product development strategy specifies the portfolios of new products and services that a company will develop. It also indicates whether development efforts will be made internally or outsourced. A marketing and sales strategy specifies how the market will be segmented and the products positioned, priced, and promoted. A supply chain operations strategy determines the nature of procurement and transportation of materials to and from the company, delivery of services to customers, along with the necessary follow up services. From a value chain perspective, supply chain strategy specifies how operations, distribution, and service will contribute to the organizational objectives. Additionally, strategies will be devised for finance, accounting, information technology, and human resources. Supply chain strategy includes supplier strategy, operations strategy, and logistics strategy. Decisions regarding inventory, transportation, operation facilities, and information flows in the supply chain are all important parts of supply chain strategy. Value chain concept emphasizes close relationships among all functional sub strategies. Each function is crucial if a company is to profitably satisfy customer needs. Various functional sub- strategies cannot be formulated in isolati on. **They are closely intertwined and must fit into and support each other for a company to succeed.**

SCM BASIC FRAMEWORK

A number of elements are brought together in order to construct the frame work of SCM. These elements are:

- Generic Activities
- Objectives of SCM Framework and
- Architecture of Supply Chain

Generic Activities

Concept of process control lies at the heart of SCM framework. By process, is meant a group of related tasks that together create a value for a customer. The value, which could be in the form of a product or service, is output of some action. On the supply chain, there are some 'generic activities', cutting across functional lines, which contribute to value experienced at the end of the chain. To understand what these activities are, we visit the conventional definition of supply chain: Flow of materials is through procurement, manufacture, distribution, sales and disposal or consumption. If we look at what actually happens in a supply chain, we could capture it in the following string:

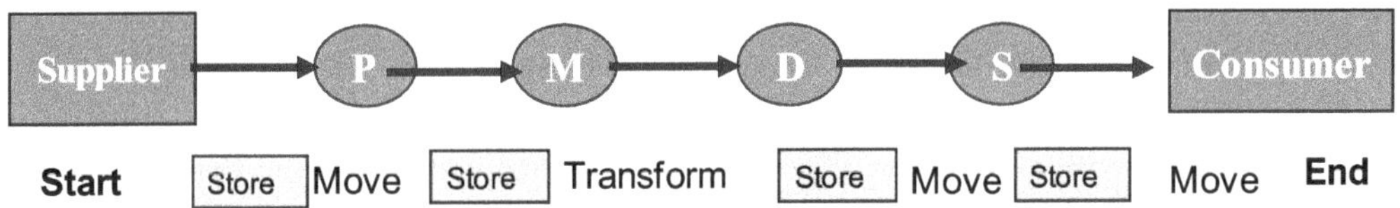

In addition to conversion activities, it is essential to view storage transportation and other activities also as a process what capability can be built up. Essentially, value is delivered on the supply chain through the following 'generic activities' that are strung together:

- Store
- Transform
- Move

The direction of movement of these activities is from left to right, i.e. upstream to downstream. However, these generic activities viz. Stores, transform and Move are triggered by information flow from left; hence a fourth value adding to generic activity can be communication.

Objectives of Supply Chain Framework

As stated earlier the objective of every supply chain is to maximize overall value generated. The value a supply chain generates is the difference between what the final product is worth to the customer and the effort the supply chain expends in filling the customer's request. For most commercial supply chains, value will be strongly correlated with supply chain profitability, i.e. the difference between the revenue generated from the customer and the overall costs incurred across the supply chain. Some critical questions that are to be asked while designing the chain to deliver its objectives are:

- What are the levels of customer service in terms of lead time and product availability?
- What is the lowest cost network of suppliers, factories, warehouses and transport links?
- What levels of inventory are required at each stock point?
- Should operations be in house or contracted out?
- What are the best logistics arrangements?
- What is the best design for information flow in the chain?

The answers to the above questions will lead to the design of value adding generic activities of the supply chain. It is here that pay off is considered among storing, moving and processing. One supply chain may decide to have strong de coupling points while other may move to flexible transforming processes and movement, thereby eliminating storing. **Ultimately, the best configuration of chain will vary from individual chain to chain, therefore the importance of concept of competing is between chains and not between individual businesses.**

Architecture of SCM

Architecture of SCM is built on three elements viz. Technology, System and Relationships. Technology enhances process, Systems link events and processes, Relationships bring alive the chain with a commonality of purpose through mutuality and truest. The above three elements must be integrated and lie at the base of an effective supply chain for achieving desired results. The way to use this framework is to identify all existing, philosophies, concepts and techniques in the grid of activities v/s desired value. The Framework is diagrammatically shown in Figure 24.3.

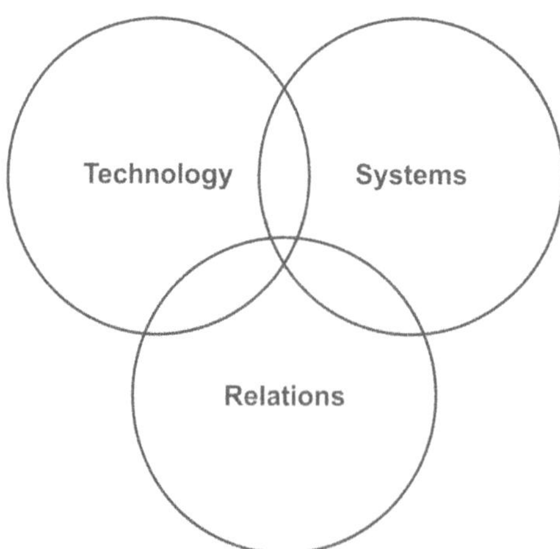

Figure 24.3 Architecture of SCM

SUPPLY CHAIN INTEGRATION

New concept of integrated management of the supply chain was a breakthrough but the practice of integrated management depended on bringing together all the earlier philosophies and techniques, and linking them. There has been a richness of continuous improvement philosophies given the widely prevalent view that future of businesses depends on the pursuit of such philosophies, practices and techniques. These, however, have addressed only parts of the supply chain and integration is attempted by just joining them together. The disadvantage of this approach is that interface raises its own problems. Most firms have not appreciated the advantage of coordinating various decisions and plans across different entities in the chain. Suppliers are optimizing locally. Plants are optimizing locally and so are the distribution channels doing. As a result, inventories remain high with working capital being tied up to for longer periods of time. Thus there are delays in delivery and overall cost across the chain remains high. Also, in some cases, a myopic view prevails that some given technique is suitable only for one given function, e.g., **Single Minute Exchange of Die (SMED)** is suitable only on the shop floor. There is a need for a framework which moves away from functional integration to generic activity integration. The framework should also highlight how each of the new techniques and philosophies, contributes to basic business objectives.

SCM THRUST AREAS

In view of the foregoing, there are several thrust areas in SCM which need to be addressed. The important among them are

Minimizing Uncertainty

Supply uncertainty due to unreliable vendors, process uncertainty due to internal processes and demand uncertainty are major hurdles to effective SCM. Supplier uncertainty can be addressed through a number of initiatives such as vendor development and certification, sharing of production planning information and joint attention to transport arrangements. Process uncertainty is due to machine breakdowns, uncertain yields and employees' absenteeism, which can be addressed through good maintenance practices, better technology, etc. Demand uncertainty can be reduced to some extent by forecasting techniques and by better communication with customers.

Reducing Lead Times

Lead times at the stages of procurement, conversion and distribution can be cut down by utilizing faster modes of transport, better planning practices use of information technology and process technologies.

Minimizing the Number of Stages

The number of stages that goods and services flow though adds to the complexity of SCM. Unification of tasks and reducing the number of stages make the coordination of decisions easier. This is also the essence of Business Process Reengineering.

Improving Flexibility

Reducing set up or changeover times in various processes and use of flexible manufacturing and assembly techniques improves flexibility of response. Use of smaller transport vehicles provides flexibility in making dispatches at short notice without being constrained by batching economies.

Improving Process Quality

Doing things right at the first time is ideal for improving process quality. The techniques for this include statistical process control, root cause analysis of poor quality and improvement of process capability.

Minimizing Variety

Variety is one of the major causes for excessive inventory in the downstream part of supply chains. One response is to modularize product designs so that variety is offered in a controlled way and some economies of scale can be exploited. Another is to standardize product and service offerings.

Managing Demand

Uncertainty and anticipated variations in demand should be dealt with by appropriate promotion and branding. This will enable a better control of the supply chain, right from demand generation.

Delaying Differentiation

Value addition through product differentiation should be postponed as far as possible, so that precise customer needs can be met without holding committed stocks in the entire chain. This can be achieved by shipping of component level goods to major points and assembling according to customer needs, postponing finishing operations like grinding and mixing of additives till near the final point of consumption, e.g. Mixing paints at retail outlets.

Kitting of Supplies

In assembly systems, a major source of delay is the staging delay where some components for assembly have to wait since matching components are not available. Vendors or internal facilities that supply components can be arranged so that all components required for an assembly are supplied to one stage where they are kitted into sets of matching components, ready for assembly and further operations. This involves restructuring of vendors or internal activities and some vertical integration.

Focusing on 'A' category

This is a well known theory of Pareto's principle or 20/80 formula. The concept of **Vilfredo Pareto** was made use if in mid 1950 in inventory management based on consumption value. This concept is applied in different areas of management such as quality control, customer's relationship management, territories that are important to accord special treatment etc.

Planning for Multiple Chains

Better SCMs require different supply chains for different customer segments based on response requirements. The tendency to club supply chain in the interest of efficiency can be counter productive for effectiveness.

Modifying Performance Measures

Multi actor performance measures focused on the supply chain are superior to single actor ones. In the context of a warehouse, retrieval time would be more in tune with SCM instead of warehouse space utilization as the primary measure of warehouse performance, since this focuses on both the warehouse and the downstream actor. Similarly, a transporter like the railways could focus more on time taken for delivering a wagon/rake to a customer from the time indent is placed, rather than wagon utilization/turnaround.

Competing on Service

Service aspects of value delivery to customers are big opportunity.

Moving from Functions to Processes

Job rotation, flatter and leaner organizations rather than functional organizations help improve supply chain practices through integrated process orientation.

Initiatives at an Industry Level

Industry level (rather than firm level) initiatives in specific product categories can focus on poor infrastructure e.g. transport and/or warehousing inadequacies and help develop appropriate service providers. There is opportunity for third party logistics services here.

SUPPLY CHAIN STRATEGY

Several principles have to be dovetailed into supply chain strategy. These include segmenting customer based on service needs, customizing the logistics network to service requirements, listening to customers, managing sources of supply strategically to reduce total cost of owning materials and service, developing a supply chain wide technology that supports multiple levels of decisions making, and adopting channel spanning performance measures to gauge success in reaching the end user effectively and efficiency.

There are three basic steps to achieving this strategic fit viz.

1. First step is to understand customers by mapping where their demand is located on the implied uncertainty spectrum.
2. Second step is to understand the supply chain and map it on responsiveness spectrum.
3. Final step is to match supply chain responsiveness with the implied demand uncertainty in the zone of strategic fit.

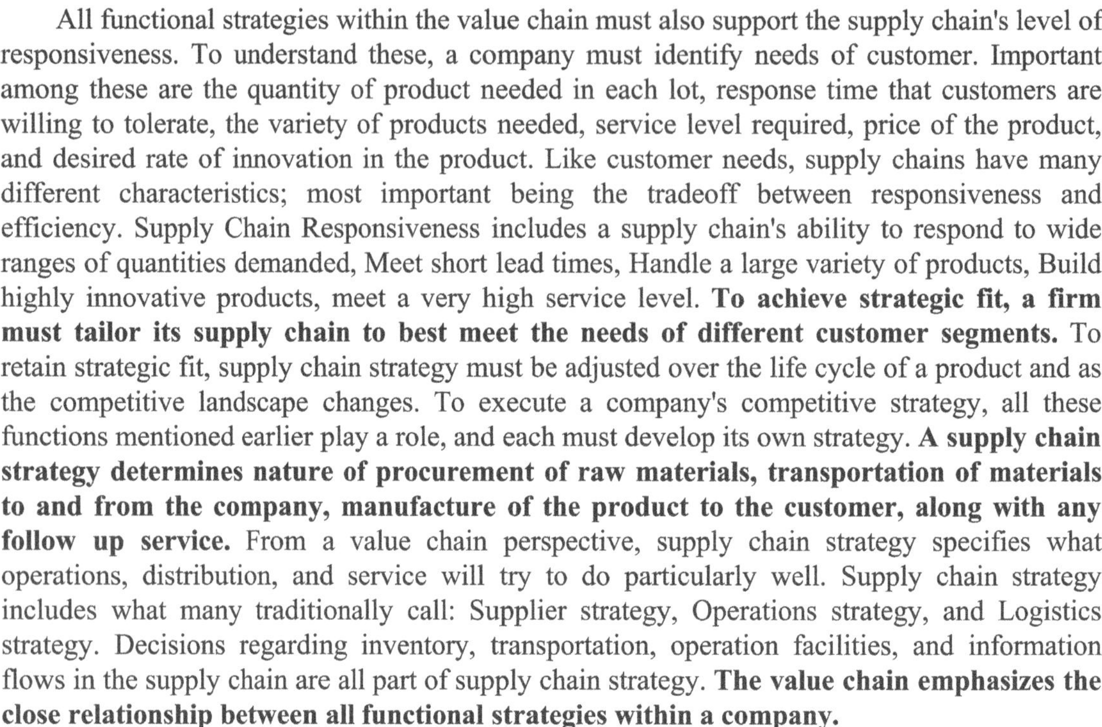

All functional strategies within the value chain must also support the supply chain's level of responsiveness. To understand these, a company must identify needs of customer. Important among these are the quantity of product needed in each lot, response time that customers are willing to tolerate, the variety of products needed, service level required, price of the product, and desired rate of innovation in the product. Like customer needs, supply chains have many different characteristics; most important being the tradeoff between responsiveness and efficiency. Supply Chain Responsiveness includes a supply chain's ability to respond to wide ranges of quantities demanded, Meet short lead times, Handle a large variety of products, Build highly innovative products, meet a very high service level. **To achieve strategic fit, a firm must tailor its supply chain to best meet the needs of different customer segments.** To retain strategic fit, supply chain strategy must be adjusted over the life cycle of a product and as the competitive landscape changes. To execute a company's competitive strategy, all these functions mentioned earlier play a role, and each must develop its own strategy. **A supply chain strategy determines nature of procurement of raw materials, transportation of materials to and from the company, manufacture of the product to the customer, along with any follow up service.** From a value chain perspective, supply chain strategy specifies what operations, distribution, and service will try to do particularly well. Supply chain strategy includes what many traditionally call: Supplier strategy, Operations strategy, and Logistics strategy. Decisions regarding inventory, transportation, operation facilities, and information flows in the supply chain are all part of supply chain strategy. **The value chain emphasizes the close relationship between all functional strategies within a company.**

EFFICIENT VS RESPONSIVE SUPPLY CHAIN

Table 24.1 Comparison between Efficient and Responsive Supply Chains

Objective and strategies	Efficient supply chains	Responsive supply chains
Primary goal	Meet the demand at the lowest possible cost	Demand to be met quickly
Product design strategy	Maximize performance at a minimum product cost	Create modularity to allow postponement of product differentiation adopt modularity concept
Pricing strategy	Lower profit margins because price is a prime consideration for customer	Higher margins, as price is not a prime consideration for customer
Manufacturing strategy	Optimum utilization of men and machinery to lower the costs	Maintain capacity flexibility to meet unexpected demand
Inventory strategy	Reduce levels of inventory to lower costs	Buffer inventory to be maintained to meet unexpected demand
Lead time strategy	Reduce but not at the expense of costs	Aggressively reduce even if the costs are significant
Supplier strategy	Vendor selection is made based on cost and quality	Select based on speed, flexibility, and quality
Transportation strategy	Greater reliance on low cost transport	Greater reliance on responsive transport

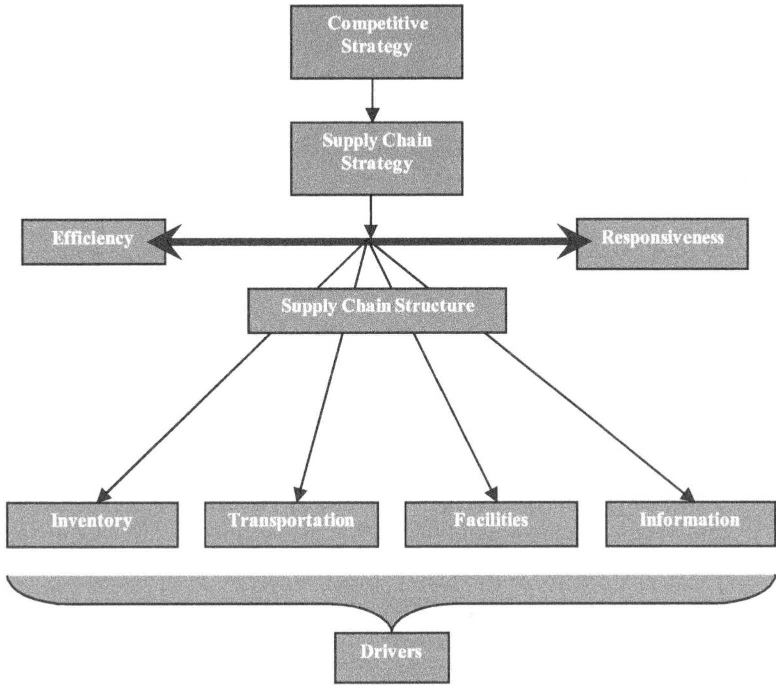

Figure 24.4 Supply Chain Decision Making Framework

The objective of supply chain is to strike a balance between two conflicting interests' viz. responsiveness and efficiency for achieving a strategic fit in the competitive strategy. Table 24.1 highlights the major differences between efficient and responsive supply chain. To reach this objective a company uses four supply chain drivers viz. inventory, transportation, facilities and information. The combined effect of the four drivers' Figure 24.4 determines the responsiveness and efficiency of Supply chain. A company will need a supply chain which is efficient as well as responsive.

ROLE OF MATERIAL MANAGERS IN SCM

The supply chain metaphor signifies connectivity and interdependence. From a conceptual viewpoint, it is difficult to determine which link in the chain is more important than the other. In human anatomy every organ in the body is important, however one or some of them e.g., heart and brain are considered as the more vital organs. Similarly, certain functions play a decisive role in the success of essential component. The MM professionals therefore have to play a crucial role in linking the supplier and the manufacturer while maintaining good relationships. MM professionals should not be content with mere vendor development and vendor relationships but extend it to customers as well. MM personnel should graduate from inventory management to integrated supply chain management. This calls for change in mindset, new attitudes and acquisition of polyvalent skills. **Receptivity to new ideas, multidisciplinary skills and teamwork become essential requirements. Purchasing professionals,** materials managers and other connected functionaries should be given exposure to a variety of jobs at the horizontal level through job rotation. Good knowledge of computers and E-commerce will enable the team to work cohesively and efficiently but will not substitute for business and customer knowledge. Some of the important key result areas where focus is needed are to minimize uncertainty, reduce lead time, improve flexibility and process quality, shorten links in the chain, setting up multiple supply chains and competing on service. Moving from functions to processes, setting new performance measures and above all taking initiatives at industry level is required. India has excellent individual professional managers. What is needed is to make management professional and excellent teamwork must be the new work ethic. Need of the hour is to quickly create greater awareness and facilities for training our managers to visualize opportunities and confidently handle the issues relating to e-commerce. Training workshops can bring about increased awareness of integrated logistical management of both material and information flows. Increased use of supply chain management in government requires both material and information flows. Inculcation of a strong customer service ethic and work culture is a prime requisite. We can and should bring about a seamless transition through appropriate restructuring of functions both in the government and industry with an integrated systems perspective.

SCM AND INFORMATION TECHNOLOGY

Shareholders want managements to take pro active action to beat the growing competition. They seek value addition, high returns as well as creation of long term shareholder value. Chief executives are hard pressed to optimize sales growth, reduce costs, secure better working capital management and improve overall performance, productivity and profitability. Production should not rely solely on sales forecasts, but instead, be synchronized closely with customer orders. It is here that Information Technology (I.T) can play a significant role by giving an edge to logistics and link individual parts with the whole chain. IT can provide competitive advantage by reducing costs and harness external drivers of change through better information sharing, connectivity and speedier communications.

SCM FUTURE TRENDS

Today is confined but tomorrow can be defined. To chart and mould our future we have to gauge, engage and manage change. Wisdom dictates that this should be done with clear sight, insight and foresight (M. Gopala Krishna). Future trends are becoming visible and we need to reckon them. The secular shift in power from the supplier to customer is clearly visible. Hitherto, the point of purchase was the mart or the shop. Today, the point of purchase is moving from the shop to the home. The ubiquitous personal computer bids to become both virtual one stop shop and a factual one click stop. Competition will spur chain innovation to seek wider global sources and markets. Sourcing will be at lowest global cost, while widespread outsourcing will create many internal supply chains. Agility, flexibility and responsiveness will be determinants of success in the market place since time

 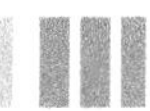

will have a premium. Environmental considerations will require "recycling" supply chains where customers return used materials for recycling. Customer relationship management all along the supply chain will become an imperative.

SUPPLY CHAIN IN HEALTHCARE BUSINESS

In healthcare business, a supply chain needs to be designed with respect to the strategy and nature of business. Across hospitals, the strategy is consistently to maximize patient care. **Hospital supply chain enables this by:**

- Ensuring product availability
- Minimizing storage space
- Reduce material handling time and costs for all medical staff (nurses, pharmacists, doctors)
- Minimizing non liquid assets (inventory)
- Maximizing patient care space

Hospitals have complex supply chains. Their product lines consist of high cost and low cost items as well as perishable and durable goods that are consumed in large and small volumes. There are highly critical as well as non critical items. Hospital supply chains handle products with all combinations of these various traits (i.e. highly critical, low volume, high cost, perishable goods). Size, geographic location, diversification, and various specializations all affect the nature of hospital business, and, hence, the requirements of its supply chain. Each ward within a hospital is unique. The number of products and demand of those products varies greatly from department to department such as Cardiac Cath Lab to Nephrology to Intensive Care Unit etc. Optimal supply chain in one ward of a particular hospital is not necessarily the best recommendation for any other ward in that hospital or any other hospital. Nor should the supply chain policy for a particular product within a ward be identical to that of other products in the same ward. Hence need for differentiating the supply chain policies within a hospital. The supply chain policy developed for a particular product should reflect the nature of that product. Differing products should have different policies. A hospital should develop its supply chain for a specific product based on that product's unit cost, demand, variability, physical size, and criticality. A hospital requires more than one supply chain policy in order to meet its strategy of maximizing patient care without incurring prohibitive costs.

DIFFERENTIATION BETWEEN MANUFACTURING AND HOSPITAL SUPPLY CHAIN

In manufacturing organizations SCM focus on movement of physical products and materials with information flow and cash flows taking a supportive role. In manufacturing organizations one can have a trade off between the cost and inventories. Supply chains are focused more towards achieving operational efficiency. In case of service organizations especially the corporate hospitals, the trade off may neither be desirable nor possible and one should ensure that the supply chains are fully responsive. The responsive supply chains must be

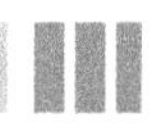

able to cope with unpredictable demands, high forecast errors and should ensure speed, timely service, delivery of customized service and volume flexibility. In order to achieve excellence in healthcare sector, the hospitals should develop and implement responsive supply chains which are crucial from the point of view of the customers as well as the hospitals. Poor supplychain performance may be the result of using wrong supply chain design such as using an efficient supply chain where a responsive chain would be needed as in the case of hospitals which need to be kept in view. In case of hospitals and healthcare SCM focus is on knowledge, information and service with associated cash flows. One needs to recognize this fact in designing and implementing SCM in hospitals and health care sectors. In designing and implementing SCM in corporate hospitals one should recognize the scope as well as the potential obstacles. Product characteristics should be used to map supply chain goals to supply chain strategies.

These involve following steps.

- More Frequent Reviews for High Value Items
- Minimize Inventory Value
- Utilize Automated Point Usage (APU) Systems
- Reduce Material Handling Time
- More Frequent Reviews for Large Items
- Evaluate Review Period Impact on Minimum Inventory
- Minimizing Storage Space
- Implement Inventory Policy
- Differentiate Service Level Based on Criticality, Demand, Demand Variability;
- Ensure Product Availability

VARIOUS FLOWS IN HOSPITAL SUPPLY CHAINS

Hospital competitive strategy defines a set of patient needs that it seeks to satisfy through its products and services. **There are three flows in a Hospital Supply chain, they are**

1. Value Flow
2. Information Flow
3. Cash Flow

Value Flow

Most obvious and visible flow in the Supply Chain is movement of goods and services largely from vendors to ultimate Customer Viz. Patient. Value chain begins with development of products and services, which create satisfaction for customers. Marketing demand forecasting

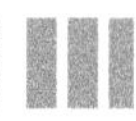

generates demand by publicizing the customer priorities that the products and services will satisfy. Marketing brings customer input back. Using new product specifications and materials flows, storage and transportation operations transform inputs to outputs to create the patient services. These are the core functions that must be performed with material, finance, accounting, information technology, and human resources support in order to facilitate the functioning of the value flow in the Supply Chain. An excellent example of value delivery network is the one that connects Apollo Group of hospitals. Figure 24.5.

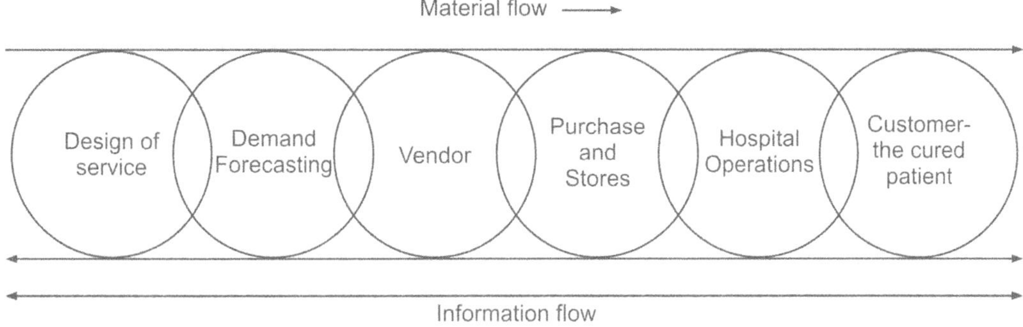

Figure 24.5 Process of Integration of Supply Chain

Information Flow

Depending on the sophistication of the data processing system and the corporate management information system (MIS), the quality and speed of the information flow varies, affecting the hospital's ability to provide fast and consistent patient services and to achieve transportation consolidations and the lowest possible inventory levels. SCM requires flow of information from one department to another, as well as referencing or accessing of several files or databases, such as creditworthiness status, inventory availability, and transportation schedules. Information system may be fully automated or manual; as on today most are fully automated. In a Supply Chain, information flow is necessary to provide management with the ability to perform a variety of tasks, including penetrating into new markets, choosing among common, contract, or private carriages, controlling inventories, determining profitability of patient services and establishing profitable customer service levels etc. Information Technology (I.T) plays a significant role by giving an edge to logistics and linking individual segments with the whole chain. It provides competitive advantage by reducing costs and harnessing external drivers of change through better information sharing and seamless connectivity. Timely and accurate information is invaluable. Information delays lengthen the order cycle. Automating and integrating the order process frees time and reduces the likelihood of information delays. Communications network is clearly a key facilitator in achieving the least total logistics cost. A typical hospital pharmacy information network is shown in Figure 24.6.

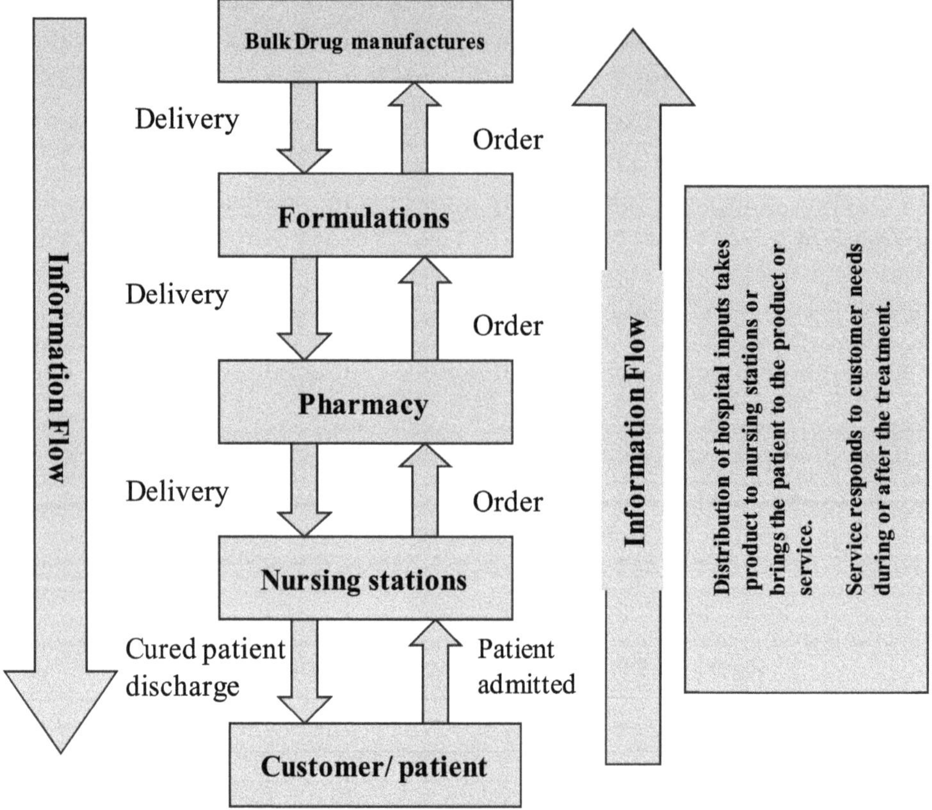

Figure 24.6 Hospital Pharmacy Information Network

Cash Flow

Cash flow is commercially significant flow in supply chain, which is largely in a direction opposite that of the major value flow of goods and services. The major part of this flow is money paid for services rendered by the hospital. However cash flow also involves some other features such as credit periods of suppliers, advances paid to vendors but still to be adjusted and credits/advances with respect to the transfer of title and/or product or service delivery in the supply chain etc. Cash flow determines how a given value flow is financed by the various parties involved in the supply chain. **Cash to cash cycle time obviously has an impact on working capital management of the hospital.** The more the cash to cash cycle time, the more will be need of working capital.

A few clinics and small nursing homes are able to manage with **negative working capital which means they get money from patients before paying their vendors.** Sometimes, they obtain 60 to 90 days credit for most of their inputs whereas they collect the money on the spot or before discharge of patient. For better supply chain management, it is necessary to view the two flows hierarchically. i.e., Value flow and cash flow. As a first step, value flow needs to be optimized and then cash flow viewed as how best to finance it. Optimal cash flow structure will be determined by the power balances between vendor, hospital and customer, the relative cost of finance and other fiscal benefits among these actors. Proper realignment of value chain means increased savings, greater access to required materials, faster patient service and this underscores the enormous value of relevant information. Supply chain management is the heart of value creation and for exploring new opportunities that add economic value.

CONTEXTUAL VIEW OF CORPORATE HOSPITALS AT APEX LEVEL

Flow of customers/patients to hospitals through different channels and also the critical functions and activities that impact the performance as well as quality of service offered depend upon the internal supply chains which are varied and vital for performance of the hospital. Performance of the supply chains may not be directly reflected in financial terms, but gets reflected in quality and timeliness of the service which have a bearing on the productivity as well as overall excellence of the organization. There is interdependence between the numerous internal supply chains which necessitates that they all work in tandem to contribute to organizational performance and excellence. Supply chains require functional and organizational integration. This assumes importance in the context of corporate hospitals. Enterprises should be prepared to undergo rigours involved in developing and implementing integrated supply chains in a progressive manner. In structured organizations, the managers normally work to optimize their own function or department. They need to follow process centric approaches and strive for organizational excellence. This transformation is essential if SCM is to be effective. SCM managers must balance the advantages of high degree of specialization and control with those of flexibility and change.

Linkage between a patient's consultation with doctors/specialist and the response of diagnostic facilities to provide timely information to Doctor/Specialist in deciding disease and treatment are of paramount importance. Logistics to move the patient from satellite hospitals to apex hospital or from patient's residence to hospital incase of emergencies is essential. Hospital SCM also must ensure availability of medicines and other requirements like IV fluids, oxygen, blood etc., in providing patient care. Admission procedures in hospitals must facilitate providing of timely treatment by ensuring that operation theaters as well as surgical facilities are available so that surgeries are not delayed or postponed.

Some other important considerations for hospital SCM are as follows.

- Ensure that emergency medical facilities like critical care units are fully geared up to meet the customer needs.
- The hospital must be fully geared up to meet or exceed the requirements of inpatients care in terms of availability of medicines, providing timely diet through catering arrangements and house keeping.
- Basic amenities must be provided to the attendants of the inpatients, who are indirect customer to hospital.

Facilities for proper and timely billing and discharge of patients must be in place.

Interdependent internal supply chains gets extended to cover external organizations like equipment suppliers, drug supplier and others to ensure that all of them are fully integrated and geared to contribute towards organizational excellence. Typical hospital supply chain is shown in Figure 24.7.

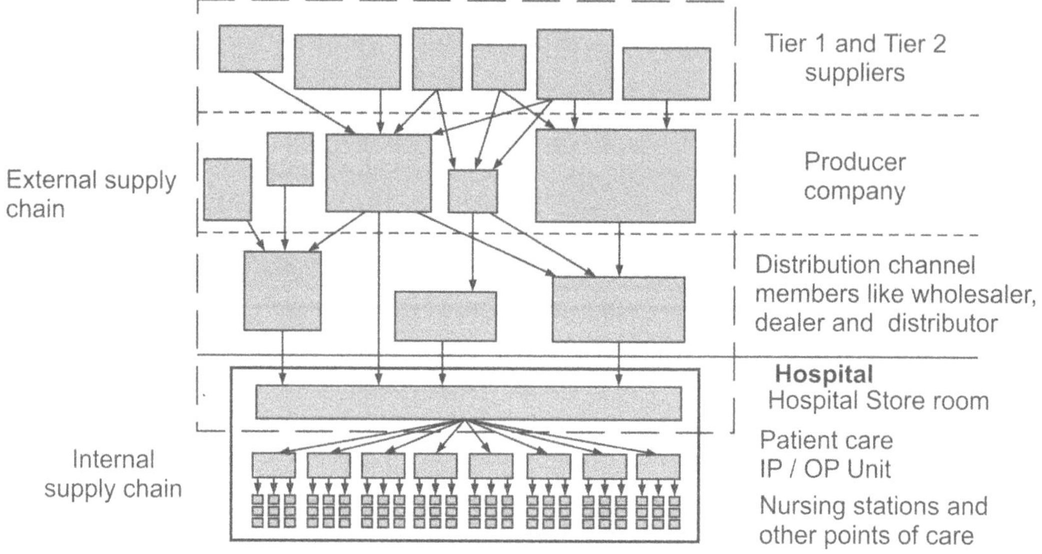

Figure 24.7 Typical Hospital Supply Chain

Many corporate hospitals have state of art equipment and facilities to provide quality and timely service to the patients. The managements of corporate hospitals must appreciate that SCM facilitates the proper up keep of the sophisticated and costly equipment by taking care of aspects like supply of consumables, spares and maintenance of equipment and facilities. It is not enough if sophisticated medical equipment is alone taken care. Even the support facilities like the computers, communication facilities, air conditioners, DG sets, Ambulance etc., need to be taken care of.

STANDARD SUPPLY CHAIN PRACTICES IN HOSPITALS

In the decade from 1985 to 1995, hospitals began implementing innovative supply chain strategies in order to reduce costs and, more importantly, improve service levels. The standard supply chain paradigms are stockless inventory, vendor managed inventory, consignment, and automated point of use systems. For clarification, this chapter will define the nature of the standard supply chain and the four emerging paradigms.

In a standard hospital supply chain, all material operations are controlled by the hospital. Material personnel include purchasers, material handlers, and stockroom personnel. Other personnel, mainly nurses, technicians, and pharmacists, also spend a considerable proportion of their time with

 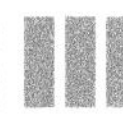

material operations. Purchasers and material handlers are typically assigned to specific wards within a hospital. Materials received from various suppliers are delivered in bulk to hospital's loading dock and transported to a main store room. Material handlers later transport those materials from main store room to various secondary store rooms located in wards throughout the hospital as the inventory in those wards diminishes. Hospitals typically do not track perpetual inventory, but rather use visual cues to decide when to place an order for more material. Various hospital employees pull inventory as deemed fit with practically no record or accountability. The standard hospital supply chain is characterized as having inflated inventories (6 - 8 weeks) and a high occurrence of stock outs (90-95percent fill rate). Medical staff generally has no incentive or time to work towards achievement of efficiency in material operations as they are much more concerned with patient care. In addition, lack of any inventory system makes it virtually impossible for the personnel to know which inventory is in excess and which is short as they have no visibility into the inventories that are scattered all over the campus.

It is estimated that inventory management accounts for anywhere between 15 to 35 percent of a hospital's total revenue. Inventory holding is defined as the cost of supplies and labor required to manage inventories and information flows. Therefore, a small reduction in inventory holding expenses can have an enormous impact on hospitals bottom line. For example, a hospital running at 5 percent profitability, with 25 percent inventory holding costs could improve profitability by 50 percent with a 10 percent reduction in its inventory costs. Hospitals can then reinvest these savings into equipment and personnel that further enhance patient care.

Some of the strategies that hospital can adopt to enhance efficiency are

- Stock less inventory
- Vendor Managed Inventory
- Consignment stocking policy
- Automated point system

Stockless Inventory

Indian healthcare industry should understand and adopt the concept of stockless inventory. In order to help hospitals reduce inventory and increase fill rates, healthcare distributors will begin to offer stockless inventory programs to their various customers. Under a stockless program, the distributor delivers product in small quantities rather than bulk. The hospital is still responsible for placing the purchase orders. Orders are transmitted from individual wards, and material is delivered directly to the respective wards, bypassing store room. Some redundant functions are removed from the supply chain as shipments are counted only once (at distributor's warehouse) as compared to the existing systems, where each shipment is counted twice (once at the distributor's warehouse and on receipt at the hospital receiving dock). In essence this system transfers to suppliers the duties of holding inventory and replenishing individual locations. Implementation

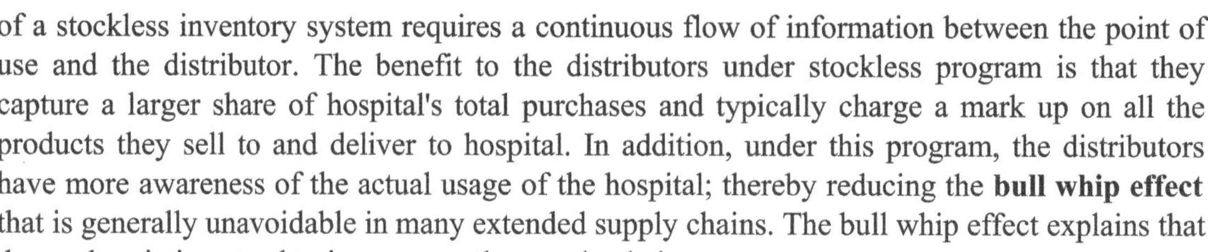

of a stockless inventory system requires a continuous flow of information between the point of use and the distributor. The benefit to the distributors under stockless program is that they capture a larger share of hospital's total purchases and typically charge a mark up on all the products they sell to and deliver to hospital. In addition, under this program, the distributors have more awareness of the actual usage of the hospital; thereby reducing the **bull whip effect** that is generally unavoidable in many extended supply chains. The bull whip effect explains that demand variations tend to increase up the supply chain.

Stockless program reduces hospital inventories, labor costs and stockouts. Some hospitals rented their stockroom space, and stockless programs allowed them to close those areas and remove those expenses. In other cases, hospitals were able to convert their store rooms into patient care units, enabling higher revenues for the hospital. Reduced expenses free up blocked investment such that the hospital can invest those amounts afresh in medical equipment and other assets. In addition, as the number of suppliers is reduced, the hospital's associated administration expenses also reduce.

Vendor Managed Inventory

Stockless inventory systems have clear benefits for hospitals with virtually no inventory control. The system reduces costs and optimizes operations within the entire supply chain channel. It removes fiscal accountability from hospital employees placing orders on the distributors. With no cost penalty, hospitals may, for example, order one piece of a particular part every day (i.e. a hairbrush) rather than consolidate to weekly shipments. However over time, many distributors increased their charges for their stockless accounts to offset these inefficiencies inherent in the system. As a result, distributors offer a service of **Vendor Managed Inventory (VMI).** Under VMI, the distributor hires employees to work in the hospital for assuming all material operation duties, including material handling, warehousing, and purchasing. The distributor not only purchases material from its own facilities, but also from manufacturers and their competitors, as directed by the medical staff. VMI stockless systems are mutually beneficial to both channel partners as they reduce costs by removing redundant functions and inventory within the channel and optimize picking, inventory control, and information processing systems. Distributors have a high incentive to focus on the supply chain efficiency. They implement inventory systems within the hospital operations and focus on optimizing order sizes and inventories. **VMI has a major impact on control of unofficial inventories also.** The Unofficial inventories has been discussed in depth in part III on Inventory management.

Consignment stocking policy

Under consignment stocking policy, vendor (i.e. distributor or manufacturer) owns the inventory until it is actually issued to the end user, termed the point of care. Consignment policies exist within supply chain strategies. The only real benefit of a consignment policy is that the hospital's inventory assets decrease and the hospital can invest the cash in other assets such as medical equipment.

Automated Point of Use Systems (APUs)

Implementation of **Automated Point of Use (APU)** systems is another improvement in hospital supply chains. These devices are placed in various wards throughout the hospital and only allow authorized users to pull inventory. Pull transactions are inputted directly on a computer or monitor or by pressing a "take" button located on the appropriate bin. APU systems keep perpetual inventory records and automatically place orders based on the established reorder and order up to points. These systems apply accountability to those using the inventory and, therefore, reduced shrinkage (i.e., wastages, pilferages etc.) and increase cost capture. **Cost capture is defined as an act of charging patients for the actual materials that were administered to them. These items can be quite effective in controlling inventory.** They are also quite costly and slow down inventory deployment, as medical staff is required to login before they can take any supplies. Therefore, it is not cost effective to place low cost, non critical items into these devices. Another benefit of APU systems is that they allow for visibility into the entire hospital's inventory. Hence, for common parts, a shortage in one ward can be mitigated with excess inventory from another ward until the next replenishment arrives. Emergency demand is a characteristic of many hospitals business model. The added visibility from APU systems increases the resiliency of the hospital supply chain under emergency demand situations. With the advent of Automated Point of Use systems, the hospital industry has become much more sophisticated in the implementation and measurement of its supply hain policies. **Data collected by APU systems can be used to automatically generate statistically appropriate inventory policies rather than the rules of thumb.** There is a wide array of products within a hospital; and therefore, there is an inherent flaw to treat them alike and measure supply chain performance at an aggregate level. Service level for critical items, such as a stent, life saving drugs etc. should be higher than that of a non critical item, such as a gauze pad or glove. Hospital part master files should be updated to go beyond the standard part number, description, unit of measure and unit price information to include attributes such as physical size, and criticality. These added attributes will enable the hospital to further meet its strategy of maximizing patient care.

OBSTACLES TO IMPLEMENT SCM

In designing and successfully implementing supply chain management in corporate hospital one should keep in view barriers imposed by cultural factors, organizational designs, suppliers, inadequate resources, skills and knowledge, and constraints of project management. Necessary steps need to be initiated to overcome these barriers, so that the SCM can contribute to hospital performance. Opening up of economies have subjected national business to international companies. Most hospital finds their margins getting squeezed as they are forced to lower the margins due to competition. At the same they have to invest more resources to ensure speed and reliability. Integrated supply chain scenario today is a tug of war pulled on one side by patients and Medi claim insurance companies ever multiplying demands and on the other by hospital's strong urge to grow and run the hospital on a profitable basis with the cooperation of referral hospitals distributors, manufacturers and other hospital material suppliers.

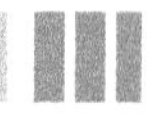

Hou L. Lee and Corey Billington identified 14 key pitfalls in supply Chain Management. If hospitals are to successfully implant SCM they need to avoid following pitfalls.

- No supply chain strategy
- Inadequate definition of customer service or patient care
- Inaccurate delivery status data
- Inefficient information systems
- Ignoring the impact of uncertainties
- Simplistic inventory stocking policies
- Discrimination against internal customers
- Poor coordination
- Incomplete analysis of shipment methods
- Incorrect assessment of inventory costs
- Organizational barriers
- Product process design without supply chain consideration
- Separation of supply chain design from operational decisions
- Incomplete supply chain strategy

SCM IS TEAMWORK

The gap between the best and average performers in healthcare industry lies in the supply chain. There is a need to develop greater capabilities characterized by deep functional excellence, ability to manage surge situations and uncertainty, develop world class IT which can leverage third and fourth party logistics services, especially for healthcare institutions which are involved in medical tourism, and effectively collaborate and coordinate extended supply chains. In short, we need to cooperate in order to operate and create a win-win situation. Only then can a hospital compete and win. Reinvention of supply chain will mean increased cost savings, greater access to customers, faster time to market and the enormous value of relevant information. **In the cyber age, cyber highways are as important as highways. Websites, E-mails and E-Commerce are the order of the day. E-commerce and IT companies create economic value when supply chains become intelligent supply chains (M. Gopala Krishna).** SCM lies at the heart of value creation for exploring new opportunities to add economic and market value. Hospitals in future will use E-commerce technologies extensively. They are working now in the direction of linking up with suppliers and service providers. E-commerce technologies can cut time and cost by cutting redundant links and intermediaries, enhance process efficiency, restructure channels, and bring about an integrated supply chain. The entire network will be on line working instantaneously, simultaneously and transparently.

SUMMARY

The challenges which organizations are facing today are vastly different from those a few years ago. Forces of globalization of economies have subjected the national businesses to international competition. Traditional business cycles are being affected by stiff competition. Time pressures and speed of change are constantly accelerating. To day, every thing in business must be faster, newer and quicker. The alignment of firms that bring products or services to market has been called the supply chain, the demand chain or the value chain. Supply chain management is the integration of all business processes from tier two suppliers to end users that provide product services and information that add value for customers. A supply chain consists of all stages involved, in fulfilling a customer request including manufacturers and suppliers, transporters, warehouses, and retailers. Supply chain management is the management of all key business processes across the various links in the supply chain. With in each organization, the supply chain includes all function such as Customer relationship management, Customer service management and Demand management etc.

SCM policies improve the hospital's service level and simultaneously reduce material management costs. Implementation of automated point of use systems enables hospitals to develop more sophisticated supply chain policies that can further increase patient care and simultaneously reduce costs. Supply chain policies should be differentiated with respect to a product's demand, variability, unit cost, physical size, and criticality. This differentiation better aligns the hospital supply chain with its strategy of maximizing patient care. Moving forward, hospitals should add attributes indicating physical size and criticality information to their product master files. This enhancement will allow hospitals to further differentiate their supply chain policies and better align supply chain implementation and measurement with the hospital's strategy of maximizing care. Unit cost, physical size, and criticality dictate the appropriate supply chain policy to be implemented. High cost, highly critical products should have very frequent review periods, tight control, and very high service level targets. Meanwhile, low cost, non critical products should have less frequent review periods, loose control, and moderate service level targets. These distinctions must be embedded into the supply chain policies and performance metrics. Supply chain should be aligned with goals of ensuring product availability, minimizing storage space, minimizing medical staff material handling time, and minimizing inventory value.

Each stage of supply chain performs different processes in accordance with its core competence and interacts with other stages of supply chain. Supply chain activities begin with a customer order and end when a satisfied customer has paid for purchase or service. The term supply chain conjures up images of products, or supply, moving from suppliers to manufacturers to distributors to customers along a chain. In the supply chain, materials and products flow downstream, funds flow upstream and information flows both ways. The Supply Chain Management is a process oriented, integrated approach to procuring, and delivering products and services to customers. SCM covers the management of material, information and funds flow. Customer satisfaction moved towards customer delight and customer surprise. Plan people and process also constitute three pillars supporting supply chain system. Supply chain encompasses over and above logistics, flow of materials and products to customers and also includes external organizations that are part of the process. Its objectives include reduced costs, improved and enhanced customer services.

A supply chain operations strategy determines the nature of procurement and transportation of materials to and from the hospital, delivery of services to patients, along with the necessary follow up services. From a value chain perspective, supply chain strategy specifies how operations, distribution, and service will contribute to the organizational objectives. Supply chain strategy includes supplier strategy, operations strategy, and logistics strategy. Decisions regarding inventory, transportation, operation facilities, and information flows in the supply chain are all important segments of supply chain strategy.

The architecture of the supply chain includes three basic elements, systems, technology, relationships. The primary objective of every supply chain is to maximize the overall value generated. The value which a supply chain generates is the difference between what the final product is worth to the customer and the effort that the entire supply chain expends in filling the customer's requests. For most supply chains, value is strongly correlated with supply chain profitability, i.e. the difference between the revenue generated from the customer and the overall costs incurred across the supply chain. Competition is between chains and not between individual businesses.

A company uses four supply chain drivers viz. inventory, transportation, facilities and information for creating a supply chain which is efficient as well as responsive. Better SCMs require different supply chains for different customer segments based on response requirements. Multi-actor performance measures focused on the supply chain are superior to single actor ones. Job rotation, flatter and leaner organizations rather than functional organizations help improve supply chain practices through integrated process orientation.

Several principles have to be dovetailed into supply chain strategy. All functional strategies within the value chain must also support the supply chain's level of responsiveness. Like customer needs, supply chains have many different characteristics; most important being the trade off between better responsiveness and efficiency. Supply Chain Responsiveness includes a supply chain's ability to respond to wide ranges of quantities demanded, Meet short lead times, Handle a large variety of products, Build highly innovative products, meet a very high service level. From a value chain perspective, supply chain strategy specifies what operations, distribution, and service will try to do particularly well. Supply chain strategy includes what many traditionally call: Supplier strategy, Operations strategy, and Logistics strategy. Decisions regarding inventory, transportation, operation facilities, and information flows in the supply chain are all part of supply chain strategy.

There are three flows in a Supply chain Value Flow, Information Flow and Cash Flow. Supply chain management is the heart of value creation and for exploring new opportunities that add economic value.

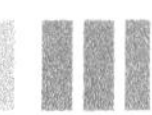

Supply chain policies should be differentiated with respect to a product's demand, variability, unit cost, physical size, and criticality. This differentiation better aligns the hospital supply chain with its strategy of maximizing patient care. This enhancement will allow hospitals to further differentiate their supply chain policies and better align supply chain implementation and measurement with the hospital's strategy of maximizing care.

Reinvention of supply chain will mean increased cost savings, greater access to customers, faster time to market and the enormous value of relevant information. E-commerce and IT companies create economic value when supply chains become intelligent supply chains.

A product's unit cost, physical size, and criticality dictate the appropriate supply chain policy to be implemented. Supply chain should be aligned with goals of ensuring product availability, minimizing storage space, minimizing medical staff material handling time, and minimizing inventory value. The supply chain metaphor signifies connectivity and interdependence. MM personnel should graduate from inventory management to integrated supply chain management. Increased use of supply chain management in government requires both material and information flows.

Hospitals have complex supply chains. Hospital supply chains handle products with all combinations of these various traits (i.e. highly critical, low volume, high cost, perishable goods). The optimal supply chain in one ward of a particular hospital is not necessarily the best recommendation for any other ward in that hospital or any other hospital. The supply chain policy developed for a particular product should reflect the nature of that product. A hospital should develop its supply chain for a specific product based on that product's unit cost, demand, variability, physical size, and criticality. A hospital requires more than one supply chain policy in order to meet its strategy of maximizing patient care without incurring prohibitive costs.

Stockless program reduces hospital inventories, labor costs and stock outs. Stockless inventory systems have clear benefits for hospitals with virtually no inventory control. The system reduces costs and optimizes operations within the entire supply chain channel. Distributors have a high incentive to focus on the supply chain efficiency. They implement inventory systems within the hospital operations and focus on optimizing order sizes and inventories. Consignment policies exist within supply chain strategies.

Implementation of Vendor Managed Inventory systems enables hospitals to develop more sophisticated supply chain policies that can further increase patient care and simultaneously reduce costs. With point of use data, hospitals can do away with antiquated methods and implement statistically appropriate inventory policies. Implementation of Automated Point of Use (APU) systems is another improvement in hospital supply chains. The added visibility from APU systems increases the resiliency of the hospital supply chain under emergency demand situations. All functions such as customer relationship management, customer service management, Demand management, flow Management, procurement product development and commercialization need to be maintained in top shape for the SCM to succeed.

REVIEW QUESTIONS

1. What do you understand by the term 'Supply Chain Management'? Explain with a flow diagram.
2. Explain relevance of SCM in healthcare industry.
3. Explain the various flows in Hospital SCM.
4. How will implementation of SCM improve patient care and profitability?
5. In healthcare scenario, how does value chain compliment Supply Chain?
6. Write short notes on
   a. Efficient and Responsive SCM
   b. Architecture of SCM
   c. Delaying differentiation
   d. Kitting Supplies
   e. Variuous flows in hospital SCM
   f. Automated point of use of system
   g. Vendor managed inventory

Information Technology (IT) Applications in Healthcare

Contents

CHAPTER - 25

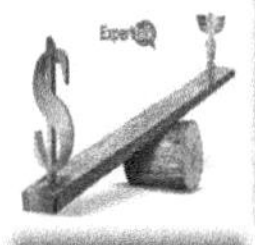
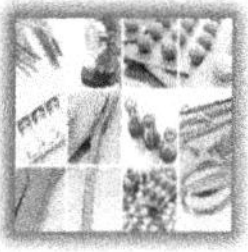
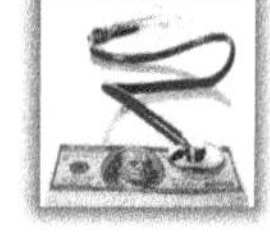
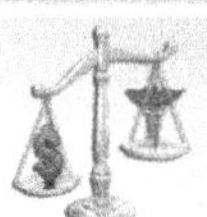

Information Technology (IT) Applications in Healthcare

INTRODUCTION

IT Systems are an integral part of the hospitals, accumulating information in chain of command control that begins with the inventory control, progresses to the material management, and ends with hospital administration. The Computer Aided Systems still require manual procedures. So the electronic data should be integrated carefully with manual information. Menus and files display variables, parameters and options that can be selected to complete a task using data. A finished computer system will provide most of the needed data. This is true whether the hospital purchases software or designs the system itself. The hospital thus should freeze what it has and add the remaining later, but only after it has received considerable return on the time and money invested.

E-HEALTH SOLUTIONS

E-Health Solutions are the most important need of the modern healthcare institutions. Clinical productivity depends on access to information, rapid, seamless data flow, and reliable data networks. Reduced complexity results in higher efficiency. E-Health Solutions provide IT infrastructure for integrated healthcare based on both clinical, networking and IT security expertise. These systems focus on Integrated Care Solutions that improve processes by featuring an electronic health record. Identity solutions enable secure access and efficient administration. This adds up to effective cooperation for healthcare providers and a better quality of patient care at reduced costs - giving relevant answers to the demands of integrated healthcare. By combining the most advanced laboratory diagnostics, imaging systems and healthcare information technology, E- Healthcare solutions enable clinicians to diagnose disease faster and more accurately, making a decisive contribution to improving the quality of healthcare. Healthcare technology offers solutions for entire supply chain under one roof - from prevention and early detection through diagnosis and on to treatment and aftercare. E-healthcare solutions range from point of care applications to automation of laboratories, producing high quality outcomes that save time, money and lives.

MATERIALS MANAGEMENT INFORMATION SYSTEMS (MMIS)

MMIS are a combination of human and computer based resources that results in the collection, storage, processing, retrieval, communication, and use of data for the purpose of cost effective

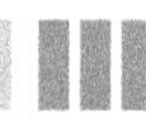

management of materials. MMIS elements must be considered in terms of both their developmental and their operational costs. Such costs must be balanced against value and use of information, and finally against its potential effect on providing cost effective care. It is necessary to collect and store all data on every transaction taking place within a hospital to allow for its retrieval in any conceivable form and to accomplish this within negligible or virtually zero time.

Data may be collected in a variety of ways from network. The choice must depend on an analysis of the value of the information and its intended use. In the area of data retrieval, there are numerous choices. It may be most economical to search the files in the archives. In other cases the data may best be retrieved through reports. At higher levels of importance, urgency, or timeliness, retrieval through on line inquiry terminals is justified.

Large healthcare institutions facilitate communication of computer provided reports, analyses, and exception messages through the use of weekly briefings for MM personnel. The most difficult aspect of effective MMIS design involves determining what data to collect; how and at what organizational or institutional level to collect it; which medium to use; what retrieval method to adopt; what analyses to perform; and which control ratios to calculate. Information cannot be generated if the supporting data are absent. Data are meaningless, and thus useless, unless interpreted, analyzed, and digested into information or operationally meaningful intelligence. At the same time, information does not exist without supporting data. These two issues deserve commensurate attention. What is needed is a way to tailor the information to the needs of the intended user in a cost effective way. In this consideration lies the framework of MMIS structure.

MMIS should be capable of supporting various studies as needed, as well as produce periodic and exception reports. Consequently, in addition to the broad question of which data to collect, which data to store, and how, there are several fundamental questions in the area of exception processing. Analysis must determine system design and processing requirements in order to provide capability to satisfy requests for any unusual analyses or reports. The difficult choices concern the borderline functions, items with a complexity of processing requirements and a low frequency of occurrence to raise the question about potential paybacks of computerization. A hospital has several choices in this regard which must be evaluated and then proper decisions should be taken.

Objectives

1. Provide cost justified and timely service
2. Obtain user input on scheduled basis
3. Develop appropriate systems
4. Develop short and long range materials plans compatible with business andstrategic plans

Characterisitics

1. Uses a common data base and avoids duplication of files

2. Consist of accurate documentation of procedures, applications, and programs
3. Permits periodic review and update
4. Ensures control of input data, accuracy, and completeness of output
5. Safeguards against intruders, fraud, etc.
6. Leaves a system audit trail.

Real Time Systems

On Line systems utilize terminals linked to the main server. Authorized personnel can call up information from the computer data base. Data is also entered through the terminals. These are Real Time Systems. Real time systems process each transaction as it occurs. Perpetual inventories in the various locations are instantaneously updated. Real time systems are the future scenario in hospital and clinic information systems. The information is entered on line into the computer and updated simultaneously. For example, open or incomplete orders will be updated based on the time the last receiving report was entered into the system. Special purpose terminals have optical mark readers, bar code printers, and printers. They are used for processing requisitions by reading optical marks and for translating marks into numbers and letters. It also can be used as a turnaround document terminal to validate the requisition or to supply additional data. A computer terminal in a department at one hospital's inventory department may share data directly with a computer at the vendor's order entry department.

Distributed Processing Systems

In Distributed Processing Systems, which are comparatively a more recent development, a major computer processing unit is linked with a smaller computer in another location, such as a warehouse. The local, smaller computer becomes an extension of the computer, the host. This system often gives the user greater control of data entry and document preparation. It relieves the host computer of some functions and reduces total operating costs. Planning functions are done at the host computer while certain operating functions are performed at local computer.

DISTRIBUTION ORIENTED VS STORAGE ORIENTED

The operations of a distribution-oriented information system emphasize the transmission of information to decision making stations throughout the organization. In contrast, the storage oriented system is more concerned with efficient storage of data, rather than its transmission to information users. A medical records library is a storage oriented information system. Retrieving information from such a system requires some effort on the part of the information user. Some health centers have already installed such systems for entering and retrieving information concerned with appointment making and with fiscal and other matters. As computer hardware and support technology becomes less expensive and more accessible, health centers will enter some if not all of their MMIS onto the interactive online mode of operation. In this way health

DATA RETRIEVAL VS DOCUMENT RETRIEVAL

Data retrieval information systems retrieve data kept in storage devices so as to manipulate data in some predefined way. Such manipulations often involve complex statistical, arithmetic, and mathematical calculations. Materials transactions data can thus be reported, arrayed according to units of physical quantities, currency or store keeping units. Averages, standard deviations and variances can be calculated, as can various control ratios such as units consumed per patient day. Similarly, reorder points and quantities can be calculated based on sophisticated mathematical relationships between usage histories, forecast of demand, lead time, cost, and other information. **Document-retrieving systems reproduce a desired document with little or no manipulation of data.** Such a system makes use of microfilm and other analog/ digital recording techniques that utilize miniaturized reproduction in order to store documents and records. Upon inquiry, such a document can be reproduced on a screen or a hard copy of the original document can be printed. These two types of systems are not mutually exclusive. It is possible to have both capabilities and the same computer configuration provided the benefits justify the costs.

CENTRALIZED VS DECENTRALIZED MMIS

Much like MM systems, the information handling and processing systems can be either centralized or decentralized. It is difficult to conceive of a centralized MMS with a decentralized MMIS. However, the reverse is sometimes possible. Thus, radiology can buy and stock its own X-ray film and report all its transactions via standardized forms to a central MMIS which in turn provides radiology and high administrative councils with reports on usage, inventories, and so on. **A centralized information system is one in which all function of the information system data gathering, processing, storage, report generation, and transmission are performed by MMIS.** All the reports and most of the forms and other documents that carry information to decision makers within the institution originate here. Similarly, all the data collecting done by the organization is done by the centralized system, where the data are then stored and used to prepare the reports required.

A decentralized information system, on the other hand, is one that involves several rather autonomous information systems serving functional departments or sub organizations within the institution. Each of these gathers its own data, produces reports as needed by the department it is serving, and stores data accordingly. Thus, in this case Oncology would keep and process its chemotherapy transactions and generate its own reports. Good decentralized management information systems have some form of centralized coordination, in order to achieve optimum institutional-level effectiveness.

Most information systems combine both manual and automated techniques in getting the work done. Institutions employing the most sophisticated computing equipment still find it necessary to buy pencils or ball point pens. Some small old fashioned hospitals or clinics still maintain information systems that are entirely manual, with all the gathering, storage, processing, and transmission of data accomplished without the use of automated devices of any kind. The degree to which an information system should be automated depends on the speed with which information must be processed, the amount of information to be processed and stored, and the value of the information to the decision maker compared with the costs of automating the system.

SCALABILITY

MMIS must be a scalable system. During the design of a system, it is important to build in maximum flexibility to anticipate future advances in equipment and methods with regard to hardware limitations. This flexibility should be limited only by the imagination and ingenuity of those participating in the system's design. The flexibility applies to basic concepts of the system, which in turn determine the programming logic. A computer programmer or system designer must not impose inflexibility which may be based on a desire to achieve simplified or conventional programming. The technical restrictions must not prevent ideas and specific needs from being designed into the system. It is possible to design and develop a system for any department but it must be tailored to the organization's needs and financial structure and the department's business objectives. Progress comes only through change. A wider range of hardware is available and this will further improve with time.

MMIS REPORTS

Periodic reports

Provided on an ongoing basis at recurring specified times throughout the year

Periodic activity reports must include the following:

1. Materials usage vs. standards report
2. Allocation of costs to user departments
3. Department year to date volume and capital invested
4. Report on turnover of items
5. Backorder and stock out report

Activity reports

To summarize activities performed over a specified time period (for example, requisitions by the department of Gynecology in the month of November).

Status reports

Snapshots taken of an entity at a particular time

(for example, inventory levels of items on Saturdays)

Exception reports

Reports to flag unusual developments threshold values are required so that situations falling above or below these performance levels are reported (for example, surgery items with actual lead times higher than the predetermined ones).

Special purpose reports

Reports resulting from special studies involving analyses of some or all of the data. To accommodate such studies the data-retrieval and information system must be flexible and responsive to most of the possible study and report types. Often these studies require ability to recall data for several years. This length of time is often necessary to determine trends or help identify usage-pattern changes. MMIS will then report timely information on the basic data categories.

Top Management Reports

E.g. Percentage of the dollar spent on supplies of physiotherapy facility with regard to the total regional Dollars spent on supplies for last year or, say, Dollar value of items used per work unit to date.

Middle Management Reports

These are produced for each facility on a departmental basis. Each facility administrator receives the report pertinent to his facility. These reports are available to top management in the form of backup or more detailed information.

Departmental Reports

These reports are generated for each department in each facility. MM in charge receives the report pertaining to his or her department. These reports are available to the facility administrator as backup.

MMIS should generate reports providing management with concise, timely, accurate, and relevant information for decision making. It should capture data to analyze the activities of the following important MMS functions:

1. Requisitioning
2. Procurement.
3. Receiving.
4. Storage.
5. Shipping.
6. Distributions to facilities.
7. Distributions within a facility.

   For the warehouse, facilities, and departments, the database should contain timely information regarding quantity on hand and location.

8. Quantity on order and location.
9. Usage

10. Expected lead time
11. Record of vendor's reliability.
12. Out of stock and/or backordered items (and items obtained from other sources).
    a. Number of stock outs.
    b. Unit prices, quantity discounts.
    c. Oversupply items.
    d. Returns to vendors (excess supplied, damages, and so on).
    e. Required cost information: Most specifically, inventory values at net prices rather than gross prices to aid in reconciliation with the general ledger. Alternatively, discounts earned should be allocated into the issue system.
    f. Actual service levels for individual items
13. Late / early deliveries by vendors.
    a. Items to be shipped to facilities.
    b. Alternative sources for urgent items.
    c. Substitutable items (identified by code).

PLANNING AN MMIS PROJECT

Before converting to or upgrading a computerized system, MM must clearly and completely define its objectives. Once this is done, the basic steps in planning, justifying, and obtaining a computer system are those in the next list. However, these steps should be modified to suit the specific environment in which the institution is working. All the steps may not be necessary, especially in a small hospital or when a minor system change is being made.

Planning an effective MMIS requires a clear definition of the basic objectives of the system and the milestones in achieving these objectives. Only a concise set of objectives can give the effort its direction. In addition, a review of the objectives and milestones provides a basis for evaluation of the success or failure. The next step is the evaluation of the means by which these objectives are fulfilled. This requires analysis of organizational structure. A determination must be made of existing patterns of information flow among various functional elements, departments, floors, and divisions. Any decentralization trends must also be studied.

The role, nature, extent of leadership, and degree of control exercised by each organizational entity must also be considered. Moreover, in introducing any new system into a healthprovider institution, recognition must be given to the credibility of the administration and the systems and procedures function from the perspectives of physicians, nurses, and other health providers. It is imperative to understand decision making processes within the institution in order to service the health providers and administration with accurate, timely, and effective MMIS.

The analyst must be sensitive to institutional plans for future growth and the means of their implementation. Effects of an expansion program in real estate buildings or in the number of beds, physicians, research, teaching, and so on should be in quantitative terms. MMIS will be required to capture and process greater volumes and at times even different kinds of data. Clearly, the effects of diversification for example, a hospital branching out into new treatment procedures or into research or teaching, or affiliating with another health maintenance organization - on the development of an MMIS are complex.

MMIS should be compatible with present organizational direction and structurally consistent with any future institutional information needs. The development of MMIS should involve administration at levels where strategic decisions are made. The plan for an MMIS cannot otherwise be realistically expected to fulfill its potential. Any effort to develop an MMIS without involving, at a strategic level, the ultimate users and managers of the MMIS is shortsighted.

Structuring the process of designing new systems and procedures for organizations uses the task force approach. Task force must include systems professionals as well as line personnel from the user departments. The design task force should include MM personnel and healthprovider personnel from the client institution, in addition to systems personnel. Moreover, task force must periodically report to committee of top institutional management, such as administrators, physicians, and nurses. These review, evaluation, and planning sessions should have as their objectives the sharing of information; planning and direction of the project; and eventually transferring project ownership from systems to user and management personnel. Such approaches tend to maximize probability of successful implementation. It is good idea to seek inputs from potential MMIS users regarding their preferences of the kind of reporting they desire. The users should be asked to convey desired content and frequency of reports.

STEPS IN PLANNING

1. **Analyze Existing System :** Evaluate existing system to identify satisfactory procedures, forms, reports, etc., as well as those that are inadequate or missing. For all unsatisfactory items, recommendations should be made concerning improvements necessary

2. **Define Purpose of MMIS :** Determine the primary problems and the desired objectives of computerization. It should be guided by the hospital objectives and policy, both overall and for MM.

3. **Project Team :** Establish a team of material and systems personnel, assisted by others such as the biomedical specialist, which will work as a group, headed by the material manager. A steering committee, consisting of higher level hospital executives, should review the work of the project team critically, approve and authorize continuing efforts. A tentative work plan should be developed that includes priorities, schedule, and work force.

4. **Preliminary system design :** Kinds of information that will be required, when it will be required, and what its unique characteristics are.

5. **Conceptual design :** A large flow chart of a generalized nature showing the inputs, reference documents, and outputs of the desired system.

6. **Justification :** Qualitative and quantitative benefits expected from the investment must include all the elements of the total system and cost benefit analysis that could be used to initially summarize the expected cost and return on the proposed system. Costs often are distributed in about three equal parts programming, equipment, and operation.

7. **The final proposal :** Project team to present the proposal to management via the task force and steering committee, stressing the advantages of the system, the time required, and the expected benefits. It is desirable to use visual aids in the presentation.

8. **System design :** It stipulates that the desired system design should expand on the conceptual flow chart and, be cost justified.

9. **System specifications :** This includes characteristics and technical details of desired system. Specifications should not be restricted to those in any particular package available, nor should they exclude desirable features because they might cost too much. Database requirements must be included.

10. **Estimated price breakdown for the vendor proposal :** Detailed costs of the subcategories such as hardware, peripheral equipment and software. A programmer should also make a cost estimate for an internal change method. Then the trade off can be studied.

11. **Requests for quotations :** (RFQ's) To be sent to hardware and software vendors, carefully describing the items required in the system for discussing proposals separately with individual suppliers.

12. **Quotation evaluation :** Use spreadsheets to list the information furnished by vendors to create a comparative matrix.

13. **Supplier selection :** Look for the least overall cost and invite the vendors with the best bids to separate meetings to discuss in depth the details of their quotations. The price on quotation is not necessarily the vendor's final price. Negotiate the final specifications, price, terms, and conditions.

14. **The schedule :** Communicate broadly plan and the rationale for it. Begin the implementation with a revised design and implementation schedule. Conduct a series of training sessions to brief MM and other personnel about the planned revisions.

15. **Install the system :** Pay attention to hardware equipment and the software programming instructions during installation. Perform necessary customizing. Remember to document the procedures in standard operating procedure manuals.

16. Debug as necessary

17. **Audit :** Check the accuracy of the original cost-benefit justification for the new system at the end of the first year of use and again at the end of three years.

MMIS DESIGN

1. Conceptual

A plan prepared by users and data processing system designers, then approved by management. It provides top level overview of the proposed system showing basic interrelationships and general procedural flow. The output of a conceptual design is: overview style flow chart and a written narrative.

2. General Design

A highly interactive description developed by the user and system designer based on approval assumptions in the conceptual design, it provides a second level of detail for each individual system, further amplifying the processing from a generalized viewpoint to assist in obtaining additional understanding. The output is a written description of each system's output reports.

3. Detailed Design

Consisting of tested and debugged programs for final user and management sign off approval, it provides a third level of detail for each system that clarifies the individual component subsystems by highlighting the essential transaction processing and their required data files. The output is: A detailed list of transactions, master files, and operating procedures.

4. Database Selection

Database is the basic collection of information. Creation of a uniform data base requires standardization of a number of elements. For the requisitioning cycle, for example, there should be ordering specifications, item descriptions, units of storekeeping, units of measurement, and commodity codes of all repetitively purchased materials and stores items Materials codification and standardization of commodity data is essential because the information is perpetuated as master files for subsequent processing in other functions.

5. Hardware Selection

Healthcare delivery institutions consider computer capability; it is generally for purposes that include MMIS needs, in addition to the information or data processing needs of functional units in the organization. Regardless of whether MM personnel are involved in the final computer-selection decisions, they should be knowledgeable in the various aspects of the selection process so that they can make intelligent contributions to the process. Various economic and technical considerations affect the choice of hardware and software systems. Costs are exclusively tangible Dollar cash flows, such as projections of payments to be made to manufacturers, software suppliers, and all those involved in the installation and continued use and the supporting facilities. This includes projections of any revenues attributable to the use of the system.

Hardware characteristics include primary memory capacity, basic instruction cycle time, and power supply. Expansion potential typically consists of factors representing either the amount of slack time in the current system, expressed on a time scale; or an indication of maximum expansion in terms of numbers of certain physical units such as printers; or add on memory. Vendor support involves programming assistance, training, and personnel loaned probably best measured on a man day scale. Maintenance and backup typically might be measured in terms of kilometers to the source, travel time, or some other measure of availability.

6. Software selection

- **Experience of software developers:** Software name, license fee, hardware required, number of terminals, query and report facility, date of first installations, number of installations, level of integration, online vs. interactive et al.
- **Specifications:** Inventory item by class codes, ABC analysis, inventory location, lead times, reorder points, safety stock, EOQ analysis, inventory status and tracking inquiry, Receiving notice, Inventory multiple storerooms, Inventory shortage report, Physical inventory, Material availability, projection, Inventory valuation, Inventory picking list, Cycle counting, Inventory adjustments, Summary of inventory activity, Item costing, Statistical measures.
- **System Elements:** Simplicity, documentation, user programs, support, standard system, training, security, stability, vendor interest, performance, processing time.
- **Overall Evaluation:** Company experience, System specifications, System elements, Total rating.

SYSTEM DOCUMENTATION

In order that all concerned will understand a set of systems and procedures in the same way, such systems and procedures must be documented. This is true both for systems and procedures in existence and for those contemplated. Such a level of understanding is necessary prior to making meaningful changes, in order to teach users as well as systems personnel, and as a means of enforcement or control. Documentation on all systems and procedures concerned with the management of materials must be maintained up-to-date.

SWITCHOVER TO COMPUTER AIDED SYSTEMS

Switchovers from manual to computer aided materials management information systems are never easy. Administrative and healthprovider personnel must be led to recognize the ultimate advantages and the short term dislocations. The strategy calls for a meaningful involvement in its process of all those who will be affected by the changeover. They must be involved all the way from the inception of the study intended to identify the optimum system for their institution, through the implementation of that system. Computers handle the paperwork while people handle the input and the materials. The manner in which the computer works is fixed. The corrections and changes required can still be made without conflicting with the computer activity.

The objectives of the changeover are to establish a perpetual inventory system that functions in an accurate and timely manner, controlling all aspects and requirements of inventory control; and produces management reports necessary for that control.

Advantages of computerized systems are:

1. Reduction of posting time.
2. Perpetual inventory calculations.
3. Easily accomplished storeroom catalog update procedures.
4. Physical inventory facilitating procedures.
5. Daily update of all records.
6. Purchase order requirement notification.
7. Notification of minimal inventory (follow up required).
8. Overstock notification.
9. Control of unserviceable inventory.
10. Centralized control for all items.
11. Timely management and/or exception reports.
12. Control of loaned and borrowed material.

INTERACTION WITH MMIS

Three methods are available to use the MMIS

1. Online inquiry, such as determining the purchase order status
2. Online entry, when it is necessary to revise the item nomenclature
3. Real time, for obtaining the latest inventory status date

The points to be covered include:

1. Menu
2. Messages
3. Security codes
4. Creation of files
5. Inquiring
6. Input data

7. Display
8. Print document

MMIS BENEFITS

- A sizable saving in inventory carrying costs
- A great reduction in paper work
- Standardization of pertinent data and terminology, with everyone using same data base
- Easier implementation of volume purchasing
- Large-scale contracts with resultant savings
- Substantial reduction in overall clerical time and time for supervision
- Centralized management without loss of utility
- Savings in equipment and floor space, principally through elimination of files
- Improved communications among all personnel in the hospital.
- Ready accessibility of data to all authorized personnel, controlled with built-in security checks
- Reduction in time required for all forms of input, retrieval, computation, and response
- Adaptability and fast response to changes in priorities, prices, and other variables of material management

SUMMARY

Computer Aided E-Health Solutions still require manual procedures, so the electronically prepared data should be integrated carefully with manual information. Materials Management Information Systems (MMIS) will provide most of the desired data. MMIS are a combination of human and computer based resources that result in the collection, storage, processing, retrieval, communication, and use of data for the purpose of cost effective management of materials. In other cases the data may best be retrieved through reports. Large healthcare institutions facilitate communication of computer provided reports, analyses, and exception messages through the use of weekly briefings for MM personnel. Information cannot be generated if the supporting data are absent. At the same time, information does not exist without supporting data. Online systems utilize terminals linked to the main server. Authorized personnel can get information from the computer database. Real time systems process each transaction as it occurs. Real time systems promise to be the wave of the future in hospital and clinic information systems. A computer terminal in a department at one hospital's inventory department can share data directly with a computer at the vendor's order entry department. In Distributed Processing Systems a major computer processing unit is linked with a smaller computer in another location, such as a warehouse. This system often gives the user greater control of data entry and document preparation. A distribution oriented

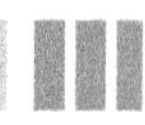

information system is one whose operations emphasize the transmission of information to decision making stations throughout the organization. The storage oriented system, on the other hand, is more concerned with efficient storage of data, as opposed to its transmission to information users. Retrieving information from such a system requires some effort on the part of the information user. Data retrieval information systems have the ability to extract data kept in storage devices and to manipulate the data in some predefined way.

Much like MM systems, the corresponding information handling and processing systems can be centralized or decentralized. A centralized information system is one in which all function of the information system are performed by the institution's MMIS. Similarly, all the data collecting done by the organization is done by the centralized system, where the data are then stored and used to prepare the reports required. A decentralized information system is one that involves several rather autonomous information systems serving functional departments or sub organizations within the institution. Each of these gathers its own data, produces reports as needed by the department it is serving, and stores data accordingly. MMIS decentralized systems still have some form of centralized coordination in order to achieve optimum institutional level effectiveness.

Most information systems combine both manual and automated techniques in getting the work done. The degree to which an information system should be automated depends on the speed with which information must be processed, the amount of information to be processed and stored, and the value of the information to the decision maker compared with the costs of automating the system. MMIS must be a scalable system.

MMIS reports on going transactions and also flag unusual developments. To accommodate such studies the data retrieval and information system must be flexible and responsive to any number of possible study and report types. Moreover, the users should be informed that the MMIS will contain timely information on the basic data categories. MMIS Reports include Top Management Reports, Middle Management Reports, and Departmental Reports

Planning an effective MMIS requires a definition of objectives of the system. It is imperative to understand fully the decision making process within the institution in order to service the health providers and administration with an accurate, timely, and effective MMIS.

Structuring the process of designing new systems and procedures for organizations typically uses the task force approach. Task force must include systems professionals as well as line personnel from user departments. An MMIS design task force should include MM personnel and health provider personnel from the client institution, in addition to systems personnel. The designing process involves conceptual design, database selection and hardware and software considerations. In order that all concerned will understand a set of systems and procedures in the same way, such systems and procedures must be documented and continuously updated.

There are ultimate advantages and short term dislocations. The implementation strategy calls for a meaningful involvement in its process of all those who will be affected by the changeover.

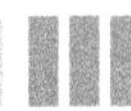

The objectives of the changeover are to establish a perpetual inventory system that functions in an accurate and timely manner, controlling all aspects and requirements of inventory control; and to produce management reports necessary for that control.

MMIS benefits include easier implementation of volume purchasing and large scale contracts with resultant savings and a substantial reduction in overall clerical time and time for supervision. Also Adaptability and fast response to changes in priorities, prices, and other variables of material management

REVIEW QUESTIONS

1. How does the information system helps Hospitals to efficiently manage inventories?
2. What are the objectives and characteristics of Hospital Material Management information systems?
3. Describe in detail different Materials Management Information system reports.
4. Planning an effective MMIS requires a clear definition, basic objectives of the system. Discuss.
5. What are the steps involved in planning the implementation of MMIS in hospitals?
6. Write short notes on
    a. Distribution oriented vs. Storage oriented MMIS
    b. Data retrieval vs. Document retrieval MMIS
    c. Centralized vs. Decentralized MMIS
    d. Types of MMIS design
    e. MMIS benefits

BIBLIOGRAPHY

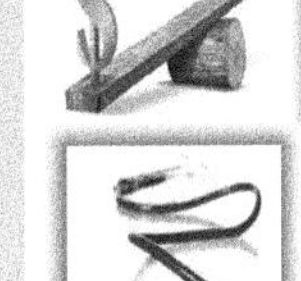
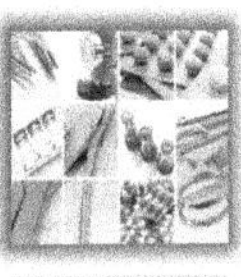
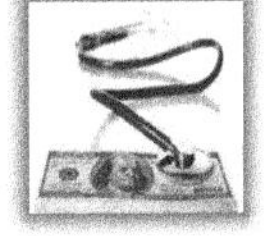
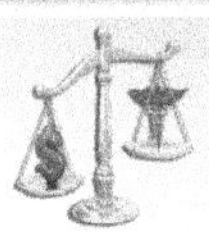

ARTICLES FROM PERIODICALS AND JOURNALS

1. Adams, Charles B. The Selection of Vendors - Management Report No.20, American Management Association, New York, 1958.
2. Amol Abhyankar. Losses from the Transformation, Materials Management Review, Jan-Feb 2000.
3. Anantapadmanabhan. Hospital Materials Management vs. Industrial Materials Management. The materials manager May-Nov 1985.
4. Anita, D.P. Materials Management in National Planning. Key note address, Indian Buyer, IIMM, Feb 1976.
5. Arabinda Tripathy. Global sourcing for competitive advantage. Materials Management Review Nov-Dec-1996.
6. Ashok K. Sharma. Purchasing marketing interface. The materials manager July-August 1988.
7. Ashok K. Sharma. Role of Materials Managers in National/International Economy. The Materials Manager, September-October 1993.
8. Balagopal S. Strategy Management An integrating tool of MM functions, The Materials Manager, 1988.
9. Bhatt H.M. Conservation of Materials Resources the need of the hour. Indian Buyer, July 1980.
10. Bhattacharya S C. Journey to World Class Materials Management, The Materials Manager, Jan-Feb-1999.
11. Bush, G.E. A New Twist on Supplier Evaluation Purchasing LV. No.5, 1963.
12. Capoor ML. Expectation from materials managers in 2000 AD. The Materials Manager May-June 1996.
13. Carl Heycl. The Encyclopedia of Management, Van Nerste and Reinhold Company, New York, 1973.
14. Chalapathi Rao G.V. Is audit impediment to Materials Management, Indian Buyer, April 1976.
15. Chalapathi Rao, G.V. Purchase Research. The Materials Manager, July 1987.
16. Chitra Iyer. Virtual Procurement very 'real' Benefits, Materials Management Review, May-June 2000.

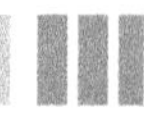

17. Coates, Joseph, F. In Defence of Delphi - A Review of Delhphi Assessment, by H.Sackman, Technological Forecasting and Social Change Vol.7.
18. Dag Ericsson. The strategic role of the purchasing function in a changing environment, The Materials Manager, 1984.
19. Dr. Hans F.Busch. Integrated Materials Management, The Materials Manager, March-April 1989.
20. Drucker, P.F. Practice of Management, Pan Books.
21. Eline M Whittington. Sub-contract Management Manual Lockhead, Missiles and Space Company, Inc., 1984.
22. Geist K.R. What other departments expect of purchasing - Purchasing, 1960.
23. Gopal Iyengar. Research Notes: Value/Cost ratio in the supply chain, Materials Management Review, Jan-Feb 2000.
24. Gopala Krishna M. Experts from keynote address on "Supply Chain Management in Cyber age", National Convention of Indian Institute of Materials Management (NATCOM XXII), Nov 1999.
25. Gopala Krishnan Nair K. Preventive repair - A new technique in spare parts management. The materials manager June-July 1987.
26. Gopala Krishnan Nair. Kanban and Just in Time Relevance to Indian Industry. The Materials Manager Nov-Dec 1988.
27. Gopala Krishnan P. Materials conservation in hospital administration, Indian Buyer May 1980.
28. Gurnani V G. Cost Reduction in Materials Management, Indian Buyer, IIMM, Dec 1975 to Jan 1976.
29. Hafer R.A. and Umhaner H.J., Vendor Rating: Get Quality you are paying for "Purchasing, XIVIII, No.4, 1960.
30. Hariharan T.V. Materials Management then and now, Materials Management Review, Jan- Feb 2002.
31. Hariprasad Rao K., Chandrashekar T S. Changing Role of Materials Manager, Materials Management Review, Jan-Feb 2000.
32. Harlod E Fearson and John Hoagland H Purchasing. Research in American Industry, AMA Research Study, 1983.
33. Heizer J.H. Effective and ineffective actions of Purchasing Managers, Journal of Purchasing, 1971.
34. Inbound Logistics, Thomas Publishing Co. Inc. Vol.4 No.2, New York.
35. Iyer V H. and Khetrapal. Cost reduction through MM in the farm sector in Nashik and nagar districts, Materials Management Review, Jul-Aug-2001.

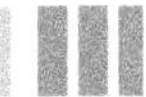

36. Jeanette Chung and Others. A frame work for measuring Healthcare Efficiency and Value, American Medical Association, August 2008.

37. John Hughes, Mark Ralf, Bill Micheles. Transform your supply chain public buying, Materials Management Review, Jul-Aug 2001.

38. John S Dawson. Materials Management in the future, The Materials Manager, Dec 1986-Jan 1987.

39. Krishna Kumar. The New Corporate Horizon, Materials Management Review, April 2000.

40. Lal L. Materials Management New perspective on tomorrow, The Materials Manager, Sept-1982.

41. Lal L. Strategy for achieving Management Excellence, Indian Buyer, June 1976.

42. Levitt, Theodore Industrial Purchasing Behaviour. A study of Communication Effects, Boston, Harvard University, 1965.

43. Madhavan S. Materials Management and its role in Corporate Management, Indian Buyer, Dec 1975-Jan 1976.

44. Madho Narain, Purchasing in India and its challenges, The Materials Manager, Sep-Oct 1991.

45. Madho Narain. Role of Materials Management in Inflatory environment. The Materials Manager, March 1983.

46. Mahendra S., Gupta, Pushkar Bhobe. Transformation of purchasing and supply chain management in next millennium- The Materials Manager, Nov-Dec 1998.

47. Malhotra B B. Simulating reduces cost, Indian Buyer, Dec 1975/ Jan 1976.

48. Manish Naik, Cost Effective Supply Chain, Materials Management Review, May-June 2000.

49. Martino Joseph P. Log Normality of Delphi Estimates - Technological Forecasting Vol.I, 1970.

50. Matthai John & Bijosh Koshy, Marketing the Purchase function, The Materials Manager, Jan-Feb 1991.

51. Measuring Purchasing Performance, Purchasing, L No.10, 1961.

52. Menon K.S. and Ashok Sharma. Inventories in the Public Sector, The Materials Manager, July-Aug 1989.

53. Menon K.S. Sharpening your negotiating skills. The Materials Manager, March-April 1988.

54. Minocha A S. Incidence and affects of statutory duties and other Taxes on Materials Cost, Indian Buyer, April 1976.

55. Mukesh Saxena. WTO ministerial conference at Doha, Emerging Issues for Materials Managers, Jan-Feb 2002.

56. Mukherjee S K. Materials Management towards next millennium, The Materials Management Review, Sep-Oct 1999.
57. Newman R.G. & J.Scordro. Price Analysis for negotiations - Journal of purchasing and Materials Management, Spring, 1988.
58. Ojha KK. Materials Management through bench marking, TMM Nov-Dec-1988.
59. Overview on performance of Public Sector Enterprises, Dept. of Public Enterprises, Govt. of India, 1999-2000.
60. Palepu Gour. Working Capital Management in relation to Inventories, Indian Buyer, August 1978.
61. Parimala Devi, Cost consciousness in engineering Industry, Materials Management Review, Mar-Apr-2001.
62. Peter F. Drucker. The Economy's Dark Continent, Fortune magazine, 1962.
63. Prasad K. Should the production bypass Purchasing Chief, Indian Buyer Dec 1975-Jan 1976.
64. Pritibusan Sinha. Materials Management in Hospitals, The Materials Manager, July-Aug 1998.
65. Prof.Joe Ezekiel. Commitment to professional integrity and Ethics in purchasing and Materials Management. The Materials Manager, Dec 1985-Jan 1986.
66. Prof.Joe Ezekiel. Problems of Materials Management in developing nations, The Materials Manager, Dec 1986.
67. Prof.Joe Eziekel. Conservation of Material Resources - The energy angle, Indian Buyer, March 1980.
68. Puri I.C. Role of Materials Management in Ancillary Development, Indian Buyer, March 1978.
69. Ram Niwas Mirdha. The Challenge of Public Buying, Indian Buyer, November 1976.
70. Rama Krishnan R V. Strategic Sourcing and Supplier Partnership for Competitive Advantage, The Materials Manager Jan-Feb 2000.
71. Rama Krishnan R.V. Kaizen - The key to Japan's competitive success, The Materials Manager, Materials Management Review, May-June 1988.
72. Rama Swamy. Changing Perspective of Materials Management, The Materials manager Jan-Feb 1992.
73. Rao D S. Project stage-Standardization and Variety Reduction through design, Indian Buyer, December 1976.
74. Ravindra Kumar. Effective Materials Management. The Materials Manager. September 1984.
75. Ravindra Shinde and Viswadeep Bose. Purchasing measurements to the size of the spend or something else, The Materials Manager, Mar-Apr-1998.

76. Roy Chowdhury. A New Approach to Purchasing Management Product Price Pre-Calculation, Indian Buyer, March 1976.

77. Samar Roy Chowdhury & Hari Kumar G. MM in Biotechnology R & D, Nov-Dec 2002.

78. Sapre P.N. Economic growth and Resources Development - The Materials Manager, Jan 1982.

79. Sardalia K S. Internet and its application in Materials Management, Materials Management Review, Sep-Oct-1999.

80. Sarika Kulkarni. Stockless Purchasing A cost Saving Device - The Materials Manager May June 1995.

81. Sathe A V, Brijesh Garg, Das P K, Rao N. Life Cycle Costing, Materials Management Review, May-June 2000.

82. Satyendra Pal, Nagesh. Transformation of Purchasing Management in the next Millennium, The Materials Manager, Sep-Oct 1999.

83. Seshadri S. Management by objectives and results in Materials Management, Indian Buyer, Dec 1975-Jan 76.

84. Shillingham, Gordon and Birton, John C. Materials Management and the Profit Centre Concept, AMA Management Bulletin 44, 1964.

85. Shivaji Basu and Somashekara H, Managing Procurement and Supply in a Global Knowledge Economy, Materials Management Review, Sep-Oct 2000.

86. Siladitya Ghosh. Materials Management Vision-2001, The Materials Manager, May-June 1996.

87. Spare Parts Management - Seminar Proceedings New Delhi Oct. 1977, National productivity Council, New Delhi, 1980.

88. Srinivasamoorthy. Good Practices in Procurement, Materials Management Review, Jan-Feb 2000.

89. Studies in Business Policy, National Industrial Conference Board Inc.

90. Subrahmanyam C. INCOTERMS-The changes from 1999 to 2000, Materials Management Review, Jan- Feb 2000.

91. Sundar N. Longterm approach to outsourcing, Materials Management Review, Sep 2000.

92. Sundar. The critical link in the Supply Chain Vendor, Materials Management Review, Mar-Apr 2001.

93. Sunder Ram S. External Tariffs - Their effect on International Purchasing, Indian Buyer, Feb 1980.

94. Surendra Deodhar. Savings, What is it all about Materials Management, Materials Management Review, Nov-Dec 2001.

95. Sushmita Chanda, Amit Mukherjee. Transportation of Purchasing and supply chain management in the next millennium, The Materials Management, Mar-Apr, 99.

96. Tom Orr, P.E. A value Analysis approach to Healthcare Revenue Improvement Atlanta GA.

97. Tony Trupiano and Others, The Benefits of a Successful Value Analysis Programme, WellStar Health System.

98. Vardan M S S. E-Commerce for effective Supply Chain Management, Material management review, Jan-Feb 2001.

99. Vardan M.S.S. Information Technology. Key to better Materials Management, The Materials Manager, May June 1994.

100. Venkata Rangan B K. Emergency reduction of Inventory, Indian Buyer, June 1976.

101. Venkat Reddy V and Kuldip Rai. Emerging Paradigms in Supply Chain Management, Materials Management Review 2007.

102. Venkat Reddy V and Kuldip Rai. Supply Chain Implementation-An Optical Network in the Intranet, Materials Management Review 2000.

103. Venkat Reddy V. Electronic Data Interchange, Materials Management Review, Jan-Feb 1999.

104. Venkata Rangan B K. An integrated Approach to Materials Management-Need of the Hour, Indian Buyer, March 1976.

105. Venkat Reddy V. How a materials Manager can become a Member of the board, Indian Buyer, April 1976.

106. Venkatesh (Lt Col) SM. How to cut Material Cost, Indian Buyer Jan 1980.

107. Vittal M.S. Cost Reduction in Materials Management, The Materials Manager, 1991.

108. Williams W H. The Purchasing Man: Manager-Business Man-Citizen, Indian Buyer, April, 1976.

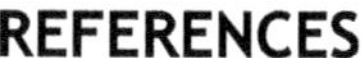

REFERENCES

1. Agarwal C B. Store keeping, Forward Book Depot, New Delhi, 1985.
2. Ahuja K K. Materials Management, CBS Publishers and Distributors.
3. Alan R.Raedels. Value focused supply chain management - Getting cost out of the supply function Vol.III the NAPM Professional Development Services. IRWIN Professional purchasing, Chicago, 1995.
4. Albert Raymond and Associates. Controlling Production and Inventory Costs, Printice Hall Inc., Englewood Cliffs, New Jersey, 1978.
5. Alijian, George W. Purchasing Handbook - 3rd Edition, Mc Graw Hill Book Co., New York, 1983.
6. Alivin J Williams and Kohelene Dukes. Purchasing handbook, Mc Graw Hills Inc., 1993.
7. Ammer D.S. Material Management and Pharmacist. Hospital purchasing management 1978.
8. Anne Osborne Kilpatrick, James A. Johnson. Handbook of Health Administration Policy, Markel Dekker Inc. 1999.
9. Anyon, Jay, G. Managing an Integrated Purchasing Process, Holt, Rinchart & Winston, Inc., New York, 1963.
10. Arnold Reisman. Materials Management for Healthcare Services Lexington Books, 1981.
11. Aswathappa K and Sridhara Bhat. Production and Operations Management, Himalaya Publishing House, Mumbai, 2000.
12. Baily P J H. Purchasing and Supply Management, London Chapman and Hall, 1973.
13. Ballot Robert B. Materials Management A Result Approach, American Management Association Inc., 1971.
14. Bharadwaj M.K. and Jain V.K. Glossary of Purchasing and Supply Chain Management, Excel Publications, 2007.
15. Bhattacharjee C. Services Marketing concepts, planning and implementation, Excel Books, New Delhi, 2006.
16. Bhattacharya S C. Modern Materials Management, Jhanan Bhattacharya, Calcutta, 1997.
17. Bhuyan, Ankush. Development of Computer - Added vendor rating system using Delphi techniques, Unpublished MS Thesis, IIT, Madras, 1976.
18. Brown, Robert G. Statistical Forecasting for Inventory Control, Mc Graw Hill, 1959.
19. Bruce L Fryman. Contribution of the Purchasing function in achieving corporate goals, The Materials Manager, 1984.
20. Burton E Lipman. How to Control and Reduce Inventory, D B Taraporvala Sons and Co Pvt Ltd, Bombay 1981.

21. Burton J.A. Effective Warehousing, The English language book society.
22. Carson F. Dye, Executive excellence, protocols for Healthcare Leaders, second edition, prentice-Hall of India Pvt. Ltd, New Delhi, 2007.
23. Chandra Bose D. Inventory Management, Prentice Hall of India Pvt. Ltd., New Delhi, 2006.
24. Charles E. Housely. Controlling Hospital Supply Inventories, Aspen publications. 1983.
25. Charles E. Housley. Hospital Materiel Management, An Aspen publication 1978.
26. Chhibber O N, Warehousing in India, Central Warehousing Corporation of India, New Delhi.
27. Christopher E Bogan and Michael J English. Benchmarking for best practices, winning through innovative adaptation, Mc Graw Hill Inc. New York, 1994.
28. Colton R. Industrial Purchasing, Columbus, Charles Meril Ohio, 1972.
29. Compton H K. Storehouse and Stockyard Management, Pitman Publishing, London.
30. Compton H K. Supplies and Materials Management, Business Book London, 1972.
31. Cynthia Hayward. Healthcare Facility Planning, PHI learning Pvt.Ltd. New Delhi, 2008.
32. Daleler S and Mansoor Ali. Industrial Engineering and Management Systems, Standard Publishers and Distributors, New Delhi, 1995.
33. Daniel Hunt V. Re-engineering the power of integrated product development, Oliver Wright Publication Inc., Essex Junction 1991.
34. Danna. John P. Inventory and Profit, AMA, 1966.
35. Datta A K. Integrated Materials Management, S Chand and Co Ltd, New Delhi, 1971.
36. Datta A K. Integrated Materials Management, S Chand and Co. New Delhi 1978.
37. Datta A K. Materials Management and Inventory Control, Jaico Publishing House, Bombay, 1982.
38. David Hutchins. Just-In-Time, Jaico Publishing House, Bombay 1995.
39. Dean S Ammer. Materials Management, Richard D Erwin Inc., lllinois, 1968.
40. Dean S Ammer. Purchasing for profit Logistic Management and Readings in purchasing edited by L Leslic waters Houghston, Mifftin Company, Boston, 1969.
41. Dean S. Ammer. Purchasing and Materials Management for Healthcare Institutions. Lexington Book, 1983.
42. Dey B R. Business Process Reengineering and Change Management, Biztantra, Dreamtech Press, 2008.
43. Donald W Dobler, Lamer lee and David N Burt. Purchasing and Materials Management Text and Cases, Tata MC Graw Hill Publishing Ltd, New Delhi 1992.

44. Edward D. Sanderson. Effective Hospital Materiel Management.

45. Evertett E Adam, Jr. and Ronald J. Ebert. Production and operation Management, Prentich-Hall Inc. Engle Wood, New Jersy, 1995.

46. Elwood S Buffa and Rakesh K Sarin. Modern Production / Operations Management, John Willy and Sons, Singapore, 1994.

47. Floyd D Hedrick, Purchasing Management in a Smaller Company, American Management Association Inc., 1971.

48. Goel S L and Kumar R. Hospital Supportive Services, Deep and Deep publications private Ltd, New Delhi, 2004.

49. Goel SL and Kumar R. Hospital support services, Deep and Deep publication, New Delhi.

50. Gokaran P.R. Essentials of Materials Management, Somaiya Publications Pvt. Ltd, Bombay-1970.

51. Gopala Krishnan P and Sandilya M.S. Stores Management and Logistics, S Chand and Company Ltd., New Delhi, 1980.

52. Gopala Krishnan P and Banerji A.K. Handbook on Contract and Purchase management, Printwell, Jaipur India, 1991.

53. Gopala Krishnan P and Banerji A.K. Maintenance and spare parts Management, Prentice Hall of India, New Delhi, 1991.

54. Gopala Krishnan P and Sandilya M.S, Purchasing Strategy Text and Cases. Sterling publications (P) Ltd. 1978.

55. Gopala Krishnan P and Sandilya M.S. Inventory Management Texts and Cases, Mac Millan Company of India Ltd, New Delhi, 1977.

56. Gopala Krishnan P and Sundaresan. Materials Management an Integrated approach, Prentice Hall of India, New Delhi, 1991.

57. Gopala Krishnan P. Cost reduction hand book, Jaico Publishing House, New Delhi, 1992.

58. Gopala Krishnan P. Handbook of Material Management, Prentice-Hall of India Pvt.Ltd, New Delhi, 2005.

59. Gopala Krishnan P. Integrated Spares Management, S. Chand and Company, Ltd. Ram Nagar, New Delhi, 1984.

60. Gopala Krishnan P. Inventory and working capital management, Macmillan India Ltd. New Delhi ,1991.

61. Gopala Krishnan P. Purchasing and Materials Management, Tata MC Graw Hill Publishing Company Ltd., New Delhi, 1990.

62. Gupta C B. An introduction to Statistical Methods, Vikas Publishing House Pvt Ltd., New Delhi, 1973.

63. Harold E Fearson, Donald W Dobler and Kenneth H.Killen, The purchasing Handbook, MC Graw Hill, Inc., New York, 1995.

64. Harold-E Fearson. Purchasing organizational relationship, Centre for Advanced purchasing studies (CAPS), NAPM, 1988.

65. Herbert H Peckhan. Effective Materials Management, Printice Hall Inc. Englewood Cliffs, New Jersey, 1972.

66. Iwao Koboyashi. 20 keys to work place improvement, Productivity press (India) Pvt. Ltd., Madras, 1994.

67. James H.Green. Production and inventory control handbook, MC Graw Hill, Inc., New York, 1976.

68. James Pilditch. The Silent Sales Man, how to develop packaging that sells, Business Books Limited, London 1973.

69. Jayaraman M.S. and Ganesh Natarajan, Business process Re-engineering, Tata N.C. Grad Hills Publishing Company Ltd., New Delhi, 1996.

70. Jha S M. Hospital Management, Himalaya Publishing House, 2001.

71. John H. Holmgren and Walter J.Wertz. Materials management and purchasing for Healthcare Facility AUPHA press 1982.

72. John P D. Anna Inventory and Profit, Taraporevala Publishing Industires Pvt Ltd., Bombay, 1978.

73. John Wornoff. Japanese Management keys fique, Neo Publishing Company, New Delhi, 1993.

74. Jon, Woronoff. The Japanese Management, mystique. Neo Publishing company, New Delhi, 1993.

75. Joseph Buchan and Earnest Koenigsberg K. Scientific Inventory Management, Prentice, Hall of India Pvt Ltd. New Delhi, 1970.

76. Joseph G Monks. Operations Management Theory and problems, MC Graw Hill, Inc. New York, 1987.

77. Joseph L.fink. Pharmacy law digest Harvard Publishing Company. 1984.

78. Kelley lee and Jeff Collin. Global change and Health, Tata Mc Graw Hill, New Delhi, 2006f.

79. Kennth H.Killen and John W.Kamauff. Managing purchasing - Making the supply team to work Vol.II and NAPM Professional Development Services, IRWIN Professional purchasing, Chicago, 1995.

80. Khare B.D. and Monga R.C. Inventory Control A - Management Guide, National Productivity Council, New Delhi, 1976.

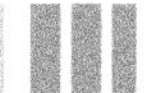

81. Lewis, Howard, T. Problems on Industrial Purchasing, Mc Graw Hill, New York, 1930.
82. Lisa M.Ellram and Launa M.Birow. Purchasing for Bottom line impact. Improving organization through strategic procurement., IRWIN Professional purchasing, Chicago, 1995.
83. Malhotra A K. Hospital Management-An Evaluation, Global India Publications, 2009.
84. Marie Carney. Health Services Management Culture, Consensus and the Middle Manager. Prentice Hall of India Private Ltd. New Delhi, 2007.
85. Mark Kobayashi-Hillary, Outsourcing to India, Second edition, Spinger publications, 2005.
86. Martin K Starer and David W Miller. Inventory Control Theory and Practice, Prentice Hall of India Pvt Ltd., New Delhi, 1981.
87. Martino and Joseph P. Log Normality of Delphi Estimates - Technological Forecasting Vol. I, 1970.
88. Masaaki Imai. KAIZEN - The key to Japan's competetive success Mc Garw - Hills International Edition.
89. Mathew P.D. Handbook of Materials Management, Mc Hartly International, Calcutta.
90. Megan London. Environment, Health and Sustainable, Development, Tata Mc Graw Hill, New Delhi, 2006.
91. Menon K.S. Purchasing and Inventory Control, A.H.Wheeler & Co., 1993.
92. Menon K.S. Stores Management, Mac Millan India Press, Madras, 1992.
93. Menon P.G. Materials Management and O.R. in India, M.M.J.Publication, New Delhi, 1968.
94. Michael D. Drobot. Hospital Materials Management, George Washington University, 1970.
95. Michael Hammer and James Champy. Re-engineering the corporation. A Manifest for Business Revolution, Nicholas Breaking Publication of London, London, 1994.
96. Michiael R Leeders and Anna E Flynn. Value Driver purchasing Vol.I, IRWIN Professional purchasing, Chicago, 1995.
97. N K Nair. Purchasing and Materials Management, Vikas Publishing House Pvt. Ltd.
98. Narayan P, Jaya Subramanian. Inventory Management, IIMM NHQ Education Wing, Mumbai, 2009.
99. Nick Goodwin, Reinhold Gruen and Valerie Iles. Managing Health Services, Tata McGraw-Hill, New Delhi, 2006.
100. NIGP. The dictionary of purchasing terms, fourth edition, The National Institute of Governmental Purchasing Inc, Virginia.

101. Nobert Llyod Enrick. Inventory Management Installation, Operation and Control, Chandler Publishing Co. San-Francisco, 1973.

102. Northcote Parkinson and Rustomji M K , Sapre S A, A Critical commentary on Peter Druckers Philosophy of Management, India Book House Pvt. Ltd. Bombay, 1987.

103. Northcote Parkinson and Rustomji M K. Excellence in Management, India Book House Pvt. Ltd. Bombay, 1989.

104. Northcote Parkinson and Rustomji M K. Watch your figures, Mac Millan India Ltd Bombay, 1984.

105. Packaging course materials for PGDMM Programme, Indian Institute of Materials Management NHQ Education Wing, Bangalore, 1994.

106. Patric MC Hugh, Giorgio Merili and William A.Wheeler. III, Beyond Business process Reengineering towards Holonic enterprise., John Willy and Sons New York, 1995.

107. Paul F. Wilson and Richard D. Pearson. Performance based assessments, Tata McGraw Hill inc.

108. Paul, Farrell V. Algians's Purchasing Handbook, McGraw hills Book Company, New York, 1982.

109. Paul, Farrell. Fifty Years of Purchasing - The story of NAPA, New York, 1954.

110. Peter Baily and David Farmer. Managing Materials in Industry, Gower Press, London.

111. Peter Baily. Successful Stock Control by Manual Systems, Gower Press.

112. Peter F. Drucker. Managing for Result, Elsevier, 2006.

113. Peter F. Drucker. Managing for the future, Elsevier, 2006.

114. Peter F. Drucker. The Practice of Management, Butterworth, Helnemann, 1955.

115. Peter P Schoderbek. Management Systems , John Wiley and Sons Inc., 1971.

116. Philip B Schary and Tage Skjott Larsen. Managing the Global Supply chain Viva Books Pvt Ltd., New Delhi, 2000.

117. Philip Kotler and Gary Armstrong. Principles of MarketPrentice Hall of India Pvt. Ltd., New Delhi, 1995.

118. Philip Kotler. Marketing Management, Prentice Hall, Upper Saddle River, New Jersey 07458.

119. Purchasing Management GDMM Course Material, IIMM NHQ Education wing, Mumbai, 2010.

120. Purusottam Behra. Hospital and Healthcare Management, Mittal Publications New Delhi, 2007.

121. Rajaram S and Siva kumar M. Total Quality Management, Biztantra, 2008.

122. Rangarajan L.N Kautilya. The ArthaSastra Penguin Books 1992.

123. Rastogi P.N. Management of Technology and Innovation, Sage Publications, New Delhi, 1995.

124. Reinhold Gruen and Anne Howarth. Financial Management in Health Services Tata McGraw Hill, New Delhi 2006.

125. Reuben Ray. Store Management, Himalaya Publishing House, Mumbai, 1997.

126. Richard J.Tersine and Johan H Cambell. Modern Materials Management, North Holland Publishing Company, Netherlands, 1977.

127. Robert B. Williams. Hospital Pharmacy Management Primer American Society of Hospital Pharmacists-1985.

128. Sarah Smith, Don Sinclair, Rosalind Raine and Barnaby Reeves, Health Care evaluation, Tata McGraw-Hill, New Delhi, 2006.

129. Schorr John. E. and Olive Weight. Purchasing in Twenty First Century, APICS.

130. Shakti Gupta. Hospital Stores Management - an integrated approach J.P. Brothers Medical Publications (P) Ltd, 2004.

131. Srinivasan R.V. Managing Modern Hospitals. Sage Publications New Delhi, 2000.

132. Stanley E Larson. Inventory systems and controls handbook, Prentice-Hall Inc., Engle Wood, New Jersy, 1977.

133. Stephen Jan and Others. Economic Analysis for Management and Policy, Tata McGraw Hill, New Delhi, 2005.

134. Stukart H.L. The Importance of Materials Management in Industries, Kalbin de papel e cellulose, SA, Sterling Publishers (P) Ltd., New Delhi, 1978.

135. Subba Rao SVR, Game plans for post GATT Era Action Agenda for Indian Pharmacentilal Industry, Panther Publication Private Ltd., Bangalore, 1999.

136. Sunil Chopra and Peter Meindl. Supply Chain Management strategy, planning and operation, Wesley Longman Singapore Pvt Ltd., Indian Branch, New Delhi, 2001.

137. Supply chain Management-An Indian Perspective-A collection of Articles, edited by Bharadwaj M K, Sagar Books, IIMM, 2011.

138. Tachiichi Ohno. Work Place Management, Productivity Press (India) Pvt. Ltd. Madras, 1993.

140. Taiichi Ohno and Setsuomito. Just-in-time for today and tomorrow, Productivity Press (India) Pvt. Ltd., Madras, 1995.

141. Taiichi Ohno. Toyota production systems, Productivity press (India) Pvt. Ltd., Madras, 1993.

142. Thomas E. Vouman, D. Clay Why Bark and William Berry Manufacturing and Control systems, Galgotia Publications Pvt. Ltd, New Delhi 1989

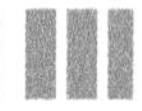

143. Tonywild. Best practice in Inventory Management Buffer Worth, Jordan Hiel Oxford, 2001

144. Varma MM. Essential of stores keeping and Purchasing, Sultan chand & Co.

145. Venkat Reddy V. Hospital Materials Management, Training Programme course Material, March 2012

146. Vittal M.S. Value engineering for cost reduction and product improvement, Systems consultancy services, Bangalore, 1993

147. Wayne Barlow C. Corporate Packaging Management, Taraporewala Publishing Industries Pvt Ltd., 1980

148. Westing J H, Fine I V and Zeng G. J. Purchasing Management Materials in Motion, Wiley Eastern Private Ltd., New Delhi, 1991

149. Wilbur B England and Michiel R Leenders. Purchasing and Materials Management, D.B.Taraporawala Sons & Co. Pvt Ltd., 1983

150. Willets, Walter, Fundamentals of Purchasing , Appleton Century - Crofts, New York, 1969

151. William Grant Ireson and Eugeru L Grant. HandBook of Industrial Engineering and Management, Printice Hall of India Pvt Ltd., New Delhi, 1971

152. William L.Scheyer. Handbook of Healthcare Material Management. An Aspen Publication 1985.

GLOSSARY

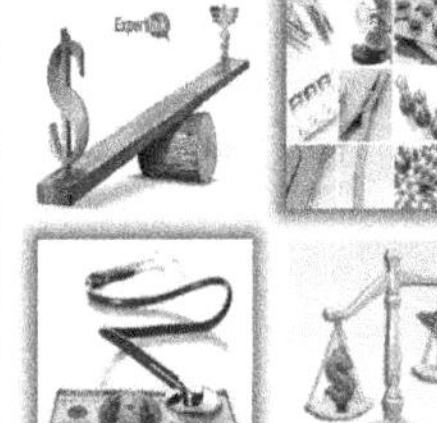

1. **ABC analysis:** Inventory items are grouped into three categories i.e., as

   A items: About 10 percent of items that account for 70 percent of the consumption value.

   B items: 20 percent of items that account for 20 percent of the rupee value of consumption.

   C items: 70 percent of items that account for 10 percent of the rupee value of consumption.

2. **ABC Classification:** The items in the inventory are arranged in descending order of annual consumption value. This array is then split into three classes viz. A, B, C classes. The class A comprises of items with highest rupee value of consumption and receives the maximum attention. The items of class B receive moderate of attention and the class C, which comprises with low rupee value, is controlled more often than not. The ABC classification is a practical function of Pareto's principle or 80/20 formula.

3. **ABC analysis report:** A statement listing all inventoried items classified into three classes A, B and C.

4. **ABC inventory control:** An inventory control approach based on ABC categorization.

5. **Absorption costing:** Valuation of finished inventory based on variable costs plus distribution of fixed costs.

6. **Acceptable Quality Level (AQL):** A term used in inspection by statistical sampling method to signify highest acceptable ratio between the number of faulty parts and total parts in a batch or delivery. For instance, an AQL of 0.98 indicates that the buyer is willing to accept shipments that have 2 percent of the items out of specification or with more characteristic properties.

7. **Acceptance:** A promise to pay by the debtor against whom a draft or bill of exchange has been drawn, usually evidenced by signing the draft or bill and writing "accepted" on its face. It is an intentional indication of offer.

8. **Acceptance of an offer:** The (formal) agreement to accept an offer. An acceptance must be unqualified assent or else it is a counter offer.

9. **Acceptance of an order:** The agreement of the seller to reassign the property in goods ordered to the buyer for a consideration. (See also the acknowledgement of order.)

10. **Accessorial service:** Supplementary or exceptional services provided in addition to essential service.

11. **Accuracy level:** A term used to indicate the extent to which the physical and 'book' or 'file' balance agree to an inventory usually in combination with stock taking programme. It is generally expressed as percentage and calculated by the following equation:

$$\frac{\text{Items to which accounts agree}}{\text{Total items counted}} \times 100$$

12. **Acknowledgement of order:** Intimation by a vendor to confirm to a purchaser that a purchase order has been received. It generally implies acceptance of the order by the supplier subject to the terms of the acknowledgement document. Such terms and conditions may vary and conflict with those stated on the purchase order and thus resulting in a counter offer.

13. **Acquisition cost:** When applied to arrive at economic order quantities, it refers to the costs which increase as the number of orders placed increases. It includes costs related to the clerical work of preparing, issuing, following and receiving orders, the physical handling of goods, inspections, and machine set up costs. Often, it is treated as the marginal cost of an additional batch of orders. Preferably, acquisition cost should be calculated on an incremental basis. When this occurs, it is termed as "internal acquisition cost".

14. **Acronym:** A word formed from the first letter of the words in a term or phrase, for example: RFID, FSN, PERT, CPM.

15. **Active inventory:** An inventory that had recent use or likely to have regular usage.

16. **Activity Based Costing (ABC):** It enables cost identification to a reasonable degree of accuracy to various products. It facilitates cost reduction by reducing or eliminating the non value adding activities. It also helps in proper determination of appropriate selling price in order to remain competitive.

17. **Adoption notice:** One carrier lawfully takes over another carrier's operations and obligations.

18. **Administrative Lead Time (ALT):** The time taken by the purchasing department to place an order for an item with the supplier after the order point has been reached or an authorized purchase requisition has been received. Administrative lead time is usually recorded as a separate figure in inventory control algorithms or in order to produce purchasing performance reports. ALT is also termed 'internal lead time' or 'purchasing lead time'.

19. **Aggregate inventory:** The sum of the inventory levels for individual items or products indicated by multiple stock keeping units (SKU).

    For example, the combined inventory would be made up of one half the sum of all the lot sizes plus the sum of all the safety stocks plus any anticipation or seasonal inventory.

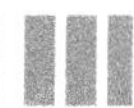

20. **Aggregate inventory management:** Establishing the overall levels of inventory that will be required and making sure that the individual replenishment techniques accomplish this overall policy.

21. **Ageing schedule:** A report showing how long accounts receivable have been outstanding. It gives the percentage of receivables now past due and the percentage past due by, for example, one month, two months, or other periods.

22. **Algorithm:** A prescribed set of well defined rules or processes for the solution of a problem in a finite number of steps. An example of it is a full statement of arithmetic procedures for determining the lot size or EOQ for an item of inventory.

23. **All or none:** A bid submitted in response to an invitation for bids (IFB) in which the bidder states, he will not accept a partial award, but accept an award for all items, services etc. This conditional offer may be accepted, only if provided for in IFB, or if the bidder has not quoted individual prices for each of the items, services etc.

24. **Allocation:** Assigning one or more items of cost or revenue to one or more segments of an organization according to benefits received responsibilities, or other logical measures of use.

25. **Alphanumeric:** A contraction of alphabet numeric, it is the system of communication employing letters of the alphabet, numerals, and other symbols such as punctuation or mathematical symbols.

26. **Alphanumeric data:** Data made up of the letters AZ, numeric characters 09 and special symbols like +, $, #, !, and so on.

27. **Amortization:** The gradual liquidation of a burden by means of sinking fund in which the principal amount of the loan is repaid in installments during the tenure of the loan period.

28. **Amount to reorder:** A predetermined quantity of material to be ordered, usually considered by some decision rule, such as the economic lot size.

29. **Analysis:** A careful and comprehensive examination, the study of offered prices, or the inspection of offered goods to determine the conformance with the requirement.

30. **Annuity:** A series of payments of a fixed amount for a specific number of years.

31. **Anticipation:** An amount taken off a bill when an invoice is paid in advance of the discount or net due date. This is granted in addition to any discounts and is calculated at a declared percentage rate for the number of days between actual payment and the due date.

32. **Anticipation inventories:** Additional inventory that accumulated for a definite, predictable trends of increasing sales, planned sales, promotion programmes, seasonal fluctuations, plant shutdowns, and vacations.

33. **APICS:** American Production and Inventory Control Society; a professional society committed to the development and advancement of the field of production and inventory control.
34. **Appreciation:** An increase in value.
35. **Appropriation:** An authorization to spend a specified amount of funds.
36. **Arbitrage:** Buying in one market and selling simultaneously in another in order to profit from price variances. See also Hedge.
37. **AS IS where IS:** In as is condition and at their current location, the purchasers responsible for all handling of transport and insurance to remove goods from their current location.
38. **Asepsis:** The methods of making or keeping free from pathogenic micro organism.
39. **Assembly:** A group of sub assemblies and/or parts that are put together; the total unit constitutes a major subdivision of the final product.
40. **Asset management programme:** A joint accountability of material and finance management and departments whereby capital equipment is ordered, received, depreciated and recorded on a systematic basis.
41. **Automatic stocking:** A predetermined quantity of one or more line items routinely issued at a specified time.
42. **Automated cart system:** This commonly used phrase is a misnomer because there is no such thing as an automated cart system. The phrase more appropriately refers to a programmed distribution system for supply cart.
43. **Auxiliary storage:** Storage that supplements the main memory section of the central processing unit. Auxiliary storage may be an on line or off line.
44. **Availability:** A term usually interpreted to mean "material available for planning" and thus includes not only the on hand inventory, but also inventory on order.
45. **Available stock:** It can signify (a) stock on hand (b) stock on hand plus replenishment orders, (c) stock on hand less known requirements or (d) stock on hand plus orders less requirements The last sense is the most useful; thus Magee defines available stock as "the algebraic sum of stock on hand and the stock already on order, less any unfilled customer demand". In this sense, it does not entail that available stock is actually in the stores, but merely that it is available for allocation against new demands. R G Brown states: "Hence available stock may be greater than, equal to or less than physical inventory and may even be negative if there are back orders."
46. **Available time:** It is used in stock control, to mean the interval between the earliest time at which a specific requirement of an item can be calculated and the time at which it is required.
47. **Backdoor buying:** The term usually commonly used to describe buying for reasons ranging from ignorance of hospital policy or lack of confidence in purchasing ability to respond to departments' "special needs".

48. **Backdoor selling:** Bypassing the purchasing by salesperson who goes directly to the function or end user of product being purchased. In hospital, this takes place where there is decentralized purchasing.

49. **Backlog:**

    i. **Of orders** – All the orders outstanding with a supplier not executed.

    ii. **Of requisitions** – Issue requisitions as yet unfilled by a warehouse or store.

    iii. **Of receiving** – Receipts from suppliers as yet to deliver to end users or placed into storage.

    iv. **Of transport** – Goods held up at an intermediate location awaiting transportation to final destination.

50. **Backorder:** The receipt of a demand for a product when there are no units on hand in inventory. These backorders become shortages, which are ultimately satisfied when a new supply of the product becomes available.

51. **Backorder quantity:** The quantity demanded which cannot be filled from currently available inventory and which will be supplied upon receipt of incoming orders.

52. **Backward scheduling:** A scheduling technique where the schedule is computed, starting with the due date for the order and working backward to determine the required starting date.

53. **Balance of stores record:** A double entry record system that shows at all times the balance of material on order and 'available' for expected orders.

54. **Balance out:** At the end of a financial year, or in anticipation of an engineering or design change, the stocks of all subordinate items can be reduced in a balanced way. Items that cannot be carried over to the next model are stocked somewhat below forecast requirements. Items that can be carried over can be stocked to a level somewhat above forecast.

55. **Bank:** Quantity of materials that are waiting for further processing.

56. **Base level inventory:** The normal inventory level made up of the lot size inventory plus the safety stock inventory.

57. **Basc pipeline stock:** Stock in transit to fill the many stocking points in the distribution system.

58. **Base stock:** A bare minimum quantity of inventory that can be identified as necessary in certain types of operations to maintain a continuing service or production.

59. **Bank guarantee:** An undertaking by a bank to creditor that it will answer for debt of a principal debtor in consideration of creditor foregoing payment of deposit or security or supplying materials without prepayment to the principal debtor.

60. **Bar coding:** A technology which uses a variety of printing or imaging techniques to encode data in a pattern of bar and spaces. This bar code is attached to parts, containers, or documents and then scanned to allow computers for instant access to information.

61. **Base stock system:** A method of inventory control that issues replenishment orders whenever an order is received for an item. Base stock orders are also used to adjust the level of the base stock for each item.

62. **Bathtub curve:** A typical shape for the failure rate curve for many parts of equipment, i.e., the conditional probability of failure that occurs immediately after commissioning the equipment, will be high because new equipment may have 'birth defects', decreases to a low fairly constant rate for a long period of time, and then starts to increase again as the equipment reaches 'old age'. The three stages in generally described as wear in period, stable period and wear out period.

63. **Basic stock:** The desired level of the average inventory.

64. **Batch:** The material and/or information required or used in one production or processing cycle.

65. **Benchmark:** An approach of testing the computer software or hardware with an actual application to demonstrate that it works.

66. **Bid:** 1. A price offer by a prospective seller. 2. A quotation given, usually in competition with other vendors, in response to a prospective buyer's request.

67. **Bill of lading:** Document issued by common carrier inventorying the containers that are shipped.

68. **Bill of landing:** An order negotiable or non negotiable document that is a contract for transportation between the shipper and the carrier.

69. **Bill of Material (BOM):** A structured list of the items used in making a parent assembly that reflects the actual manufacturing process in terms of timing and quantities consumed. A BOM may optionally include information relating to back flushing, use of alternate and optional components, tie between the components and the operations that use them, and other data. BOMs are used by the MRP function to estimate component requirements when given a parent demand, and in building product costs.

70. **Bill of sale:** A written agreement transferring ownership of a property from one party to another.

71. **Bin cards:** A bin card is kept in along with a particular item to record receipts, issues, and stock balances, held in the stores in which the items are stocked although not necessarily in the bins. These cards are usually simple, giving description of the item, including its code number. The essential difference between a bin card and a stock card is that the main purpose of the stock card is to provide information as a basis for placing replenishment

 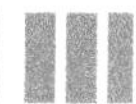

orders. A bin card is just a local record of what is currently in store, and may also carry its location. Bin cards and allocation cards can be combined.

72. **Bin location:** A storage segment within the store or warehouse, used to locate and store warehouse stock, generally of the small variety.

73. **Bin location file:** A list that specifically identifies the physical location of each item stored in inventory.

74. **Bin tally:**

    i. A type of perpetual inventory, designed for storekeeping purposes, maintained at the store area for each inventory item on which the balance of stock on hand is recorded.

    ii. A card or tag maintained at the storage location of an item of inventory and on which the balance of stock on hand is recorded.

75. **Bin tag:** Card or tag maintained at the storage location of an item of inventory and on which the balance of stock on hand after each transaction is recorded.

76. **Bin trips:** The number of times (per annum) that an item is ordered by separated customer transactions, irrespective of the number of units ordered.

77. **Blanket order:** Sometimes referred to as Master Contract for reducing number of small orders. It provides the supplier to furnish special commodities for certain period of time at a determined price or on the basis of a formula for prices based on market or other conditions.

78. **Book inventory:** A definition of inventory units or value obtained from perpetual inventory records rather than by actual count.

79. **Book value:** The accounting value of an asset. Normally, it is the original acquisition cost less all depreciation taken.

80. **Break even analysis:** An analytical technique for studying the relationships among fixed costs, variable costs, and profits. A break even chart graphically depicts the nature of break even analysis.

81. **Breakeven point:** The level of manufacture or the volume of sales at which operations are neither profitable nor unprofitable.

82. **Bridging run:** The quantity ordered when tooling is to be changed or when the unit cost of the materials is to be changed. The quantity ordered will last longer than usual and will bridge over the period when the source cannot supply more, because the plant is being retooled.

83. **Budget:** A plan that includes an estimate of future expenditure and revenues related to expected activities over a specified period of time say an year.

84. **Budget variance:** The discrepancy between the actual amounts and the budget figure.

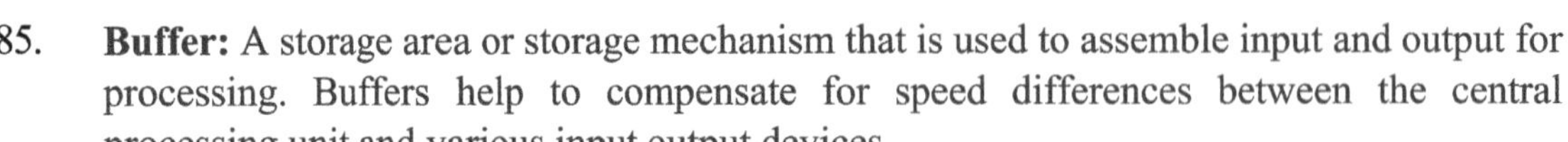

85. **Buffer:** A storage area or storage mechanism that is used to assemble input and output for processing. Buffers help to compensate for speed differences between the central processing unit and various input output devices.

86. **Buffer stock:** A stock allowance to cover errors in forecasts of demand during the procurement period (lead time) or to cover for a production facility maintenance shutdown.

87. **Bulk stores:** In bulk store, area supplies are stored as is received in manufacturing state. These quantities are broken down into small quantities for distributing to user departments from central stores or central supply.

88. **Bulk order quantity:** A quantity bigger than the EOQ, which may be ordered in order to get a lower unit price.

89. **Bullwhip effect (whiplash):** The observation in multi-echelon inventory systems that a small variation in the demand for each period at the retail end may result in a remarkable fluctuation in the amount demanded at the manufacturer, analogous to how small flick of the wrist will cause the tip of the bull whip to move a great distance. This effect was called Bullwhip effect by Prof. Hane Lea of Stanford University. The fluctuations in demand by the retailer on the supplier may be due to a number of reasons. Important among them are demand forecast updating and order batching driven by each member of supply chain trying to optimize internal operation of inventory management. Fluctuations and rationing and shortage gaming are causes on account of members reaction to market dynamics.

90. **Business analysis:** A stage in new product or service development in which detailed forecasts of probable sales, income, and expenses are prepared.

91. **Business cycle:** A diagramme of fluctuations in the levels of economic activity in country overtime.

92. **Business risk:** The basic risk inherent in a firm's operations. Business risk plus financial risk resulting from the use of debt equals total corporate risk.

93. **Buy back:** A type of counter trade in which an organization builds a plant in a foreign country (or supplies technology, equipment, training or other services) and agrees to take a certain share of plant's output as a part payment for investment. See also counter trade.

94. **Buyer:** An individual who is a member of materials management function, whose primary duty is processing materials of specified category. His position is a key line function without supervisory responsibilities.

95. **Buyer's market:** A market condition favourable to purchasers existing when the forces of supply and demand keep prices relatively low.

96. **Buyer's risk:** The probability that a sample will contain fewer defects than the rest of the lot.

97. **Buying:** The functions of finding sources of supply, obtaining quotations, placing purchase orders, issuing delivery schedules to suppliers and progressing supply of goods.

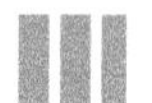

98. **Buying centre:** The managerial members actually involved in purchase decisions. This could include users, buyers, influencers, and decision makers.

99. **Calendar time:** It refers to the passage of days or weeks, as in the definition of lead time or scheduling rules, in contrast to running time.

100. **Call off quantity:** On a delivery schedule sent to a supplier, the quantity specified to be delivered at one time (and paid for) against a covering order for a larger quantity.

101. **Capacity:** The highest sustainable output rate that can be achieved with the current product specifications, product mix, worker effort, plant, and equipment.

102. **Capital asset:** An asset with a life of more than one year that is not bought and sold in the ordinary course of business.

103. **Capital budgeting:** The process of planning expenditures on assets whose returns are expected to extend beyond one year.

104. **Capital costs:** Cost of monies tied up for certain period, normally for one year. This is usually expressed as a percentage and may be based upon factors such as the average expected return on alternative opportunities for investment of comparable funds. The cost of borrowed funds would represent the lower limit.

105. **Capitalization rate:** A discount rate used to find the present value of a series of future cash receipts; sometimes called discount rate.

106. **Carrier:** Any individual, company, or corporation engaged in transporting goods.

107. **Carry back, carry forward:** For income tax purposes, losses that can be carried backward or forward to reduce income tax burden.

108. **Carrying cost:** It is cost of carrying inventory, consisting of cost of capital, taxes and insurance, obsolescence and spoilage, and space costs. See also holding cost.

109. **Cartage:** Intra city hauling.

110. **Cart exchange system:** A type of supply distribution whereby supplies for a unit or department are depleted and replenished via a mobile cart.

111. **Cascaded systems:** Multi storage operations where the input to each stage is the output of a preceding stage.

112. **Cash budget:** A schedule depicting cash flows (receipts, disbursements, and net cash) for a firm or institutional unit, such as a pharmacy, over a specified period.

113. **Cash cycle:** The length of time between the purchase of various inputs for production of goods and services and the collection of accounts receivable generated by way of sale of the final product.

114. **Cash discounts:** Cash discounts are designed to encourage prompt payment of bills. A policy such as "2/10 net 30" means the purchaser can deduct 2 percent of the list price if he pays for the order within the first ten days of the month following receipt of the bill. Payment is expected within thirty days, even if the discount is not utilized. Vendors offer cash discounts to improve their cash flow positions and thus to reduce the need for borrowing money to pay their bills on time.

115. **Certified cheque:** A cheque endorsed by a bank, guaranteeing its payment.

116. **Caveat emptor:** 'Let the buyer beware'. The sale is at buyer's risk.

117. **Caveat venditor:** 'Let the seller beware'. In some cases, vendor is liable to the buyer if the goods delivered differ in kind, quality, use and purpose from those specified in the contract of sale.

118. **Centralized system:** A set of functions or programs processed by or in a single centre and servicing several locations.

119. **Central Processing Unit (CPU):** The main unit of the computer system where all control and processing work is done like processing of data, movement of data, and execution of instructions. Sets of circuits that together make up the control unit, the arithmetic/logic unit, and the main memory unit.

120. **Certificate of compliance:** A supplier's written assurance to the effect that the supplies or services delivered fulfill specified requirements. This is akin to self certification by vendors.

121. **Chain of distribution:** The path of an item from producer to final user.

122. **Change order:** A formal notification that an order must be changed in some form. This may result from a changed date or specification by the customer, engineering or design change, a change in inventory requirement date, or some other changes.

123. **Changeover cost:** Setup cost and tear down cost.

124. **Christmas tree:** A bill of material in the form of graphic product; structure chart showing how the assembly is made up of sub assemblies, the sub assemblies made up of lower level components, and so on.

125. **Classification of goods theory:** A breakdown of goods and services based on product or service characteristics and consumer purchasing behaviour; the three general categories are convenience, shopping, and speciality goods.

126. **Closed loop system:** A system in which the computer directly controls an external process without human intervention. In a closed loop process control system, for instance, the computer may be connected directly to instrumentation through a digital to analog converter. The computer can then apply control action directly to the process by actuating valves, setting controls, and so forth.

127. **Closed short:** An order is closed short when less than the quantity ordered will be delivered to stock. This may be the result of scrap losses or unavailability from the vendor.

128. **Code:** A verb denoting the assignment of a number or letter to identify and designate a specific character or group of characters to make available a tool for supply management.

129. **Cognitive dissonance:** Buyer's discomfort caused by post purchase conflict of product or products.

130. **Collate:** To combine parts or all of two or more ordered sets (files) of information in any way so that a similar sequence is observed in the combined set.

131. **Collateral:** Assets that are used to secure a loan.

132. **Commercialization:** The final stage of new product development, that is, fullscale introduction and marketing.

133. **Commodity records:** Extensive card indexes showing where to buy goods and materials.

134. **Common carrier:** A transportation company operating under a certificate of convenience and necessity, which provides service to the general public at published rates.

135. **Company managed inventory:** A support arrangement alike to vendor managed inventory, however replacement orders for the vendor owned stock are agreed by the user prior to delivery.

136. **Compatibility:** Capacity of interchangeability among products, programmes, and media.

137. **Complementary product:** When demand for one product increases with demand for another, they are complementary.

138. **Component:** An inclusive term used to describe a subassembly or part that goes into higher level assemblies.

139. **Component parts:** An inventory grouping that comprises items that are either purchased or manufactured from raw material and stored for use in assemblies or for sale to customers as repair or replacement parts. (Parts may be held in component parts stores and still require further processing or finishing at final assembly.

140. **Condition sales contract:** A contract for the financing of new equipment that calls for paying off the loan in installments over a one to five year period. The seller retains title to the equipment until payment has been completed.

141. **Consignment goods:** An inventory of materials or sales parts held by an agreement with the supplier in the warehouse of purchasing organization and which whilst under the physical custody of the purchaser, remains the property of the supplier until issued for use by the purchaser at which point payment becomes due.

142. **Consolidation:**

(i) Of goods (cargo) the receipt of goods at an offsite depot, the segregation of such goods according to most economic and/or timely transport mode and the repacking, storage utilization and protection of goods in a method most suited to the economic and safe use of selected transport mode.

(ii) Inventory terms (a) Warehousing The reorganization of storage to bring like items into storage layout. (b) Cataloging The bringing together of similar items under common stock number or group/class and deletion of redundant items from file.

143. **Constant demand rate:** An assumption of many inventory decision models, which states that the same number of units are taken from inventory in each period of time.

144. **Constant supply rate:** The situation in which the inventory is built up at a constant rate over a period of time. This assumption is used in many production and economic lot size models.

145. **Constraint:** The limitations placed on the maximization or minimization of an objective function, as in mathematical programming.

146. **Constraints:** Restrictions or limitations imposed on a particular problem or situation.

147. **Consumables:** Consumables are those items which after use cannot be cost-effectively restored to a serviceable condition.

148. **Consumerism:** A general term referring to identification and resolution of problems that consumer's experience.

149. **Consumer product safety forum:** A regulatory agency charged with identifying and investigating products that may harm consumers.

150. **Containerized freight:** Shipments packaged in standard size and shape containers for transportation by truck, train, or ship.

151. **Continuous budget:** A budget that perpetually adds a month or quarter into the future as the month or quarter that just ended is dropped.

152. **Continuous stock taking:** Checking recorded stock balance against physical counts all the year. Instead of once or twice a year typically, a selection of items are checked every week; at times called perpetual stock taking. The alternative is periodic stock taking.

153. **Contra cyclical buying:** Buying goods during the "off" season for a particular industry. The incentives for the buyer are usually major price concessions.

154. **Contribution:** In marginal analysis, contribution is the difference between price per unit and variable cost per unit. It is the amount left over to cover fixed costs and provide a profit.

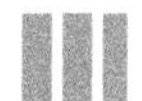

155. **Control board:** A visual means of showing machine loading or project planning. Usually, it is a variation of the basic Gantt chart.

156. **Convenience goods:** A classification of consumer goods. These are usually low-cost items for which substitutes are available.

157. **Conversion cost:** The cost of converting prime goods to finished goods. These costs also include overhead and indirect labour.

158. **Cooperative purchasing:** An approach in which several organizations jointly buy selected items. They may form or utilize a centralized buying service that purchases specified types of items for all members of the group or cooperate informally. The consequential volume buying usually produces significant cost savings for group members.

159. **Corporate prime supplier agreement:** A type of purchasing whereby the hospital can buy entire categories of applicable supplies from a parent company and all of its subsidiaries, branches, franchises, etc. at the same negotiated levels of price, quality, and service. The total corporate purchases are combined for volume price and service considerations.

160. **Corrective action:** Action that must be taken to get actual inventories or production back on plan, such as expediting

161. **Cost Insurance and Freight (CIF):** This INCOTERM TERM is essentially same as C and F but with addition that seller has to acquire marine insurance, against risk of loss of or damage to goods during the transit. The seller contracts with insurer and pays the insurance premium

162. **Cost benefit analysis:** A method of assessing the impact of projects, new systems, procedures, products, and/or information systems in organizations to identify the costs and benefits of acquisition.

163. **Cost centre:** A sub division of the institution established for the purpose of assigning or allocating costs. The unit may be division department or section, a group of plant and machinery or group of employees or a combination of several units. Also, occasionally called as budget centre.

164. **Cost containment:** Cost control in a hospital involves utilization of manpower and physical assets in a way that ensures economical delivery of high quality healthcare. The true goal of a cost containment effort in a hospital are to evaluate whether the institution is obtaining optimum quality and quantity of goods and services for its money and to seek improved ways of acquiring those goods and services, all within the parameters of the institution's recognized standards of patient care.

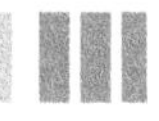

165. **Cost effectiveness:** The correlation between cost calculated in terms of rupee value (foregone opportunities, and so on) on one hand, and effectiveness measured in terms of specified performance characteristics on the other. Cost can be held constant and effectiveness varied, or effectiveness held constant and cost varied in order to arrive at a specified cost effectiveness relationship. Similar to cost benefit.

166. **Cost factors:** The units of input that represent costs to the materials management system, such as labour hours and purchased material, freight costs and storage costs.

167. **Cost of capital:** The discount rate that should be used in capital budgeting and/or establishing the cost of holding inventory.

168. **Cost of holding inventories:** The cost incurred over a time because the inventory exists. See holding costs.

169. **Cost plus:** A pricing method allowing the vendor to charge his costs plus a fixed proportion of those costs.

170. **Cost reduction:** The act of lowering the cost of goods or services, by securing a lower price etc. In cost reduction, the item usually isn't changed, but rather the circumstances around which the item is secured are changed.

171. **Critical Path Method (CPM):** Project management expression to analyze all stages in a complex project to identify the shortest path in which any segment delay would delay the final completion of entire project. The shortest route is called critical path.

172. **CPD:** Acronym for Central Processing Department, where most of the hospital's processing and reprocessing is performed.

173. **CPU:** The Central Processing Unit of a computer.

174. **Crashing:** In CPM, the process of reducing an activity time by adding resources and hence usually costs.

175. **Creeping inventories:** The gradual increase in inventories often owing to suppliers shipping ahead of schedule and/or users hoarding.

176. **Criticality analysis of drugs in pharmacy:** In a hospital, the criticality of a drug is identified on basis of the recommendation by a panel of doctors. Drugs which simultaneously appear in all categories are to be classified as vital. The drugs, which emerge in both vital and essential categories, are classified as vital. If some doctors classify a particular drug as vital and others as essential, it is treated as vital. Likewise, if some doctors classify it as essential and others as desirable, it is classified as essential. The degree of importance in procurement and control procedures reduces from vital drugs to desirable drugs.

177. **Cross functional teams:** Groups of individuals from a range of organizational functions who are brought together to achieve clear, worthwhile and compelling goals that could not be reached without a team. Purchasers typically participate on teams dealing with sourcing commodities, quality and new product or service development.

 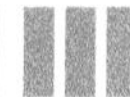

178. **Cross rate:** The exchange rate between two countries based on the exchange rate of each currency against a trend currency usually the US dollar

179. **Cross functional:** An activity system or a team that contains more than one functional area with in an organization and may involve balancing conflicting objectives.

180. **Cross docking:**

    1. The direct flow of merchandise through a ware house facility known receipt to dispatch with no intermediate storage.
    2. A distribution system in which freight moves in and out of distribution centre or point with out ever being stored there.

181. **Criticality:** Degree to which an inventory item's availability is critical to the continuity of production or operations. Generally issued as the basis of establishing service levels for items or group of items. See also critical value analysis.

182. **Critical rate:** A priority factor for workshop scheduling, which measures the ratio of the proportion of stock on hand relative to the order point to the proportion of time remaining relative to the total lead time.

183. **Critical value analysis:** A modified version of ABC analysis concept in which a subjective value of criticality as opposed to actual rupee value is assigned to each inventory item.

184. **Culture:** The distinctive way of life of a group of community often used to describe social heritage of a society, including living habits, arts, aspirations, and the distinctive "style" of a collective of people.

185. **Cumulative lead time:** The longest length of time to complete the activity in question.

186. **Cumulative scheduling:** Scheduling production on an aggregate basis to achieve economical run lengths

187. **Current purchase unit price:** The current purchase price of a single item or unit of issue of that item. It is used as an input in choosing the quantity to be purchased and in evaluating vendors.

188. **Customer service costs:** They include cancelled or lost orders, both current and future, expediting costs, extra freight, more expensive substitutes, and special handling charges.

189. **Cycle:** The time interval during which a system returns to similar initial conditions, for example, the length of time between replenishment shipments.

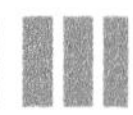

190. **Cycle stock:** The active portion of inventory; that part of inventory which is depleted through regular withdrawals of use, and is replaced through repetitive orders.

191. **Cycle time:** The length of time between cycles, for example, between placing two consecutive orders for replenishing inventory.

192. **Cycle inventory:** An inventory system where counts are performed continuously which often eliminates the need for an annual overall inventory. The usual practice is that 'A' items are counted frequently, say once in a month, and 'B' items once in two to three months, and 'C' items once in a year. (See also perpetual stock taking.)

193. **Cyclical inventory count:** A physical inventory checking technique whereby inventory is counted continuously rather than once a year at predetermined intervals, depending upon their ABC classification. Thus the physical inventory counting goes continuously without interrupting operations or store room activities. Also referred to as "Continuous inventory".

194. **Damages:** Compensation demanded by the buyer as for a late delivery.

195. **Data administrator:** Person (or group) responsible for control and integrity of a set of files.

196. **Database:** A collection of records or units of information normally stored together with controlled redundancy to serve one or more applications.

197. **Data processing:** Preparation of data or basic elements of information, and their handling, according to precise rules of procedure to accomplish such operations as classifying, sorting, calculating, summarizing, and recording. *Synonymous with* Data handling.

198. **Decentralized dispatching:** Organization of the dispatching function into individual departmental dispatchers.

199. **Decrement:** The quantity of inventory reduction. Example: When a user department requisitions certain items. Upon computer processing, these items are immediately recorded as a reduction of inventory and charged to that department. This reduction of inventory is called as decrement.

200. **Dedicated:** Pertaining to a mode of operation in which a procedure requires all the resources of the system.

201. **Deliver to:** Denotes the final destination of materials shipped or distributed.

202. **Delivery date:** The expected date of arrival of shipment.

203. **Delivery leads time:** The time that elapses between the placement of an order and the time of receipt by the order placing agency.

 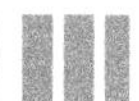

204. **Delivery period:** The time from receipt of a customer's order to dispatch of the goods.

205. **Demand:** 1. The requirement rate of any item during particular horizon time. 2. The interactive processing mode usually to and from the computer and remote terminals. 3. The expected demand for a particular commodity or service in a particular industry or market.

206. **Demand distribution:** A relative arrangement of a set of demand data. Demand during a lead time. The expected demand over the lead time period.

207. **Demand filter:** As total demand is posted during a forecast review period, it is compared with the most recent forecast for that period. If the difference is large purpose compared to the standard deviation, the demand filter creates an exception report, in case something is wrong with the value being posted. The objective is to catch very grave errors in entry or in coding special orders as normal.

208. **De marketing:** A firm's attempt to discourage consumption of a product or service, particularly when shortages of necessary resources occur.

209. **Demographics:** A set of objective data about a group of people. Generally, the data includes such factors such as age, sex, marital status, mobility, income.

210. **Demurrage:** Charges assessed by the carrier against the shipper or consignee for delay of a car, vessel, or vehicle beyond a specified time allowed for unloading or loading and releasing the same to the carrier.

211. **Departmental stock:** An informal system of holding stock in a production or service department.

212. **Dependent demand:** Demand (typically for components) that is dependent on requirements generated by higher level sub assemblies and assemblies.

213. **Depreciation:** Decrease in value of a capital asset because of use, deterioration, inadequacy, obsolescence, and/or applicable tax laws.

214. **Desirable drug:** In a hospital, the desirable drugs are those, which have readily available substitutes. In case of such items, the stock outs longer than 48 hours could be tolerated well by patient care process.

215. **Detail persons:** Salespersons who do not attempt to make immediate sales, but who foster "goodwill," make informal presentations, and/or leave samples.

216. **Detention:** Penalty against shipper or receiver for delaying beyond the allowed time in the transport industry.

217. **Deterioration:** Product spoilage or damage which may occur over time in storage or due to environmental factors in storage or during transport.

 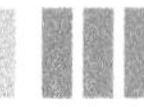

218. **Direct cost:** Cost that can be directly attributed to a particular job or operation.
219. **Direct costing:** The type of product costing that charges fixed manufacturing overhead immediately against the revenue of the period in which it was incurred, without assigning it to explicit units produced.
220. **Direct pickup:** Method of dispatching materials from stores to the requisitioner or user in which the person or department requisitioning the material either waits for the requested material or arranges to pick up the material as soon as it is ready.
221. **Discount order quantity:** The order quantity based on a discount that the vendor will give if a fairly large quantity is ordered.
222. **Discounts:** An allowance or deduction granted by seller to buyer on list price offered to final consumers and/or middlemen who perform some service or marketing function for the manufacturer.
223. **Disposable:** A product designed for one time use.
224. **Distribution:** A materials management function whereby supplies and equipment are delivered from receiving and/or storage to their point of utilization either manually or by automated means.
225. **Distribution system:** An organization of administrative procedures, transport facilities and warehousing or storage facilities used to move materials.
226. **Distributor:** A business that purchases and resells its products, usually maintaining a finished goods inventory.
227. **Diversion:** A change in routing of a shipment.
228. **Documentation:** The process of recording explicitly and in operationally meaningful ways every step in a process, procedure, or system, so that it can be completely replicated or understood in the future if need be.
229. **Double bin system:** A control method for issuing materials in which the area or bin space allocated to an item is approximately twice the amount required for a standard lot or shipment. As each new lot is received, it is placed in the empty space and not used until the older items have been used.
230. **Downtime:** Time when the needed equipment is unavailable for use for any reason.
231. **Drop time:** Amount of time needed to unload a vehicle and take goods into the receiving dock.
232. **Due date:** The date by which an operation or order is expected to be completed.

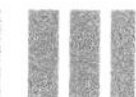

233. **Earmarked material:** Reserved material on hand that is physically identified rather than reserved in a record.

234. **Echelon:** Any stage in the physical distribution system, such as a vendor, the manufacturing plant, finished goods at a master warehouse, regional warehouses, or local stocking outlets.

235. **Economic Order Quantity (EOQ) :** The quantity to be purchased or manufactured in one lot in order to minimize the sum of cost of holding inventory and of ordering and/or of setup for manufacturing. A lot size model attempts to balance the costs associated with placing individual orders with costs of carrying inventory.

236. **Economic run length:** The equivalent of EOQ when the material ordered is produced in house.

237. **Economic time cycle:** The number of periods of demand that corresponds to the economic batch quantity over the planning horizon.

238. **Effective date:** The date when demand is expected to start being recorded, as when the item is released for sale to customers or when it appears in the bill of materials of some parent item.

239. **Eighty twenty rule:** It is a rule of thumb states that about 80 percent of an organization's total demand or usage is accounted for by 20 percent of the items.

240. **Electronic Data Processing (EDP):** A term used to identify both the manufacture and use of computing equipment and the function of processing and/or manipulating data by electronic means.

241. **Emergency orders:** Some companies provide different services and different payment terms for "emergency" orders from customers, such as to repair a machine that is out of operation, in contrast to stock orders, which may take longer to fill but have more attractive payment terms.

242. **Essential drug:** In a hospital, essential items are those, which have readily available substitutes, but those substitutes are not as satisfactory as the original products and any stock out lasting longer than 48 hours could compromise patient care process.

243. **Exception reports:** Reports that list or flag only those items that deviate from plan or fall above or below some prescribed standards or criteria.

244. **Excess material requisition:** A requisition to authorize withdrawal from stores of material, or parts for assembly, in excess of the planned quantity.

245. **Exchange value:** A monetary measure of the qualities and properties of an item that enables it to be exchanged for something else.

246. **Exclusive distribution:** A pattern usually used for speciality goods, which are made available by only a few outlets, or possibly only one, in a given area.

247. **Expected demand:** An estimate of the average demand that should occur during some future period of time.

248. **Expediting:** The follow up of deliveries against purchase orders which are overdue or are required by a prescribed dead line. The process or systems by which suppliers are encouraged to meet due dates for delivery of outstanding purchase orders or to effect immediate delivery of even due orders.

249. **Expendable item:** An item that is consumed in use, losing its original identity, or the cost of which does not merit approval by some higher body such as the equipment committee.

250. **Explosion:** An expansion of a bill of materials into the total of each of the components required to manufacture an assembly or subassembly quantity.

251. **Exponential decay:** A fixed fraction of stock on hand that is lost at the end of each period.

252. **Express warranty:** A specific assurance made by seller concerning the performance, quality, or nature of goods sold. An express warranty often delineates the rights and obligation of the parties in the event of defective items. This term is sometimes used interchangeably with "guarantee" but it is not a precise usage.

253. **External storage:** Storage facility that is removable from the computer itself but that holds information in a form acceptable to the computer (magnetic tape, punched cards, and so on).

254. **Factor:** An agent for the sale of merchandise who may hold custody of the goods in his own name or that of his principal. He is allowed to sell and to collective payment for the goods.

255. **Failure rate:** It is the number of items failing a test, divided by the number tested.

256. **Feedback:** The flow of information back into the control system so that actual performance can be compared to planned performance.

257. **FIFO (First-In-First-Out):** (i) A method of inventory valuation which assumes that the oldest units in are the first units out. (ii) A policy for scheduling work.

258. **Fixed charges:** Costs that do not vary with the level of output, especially fixed financial costs such as interest, depreciation, lease payments, and sinking fund payments.

259. **Fixed cost:** Costs that are not related to volume.

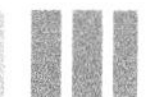

260. **Fixed interval reorder system:** A periodic reordering system in which the time interval between the orders is fixed but the size of the order may vary according to usage.

261. **Fixed order cycle:** Any system of stock control in which an order can be placed only at fixed review times.

262. **Fixed order system:** An inventory control system in which the size of the order is fixed but the order frequency varies depending on actual demand. This system involves placing an order for a fixed quantity (usually EOQ) whenever stock on order and stock on hand (virtual stock) fall below a periodically or dynamically calculated reorder point.

263. **Fixed period control system:** The time between orders is kept fixed in this system. At each ordering time, an amount is ordered to bring the stock on hand and on order (virtual stock) up to the targeted stock level required over the replenishment lead time.

264. **Flexible budget:** A budget, usually referring to overhead costs only, that is prepared for a range, rather than for a single level of activity; one that can automatically be adjusted to changes in the level of volume.

265. **Floating order point:** An order point that is responsive to changes in demand and/or lead time.

266. **Floor stocks:** Stocks of inexpensive production parts held in the production facility from which production workers can draw without requisition.

267. **Flow chart:** A graphic illustration of processes and procedures for operation on data. A diagram that describes documents, procedures, processes, and equipment used in processing data in a specific application.

268. **Flow process chart:** A graphic presentation of the sequence of operations, transportation, delays, and storages occurring during a process.

269. **FOB (Free on Board):** A term which represents how supply, delivery or transportation is to be paid. FOB in a hospital means that the cost of the item includes transportation to the hospital. A pricing strategy in which the seller bears all costs up to the point of placing the product on board a carrier at the point of the product's origin.

270. **FOB destination:** The seller bears the cost of freight and title passes to the buyer at the destination.

271. **Follow up:** Monitoring of job progress to see that operations are performed on schedule or that purchased material or products will be received on schedule. *See* expediting.

272. **Forecast:** A forecast is the extrapolation of past into the future. It is an objective estimate incorporating management's anticipation of changes or new factors influencing demand.

273. **Forecast error:** The discrepancy between actual and forecast demand.

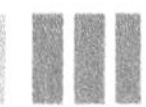

274. **Forecast interval:** The length of time into the future for which the fore cast is computed.

275. **Forecasting:** The mechanism of arriving at measures for planning the future. This covers such things as product demand, supply, cost, prices, and lead times.

276. **Format:** The arrangement of data for computer input or output and/or the arrangement of any information as in a report.

277. **Free stock:** Physical stock fewer requirements allocated, usually used as part of a shortage control procedure.

278. **General Agreement on Trade and Tariffs (GATT):** Multi lateral agreement created in 1947 to reduce barriers to world trade. It is succeeded by the World Trade Organization (WTO).

279. **Generator:** As in programme generator, a programme that permits the computer to write other programmes automatically.

280. **Global sourcing:** The procurement of goods or services outside the continental limits. In many business organizations, the term global infers the developments of a longer term continuing relationship with international suppliers to achieve the benefits of consolidation and leverage.

281. **Goingrate pricing:** It is used for homogeneous products, where prices tend to be the same for all products.

282. **GOLF classification**: Government, Ordinary, Local, Foreign (GOLF) classification is based on general nature of suppliers. The nature of suppliers determines the quality, quantity and continuity of supply, lead time, payment terms and clerical work involved.

283. **Goods in process inventory:** Goods (or work) in the process of being manufactured, which when complete will be finished goods inventory.

284. **Goods in transit:** Goods which have left the supplier but have not arrived at specified destination. *See also* pipe line stock.

285. **Goods received note:** A document used to record particulars of a consignment of goods upon arrival.

286. **Goods receiving:** The operations of receiving goods as they arrive in a hospital, comprising checking the quantity against the order and/or advice note, recording details of the consignment on a goods received note, and releasing the goods for storage or hospital operation. Goods inwards inspection, in which the quality is also checked, may be included.

287. **Goodwill cost:** A cost associated with a backorder, a lost sale, or any form of stock out or unsatisfied demand. This cost may be used to reflect the loss of future revenues because a customer experienced an unsatisfied demand.

 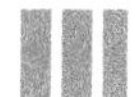

288. **Graphics:** Output displays embodying graphs or other pictorial symbols, as contrasted with output of information in strictly digital or alphanumeric form.

289. **Gravity feed:** This system requires special equipment such as either gravity feed storage bins or double access bins. In either case, incoming material is sequenced behind the old stock. Thus the old stock is removed first either from the front of the bin or from the lower end of the rack or incline.

290. **Gross Domestic Product (GDP):** A measure of a nation's domestic output, which is the total value of all finished goods and services produced within the country during a specified time period (typically one financial or calendar year).

291. **Gross requirements:** The total requirements for a particular component, not taking into account any inventory of that component which is currently on hand.

292. **Grouping orders:** Combining orders for a number of items from one vendor to take benifit of cost reduction.

293. **Group purchasing:** Buying common items for a group of individual units, not part of centralized purchasing authority but anticipating large enough requirements to earn potential price discounts for quantity purchasing. In group purchasing, hospitals combine their volumes of certain categories of supplies to get better price or supply service or both.

294. **Handling and storage costs:** Some incremental costs vary directly with the size of inventories. There are handling costs when materials must be placed in an inventory or issued from the inventory. Included also are costs associated with storage, such as rent or prorated space costs, insurance, taxes (in proprietary institutions), obsolescence, spoilage, and capital costs. If average inventories increase, these costs will also increase and vice versa. *See also* holding costs.

295. **Hedge:** Purchase or sale transaction with the purpose the elimination of profit or loss arising from price fluctuations; specifically, a purchase or sale entered for the purpose of balancing a sale or purchase already made, or under contract in order to offset the effect of price fluctuation.

296. **Hedge inventory:** Inventory created to protect against a potential future event or interruption in supply, such as a strike, major vendor shutdown, prospective trade or change in government programme, or a similar situation.

297. **Heuristic:** Pertaining to exploratory methods of problem solving in which solutions are discovered by evaluation of the progress made toward the final result. *Contrast with* algorithm.

298. **Hidden quality:** Product or service characteristics that are not immediately obvious to potential purchasers but that may differentiate the item from competitors sufficiently to encourage purchase.

299. **HML analysis:** This method is similar to ABC classification. But in this case instead of "consumption value" of items, unit price of the item is used as a criterion. Materials are classified according to their unit price as high, medium and low; the cut off point will depend upon the individual units.

300. **Holding or carrying cost:** All costs associated with maintaining an inventory, including the cost of the capital invested in the inventory, insurance, taxes, warehouse overhead, and so on. This cost is often stated as a percentage of the cost of the units stored in the inventory.

301. **Hold order:** A written order directing that certain operations or work be interrupted or terminated, pending a change in design or other disposition of the material.

302. **House accounts:** Customers who are called on by upper level sales executives rather than by field representatives.

303. **Ideal capacity:** The absolute maximum number of units that could be produced in a given operating situation, with no allowances for work stoppages and repairs.

304. **Idle time:** Time when operators or machines capable of producing but are not producing because of setup, maintenance, lack of material, tooling. *See also* down time.

305. **Impact:** An acronym for Inventory Management Program and Control Technique. This term refers to an application developed by IBM Corporation for determining when to order and how much to order

306. **Import:** Is a process of procuring goods and materials from countries abroad. It presupposes a contract between the importer (Buyer) and the overseas supplier. It involves out flow of foreign exchange from India. An import transaction is subject to the laws and regulations of Foreign trade (development and regulations) Act of 1992 as regards importability.

307. **Imprest stock control:** Also called as topping up system. It is a method of stock control in which imprest level, after reviews at regular intervals, is replenished with no running stock records being kept.

308. **Impulse goods:** Goods or services that consumers tend to purchase impulsively, with little planning or consideration.

309. **Inactive inventory:** It designates the stocks that are in excess of the contemplated or actual consumption within the budgeted period.

 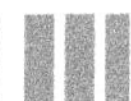

310. **Incoterms:** A series of internationally standardized contract terms which determine whether the buyer or seller of goods moving internationally will arrange and pay for transport and assume the risk for loss or damage.

311. **Increment:** The quantity of addition to inventory. Example: One hundred boxes or units of issue of tongue depressors are checked in by the receiving department. When the one hundred boxes are entered into the computer inventory, this action is called increment.

312. **Incremental cost of capital:** The average cost of the increment of capital raised during a given year.

313. **Independent demand:** Demand that is directly related to customer demand and as such must be forecast. (The demand for finished goods inventories is typically an independent demand, whereas the demand for components is dependent and may be calculated.)

314. **Independent demand items:** Distribution inventory from which any buyer may order.

315. **Index:** A computer stored table containing the addresses of records in a data base. There may, for example, be a par tnumber index used to refer to a file of inventory records. Also referred to as a list.

316. **Indexed sequential:** A method of data retrieval where information is acquired based on some group of unique identifying characters on the input record matching a similar field on the stored record.

317. **Indirect cost:** Any cost not directly identified with specific products or services but related to the normal operations of an organization. Also referred to as overhead, indirect costs are composed of fixed costs, variable costs and semi variable costs.

318. **Indirect materials:** Raw materials that become part of the final product but in such small quantities that their cost is not applied directly to the product. Instead their costs become part of the overhead associated with producing goods or services.

319. **In process inventory:** Unfinished goods awaiting completion.

320. **Insistence:** The final level of consumer brand acceptance; the consumer has become so loyal to the brand that he will not accept any substitute.

321. **Integrated system:** The system characteristic in which input data can be directed to service all required users with minimal duplication of process.

322. **Intensive distribution:** Placing goods or services in multiple outlets; mainly used for impulse or convenience goods.

323. **Intrinsic forecast:** A forecast based on past history, such as a forecast made from a moving average.

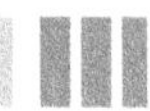

324. **Inventory:** A dictionary definition is "a detailed list of goods; stock of goods". Some people try to distinguish the words "inventory" and "stock" feeling that either inventory includes work in progress or inventory is managed scientifically. Or Americans have inventory, the British just have stock; such attempted distinctions are confusing because common usage of inventory means exactly same as stock.

325. **Inventory analysis:** Determination of the levels of investment in inventory that are necessary to support various commercial, institutional, and production policies on delivery periods, service levels, plant utilization, and the extent to which the output required from the production facility is to be allowed to fluctuate.

326. **Inventory carrying costs:** One type of cost involved in planning and controlling inventory. Factors included in inventory carrying costs are cost of money invested, obsolescence, deterioration, shrinkage or loss, taxes, insurance, space charges, and handling costs. *See* holding costs.

327. **Inventory classification:** The use of a code to group items with in an inventory according to defined characteristics such as : Nature of frequency of demand, turnover value, general or specific end user commodity group accounting or valuation method The use of the code permits the use of particular inventory management techniques to be used on groups of items which display or are subject to particular circumstances of use, nature demand, and accounting or procurement cycles. *See also* inventory specification.

328. **Inventory control:** The control of inventory, and chiefly tradeoffs between the various associated costs on the one hand, and the service level or stock out rate on the other.

329. **Inventory cost method:** To apportion the cost of goods available for sale or use between the cost of goods sold or used and ending inventory.

330. **Inventory data base:** A record of all the information relevant to each item carried in stock.

331. **Inventory file:** A record containing the net quantity of all parts and subassemblies normally maintained in inventory.

332. **Inventory investment:** The money that is tied up in inventory.

333. **Inventory models:** Models relating to inventory management that answer the questions "How much?" and "When?" They permit the manager to determine the point at which orders should be placed for repeat goods, and the quantity of each order.

334. **Inventory policy:** A definite statement of the philosophy of management on inventories.

335. **Inventory reduction:** A planned process through which supply quantities are decreased to adequate quantities to more appropriately reflect the inventory turnover rate and usage patterns. It is an achievable cost containment objective.

336. **Inventory shorts list:** A listing of all items that are low or out of stock.

337. **Inventory shrinkage:** Losses resulting from scrap, deterioration, breakage, pilferage, and so on.

338. **Inventory simulation:** The use of simulation to determine how different inventory control techniques will work.

339. **Inventory standard:** A standard level, expressed in monetary value, for any class of inventory (material, parts, work in process, and so on) calculated realistically to take account of operating policy and decision rules to be used in stock control and operation scheduling.

340. **Inventory stratification:** Analysis on inventory items into a descending order of predetermined parameters (e.g., ABC classification of items based on value of consumption). The results of this analysis may be used to amend other parameters applying to inventory items. *See also* inventory classification.

341. **Inventory team:** Team for taking physical inventory, consisting of one or two counters, a checker, and a writer.

342. **Inventory turnover:** The number of times that an inventory cycles during the year. The inventory turnover is arrived at by dividing the annual sales or usage with the average inventory level. Higher turns indicate a more efficient use of inventory. Absolute targets can only be set based on relevant industry figures, as the turn over for grocery chains is vastly different than for capital goods manufacturers.

343. **Inventory usage:** The value or the number of units of an inventory item consumed over a period of time.

344. **Inventory valuation:** The value of the inventory at either its cost or its market value. Because inventory value can change with time, some recognition must be taken of the age distribution of inventory. Therefore, the value of inventory items is usually based on average price on first in first out (FIFO) or last in first out (LIFO) or a standard price.

345. **Inventory value:** The sum of the number of units of each item on hand or in storage in the storerooms and elsewhere of each line item times its current purchase unit price or market value.

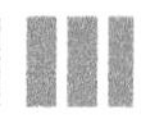

346. **Inventory velocity:** The speed with which inventory moves through a defined cycle (i.e., from receiving to shipping).

347. **Invoice:** An invoice is a notice from a seller to a buyer that goods ordered have been delivered or shipped and that appropriate payment is expected. It indicates the purchaser, seller, amount to be paid, discounts, and other terms of payment.

348. **Inventory writes off:** Deduction of inventory value from the financial statement because the inventory is no longer usable or because it has been disposed of or lost.

349. **Issue time:** Time required for responding to a material requisition by taking material from an inventory location and moving it to its destination. Sometimes called "issue cycle".

350. **Job order costing:** A system of applying manufacturing costs to specific jobs or batches of specialized or unique production in proportion to the amounts of materials, attention, and effort used to produce each unit or group of units.

351. **Judgement items:** Those inventory items that cannot be effectively controlled by mechanical means because of age (new or obsolete product) or management decision (promotional product).

352. **Just-In-Time (JIT):** System in which materials are purchased, transported and processed "just in time" for their use in a subsequent stage of the manufacturing process. An operations management philosophy whose objectives are to reduce waste and cycle time. Operationally, JIT minimizes inventory at all levels.

353. **Kaizen:** Japanese term for continuous improvement. The understanding that process and product quality can improve as a result of numerous small improvements made continuously over a period of time.

354. **Kanban:** Communication devices for transmitting information within a process or to a supplier about what products to supply and in what quantity. They are an order release mechanism.

355. **Kanban system:** Inventory control system generally associated with JIT. Kanban means the travelling requisition cards on which the system depends. Kanban is similar to materials requirements planning except that in order to make the Kanban system work master schedules are smoothed so that every product is made every day and from day to day, the same mix of end products is produced giving a smooth and continuous flow of parts through all areas to the final assembly line. Safety stocks are not provided, the object being to highlight bottlenecks, not hide them.

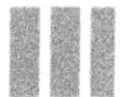

356. **Kitting:** The process of pulling a set of component items from stock and grouping them for production or for movement to another area. Kitting is usually done for a specific production or sales order.

357. **Knocked down (KD):** Goods disassembled and shipped in kit form to reduce the space required in transportation and storage and/or fulfill domestic content requirements by employing labour in the country of destination for reassemble.

358. **Landed price:** Vendor's price, which includes the cost of the goods, transportation, and other costs relating to delivery to the location specified by the purchaser. *See* free into store.

359. **Last in first out (LIFO) inventory accounting:** 1. Valuation of inventory by assuming that the items most recently received are used first. 2. Policy for scheduling work.

360. **Late bid or proposal:** Any bid, proposal, withdrawal, or modification received after the established due date and time at the designated place. Late bids may be considered or rejected as prescribed by the rules applicable to the purchasing officers.

361. **Layout:** The kits of components ahead of the assembly department waiting to be put together.

362. **Lead time:** The time interval needed to complete a portion or all of the activities in a replenishing cycle. It includes the time needed to identify a replenishment obligation, process the order, and receive the item in stock ready for use. It includes both administrative (internal) and supplier lead times. Sometimes termed as "Total lead time".

363. **Lead time demand:** The number of units demanded and removed from inventory during the lead time period.

364. **Lead time demand distribution:** In probabilistic inventory models, this is the probability distribution that describes the possible number of units required during the lead time period.

365. **Lead time offset:** A term used in time series planning where a requirement at one time period will require release of an order at some earlier time period based on the lead time for an item.

366. **Learning curve:** An empirical relationship between the number of units produced and labour hours required. A job takes longer to perform at first than after a similar job has been repeated several times. The time per job is reduced frequently by the same percentage every time the total number of jobs completed has doubled. Hence, at the beginning of a new production run, there will be some increase in efficiency compared with a standard based on earlier runs.

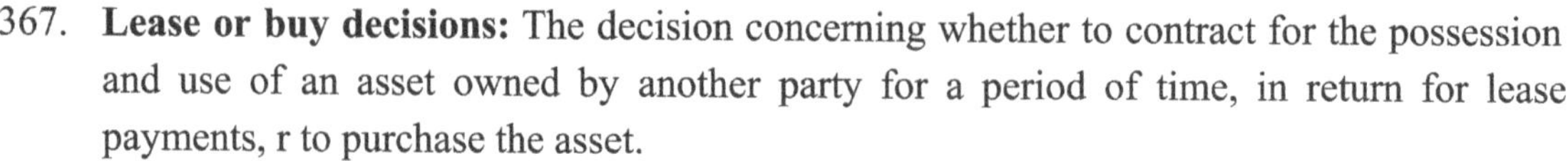

367. **Lease or buy decisions:** The decision concerning whether to contract for the possession and use of an asset owned by another party for a period of time, in return for lease payments, r to purchase the asset.

368. **Letter of intent:** A pre contract document used to enter into preliminary agreements requiring further negotiation to develop definite contract.

369. **Letter of credit:** A document that assures the seller that payment will be made by the bank issuing the letter of credit upon fulfillment of the term of the sales agreement.

370. **Level by level planning:** A term used in materials planning to describe a technique that involves the determination of gross requirements at the highest level and the comparison of this gross requirement with available inventory, which then determines the net requirements at that level. The net requirements at that level are the gross requirements for the next level of inventory down. Level by level planning takes into account available inventory of components at all levels.

371. **LIFO (Last-In-First-Out):** In cost determination, a pricing technique used in the issuance of materials that requires the cost of materials last acquired to be recorded first for current issues. Also, a policy for scheduling work.

372. **Life cycle analysis:** Analysis and forecasting of new product growth rates based on S curves. The phase of product acceptance by such various groups as innovators, early adopters, early majority, late majority, and laggards are central to the analysis.

373. **Life Cycle Costing (LCC):** Costing system which is concerned with the cost of cycle ownership. It includes costs associated with acquiring, using, caring for and disposing of physical assets, including feasibility studies, research, development, design, production, maintenance replacement and disposal, commissioning and training costs and operating costs. *See also* Life cycle analysis.

374. **Line management:** Those managers in an organization whose duties are concerned with direct executive control of the institution's main operations. It is contrast to staff functions.

375. **Liquidated damages:** A sum agreed on between the parties to a contract as damages for breach of contract, to be paid by the person breaching the contract or non performer.

376. **List price:** The basic price the manufacturer asks final consumers to pay for a product or service.

377. **Loading:** Comparing the hours required for each operation with the hours available in each work centre in the time period scheduled for the purpose of allotting jobs to individual machines.

378. **Locator file:** A file used in the stockroom where each item does not have a specific location. The locator file records where the product has been stored.

379. **Logistics management:** A segment of materials management concerned with getting the material to the right place at the right time. The basic problem in logistics management is to determine optimum investment and location of materials.

380. **Lot size:** The quantity of goods purchased or produced in anticipation of demand.

381. **Lot size inventory:** Inventories which are maintained whenever quantity price discounts, shipping costs, etc., make it more economical to purchase or produce in large quantities than are needed for immediate purposes.

382. **Less than Truck (LTL) Load Quantity:** A shipment which is less than the quantity required to be eligible for truck load rates.

383. **Lumpy demand:** Demand pattern with large fluctuations from one time period to another (compared to continuous demand).

384. **Machine utilization:** The percentage of time that a machine is running or producing as opposed to running time plus idle time.

385. **MAD (Mean Absolute Deviation):** Calculation used in measuring and updating forecast error.

386. **Magnetic tape:** A device used to record and store the information digitally mostly for backup purposes.

387. **Main frame:** The central processing element of a computer, containing the main memory, arithmetic units, and registers.

388. **Maintenance Management System (MMS):** System which utilizes the planning, scheduling and management of resources (men, material and time) to perform those actions which contribute to the uninterrupted functioning of equipment within its design characteristics. MMS computer systems are frequently integrated with purchasing/supply systems. See also Management Information System.

389. **Make to order:** Manufacture only as per customer explicit orders.

390. **Make to stock:** Manufacture in anticipation of demand and carry in a finished goods inventory for sale "off the shelf".

391. **Management by exception:** The practice of focusing attention mainly on significant deviations from expected results.

392. **Management by Objectives (MBO):** A form of participation management where a purchaser and his/her supervisor discuss, negotiate and agree on the purchaser's personal objectives for the coming year. These should include performance and professional development objectives as well as the resources needed to achieve them.

393. **Management Information System (MIS):** A system designed to provide the information that management needs to make decisions.

394. **Manifest:** A statement listing the particulars of all shipments loaded in a car, ship, truck, and so on. Usually refers to the ship's manifest.

395. **Marginal cost:** Additional cost incurred when level of output of some operation is increased by one unit.

396. **Markdown pricing:** A pricing strategy designed to "move out" surplus inventory by cutting product price.

397. **Market:** A set of all actual and potential buyers of a product or service, who have the means to purchase, and whom a marketer can profitably serve.

398. **Market share:** The percentage of a given market controlled by an individual seller; obtaining a specific share of the market is a standard pricing objective.

399. **Market stability:** A basic marketing strategy in which a firm tries to maintain a less competitive, steadier price structure, in times of high and low demand.

400. **Marketing:** A social and managerial process by which individuals and groups obtain, what they need and want through creating and exchanging values with others.

401. **Marketing concept:** A marketing management philosophy that accepts as its basic premise that firms must first begin to understand their consumers, needs and wants of target markets and delivering the desired satisfaction more effectively than do competitors.

402. **Marketing research:** Systematic gathering, recording, and analyzing of data related to marketing.

403. **Master procurement plan:** A schedule of those items that must be purchased in future time periods.

404. **Material:** Any commodity used directly or indirectly in producing a product, raw materials, component parts, subassemblies, and supplies.

405. **Material budget:** It contains estimate of materials to be purchased which are necessary for the manufacture of goods. It also provides a basis for the establishment of a purchasing programme.

406. **Material control:** This term is sometimes used synonymously with stock control and sometimes to cover one or more of the following: calculation of requirements, ordering and stock control, store keeping, goods receiving, and probably buying. The activity of material control is to maintain a constant available supply of raw materials, purchased parts, and supplies that are required for the manufacture of products or for the performance

 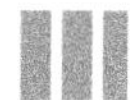

of a service. Functional tasks include the requisitioning of materials for purchase in economic quantities at the proper time, and their receipt, storage, and protection; issuing of materials or use upon authorized request; and the maintenance and verification of inventory records.

407. **Material flow process chart:** A vivid illustration of the sequence of operations, transports, delays, and storages occurring during a process. The material flow process chart presents the process in terms of the events which occur with regard to the material such as distances moved and the time required to move it.

408. **Material hold tag:** Form used to identify and hold certain materials in store for specific orders.

409. **Materials management:** A managerial and organizational approach used to integrate the supply management functions in an organization. It involves the planning, acquisition flow and distribution of production materials from the raw material state to the finished product. Activities include procurement inventory management reviewing stores and warehousing, in plant materials handling, production planning and control, traffic and surplus and salvages. In spite of a slight difference in meaning, this term is often used interchangeably with "supply management".

410. **Material obsolescence report:** A report showing slow moving and inactive items prone to obsolescence.

411. **Material requirement plan:** A schedule that outlines the time phased priority plan for assemblies, necessary to support the master schedule.

412. **Material requisition:** A document issued by an authorized person instructing a store keeper to issue certain items from stock.

413. **Material transfer:** Document used to affect the transfer of material between stock rooms and/or divisions of the institution or company.

414. **Materials Management Information System (MMIS):** The combination of human and computer based resources that results in the collection, storage, retrieval, communication, and use of data for the purpose of cost effective management of materials and for planning of materials related operations.

415. **Materials ordering system:** System used in the development and monitoring of ordering quantities to optimize inventory related costs and service levels.

416. **Materials planning:** In manufacturing, the planning of requirements for components based on requirements for higher level assemblies. The production schedule is exploded or extended through the use of the bill of materials, and the results are netted against inventory.

417. **Materials schedule:** A listing of the specifications, quantities, and deliveries of the materials to be purchased during the next period.

418. **Matrix:** A rectangular arrangement of elements in rows and columns. Matrix bill of material. Bills of material for groups of products in families having common components that are arranged in a matrix so that all requirements for common components can be readily totalled.

419. **Maximum level:** The largest amount of stock permitted to be on hand for an item at any one time.

420. **Mean Time between Failures (MTBF):** A quality and maintenance measure of the average time between failures for a resource or product that causes them to be non usable. E.g., suppose a machine works properly for six weeks, then fails and needs one week to repair, then works well for six weeks, again fails and needs one week to repair, etc. Its MTBF is six weeks, not seven.

421. **Mean time to failure:** Expected average interval between periods of equipment inoperability.

422. **Merchandise inventory:** Goods held for resale, acquired through purchase without further processing.

423. **MICR (Magnetic in Character Recognition):** A device that detects the presence or absence of a magnetic ink character.

424. **Microinstructions:** Instructions consisting of a small, single, short command, such as add or shift or delete.

425. **Minimum stock:** This term is sometimes used variously to mean the alarm level, the reorder level, or the buffer stock of an item.

426. **Mnemonic:** A technique used to assist human memory. A mnemonic represents and resembles the original word by using several letters of the original word in sequence; for example, "mlpy" for "multiply."

427. **Modular bill of materials:** Capital goods have a large variety of options and accessories and are usually assembled to order. Each of the stockable subassemblies can be forecasted and planned, so that there are reasonable stocks available to meet customer requirements. In that case, the end product is made up from modular bills of materials; and the particular mix of features is specified as firm orders are received from customers.

428. **Modularity:** A consideration in the design of systems and programs. A system has modularity when its constituent parts can be readily identified altered, or augmented.

429. **Modulation:** The process by which business machine codes are made compatible with communication carrier transmission facilities.

430. **Monitoring report:** A non decision oriented report that summarizes or describes events that have taken place.

431. **Monte carlo:** A method to derive statistically valid conclusions about the entire span of outcome of a process, one or more of whose components are characterized by numbers that can only be specified within limits. The technique consists of selecting, repeatedly and independently collections of numbers that represent the individual characterizations of one or more components such that, together. These selections duplicate the quintessence of the process as a whole.

432. **Movement analysis:** Items are classified as fast moving, slow moving and non moving based on their consumption pattern. To conduct the analysis, the last date of receipt or the last date of issue, whichever is earlier, is taken into account and the period in terms of months that has elapsed since last movement is recorded. If there is rapid change in technology, the classification will have to be updated more often. FSN analysis is especially useful to control obsolescence.

433. **Move order:** The authorization to move a particular item from one location to another.

434. **Move ticket:** A card used in dispatching to authorize movement of a job from one work centre to another and report the progress of the job toward completion.

435. **Move time:** The actual time that a job spends in transit from one operation to another in the shop.

436. **Movement inventory:** A type of in process inventory that arises because of the time required to move goods from one place to another.

437. **Moving annual total:** Total inventory throughout the previous twelve months.

438. **Moving weighted average:** A moving average is commonly used with time series data to smooth out short term fluctuations and highlight longer term trends or cycles. The threshold between short term and long term depends on the application, and the parameters of the moving average will be set accordingly.

439. **MRP (Materials Requirements Planning):** A system used to determine the quantity and timing requirements of dependent demand materials used in manufacturing operation or providing service. Material can be purchased externally or produced within the organization. Usually the term includes explosion of net requirements from a parent schedule to dependent requirements on subordinate items.

440. **Multilevel bill of materials:** A bill of materials that shows all the components going into the assembly at the various assembly levels.

441. **Need date:** The date at which net requirements become positive; there is no sufficient stock on hand and on order to cover gross requirements. *Contrast is* schedule date.

442. **Negotiation:** In a more general context, the bargaining process between two or more parties, each with its own viewpoints and objectives, seeking to reach a mutually satisfactory

agreement on, or settlement of matter of common concern. In purchasing perspective, the process of arriving at an agreement on the essentials of a purchase contract, through discussions between buyer and seller.

443. **Net change:** A materials planning system in which the materials plan is not recalculated periodically but instead is updated as each requirement change occurs.

444. **Net requirement:** The actual manufacturing or purchasing requirements for a particular component. The net requirements are calculated by deducting the available inventory from the gross requirements.

445. **Network:** A complex of data terminals all eventually able to communicate with a central server across data lines, telephone lines, tele communication lines, or other means.

446. **Non conformance bid (Non responsive bid):** A bid that does not conform to the essential requirements of the invitation of bids.

447. **Non inventoried item:** Normally, a supply item purchased and received but whose on hand quantity is not taken into account.

448. **Non patient charge item:** An item charged to a department overhead account and not directly to a patient, for example, pencils, batteries and tongue depressors.

449. **Numerical analysis:** The construction of effective methods to calculate quantitative solutions to mathematical problems that may or may not have analytic solutions, and the specification of the errors and the ranges of errors in obtaining such solutions.

450. **Obsolescence:** The degradation in the value and usefulness of a resource based on its age, replacement by newer technology, lack of demand or other factor that may require a partial or total write off of its currently stated value. The obsolescence results from a model or style change or technological development.

451. **Obsolescent:** Status of an item or an equipment, system which indicates that it is no longer to be provisioned although it may remain in use until worn out or declared obsolete.

452. **Obsolete stock (Inventory):** Existing inventory items where the total stock on hand has no potential for further use. They have been replaced by an alternative but may still be useful until stock is exhausted.

453. **Official inventory:** A classification of supplies or inventory that is brought into a storage space or unit, counted, and controlled until dispensed to a using department of the hospital. It is assigned to an official inventory account number and when it is dispensed, the inventory account is relieved of the amount which is charged off to the receiving department. This type of inventory is found most often in central stores, central sterile supply, dietary, and pharmacy.

454. **Off line:** The condition of not being in direct communication with the computer, machines, or devices those are under the control of the central processing unit.

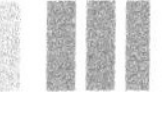

455. **Oligopoly:** Situation where there are only a few sellers of a product. The automobile, steel and cigarette industries are examples of oligopolies. Oligopolistic firms generally produce relatively few diverse products.

456. **On hand:** The balance shown in perpetual inventory records as being present at the stocking location.

457. **On order:** The stock on order is the quantity represented by the total of all pending replenishment orders.

458. **Open account purchase:** A purchase made by a buyer who has established credit with the seller. The transaction is charged to the purchaser's account, payment for which is to be made at some future date agreed on between buyer and seller.

459. **Open insurance policy:** A type of insurance covering shipments for a designated time or a stated value and not limited to a single shipment.

460. **Open ended order:** This type of order generally specifies all terms except quantity. Shipments are made against the buyer's release orders as per the contract; akin to a blanket order. Also referred to as a standing order.

461. **Open to buy:** 1. A retailer's term referring to the largest total value or volume of an item available for purchase. 2. The quantity or total value of goods remaining to be purchased against a specific requisition.

462. **Operating level:** The maximum level of stock in a minmax system. The order quantity is the difference between the operating level and the available stock when a replenishment order is triggered.

463. **Operation card:** A document printed for each operation to be done. It shows some or all of the following: product, part or assembly number, operation number, work centre, tool number, standard times, batch quantity, and start and completion date for the operation.

464. **Operations research:** A profession or discipline devoted to the application of science based methods to solving problems in which there is a choice of a number of cost effective or optimum solutions.

465. **Opportunity cost:** The return on capital that could have resulted, had the capital been used for some other purpose.

466. **Optimal:** Giving rise to the best combination of values for all the variables involved. Computer processes are optimized by rearranging the instructions or data in storage in such a way that the programme can be run with a minimum number of time consuming jumps or transfers.

467. **Optimization:** The process of determining those values for the variables in a system that will give the best or most desired values for the output variables.

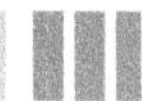

468. **Order:** A request from a customer for goods to be delivered or services to be performed.

469. **Order backlog:** Orders that have been received for which goods are not yet made available.

470. **Order cost:** Procurement costs that originate from the expanse of issuing an order to an outside supplier or due to internal production setup costs. Order costs include the fixed cost of maintaining purchasing department and the variable costs of preparing and executing purchase requisitions. Even when orders are delivered from other parts of the same institution, order costs still apply. The same purchasing routine of checking inventory levels, issuing orders, follow-up, inspection, and updating inventory records pertains to internal procurement.

471. **Order number:** Exclusive number which identifies the purchase order linking to a purchase transaction.

472. **Order point:** The level of total stock on hand and on order at which action is taken to replenish the stock.

473. **Order quantity:** The quantity ordered. The term is frequently used to mean batch quantity.

474. **Ordering:** The function of specifying what shall be made or bought, in what quantity, and by what date it is to be available.

475. **Ordering cost:** The fixed cost (salaries, paper, transaction, and so on) associated with placing an order for an item. *Also see* Order cost.

476. **Original Equipment Manufacturer (OEM):** The term used to identify prime manufacturers of the equipment. OEM repair parts are supplied by the manufacturers of the equipment or agent.

477. **Orphan technology:** Technology rendered obsolete as a result of being bypassed by another technology.

478. **Outgoing materials systems:** A system used in the receipt and control of the finished product from production, the warehousing of the product, and shipment of the finished product to the customers. This might run the whole gamut from the proper recording and handling of a single item of a finished product to be shipped against a specific customer order, to a whole elaborate system of branch warehouses located in various geographical locations, with inventories to support orders of various finished products for many customers.

479. **Out of pocket costs:** The net additional costs incurred when some change is made in business operations.

480. **Output:** Data that has been processed; the device or collective set of devices used for taking data out of a device; the information transferred from the internal storage of a computer to a secondary or external storage, or to any device outside the computer.

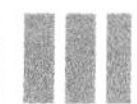

481. **Outsourcing:** A version of the make or buy decision in which an organization elects to purchase an item that previously was made or a service that was performed in house; often utilized for services. It involves sourcing and using a supplier that provides the completed item or service rather than buying the material and manufacturing them in house.

482. **Overhead:** Costs or expenses that are not directly identifiable with or chargeable to the manufacture of a particular part or product.

483. **Overhead account:** Fixed expenses required to operate a department.

484. **Overlapped schedule:** The "overlapping" of successive operations, where by the completed portion of a job lot at one work centre is processed at succeeding work centers before the pieces left behind are finished.

485. **Overrun:** 1. To make or manufacture more than the desired or specified quantity product. Many organizations set standard quantity variance limits (10%) is common. 2. Under the cost reimbursement type contracts, costs in excess of the estimated cost.

486. **Par level:** A maximum supply volume, usually applicable to unofficial inventory in the nursing units and departments, based on predetermined quotas which are established from previous use for that particular supply in that area for a specific time interval.

487. **Pareto chart:** A graph showing the incidence with which events occur, arranged in order of descending frequency. It is used to rank order the issues so that resources can be applied first to those with largest potential return.

488. **Pareto's law (Principle):** Concept developed by Vilfredo Pareto, an Italian economist that states that a small percentage of a group accounts for the largest fraction of the effort, value etc. For example, twenty percent of the inventory items comprise eighty percent of the inventory value.

489. **Part:** Part means an element of a subassembly or assembly not normally useful by itself and not amenable to further disassembly for maintenance purposes. A part may be a component or on accessory.

490. **Partial order:** Any shipment received or shipped that is less than the quantity ordered.

491. **Passage of title:** Title to goods passed when the goods reach the point designated by seller as the FOB destination or shipping point.

492. **Past due:** An order that has not been fulfilled on time.

493. **Patient charge:** A supply item which has been properly reviewed and determined to be one that should be individually charged to the patient. This supply item is appropriately marked up to reflect the direct and indirect costs and is considered to be under controlled conditions in most supply systems.

494. **Patient charge item:** A specific item used for one (only one) patient, such as a heart valve or sent.

495. **Payback period:** The length of time required for the net revenues of an investment to return the cost of the investment.

496. **Payment against documents:** The shipper does not release goods or bill of landing on arrival until full payment has been made.

497. **Payment flow:** It describes flow of cash payment from one organization to another.

498. **Pegging:** Tracing the source of requirements in a materials plan, caused by dependent demand from a customer or interplant order, or to replenish a desired inventory stock level.

499. **Percent of fill:** A measure of the effectiveness with which the inventory management system responds to actual demand. The percentage of customer orders filled off the shelf can be measured in either units or dollars.

500. **Periodic inventory:** Accounting method to determine inventory by (i) periodically taking a physical count of merchandise on hand and (ii) valuing the inventory by multiplying the quantity by the appropriate price and costs of shipment.

501. **Periodic inventory system:** No detailed record of inventory is maintained. However, at the end of a period a physical count is made to determine the amount and cost of the goods sold.

502. **Perpetual inventory:** Usually used to describe an inventory record keeping system in which each transaction in and out is recorded and a new balance is computed.

503. **Perpetual inventory record:** A record of specific items, containing an updated history of all inventory transactions, including receipts and issues of some specific items.

504. **Perpetual inventory system:** For each type of goods stocked, a detailed record is maintained that shows 1. units and cost of each purchase, 2. units and cost of the goods for each sale and 3. the units and amount on hand at any point in time. The system is in opposition to periodic review system for inventory control.

505. **Perpetual stock checking:** A method of checking recorded stock balances against a count of the physical stock which is operated continuously, a proportion of the balances being checked each week. The balance is continuously updated.

506. **PERT (Programme Evaluation and Review Technique):** A network of activities showing their precedence and time relationships. It is used to plan and control work on large, complex, one of a kind projects. *See also* CPM.

507. **Physical distribution:** Grouping of order processing, packaging, materials handling, inventory control, and warehousing, and transportation activities associated with the movement of materials, components and finished articles from production to consumer. In several cases, this movement is made through one or more levels of warehouses in varying modes to transport.

508. **Physical inventory:** The verification of on hand inventory quantities by taking an actual count. Often refers to the annual or quarterly process of counting all items, rather than the physical verification of selected groups of parts on a continuing basis (a cycle count).

509. **Picking list:** An order bill of materials, used as the basis for the stock room to actually select and withdraw from the shelves or bins the components to make up a product or the finished goods to ship to a customer.

510. **Picking sheet:** List of items to be packed and shipped on one order to one destination.

511. **Pipeline:** A system of pipes, valves, pumps, or compressors for transporting gases or liquids. Also used in describing the entire physical distribution system (trucks, railroad cars, storage in transshipment points, and so on) of rigid materials.

512. **Planning:** A statement of goals and of means for reaching them.

513. **Planning horizon:** The period of future time for which plans are formulated.

514. **Pledging of accounts receivable:** Shortterm borrowing from financial institutions where the loan is secured by accounts receivable; also called discounting of accounts receivable.

515. **Post inventory review:** A procedure used to recount the mistakes so that they can be documented and avoided the next time in order to improve inventory taking quality.

516. **Preferred supplier:** A supplier that a customer organization prefers to do business with because it provides the right combination of quality, service and cost.

517. **Prepaid expenses:** Expenses entered in the accounts for benefits not yet received.

518. **Present Value (PV):** The value today of a future payment or stream of payments discounted at the appropriate discount rate.

519. **Price breaks:** Changes in the unit price of a purchased item as the order quantity or batch quantity is increased.

520. **Price in effect at time of shipment:** An agreement between the purchaser and the supplier that the price of the goods is subject to change at the supplier's discretion between the date of purchase order and the date on which the supplier makes shipment often used in precious metal markets.

521. **Price prevailing at the date of shipment:** An agreement between purchaser and vendor that the selling price may be modified by the vendor between the order and delivery dates.

522. **Price maintenance:** A price established by a manufacturer or wholesaler below which the product will not be allowed to be sold.

523. **Price protection:** An agreement between purchaser and vendor granting purchaser any discount established by the vendor, generally prior to shipping date.

524. **Price variance:** The difference between the actual price and the standard price, multiplied by the total number of items acquired.

525. **Prime cost:** The sum of direct material and direct labour costs.

526. **Prime operations:** Critical or most significant operations whose production rates must be planned.

527. **Prime rate:** The lowest rate of interest that commercial banks charge to very large, strong corporations.

528. **Prime supplier agreement:** A type of purchasing in which entire categories of supplies are bought from a single vendor. This term is synonymous with prime vendor, contract purchasing, systems contracting, and solo vendor.

529. **Priority list:** A list of tasks arranged with the most urgent at the top. Priorities can be assigned by latest start date, slack time, critical ratio, or any of the several other techniques.

530. **Pro forma invoice:** An invoice received before a sale is consummated, informing the buyer of the price and terms of sale.

531. **Procedure oriented language:** A higher level language that is used to formulate computer programmes by specifying the procedures or algorithms that are to be executed.

532. **Procurement time:** The times from the decision to place an order until the goods are available for use.

533. **Product:** A tangible want satisfying unit, with a definable lifetime, which can be stored, transported, and resold; something someone makes for someone else.

534. **Product life cycle:** The idea that product or service items, like people, are mortal; they are born, grow, and decline.

535. **Product line depth:** The variety of product or service items offered.

536. **Product orientation:** A view of business that holds that "the firm knows what customers want," and that views the role of marketing as being limited to selling.

537. **Product/service deletion:** The process whereby weak product or service items are eliminated from the firm's or institution's product or service mix.

538. **Product/service development system:** A structured set of activities for developing, analyzing, screening, and ultimately producing new products and services.

539. **Product specification:** A document or documents that completely define the content and form of a product and its components and specify all the quality standards to be met.

540. **Production cycle:** The overall time required from the start of manufacture or from an earlier stage to completion of the product. Thus the production cycle may include the time required for specification of a customer's product, ordering, and procurement of special items.

541. **Production order:** A production order instructs a "production" facility to produce something. It will indicate what is to be manufactured or otherwise produced, how much to make, and when the production should be completed.

542. **Production rate change costs:** These comprise overtime, hiring, laying off, training, extra outside material procurement, temporary labour premiums, and increased scrap and rework costs.

543. **Productivity:** It refers to a relative measure of output per labour or machine hour.

544. **Profit centre:** A unit of a large, decentralized firm that has its own investments and for which a rate of return on investment can be calculated.

545. **Programme:** 1. A sequence of instructions used in a computer to solve a problem or to perform a function. 2. A series of actions proposed in order to achieve a certain result.

546. **Protection time:** A number of days used as a safety buffer between the date on which demands are due and that on which supply orders are to be completed.

547. **Provisioning:** The act of providing and particularly the steps taken before hand to lay in provisions.

548. **Prudent buyer concept:** A section of the Medicare regulations which stipulates that the prudent and cost conscious buyer not only refuses to pay more than the going price for an item or service, but seeks to economize by minimizing cost. This is especially so when the buyer is an institution or organization which makes bulk purchases and can, therefore, often gain discounts because of the size of its purchases. In addition, bulk purchase of items or services often gives the buyer leverage in bargaining with suppliers for other items or services. Any alert and cost conscious buyer seeks such advantages, and it is expected that Medicare providers of services will also seek them.

549. **Pull approach:** Inventory control method which views each stocking point as independent of all others in the systems. Forecasting and setting the inventory policy are done by considering only the circumstances particular to a given stocking point. Stocking levels are decided independently for each stocking point.

550. **Pull and push systems:** If replenishment of stocks in one location can be determined without reference to the stock status elsewhere, that is essentially a pull system of field replenishment. In a push system, the total stock status is taken into account in computing fair shares for all locations from the stock of a given product.

551. **Purchase journal:** It is used to accommodate the entry of all purchases made on credit.

552. **Purchase order:** 1. A purchaser's formal written order to a vendor containing all terms and conditions of a proposed transaction. 2. An offer to buy goods and services. A purchase order is prepared by an authorized executive, buyer, or other person to obligate the establishment to pay for the merchandise ordered. Prepared in response to an approved purchase requisition, purchase orders contain much the same information as that found on the requisition.

553. **Purchase requisition:** A purchase requisition is prepared by a department or employee of an organization to indicate that goods or services should be purchased. Usually, the preparer does not have the authority to order the merchandise directly from the vendor, hence the term "requisition". Purchase requisitions normally indicate a suggested vendor, the quantity of goods required, estimated price, and shipping instructions.

554. **Purchasing specifications:** Documents giving quality standards required in purchased materials, laid down as part of the function of product specification.

555. **Push approach:** Inventory control method in which inventories are allocated within the distribution system based on projected need, available space, or some other criterion. Inventory levels are set across the entire warehousing system by a single authority.

556. **Push strategy:** A promotional strategy intended to encourage middlemen to stock and sell a product, rather than to rely on consumer demand.

557. **Pull strategy:** A promotional strategy intended to develop consumer demand for a product or service and thus to "pull" it through the channel.

558. **Quantity discounts:** Discounts or lower unit costs offered by a manufacturer whenever a customer purchases larger quantities of the product.

559. **Quarterly ordering system:** A periodic inventory replenishment system whereby all requirements are reviewed and replenishment orders placed four times a year.

560. **Queue:** 1. A sequence of elements, one waiting behind the other. 2. A waiting line of jobs available to go through an operation in the shop or service facility.

561. **Queuing time:** The time after which a batch is available for an operation; the time during which it waits for a machine or an operator to become available.

562. **Quotation:** A statement of price, terms of sale, and description of goods or services offered by a vendor to a prospective purchaser; a bid.

563. **Random access:** The process of obtaining data from or placing data into storage, in which the time required to obtain or place any one element, is the same as for any other, being independent of the particular location in storage.

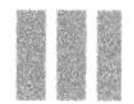

564. **Random or direct access devices:** A device in which time required for access to a stored record is not dependent on the position of that record within the storage media.

565. **Random use item:** Any item whose usage does not conform to an average quantity.

566. **Random variable:** A variable for which the occurrence of any one value within the specific range is as likely as any other.

567. **Range of items stocked:** The list of items carried in a particular location without regard to the quantity of each actually in or planned to be in stock.

568. **Raw materials:** Items that are purchased and converted by processing into finished or component parts.

569. **Reaction time:** The period of time from the moment at which a decision is made to do something, until that act is actually accomplished.

570. **Read:** Transfer information from a source, such as a memory to a part of the computer; electronic impulses for magnetic storage. The process of reading may sometimes include translation.

571. **Receiving:** This function is generally responsible for the following activities: physical report of incoming materials, inspection of shipment, identification and delivery to destination, and preparation of a receiving report.

572. **Receiving record:** A receiving record or receiving report is prepared when goods are received from a vendor. A receiving clerk uses it to list the items received, their quantities, and their condition. It is then sent to other parts of the organization requiring this information.

573. **Reconciling inventory:** Comparing the physical inventory figures with the perpetual inventory record and correcting the record.

574. **Re consignment:** A change of consignee for a particular shipment.

575. **Record:** An organized collection of information (elements) about a single subject treated as a unit. Two or more records form a file.

576. **Release:** The authorization to produce or ship material that has already been ordered.

577. **Release date:** The date on which new items are released for sale to customers.

578. **Reliability:** The consistency with which a material or data will be within certain quality parameters after passage of stipulated time.

579. **Remote batch processing:** A data processing mode combining the features of online communications and batch processing. Batches of data are entered into a system from a remote terminal, and then communicated to a central computer for subsequent processing.

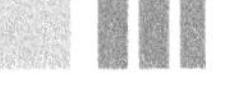

580. **Reorder quantity:** In a fixed order system of inventory control, the fixed quantity that should be ordered each time the available stock falls below the order point.

581. **Reorder report:** A listing of all items that are being reordered because the stock level is below the reorder level.

582. **Replenishment lead time:** The total period of time that elapses from the moment it is determined that a product is to be reordered until the product is back on the shelf, available for use.

583. **Requirements scheduling:** Calculation of gross and net requirements. The task includes summarizing, that is, combining individual requirements of the same item for different products or customers' orders.

584. **Research and development:** A functional area in business which conducts ongoing research designed to develop and improve a firm's product or service offerings.

585. **Reserved material:** Material on hand or on order that is assigned to specific future production orders.

586. **Response time:** The amount of time that elapses between a request for data or for processing and the receipt of the data or processing results.

587. **Retrieve:** To find and select specific information, especially a record or group of records from a data base.

588. **Return on Assets (ROA):** The ratio of operating income divided by total assets employed that indicates the relative operating efficiency of an organization.

589. **Return on Investment (ROI):** The ratio of income produced by an asset divided by its investment cost.

590. **Reverse distribution:** A form of distribution in which user or consumer of the supply has the burden of obtaining the supply from the provider (the supply area).

591. **Review interval:** The time period between successive inventory checks.

592. **Review period:** In a fixed order cycle system of stock control, the time interval between reviews at which replenishment orders may be placed.

593. **Risk premium:** The difference between the required rate of return on a particular risky asset and the rate of return on a riskless asset with the same expected life.

594. **Rolling forecast:** A forecast that is recalculated periodically and extended one period further into the future.

595. **Routine:** In computer terms, a set of coded instructions arranged in proper sequence to direct the computer to perform a desired operation or sequence of operations. A subdivision of a programme consisting of two or more instructions that are functionally related, therefore, a programme. *Also see* Subroutine.

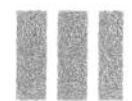

596. **ROP:** An acronym for re order point. It basically represents a minimum level at which point the supply should be ordered.

597. **Running parallel:** The running of a newly developed system in a data processing area in conjunction with the continued operation of the current system; or the final step in the debugging of a system. This step follows a system test.

598. **Rush order:** An order that for some reason must be filled in less than normal lead time.

599. **Safety stock:** The buffer or cushion of stock kept on hand to protect against stock outs caused by uncertainty of future demands or lead time.

600. **Safety time:** In a time series planning system, material is frequently ordered to arrive ahead of the forecast requirement date to protect against forecast error. The difference between the forecast requirement date and the planned in stock date is safety time.

601. **Salvage:** Material that cannot be used for its original purpose, but some part of which can be reconditioned or reused.

602. **Salvage and supplies disposal:** Arrangements for the disposal or reuse of supplies, redundant waste, obsolete materials, or plant and equipment.

603. **Salvage value:** The value of a capital asset at the end of some specified period. It is the current market price of an asset being considered for replacement in capital budgeting problems.

604. **Satiety:** Availability of as much of the product as can be used. Saw tooth diagram. A quantity versus time graphic representation of the order point, order quantity inventory system showing inventory being received and then used up and reordered.

605. **Schedule date:** The date when a production lot is due to be completed. Later, if there are limitations on material or capacity.

606. **Scheduled delivery:** Method of dispatching materials in which the storeroom provides regularly scheduled deliveries throughout the plant dates.

607. **Schema:** A description of a data base, including a statement of the characteristics of the data and the relationship between different data elements. *Contrast with sub schema.*

608. **Scientific inventory control:** The use of statistical techniques to determine proper reserve stock levels.

609. **Scrap:** Material that is of no further use to the institution or company and that should be sold for whatever price can be obtained for it.

610. **Scrap allowance:** An allowance of additional items or material over and above the quantity theoretically required, to cover, to a predetermined extent, the likelihood of scrap being produced.

611. **Scrap note:** A document that authorizes disposal of goods as scrap.

612. **Scrap rate:** The ratio of the difference between the amount or number of units of product started in a manufacturing process and that amount or number of units that are complete at an acceptable quality level, divided by the latter.

613. **SDE classification:** In SDE classification, the purchased items are classified as **scarce** to obtain, **difficult** to obtain and **easy** to obtain. SDE analysis is employed by purchase department to decide the method of buying, and fix responsibilities for buyers.

614. **Sealed bid pricing:** Competitive pricing where suppliers compete for jobs on the basis of bids.

615. **Seasonal inventory:** Inventory built up in anticipation of a peak season in order to maintain production level.

616. **Secured account:** An account on which the purchaser assumes liability for the debt incurred by a purchase transaction by signing a negotiable instrument at the time the transaction is settled or at the time of delivery.

617. **Selective inventory control:** Selective inventory control indicates where the manager should concentrate his efforts. The fundamental idea behind selective control techniques is to put the efforts where results are. All selective controls are based on the principle of Management by Objectives. In fact, the very pyramidal structure of any organization is a reflection of the principle of selective control.

618. **Seller's market:** A market condition favourable to vendors, which exists when the forces of supply and demand keep prices at a relatively high level.

619. **Seller's option:** Seller's privilege to require the buyer to purchase at an agreed price and within a given period of time.

620. **Seller's risk:** The probability that a sample will contain more defects than the rest of the lot.

621. **Selling agent:** A wholesaler responsible for selling a company's entire line of goods.

622. **Selling on consignment:** An arrangement whereby the seller takes possession of the goods from the producer but does not take title to them. Ownership passes directly from producer to buyer.

623. **Semifinished goods:** Products that have been stored uncompleted awaiting final operations that adapt them to different customer specifications.

624. **Service:** An intangible want satisfying unit, which has a short life and cannot be transported, stored, or resold; it is something someone does for someone.

625. **Service level:** The proportion of total demand of an item that is met from stock. It is sometimes expressed as the proportion of total demand Vs that which is met from stock.

626. **Service time:** The time required to serve the customer after he places a demand on an inventoried item.

627. **Setback time:** The expected lead time requirements that are deducted from the required finish date to set the start date.

628. **Setup:** Preparing a machine or workplace for the performance of an operation on a batch. It usually includes production of the first few items and may include procurement of signature for first off inspection.

629. **Setup costs:** Setup costs account for the physical work incurred in preparing for a production run (setting up equipment and adjusting machines) and include the clerical costs of shop orders, scheduling, and expediting. External orders, internal procurement, and setup costs remain relatively constant regardless of the order size.

630. **Setup time:** Time required to adjust a work station or a machine and/or to attach the proper tooling to make a particular product.

631. **Shelf life:** The length of time a material may be stored without affecting the usability or salability of the material.

632. **Shortage:** The quantity of an item that is shown to be required, beyond what is available.

633. **Shortage control:** The process of checking, either clerically or physically, the availability of materials a few hours, days, or weeks before they are due to be issued from stores. When the goods are received, the process ensures that shortages are cleared before the goods are put into storage.

634. **Shortage costs:** Costs incurred when stock outs occur, such as the incremental cost of more expensive items used as substitutes, (for example, a larger than necessary X-ray film). A part shortage can also be the cause of idle "labour" in a radiology department and of incremental labour cost to perform operations out of sequence. The magnitude of the opportunity cost incurred when patients are referred out for some service because of stock shortages. Shortage costs also include emergency measures to expedite a rush delivery. This cost is easily identified as the difference between the usual cost of procurement and the extra cost for accelerated service. When emergency procedures cannot provide a wanted item, the client is left unsatisfied. The only apparent costs are billings lost from the potential service. The reaction of a dissatisfied patient in terms of future "business" is a cost that can only be estimated.

635. **Shortage note:** A document sent to all concerned to notify them of the existence of a shortage.

636. **Short date:** A replenishment order that is scheduled for the end of the freeze period but is needed earlier.

637. **Shrinkage:** Loss of materials due to theft pilferage etc.

638. **Simulation:** Generally a computer based imitation of the operation of an actual or real world system, so that one may study its behaviour and its reaction to specific changes.

639. **SKU (Stock Keeping Unit):** A particular part number at a particular location.

640. **SMED (Single Minute Exchange of Die):** A philosophy and methodology developed by Shigeo Shingo of Toyota car manufacturing company for fast changeover of a machine from production of one product to production of another. The phrase "single minute" is slightly misleading because Shingo really meant "single digit", i.e., he interpreted any change over of 9 minutes or less as a single minute exchange. Changeover times that once were hours were reduced to minutes.

641. **Sort file:** A temporary file used for sequencing or placing data into order in a transaction or master file.

642. **SOS classification:** Seasonal, off seasonal; Agricultural products have seasonal availability pattern depending upon the monsoons. The prices will be lower at the time of harvest and hence the inventory system will have to balance between holding cost and lower prices at which it will be available. In dealing with the levels of these items, one cannot apply EOQ.

643. **Source document:** The original record of a transaction.

644. **Source programme:** A programme written in other than machine language that must be translated into machine language before use.

645. **Spare parts:** "Spare" means a part or a subassembly or assembly for substitution, that is ready to replace an identical or similar part or subassembly or assembly. Spare include a component or an accessory.

646. **SPD:** An acronym for three important material functions: Supply, Process and Distribution.

647. **Special delivery:** Unscheduled delivery of materials direct to the requisitioner to meet emergency demands for materials and supplies, or to deliver material to areas not normally serviced by a scheduled delivery plan.

648. **Specific identification:** Inventory valuation method where each good purchased is identified. When a sale is made, the cost of that unit is identified and recorded.

649. **Specifications:** Comprehensive and accurate statements of the technical requirements descriptive of a good or service, and of the procedure to be followed to ascertain that the requirements are met.

650. **Split lots:** A replenishment order initially issued under one reference number may be split into smaller pieces to get some material through a bottle neck quickly or to allow for better materials handling in the shop.

651. **Spoilage:** Products lost due to defects in workmanship or in the material.

652. **S.s inventory policy:** A two level control system in which a replenishment order is issued if the available stock is equal to or less than the order point s, (the lower level), and in which the amount ordered is equal to S (the upper level) minus the available stock.

653. **Staff functions:** Those activities that are not a part of line management but which assist line management by providing specialized advice or services.

654. **Staging:** Pulling of the material requirements for an order from inventory before the material is required.

655. **Standard:** A quantitative target that is expected to be achieved or surpassed by a predetermined margin.

656. **Standard cost:** The cost of an operation, process, or product, including labour, material, and factory overhead, calculated on the basis of standard performance and prices.

657. **Standard deviation:** A statistical measurement of the variability of a set of observations from the mean of the distribution.

658. **Standard purchase order:** A purchase order tailored to the kinds and types of materials and services being purchased by a specific company or institution.

659. **Standard purchase unit price:** Set pricing for a fixed period of time until a total issue unit price revision is instituted.

660. **Standard times:** The total time in which a job would be completed at a standard rate of working.

661. **Start date:** The date that on which an order should be placed into the shop based on some form of scheduling rules.

662. **State preference model:** A framework in which decisions are based on probabilities of payoffs under alternative scenarios or "states of the world."

663. **Stock:** Stored goods, products, or service parts ready for sale or use.

664. **Stock card:** A document showing all transactions that affect the balance of physical stock. Also, computer records identifying a particular stock item by catalogue number and other pertinent data.

665. **Stock check:** A reconciliation of a stock balance on record with counted physical stock.

666. **Stock control:** A means of deciding when an item should be ordered, made, or bought and in what quantity. The alternative to direct ordering. Also, the clerical control of movement of goods into and out of stores and the level of stocks at all times.

667. **Stock out:** Lack of materials or products that are normally expected to be on hand in stores or stock.

668. **Stock out costs:** The opportunity costs that the companies associate with not having supply sufficient to meet demand. The stock out cost comprises of tangible cost like loss of revenue and intangible costs such as goodwill costs. *See* Shortage costs.

669. **Stock records:** Records maintained for items of inventory that indicate the quantity on hand, the quantity level at which more of the item should be ordered, the vendor or supplier, receipts of stock, and issues of stock. When used, they serve as perpetual inventory records that indicate the quantity of the item on hand at any time.

670. **Stock status:** A periodic report showing the inventory on hand and usually showing the inventory on order and some sales or usage history for the products that are covered.

671. **Stocked item:** An item ordered on the basis of stock control.

672. **Stocking location:** Any warehouse that carries a particular item in its range of products. Distinguished from *bin location,* which is the place within a warehouse where the item is stored.

673. **Storage bins:** Storage facilities generally used for solids.

674. **Storage, buffer:** An element between two devices, for example, external and internal, that temporarily compensates for the difference in their respective rates of throughput.

675. **Storage, bulk:** Storage for larger amounts of programmes or data. The contents of the bulk storage first must be transferred to the main storage before they can be processed on a computer.

676. **Storage cost:** The cost of facilities, personnel, taxes, and so on to provide physically for the storage of inventory. *See* Holding cost.

677. **Storage tanks:** Storage facilities generally used for liquids and gases.

678. **Store:** A place where objects are kept and protected against unauthorized removal.

679. **Storeroom:** Any area where inventory is maintained.

680. **Stores:** Stored materials used in making a product.

681. **Storing:** The supervision, identification, and storage of materials and goods in sound condition for safety and readiness for use when needed.

682. **Strategy:** A method or plan of action designed to accomplish objectives.

683. **String:** A linear sequence of entities such as characters or physical elements.

684. **Sub assembly:** An assembly that is used at a higher level to make up another assembly.

685. **Subjective probability distributions:** Probability distributions determined through subjective procedures.

686. **Sub optimization:** (i) The achievement of the best combination of values for only a part of the total number of variables involved in the system. (ii) Optimization of one subsystem at the expense of another, for example, optimizing production costs at the expense of inventory costs.

687. **Subroutine:** A subunit of a routine. The smallest unit of a programme that can be named and run apart from another subroutine.

688. **Substitute products:** Products whose demand decreases as demand for another product increases.

689. **Sub storeroom:** A secondary storage area where a portion of the total inventory is maintained.

690. **Supplies:** Materials used in providing higher order services or in production of other products. Supplies are not readily charged to the client or to finished production (for example, tongue depressors, lubricating oils, repair parts).

691. **System:** 1. An assemblage of parts into a meaningful whole. 2. A set of resources personnel, materials, facilities, cash, time, and/or information organized to perform designated functions, in order to achieve desired results. 3. EDP systems are of two kinds: units of equipment or hardware called *computer systems* and units of programmes called *computer applications systems* or software.

692. **Tactics:** The specific means used for accomplishing objectives, as opposed to strategy.

693. **Tangible assets:** Physical assets, as opposed to intangible assets such as goodwill or the stated value of patents or copyrights.

694. **Tape drive:** Sequential access storage device used to read a magnetic tape.

695. **Target Inventory Level (TIL):** The target inventory is equal to the order point plus the order quantity. It is often used in a periodic review system.

696. **Taxonomy:** The systematic distinguishing and naming of types or categories that group similar objects or ideas.

697. **Term discount:** Synonym for cash discount.

698. **Term loan:** A loan with a maturity greater than one year, generally obtained from a bank or an insurance company. Term loans are usually amortized.

699. **Terminal:** A device capable of transmitting input to and obtaining output from the system of which it is a part of.

700. **Throughput:** The flow of materials, people, and/or information through a system. Also a term describing the total elapsed time in the performance of a computer job.

701. **Throughput rate:** A rate that applies from origin to destination.

702. **Tool order:** A document authorizing withdrawal or issue of specific tools from the tool crib or other storage.

703. **Total cover:** The total of the stock and outstanding order balances.

704. **Total inventory report:** A listing of all items in inventory with quantity, price, and lead time information.

705. **TPOP (Time Phase Order Point):** A technique to determine when to order independent demand items and when to reschedule to adjust to changes in demand.

706. **Trade credit:** Inter firm debt arising through credit sales and recorded as an account receivable by the seller and as an account payable by the buyer.

707. **Trade discount:** Deductions from list or catalogue price offered to channel members for performing certain marketing functions for the manufacturer.

708. **Traffic:** An organizational unit charged with responsibility of arranging the most economical classification and method of distribution or shipment for both incoming and outgoing materials and products.

709. **Traffic control:** Supervision of a firm's or institution's use of transportation facilities in order to obtain their optimum use.

710. **Transaction:** An event that involves or affects a business or organization. Events taking place during the course of routine business activities (for example, user's replenishing of stocks or central ordering of materials from a supplier).

711. **Transfer price:** The price charge by one segment of an organization for a product or service that it supplies to another segment of the same organization.

712. **Transit time:** The time required to move a batch from the completion of one operation to its availability for the next.

713. **Translator:** A software programme that operates on or uses as data other computer programmes to translate higher level instructions into machine executable instructions.

714. **Transportation costs:** These costs are primarily a function of four basic elements: the distance a shipment must travel, the weight volume of the shipment, the nature or type of product, and the mode of transportation utilized.

715. **Transportation inventories:** Inventories that exist because materials must be moved.

 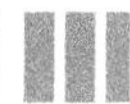

716. **Transshipment:** Shipment of material to an intermediate location from which it is then shipped to its ultimate destination on another vehicle or carrier.

717. **Travelling requisition:** A purchase requisition that is made up once and then used each time the raw material or product is reordered.

718. **Turnaround time:** The elapsed time between generation of input by a user entering it into some process and the receipt of the results of that processing by the user.

719. **Turnover:** The number of times inventory is replaced during a time period.

720. **Twobin system:** A type of fixed order system in which inventory is carried in two real or imaginary bins. A replenishment quantity is ordered when the first bin is empty.

721. **Ultimate consumer:** The buyer who is the last user of a good or service.

722. **Uniform delivered price:** A pricing strategy in which delivery price charged to all buyers, regardless of location, is the same. The delivery charge is included in the net price of the product.

723. **Unit load:** A number of items or bulk material arranged and restrained so that the combination can be picked up and moved as a single object too large for manual handling.

724. **Unit of issue:** The unit in which the inventory is maintained and the charge to a department is determined.

725. **Unit of purchase:** The packaging routinely supplied by the vendor (case, box, carton, and so on).

726. **Un official inventory:** Those supplies that have been expensed and dispensed to the various departments and units where they are temporarily stored until use.

727. **Update:** To modify a file or report with current information according to a specified procedure.

728. **Usage:** The number of units of an inventory item consumed over a period of time.

729. **Usage value classification:** Division of the stocked items into categories according to the value of an average period's consumption or usage of each so that appropriate stock control procedures can be devised for each category.

730. **Use value:** A fiscal measure of the qualities of an item that odd to its performance.

731. **Utilization factor:** In waiting line systems, the ratio of the mean arrival rate to the mean service rate. It indicates the proportion of the time the service facilities are in use.

732. **Values:** Criteria by which people evaluate and/or conduct their own and others' behaviour.

733. **Variable:** A quantity that can assume any of a given set of values.

734. **Variable costs:** Expenses like labour, raw materials, and packaging, which vary depending on the number of units being produced or sold.

735. **Variable length record:** A record that can contain a varying number of characters or data items. *Contrast with* fixed length record.

736. **Variance:** The difference, positive or negative, between actual performance and a preset standard, budget, or target.

737. **VED classification:** Spares are classified as vital, essential and desirable. VED classification is resorted to for spare parts management. Absence of vital spares can cause havoc and bring the wheels to a grinding halt. Some risk can be taken in case of 'E' class spares. Stocking of desirable (D) can be dispensed with, if the lead time for procurement is low.

738. **Vendor file:** A file including complete addresses of all specific vendors to which requests for bids and/or purchase orders are submitted.

739. **Virtual stock:** Sum of stock on hand and stock on order.

740. **Versatility:** An indication of the number of different applications for which a material can be used.

741. **Virtual access:** A data access method used when data is stored at a specific address which might be different from its physical address.

742. **Visual review system:** A simple inventory control system whereby the inventory reordering is based on actually looking at the inventory on hand.

743. **Vital drugs:** Vital drugs in a hospital are those, which have no acceptable substitutes, and for which, stock outs are not tolerated in patient care.

744. **Volatile storage:** A storage device in which stored data are lost when electrical power is removed.

745. **Volatility/stability:** An indication of the ease and/or speed at which a material may change states.

746. **Wait time:** The time a job spends waiting to be moved or waiting to be worked on in the shop; the time during which an operator is not usefully employed.

747. **Wall to wall inventory:** Raw materials, parts, or assemblies that may enter the plant at one end and are processed through the plant into end products without ever having entered a formal stock area.

748. **Warehouse:** Indoor storeroom facility.

749. **Waybill:** A transportation line record issued for each shipment, showing all details and with copies sent to all interested parties.

750. **Week supply:** Amount of inventory on hand divided by the weekly usage rate.

751. **Weighted cost of capital:** A weighted average of the component costs of debt and/or favoured stock and of common equity. Also called the composite cost of capital.

752. **Where used:** A method of retrieving all "parents" that show a given material in their product structures, used for engineering or technical changes and for coping with shortages and substitution.

753. **Wholesaler:** An intermediary connecting the producer and the retailer.

754. **Wide Area Telephone Service (WATS):** A service provided by telephone companies that permits a customer, by use of an access line, to make calls to telephones in a specific zone on a dial basis for a flat monthly charge.

755. **Word:** A sequence of characters treated as a unit and capable of being sorted in a single computer location.

756. **Work centre:** A subunit of a production or service department to indicate either a group of people or of specific machines those are more or less interchangeable.

757. **Work in process:** Product in various stages of completion throughout the production facility or factory. *Also* Work in progress.

758. **Work in process inventory:** The cost of uncompleted goods still on the production line.

759. **Work measurement:** The establishment of the work content of an operation, expressed in standard minutes or standard hours, by time study, work sampling, or use of synthetic data.

760. **Work order:** A requisition sent by the sales department to the production department specifying that a product or batch of products shall be made. It may correspond with a customer's order or may be for finished stock replenishment.

761. **Work station:** The assigned location where a worker performs his or her job. Its object is to enable best use of material, human, and plant resources.

762. **Working capital:** The part of the capital of a business that is used to disburse for materials, wages, and services and is being continually recovered in the selling price of the product. It represents all the capital of the company other than that which is invested in fixed assets.

763. **Working stock:** That element of the stock of an item which fluctuates between zero and the batch quantity, the other element being buffer stock.

764. **XYZ analysis:** While ABC classification has the value of consumption as the basis, XYZ has the value of inventory stored as basis on a particular date. This study is under taken once a year during the annual stock taking exercise. X items are those items whose stock values are high while Z items are those items whose stock values are low. As expected, Y

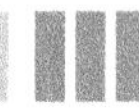

items fall in between the two categories. This classification helps in identifying the items, which are being excessively stocked. If the management is caught napping, one can expect 'C' items in X category.

765. **Yield:** The rate of return on an investment; the internal rate of return.

766. **Yield factor:** The ratio of the average good quantity at the end of the production process to the quantity intially scheduled.

767. **Zoning:** Division of warehouse stock into zones to ease order picking.

Index

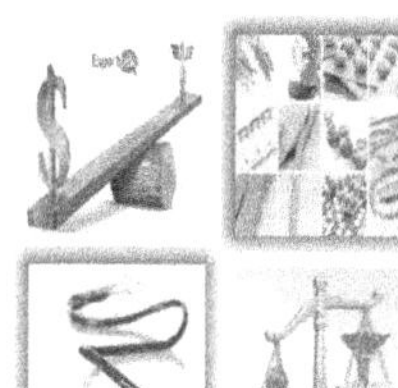
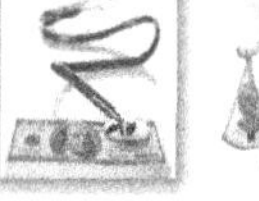
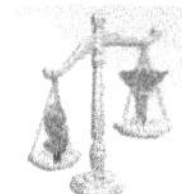

G

H

I

N

Q

R

S

T

U

V

W

X

Author Index

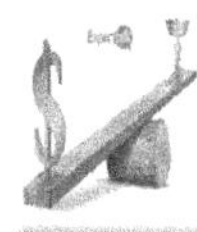
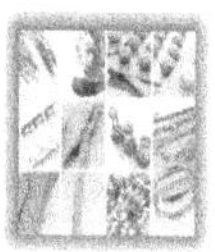
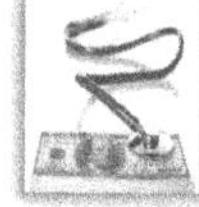
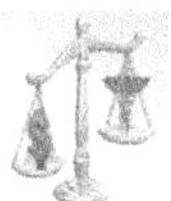

Organization Index

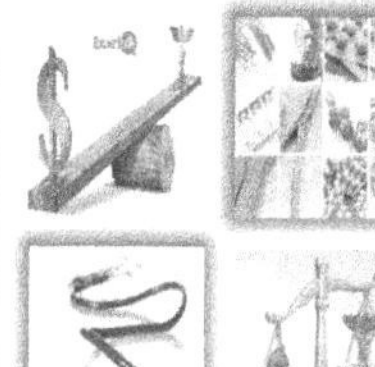

I

J

M

N

P

S

T

U

W

Y

www.ingramcontent.com/pod-product-compliance
Ingram Content Group UK Ltd.
Pitfield, Milton Keynes, MK11 3LW, UK
UKHW061535190726
13845UKWH00005B/109

9 789352 301058